FOODSERVICE MANUAL FOR
HEALTH CARE INSTITUTIONS

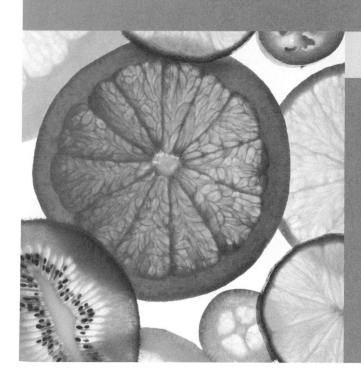

FOURTH EDITION

RUBY
PARKER
PUCKETT

Foreword by L. Charnette Norton

JOSSEY-BASS
A Wiley Imprint
www.josseybass.com

Published by Jossey-Bass
A Wiley Imprint

One Montgomery Street, Suite 1200, San Francisco, CA 94104-4594

www.josseybass.com

Jossey-Bass books and products are available through most bookstores. To contact Jossey-Bass directly call our Customer Care Department within the U.S. at 800-956-7739, outside the U.S. at 317-572-3986, or fax 317-572-4002.

Wiley publishes in a variety of print and electronic formats and by print-on-demand. Some material included with standard print versions of this book may not be included in e-books or in print-on-demand. If this book refers to media such as a CD or DVD that is not included in the version you purchased, you may download this material at http://booksupport.wiley.com. For more information about Wiley products, visit www.wiley.com.

Library of Congress Cataloging-in-Publication Data

Puckett, Ruby P.
  Foodservice manual for health care institutions / Ruby Parker Puckett ; foreword by L. Charnette Norton. – 4th ed.
    p. ; cm.
  Includes bibliographical references and index.
  ISBN 978-0-470-58374-6 (pbk.); ISBN 978-1-118-22052-8 (ebk.); ISBN 978-1-118-23411-2 (ebk.); ISBN 978-1-118-25886-6 (ebk.)
  I. Title.
  [DNLM: 1. Food Service, Hospital. WX 168]
  642'.56–dc23
                          2012027911

Printed in the United States of America
FOURTH EDITION

PB Printing   10 9 8 7 6 5 4 3 2 1

Cover Photo: © Valentyn Volkov/iStockphoto
Cover Design: Michael Rutkowski

CONTENTS

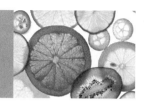

TABLES, FIGURES, AND EXHIBITS

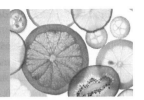

TABLES

FIGURES

EXHIBITS

FOREWORD

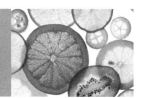

IT IS AN immeasurable honor to write this foreword for Ruby P. Puckett. I have known Ruby for more than 30 years and observed her as she became an icon in the health care foodservice industry.

As a former food and nutrition service director, I looked to Ruby as a leader in health care foodservice who was willing to share her vast knowledge with her peers. I have had the opportunity to serve on professional boards and committees with Ruby where her contributions were invaluable to the success of the outcomes to further the profession of dietetics.

After retiring as director of food and nutrition services at the University of Florida Shands Hospital, Ruby became a sought-after consultant. I have had the privilege of working with her on multiple projects. The most notable assignment was at UCLA Medical Center where her professional advice for performance measures and peer comparisons resulted in improving the department from the lowest percentile to the top percentile in cost containment and patient satisfaction. Her guidance contributed to reducing operational costs by $11 million and increasing revenues by 48 percent. She assisted in enabling the clinical team to become one of the finest in the nation.

Her commitment to continuing education has been instrumental in developing competent leaders in the field of health care foodservice management. Her former students have become leaders in the management and clinical areas. She has tackled the most difficult and intractable problems and has written or spoken about them to train current and future leaders.

Based on the numerous books, pamphlets, CDs, DVDs, online material and eLearning modules, it is imperative that readers know the author(s) to evaluate accurately the credibility of the provided information. Ruby has been a prolific writer so when people are seeking knowledge, they can be assured that her information is accurate and the most current available to the reader.

Professionals in foodservice management and health care facilities who are looking for management ideas, plans, policies, forms, charts, equipment recommendations, and the latest information on a wide range of managerial and operational ideas will find this book beneficial as they increase their knowledge. This book is a practical guide for the total operation of a foodservice department. The book is written in a manner that will benefit students in the dietary man-

ager's training program, college students, plus the seasoned foodservice manager.

This revised book is well organized, with stand-alone chapters for quick references. Each chapter includes an introduction, a summary, and a list of key terms. With the numerous charts, figures, and tables, the text can be considered a "how-to" book that allows readers to use the information to improve their operations.

Readers can be assured that this book is one of the most thorough reference books for foodservice management and includes references from authors who practice in areas besides foodservice management. Detailed information is presented on such topics as hazard analysis critical control point (HACCP), Occupational Safety and Health Administration (OSHA) regulations, disaster or emergency planning, newest concepts in marketing, continuous quality control, fire safety, equipment selection, presentation methods for menu service, layout and design, and an improved chapter on clinical nutrition management. Because communications and human resource issues involve most of a manager's time, these chapters have been updated to present the latest information available. A chapter devoted to information management and chapters on product selection and purchasing have been revised and contain new material. This book is a management and operational handbook.

Ruby writes in a style that is descriptive but not diffuse; that is, thorough but not rambling. This book will be a valuable addition to a foodservice operation's library.

Ruby is the owner of Foodservice Management Consultants and is the program director for the Dietary Manager Training Program through Professional Learning at the University of Florida. Ruby has had a variety of experience in foodservice—she has been the only dietitian in a small charity hospital, director of foodservice in private and university hospitals, a consultant, educator, and author. She has written 13 books, six chapters in other books, published more than 450 articles in peer-reviewed journals and trade/association magazines, and given more than 425 speeches—some on an international level. She presents workshops on HACCP, food safety, and emergency preparedness.

Ruby developed the award-winning Correspondence Course for Dietary Managers Training. Since the inception of the course Ruby has served as the program director for more than 40,000 students who have enrolled. She received the (IFMA) International Foodservice Manufacturers Association) Silver Plate for Health Care Operations. She has been awarded the ADA Excellence Award in Management, the ADA Medallion, and the highest honor given annually to a dietitian—the Marjorie Hulsizer Copher Award. Other awards include the Distinguished Service Award from the Dietary Manager Association and the Foodservice Consultants Society International Robert Pacifico award for her many years of service, not only to the foodservice industry, but also to other organizations, communities, and churches. The Management in Food and Nutrition Systems Dietetic Practice Group of the American Dietetic Association honored Ruby with the Ruby P. Puckett Leadership award, establishing the Ruby P. Puckett scholarship for a Nutrition and Foodservice Professional. In addition, Ruby was honored twice by ASHFSA with the Jim Rose Publication Award. Some of her writings have been translated into Spanish, Chinese, and Japanese. In April 2012, she was only the third woman to be inducted into the Council of Fellows of the Foodservice Consulting Society International. She was the first woman to be inducted into the 1905 University of Florida Athenaeum Society.

In closing, Ruby has been a mentor to me in my career as well as a close personal friend. She continues to graciously mentor many aspiring leaders, most likely contributing to others more than any single person in the foodservice. My life has been enriched by my close association with Ruby P. Puckett and by watching her inspire others to achieve their potential.

L. Charnette Norton, MS, RD, FADA, FFCSI, FHCFA
President, The Norton Group, Inc.

PREFACE

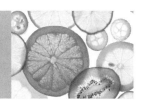

THE COMMERCIAL AND noncommercial foodservice environment continues to change, offering challenges for leadership/management skills, food and nutrition knowledge, fiscal accountability, and human resource practices. Internal and external environments require continuous learning, adapting, and assurance to the stakeholders and the public, in general, that the people who are rendering the services are competent to perform their duties. The United States is currently experiencing the worst economic crisis since the great depression of the 1930s. The unemployment rate has reached a new high, millions are without jobs, and the mortgage crisis has left many families homeless, and the political, social, and technological changes continue to have long-term effects. Health care organizations are dealing with shortages of qualified staff and reduced funds at a time when supply, labor, and operating costs continue to increase.

The passage of President Obama's health care plan, which was to provide health care insurance for millions of uninsured people, has divided the nation, due to the cost not only to employers but also to employees, and due to the question of which treatments are or are not covered. As the new Congress is being seated, there is much discussion for possible changes or repeal of the Bill. Accreditation agencies are placing more emphasis on quality, safety of the customer and the staff, and customer satisfaction. Federal regulations for health care organizations have resulted in increased regulations (especially paperwork and reporting) that organizations *must* follow. There is a shift in the delivery of health care from inpatient to outpatient, in many cases to specialty centers such as orthopedics. These changes and events continue to place an additional burden on the organization and staff for leadership and fiscal responsibility.

Today individuals seeking a career in commercial and noncommercial (health care) foodservice management are experiencing challenges and opportunities that have never before been present. These individuals must possess leadership, managerial, and technological skills. Customers are demanding that their needs, wants, and perceptions be met, which brings new opportunities and challenges to enhance the abilities and skills of the workforce. There are many new changes that must be addressed, which include the emphasis on wellness and prevention, programs to reduce obesity in all ages, reimbursement for medical nutrition therapy, exercise programs for the aging population, and methods to provide care due to the increase in diabetes and heart disease. The shift to the protection of the environment, sustainability, use of farm-grown organic foods, equipment technology, meal delivery systems, and (for the first time in history) four generations of employees working side-by-side in the organization will give the manager the opportunity to use advanced practice standards. The manager *must* be able to adapt, improve existing skills, and think outside of the box to survive in this atmosphere. These changes will affect all systems and subsystems in food and nutrition service. Managers and employees will be challenged to be more efficient and effective in the delivery of service.

Because of these ongoing and continuous changes, I have been challenged to upgrade this fourth edition of this book. As you read the book, you will find many new ideas and upgraded information.

A note: There must be a degree of acceptance and understanding of diversity among employees and customers and family and friends. People differ by race, ethnicity, social status, education, and ancestry and in their hopes and desires for the future. The following philosophy of life was written by Larry Willard Puckett, retired counselor and administrator, and has hung as a plaque in our home for 40 years.

> I Offer My Hand
> If you can accept it
> without regards to its
> color, without asking what
> political philosophy it defends,
> what religious doctrine it
> embraces, or what labor
> it undertakes, then you
> and I have taken the
> first step toward mutual
> understanding—toward
> the ultimate dream—
> universal peace.

Larry Willard Puckett© 2012. Used by permission.

Ruby P. Puckett
Gainesville, Florida

ACKNOWLEDGMENTS

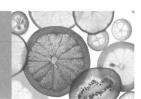

THE FOLLOWING INDIVIDUALS provided valuable assistance in obtaining resources, or providing technical assistance (or both): Laurel P. Brown, marketing and program coordinator, TREEO, University of Florida, for formatting a number of figures and charts; Keith R. Brown, safety and health consultant, University of South Florida Consultation Program, Tampa, Florida, for providing the latest information on OSHA and answering a number of questions on safety, especially during an emergency; and L. Charnette Norton, MS, RD, president of the Norton Group, for support, for the Foreword to this book, information on room service, and suggestions on other topics. A special thanks goes out to students, preceptors, dietitians, and instructors for your evaluations and helpful comments. Many of them are included in this fourth edition. Some of the latest equipment trends were provided by Robert Giele, Hobart Consultation Services. Data and "lean cell system" illustrations in Chapter 21 were provided by Roger Skillman and the Burlodge USA Co. I thank Beth Lorenzini, editor of FCSI's *The Americas Quarterly,* for ideas and encouragement. Mitch Mallard, computer assistant tech, was available at all hours when I called for help ("Someone bugged my computer!"). Mitch retrieved and saved an entire chapter and hours of additional processing. Thanks to CBORD for the computer printouts in Chapter 11. A special thanks also to Larry W. Puckett for permission to reprint the philosophy statement, "I Offer You My Hand," in the Preface. Thank you all.

The definitions of organization culture in Chapter 6 were reprinted from Robbins and DeCenzo's *Fundamentals of Management* (2001), by permission of Pearson Education. Some of the data in Chapter 11 of the 2004 edition of this manual was an update of the 1988 edition (edited by myself and Bonnie Miller, and published by the American Hospital Association). This material has been further updated for Chapter 12 in this edition.

Thanks to all of the employees, students, and colleagues who have kept me on my toes. It has been my pleasure to teach, mentor, and work with you as I strive to promote the importance of food and nutrition systems management.

I would also like to thank reviewers Carlton Green and Sharon Sweeting for their thoughtful and valuable feedback on the draft manuscript.

I am especially grateful to be able to work with such a talented group of people at Jossey-Bass/Wiley, especially my editor, Andy Pasternack, and associate editor, Seth Schwartz. Thanks for the journey.

Ruby P. Puckett

THE AUTHOR

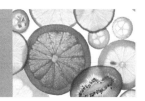

RUBY PARKER PUCKETT retired from Shands Hospital at the University of Florida after serving 27 years as the director of food and nutrition services, while working with dietetic interns and teaching food systems management to undergraduates on the University's main campus. In 1994 she opened her own foodservice management consulting company. Since 1972 she has been the program director of the twice award-winning University of Florida's Professional Education, Dietary Manager Training Program, which she developed and has revised 12 times. To date approximately 40,000 students have enrolled.

Ruby is the prolific author of 13 books (four with coauthors) and has contributed six chapters to other textbooks. Her publications include 460 articles, many of them peer reviewed. She has given more than 425 presentations to professional, educational, civic, and religious organizations. She has held elected offices as well as appointments to numerous committees and has held task force responsibilities in local, state, and national professional organizations in addition to appointed and elected positions in educational, charitable, government, and financial organizations.

In 2003 Ruby was honored with the Marjorie Hulizer Copher Award, the highest honor annually bestowed on a dietitian by the Academy of Nutrition and Dietetics (AND; formerly the American Dietetic Association [ADA]). That organization has also honored Ruby with their Excellence in Management Practice and Medallion awards for contributions to the profession.

Ruby's other awards and honors include the Jim Rose Publication Award (twice); International Food Manufacturers Association Silver Plate Award in Healthcare Foodservice; the Ivy Award of Restaurateurs of Distinction; and the Distinguished Pacesetter award from the Roundtable of Woman in Foodservice. Auburn University's College of Human Science has presented Ruby with three awards, including Alumni of the Year. In 2005 she was the first woman inducted into the University of Florida Athenaeum Society since its founding in 1905 and in that same year the University initiated the Ruby P. Puckett Leadership Award enabling a Certified Dietary Manager to attend the Association of Nutrition and Foodservice Professionals (ANFP; formerly Dietary Manager Association [DMA]) multiday leadership conference.

In 2006 the DMA presented Ruby its highest award, the Distinguished Service award for outstanding service to DMA. In 2010 the Foodservice Consultant Society International recognized Ruby with the Robert Pacifico annual award, "Doing Well by Doing Good," for dedication to her profession, the community, and to religious organizations. Also in that year the Ruby P. Puckett Legacy Leadership Award for energizing leaders was established by the Management in Food and Nutrition Dietetic Practice Group of the ADA.

Most recently, in April 2012 Ruby was inducted into the Council of Fellows of the Foodservice Consultant Society International (FCSI).

In addition, Ruby has traveled worldwide with three branches of the U.S. military (Navy, Marines, and Air Force) as an evaluator of military foodservice for the Ney-Hill and Hennessey Award.

Ruby is listed numerous times in the Marquis Directory of Who's Who in America.

*I lovingly dedicate this book to my family,
my husband, Larry Willard Puckett; our daughters,
Laurel P. (Keith R.) Brown and Hollie P. (Reed) Walker;
our six grandchildren and four great-grandchildren;
and to all the foodservice employees
who daily strive to meet the wants and needs
of the millions of people they serve.*

INTRODUCTION

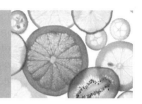

THIS FOURTH EDITION of *Foodservice Management for Health Care Institutions* is written to meet the changing needs and to explore trends and demands of today's foodservice managers by providing the latest information on systems management and operations. This edition continues to provide information on all aspects of foodservice operations, by dividing the book into areas of operation. As appropriate, quality, ethics, regulations, and customers are incorporated in many of the chapters. Each chapter for this edition contains:

- Major learning outcomes
- Introduction to chapter
- Chapter information
- Chapter summary
- Key words
- Discussion points

The purpose of this edition is to assist students, and new or seasoned managers, to use the latest information, charts, forms, formulas, policies, techniques, and references for operating in the ever-changing and challenging environment of foodservice. Whether for managers or students preparing for careers in foodservice management, this book will contribute to an understanding of foodservice operations.

The book contains 22 chapters divided into major parts, management, and operations of a health care foodservice. There are numerous charts, forms, and exhibits, tables, and formulas to assist in the understanding of the concepts presented. An appendix provides a glossary of culinary terms. The chapter on nutrition and medical nutrition therapy has been deleted from this edition. Customer service, quality improvement, and change may be found throughout the text.

Chapter 1 is among the most important chapters in the book. It is an introductory chapter which provides an overview of the entire book and identifies issues relevant to the ongoing changing environment. The fourth edition has been enlarged to include a brief history of foodservice, professional membership, ethics and social responsibilities, challenges related to the workforce, diversity, and regulations. Foodservice departments can be one of the most stressful environments for employees; suggestions on dealing with stress have been included. A comparison of the advantages and

disadvantages of contract management versus self-operated departments is noted. Political ramifications and regulatory regulations are discussed. The material in this book is written for the health care foodservice operation; however, the information is applicable to other foodservice operations such as schools, universities, and correctional facilities. Much of the information is also applicable to commercial operation.

Part One (Chapters 2 through 11) provides information on management and leadership, motivation, participative management, marketing, empowerment of employees, quality management planning, organization and time management, decision making, communications, human resources, information systems, and financial controls. Materials on how the foodservice image affects the department are added.

Chapter 3 deals with marketing, market segmentations, advertising, promotions, merchandising, with examples on how to promote the department and increase revenue, especially through catering. Methods used for merchandising and packaging of products can increase sales.

Chapter 4 discusses continuous quality improvement (CQI), quality assurance (QA), and total quality management (TQM). The use of team management to improved quality is discussed. Regulatory agencies such as The Joint Commission, (TJC), Center for Medical Services (CMS), and their standards are described. Involving and empowering teams to participate in quality assurance is described. Various tools used in TQM are outlined and examples of each tool are included. Quality is also discussed throughout the book.

Information on planning and decision making includes new materials found in Chapter 5. Various types of plans used by managers are identified. Missions, values, and methods used in strategic planning (SWOT), goals, objectives, and plans are carefully detailed. Examples of policies and procedures and a revised business plan are included. Decision-making and problem-solving procedures are outlined.

For foodservice managers to be more efficient and effective they must be able to organize their work, the work of others in the department, and to use good time management. They will need to build teams to accomplish the work and provide an organizational structure that is appropriate to their department. Job descriptions, job analysis, productivity, scheduling, and work schedules are all a part of the manager's responsibility. Information on how to accomplish these duties is described in Chapter 6.

Foodservice managers must communicate every day using written, verbal, body language, and listening skills. Chapter 7 deals with all types of communications (such as the "sender and receiver"), all types of barriers that hinder effective communications, conducting meetings, and the use of various agendas. Listening is an important function of communicating, and a discussion is included on how to listen. Foodservice managers frequently give presentations, so new materials to help the managers to be successful presenters are added. There will always be a grapevine in departments: tips on how to use this method of communicating are included.

Chapter 8 from previous editions has been split to make two separate chapters: Chapter 8, Human Resources: Laws for Employment and the Employment Process, and Chapter 9, Human Resource Management: Other Needed Skills. Foodservice managers spend more than 60 percent of their time on human resource issues. In Chapter 8, the discussion centers on federal laws and surveying agencies' standards. The remaining portion of the chapter deals with the employment process, orientation, and in-service requirements. Chapter 9 describes the evaluation of performance of employees, the right to unionize, corrective action, coaching, mentoring, the employee assistance program (EAP), and the need for an employee handbook. Turnover and absenteeism cost the department additional money. Formulas to calculate these rates and the use of the information help to achieve a more efficient department are included. Employee recognition programs are suggested.

In Chapter 10, the use of management information in foodservice operations is explored. New printouts of the use of information in foodservice have been added, as well as a warning of the consequences of inappropriate use of electronic mail and web surfing using the organization's time and computers that may lead to termination.

Chapter 11 on financial management includes new information on controlling a foodservice department's finances. Controls need to be in place to control all expenses—food, labor, supplies, and so forth. Budget procedures are used as a tool for management control and management. Various reports for food, labor, and so forth must be maintained through journaling. This chapter contains many examples of charts and forms used to control financial management. Cash handling has been elaborated.

Part Two includes Chapters 12 through 22. These chapters give the readers a road map of how to operate a foodservice operation using the system approach. Chapter 12 deals with environmental issues such as waste control, sustainability, and the 4Rs—reuse, recycle, reduce, and rethink—for the protection of the environment. This chapter is so important that plans need to be made to strive for "zero waste." Because of ongoing conflicts and concerns in areas of the world where most fossil fuel is produced, this chapter offers recommendations and suggestions for energy conservation. Clean air legislation and water conservation round out the concern for protection of the environment.

Chapter 13 and Chapter 14 make up what was Chapter 13 in the third edition of this text. Chapter 13 deals with microbial, physical, and chemical hazards, the need to use the appropriate temperature measuring devises to ensure the safety of food. The chapter was rearranged to include information that deals with emerging pathogens, food-borne illness, their causes, cost, and number of illnesses and deaths each year.

Chapter 14 thoroughly discusses the Hazard Analysis Critical Control Point Principles (HACCP), health inspection to include a form of what sanitarians are checking, cleaning, and sanitizing, pest control, and suggestions for self-evaluation of the conditions and practice completed by the foodservice management and employees.

Chapter 15 explains safety and security to include the cost and the events that cause most problems. The Occupational Safety and Health Administration (OSHA) revisions are included in material safety data sheets, and methods to use in providing orientation and training employees on safety in the workplace to include the use of personal protective equipment (PPE). This chapter has additional information available on disaster-emergency preparedness. The author has included a new form to assess the department readiness in case of a disaster. With everyday concerns about terrorism—nuclear, biological, and chemical threats—the author has included what they are and what to do in case of an attack. The different types of fire extinguishers and their use are described and instruction is given on what to do in case of a fire as well as other safety and security measures.

Chapters 16 to 22 detail how to operate a foodservice operation. Chapter 16 has been revised to provide more information on the menu planning process; it emphasizes the menu as the key to the entire operation. Various menu options are outlined. Room service as the latest innovation for foodservice to the customer is discussed.

Chapter 17 and Chapter 18 explain product selection and purchasing; new material has been added to include several new forms. Specifications for all food, supplies, and small equipment are provided including exotic fruits and vegetables. Organic, irradiated, genetically modified, cloned foods, and game meats are discussed as these foods are available on the market. The types of food in categories (meat: pork, beef, lamb, and so forth) contain examples of specifications. Ethics in purchasing is discussed.

Chapter 19 is a discussion on receiving and storage and inventory control. Receiving techniques are reviewed to ensure that what is ordered is what is received. Storage method and temperature control measures are needed to provide safe food to the customer. A number of inventory control tools are available to account for the inventory. Once food and supplies are received and stored an accounting and payment system needs to be in place.

Chapter 20 is on methods of food production to conserve nutrients. Using ingredient control rooms allows less skilled personnel, rather than cooks, to do the preparation. As a further benefit of using ingredient control rooms, the products are always consistent. Recipes are the heart of food production and a method to decrease or increase the servings of various items is essential; this chapter explains how to do this. All of the methods used to produce food are explained. A culinary glossary is at the end of the chapter.

Chapter 21 is on distribution and service and includes the four basic systems of distribution to patients. Improved tray lines and tray assembly are discussed to include drawings to depict this system. Room service is discussed as an alternative to other distribution systems. There are many delivery systems for distributing food to nonpatients including the new concept of "food truck food." Customer satisfaction allows the foodservice direction to benchmark with peer groups. A number of quality standards are available to be used to determine if standards are being met.

Chapter 22, the final chapter, gives information on the use of a team approach in planning a renovation or a new building project. When individual team members carry out their roles, the system works. Using an industrial engineering approach (Gantt and PERT methods) keeps the project on time and usually on budget. Equip-ment selection must be carefully evaluated and justified. Records for preventive maintenance schedules, cleaning procedures, and repairs and replacement *must* be kept. In designing a new area, avoiding cross-contamination and cross-traffic is vital.

This book may be read chapter to chapter when used in an academic setting. Because each chapter introduces a specific topic, the book may be used in a skip-around fashion. If specific information is needed, choose that chapter. If necessary, check out the back-of-book references for additional information on the subject.

CHAPTER 1

FOODSERVICE INDUSTRY
An Overview

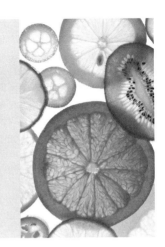

LEARNING OBJECTIVES

- Develop methods, procedures to identify a diverse and generational workforce.
- Learn who the customers are and how to meet their needs and wants.
- Accept ethical challenges and social responsibilities for all areas of foodservice operation.
- Define and apply changes, trends, and regulatory standards.
- Identify and utilize technology as a tool for effective and efficient operation of a foodservice operation.
- Discuss political issues affecting foodservice operations.
- Analyze changes in demographics—aging of the population, role of women and culture and how it is affecting services.

HEALTH CARE IS being met with increased public awareness associated with the cost of, and equal access to, high-quality care and the passage of a national health care bill that is causing much discussion with the possibility of deletion of parts of the bill or completely discarding the entire bill. If the bill is discarded, a new bill may be introduced in Congress at a later date. The percentage of the national budget spent on health care is still rising at an alarming rate and will require persistent emphasis on cost-effective management. Past cost-control efforts include rightsizing the workforce by staff reductions, flattening management levels, using multidepartment management, heightening productivity, outsourcing various activities such as environment and grounds-keeping, and participating in purchasing groups. Changes occurring within health care are affected by the economy and by business and industry trends. In addition to their effect on health care costs, these trends will affect methods of operation, especially as those methods relate to quality, customer satisfaction, and management style.

Health care of the future will experience increases in patient age and acuity level and a continued population shift from inpatients to outpatients. Responses to these changes have caused hospitals to add extended-care services such as rehabilitation units, skilled-nursing units, and behavioral health centers to increase inpatient census. Hospital-owned home care services now extend services for patients after discharge while they increase revenues. Once the primary health care facility, hospitals now face competition from a growing number of alternative health care facilities. These competitors include nursing homes, adult day-care centers, retirement centers with acute care facilities, freestanding outpatient clinics, and independent home care agencies.

There is continuing concern about the millions of people who do not have any form of health insurance or access to health care, as well as for the millions of others who have severely restricted or inadequate protection. The health care field still faces other concerns. President Obama's health care plan will impact the delivery of care as more people may be covered by insurance. It is imperative that all health care employees gain knowledge on how the plan works and its effect on the foodservice operation. This knowledge includes the obesity crisis of all ages, but especially children, autism, cancer, heart disease, diabetes, Alzheimer's disease, the increased number of people with tuberculosis (TB), the increased prevalence of child and adult drug abuse, the aging of the population, diabetes, few medically trained personnel in geriatric medicine, and the emotional stress of daily living and working that takes its toll on health care providers.

These external factors affect the internal operation of health care organizations. Many of these organizations are faced with shorter lengths of stay, reduced census, increased use of the emergency room (ER) as the primary care "physician," influx of immigrants, fewer payers, shortage of qualified personnel, increased paperwork and verification of services, and competition for customers. They are also faced with meeting the increasing cost of providing quality service while still meeting the needs, wants, and perceptions of the customers. As a result, many health care organizations are engaged in cost-effective programs that downsize the number of personnel, implement cross-functional training for the realignment of job duties, and combine elementary functions that may not meet the mission of the organization (therefore reducing expense cost). This includes more outpatient procedures, less invasive procedures, and the increased use of technology. The aging of the population and the increased number of sophisticated older adults in residential health care services are additional causes for concern. The implementation of continuous quality improvement processes or improved organizational performance as required by TJC is also tied in with cost-effectiveness.

This chapter is important because it gives an overview of food-service in health care today and in a number of instances projects problems that will need attention in the future. Read it carefully.

ISSUES: CHANGE

Changes are occurring almost minute by minute all across the world. Changes must happen for society to progress. Not all changes are due to the discoveries of scientists and advanced technology; some are due to the economic climate of the time, the desire for social equality, wars, and catastrophic disasters. *Change* is the result of substitutions, disruptions, competition, or new developments; it is a difference in the way that things are done.

A change in health care organizations may be seen in the way that care has shifted from a hospital base to outpatient departments, home health care providers, and other outreach centers. As these changes in organization take place, specialists who deliver care in hospitals are refocusing the way they deliver this care. Many physicians are being trained to perform cross-functional job duties. *Cross-functional* training is the integration and progressive sequence of learning experience whereby employees are provided with the knowledge and skills needed to perform more than one function.

Socioeconomic changes are taking place on a worldwide basis. The former Eastern Bloc nations are still seeking not only independence but also improved financial and technical assistance from the more prosperous nations. War in Iraq, Pakistan, and Afghanistan has cost many billions of dollars and the deaths of many U.S. soldiers and civilians. Problems still exist in other parts of the world, and changes are occurring now in the former Eastern Bloc. Wars and rumors of wars that use technological advances in weaponry are present. Daily across the world, thousands of people die of malnutrition, natural disasters, emerging pathogens, and major diseases and wars. Transportation and communications are almost instantaneous. When an event happens on the opposite side of the world, we are able to see and hear about it as it is happening. The length of time it takes to transport goods and people to a different location has been reduced from weeks to days (even hours). It has become impossible for any nation to remain isolated. Every developed country has experienced numerous problems: rapidly rising health care costs, increased and fluctuating gas prices, depressed or failing economy, high unemployment, sluggish home sales, increased workplace violence, homelessness and hungry people, especially children.

In the twenty-first century, health care providers face the following factors:

- Consumer movements (protection of patient rights, informed consent, reporting, privacy)
- Managed care (prepaid health care, reshaped health care)
- Increased use of ambulatory centers (may be stand-alone centers)
- Integration of health care organizations, departments within the organizations
- Health maintenance organizations (HMOs)
- The aging of the population
- A prospective payment system based on classification of patients' diagnoses and the use of resources
- Quality of care (the longer patients stay in the hospital, the higher the risk for serious slip-ups, rising 6 percent for each extra day in the hospital)
- Worker's compensation laws
- Financial woes (decreased profit margins)
- Competition, mergers, and consolidations (especially of management teams)
- Social litigation that includes:
  - Sexual equality
  - Maternity leave
  - Length of workweek
  - Flexible scheduling
  - Cultural diversity, generational difference in the workforce.
  - Increased technology
  - Ethics
- Economic downturn, high unemployment, and increase in number of people receiving workmen's compensation

  Public health: Approximately 1.3 million women and 835,000 men are physically assaulted by an intimate partner annually in the United States; many of the assaults include rape, physical injury such as gunshot and knife wounds, which result in an emergency room visit or admission to a health care facility as a result of the attack. Violence against ER nurses and other health care providers by patients and family members is on the increase.

Other Changes in Delivery of Care

Other changes in the delivery of care have been labeled *clinical pathways, empowering, restructuring, cross-functional training, decentralization, care paths, interdisciplinary team approach*, and *integrated systems approach*. Regardless of the labels placed on these changes, all of these approaches have some of the following commonality:

- Flattening of organizational structure, from the familiar pyramid-shape organization with six or more levels of management to a structure with just three or four levels may be necessary

- Redesigning of technological content and services to prevent hawking of employee personnel records and patients medical records
- Improvement of the admission and discharge procedures
- Training people to do more than one function, foodservice managers may be responsible for multioperations or departments
- Reducing the lengths of stay (quality may not be better despite shorter stay)
- Maintaining a stable, fiscally viable organization
- Building high-performance teams that empower personnel to do their jobs and take necessary risks
- Implementing standards and rewards to give control of care back to patients
- Benchmarking internally and with competitors
- Lacking qualified health care employees in some areas of the United States, especially family physicians
- Changing surveyors regulations

Many of these changes will also dovetail with the implementation of TJC's and other regulatory agencies' mandated improvement of organizational performance. Some of the changes need to be defined:

• *Empowering personnel.* Giving authority and responsibility to personnel to define problems and identify solutions that may involve resource allocation or interdepartmental coordination; giving employees the power to set their own work schedules, rotate jobs, and have a larger measure of control over the job—a greater sense of responsibility and authority. W. Edward Deming, who is credited with bringing quality control to Japan in the 1950s, is generally regarded as the intellectual father of total quality management. His concept of total quality is based on the 14-point system. These points were such that, when implemented, they improved quality, provided on-the-job training, broke down barriers between departments, and focused on zero defects.

Empowerment provides employees with the tools, authority, and information to do their jobs with greater autonomy. It also broadens the knowledge base, causing a shift in power; encourages creative open communications; and provides for access to data, the ability to cut through corporate bureaucracy and to communicate with shareholders, and the ability to implement solutions.

• *Clinical pathways.* This is a method or approach to improve care of patients from preadmission through inpatient stay and after discharge, with delineation of nutrition service for each practitioner involved. Information is provided among other providers such as physicians, home health care providers, and long-term care agencies. It is a multilevel, multidiscipline, multidimensional, long-term approach to care that "flattens" the organization, eliminates redundancy of bureaucratic functions, redesigns work, allows for creativity, allows empowerment of personnel, and gives employees the ability to take the initiative and, if needed, take risks. The facility environment must be one of support for change.

• *Interdisciplinary health care providers.* These providers have been cross-functionally trained. They are personnel who have been educated or trained to provide more than one function or job duty,

often in more than one discipline. They are multiskilled, competent, and cross-trained. The day of the generalist has come, as has the "preventive" approach to health care. Health care institutions are focusing on the interdependence of the various functions that must be completed to meet their organizational goals. *Cross-functional training* will also result in "broadbanding" (that is, combining multiclassifications of jobs under one occupational category). These changes will alter the roles of nutritional care providers. The director will assume more of the responsibilities of middle managers. Employees will play an increased and more visible role in the organization. Clinical registered dietitians will be involved in more nontraditional health care jobs, including entrepreneurial activities and consultation with pharmaceutical companies and home health care agencies as nutrition support directors, educators of the public, and major players in the critical pathway of care to patients. In-service teams can work together to cut costs and increase quality.

POLITICAL ISSUES

The future direction of health care will be influenced by *political* and *governmental* intervention as a direct result of increased public awareness and demands. Regulation of the health care industry is likely to continue, even intensify, as access to care becomes a concern of politicians and consumers alike (see the Obama health care plan). Health care foodservice departments will feel the effects of the political environment as it shapes and regulates the way service is delivered. In addition to regulation, managers will see the effects of more emphasis on environmental safety, the protection of the environment and sustainability, while they struggle to provide accurate nutrition information to consumers.

Regulation and Legislation

The nature of this text precludes a comprehensive discussion of legislation as it pertains to health care nutrition and foodservice delivery. Even so, legislative effects and subsequent regulations must be taken into account when foodservice directors plan the direction of their departments. This section briefly reviews various governmental and private sector regulations that affect foodservice delivery. In addition to those covered, the 12-week family leave legislation (Family and Medical Leave Act of 1993) should be scrutinized closely to determine what, if any, modifications are required in work methods and staffing patterns (discussed in full in Chapter 9). Another concern is the return of military personnel and the lack of medical care and job opportunities.

Most of the surveying agencies (TJC, Centers for Medical Services [CMS], Occupational Safety and Health Administration [OSHA], and *Omnibus Budget Reconciliation Act* [OBRA]), as well as local and state public health agencies, have updated and made changes in the surveying system.

Medicare and Medicaid

The regulations that currently have the greatest effect on health care are those dictated by *Medicare* and *Medicaid*, the largest managed-care providers in the United States. Reimbursement rates for services have been set by Medicare and embraced by other managed care systems. Although most foodservice managers recognize their responsibility to provide a high-quality and safe food delivery system, Medicare regulations continue to ensure these entitlements for consumers. The Obama health care plan has made a number of changes in the Medicare and Medicaid regulations that need to be noted. These plans may not affect the nutrition services offered, those services for which a fee is charged, and the quality of care delivered through meal service. Emphasis is on adherence to medically approved diets, written prescriptions, and the service of wholesome food. Medicaid coverage continues to be an ongoing problem, with various bills awaiting action in both the House and the Senate. In 2007 21.9 percent of all federal movement expenditures were spent on Medicare and Medicaid. In 2008 Medicare provided coverage to 44.8 million Americans over the age of 65 and by 2030 is expected to cover 78 million as the baby boomers retire. Federal Medicare expenditures went up steadily in the past three years. In 2006 the expenditure was $378.6 billion and in 2008 $432.6 billion, and Medicaid spending grew to $203 billion in 2008, reaching $216 billion for the federal government cost, plus more than $100 billion or more paid by states. *Medicaid* is the largest and fastest growing part of state budgets, comprising 20 percent of all state expenditures. The number is expected to grow as the population ages, the need for long-term care increases, and older people enter nursing homes. Medicaid is the largest purchaser of nursing home services and maternity care in the nation. Much of the anticipated increase in spending will go to purchasing prescription drugs. On March 20, 2010, the Congressional Budget Office estimated that the new health care bill will cost $940 billion over the next 10 years; however, the actual amount is estimated to be several trillion dollars. Two major changes in the Medicare bill are the reduction in physician payments and the reduction in the cost of drugs after a specific amount has been spent. (It is important to keep informed on the cost, as it will affect you personally as well as the foodservice operation.)

Omnibus Budget Reconciliation Act of 1987

Foodservice departments that serve hospital extended-care units and long-term care facilities also must comply with the Medicare and Medicaid Requirements for Long-Term Care Facilities. These requirements, finalized in September 1992, implemented the nursing home reform amendments enacted by the Social Security Act by Omnibus Budget Reconciliation Act (OBRA) of 1990, as published by the Health Care Financing Administration. It is estimated that nearly 50 percent of the OBRA regulations relate directly or indirectly to nutrition and foodservice departments. The OBRA standards pertain to dignity and independence in dining, initial and annual nutrition assessments, nutrition care plans, and participation of a dietitian in family conferences. Anticipate additional changes in this act.

The Joint Commission

Medicare and Medicaid regulations are government-imposed, but some facilities choose to further their compliance efforts by follow-

ing standards set by independent organizations. *The Joint Commission* (www.jcaho.org) is one such organization. Standards set by TJC are similar to those set by Medicare; however, TJC surveys tend to place more emphasis on the systems, processes, and procedures that influence quality of patient care and outcomes. More recently, publications by TJC report that future emphasis will be on the education and training of patients and their families; orientation, training, and education of staff; leadership roles of directors; work place violence, and approaches and methods of quality improvement. They also have announced increased standards for safety, infection control, pain management, and emergency readiness. They will no longer announce the date or time of the surveys. Because TJC guidelines are updated and published annually, they must be reviewed annually to ensure compliance.

Americans with Disabilities Act

In addition to significantly influencing operations, legislation continues to dictate employment practices. As the labor force shrinks and alternative labor sources are explored, Americans with disabilities are one solution to some of the problems associated with inadequate staffing. Furthermore, ensuring equal employment opportunities for this segment of the population is mandated by federal law. In 1990, President George H. W. Bush signed the *Americans with Disabilities Act*, which prohibits employment discrimination against the disabled. The act mandates that employers with 25 or more employees are prohibited from discriminating against qualified individuals with disabilities with regard to applications, hiring, discharge, compensation, advancement, training, or other terms, conditions, or privileges of employment. The act affects both the selection of employees and the service of meals to consumers. Reasonable accommodations have to be made for both groups. Further explanation of the Americans with Disabilities Act is found in Chapter 8.

Health Care Affordability

Given the alarming rate of increases in health care costs and in an aging population, alternative health care options will be necessary. In 2008 U.S. health care costs were about $7,681 per resident and accounted for 6.2 percent of the nation's Gross Domestic Product (GDP); this is among the highest in industrial countries. The new health care law, the *Patient Protection and Affordable Care Act*, and the amendment *reconciliation bill*, requires all U.S. residents to have insurance or pay a tax penalty. The Obama health care plan will provide coverage for most uninsured workers. This is extremely important and directors and managers must keep up to date on these changes.

Extended-Care Facilities

The concept of seamless delivery of care is demonstrated by hospital-based, long-term-care beds, with patients being moved to skilled-nursing beds or rehabilitation units designed to assist them in becoming self-sufficient. Moving from the higher-cost acute care setting benefits patients, hospitals, and payers. Meals and menus continue to increase in complexity (such as the introduction of the "spoken menu," room service, and gourmet menus) and diversity to meet the needs of inpatients in skilled-nursing and rehabilitation units. Although hospitals continue to convert unused beds to long-term care beds, most growth in long-term care is occurring in outside facilities. The elderly population, aged 85 years and older, will be about 17.6 million in 2050, with about 66 percent of this number being women. Assisted living continues to increase as more facilities become available. Extended-care facilities are becoming more innovative in meeting their patients' mealtime needs. Many such facilities now provide selective menus; others have experimented with wait service and restaurant-style menus (that is, a number of selections per category per meal). Providing meals that meet the required nutrition modifications for elderly patients is becoming easier with the use of general diets that are lower in fat, sodium, and sugar; the liberalization of other diets; and the increased number of products on the market that meet texture adjustment needs.

Extended care facilities include:

Skilled nursing care
Residential care
Adult day care
Elder care
Rehabilitation care
Personal/boarding care
Congregate/semi-independent living
Independent living
Life care
Home care service

Patients' lengths of stay vary from one institution to another and from one geographical region to another. The length of stay for hospitals (excluding psychiatric and rehabilitation facilities) in 1996 was 6.9 days; by 1998 it had decreased to 5.9 and has stayed in this range, with the exception of patients with acute problems such as heart disease and cancer and has continued to have slow decline since this date. In 1998 the mean occupancy rate had dropped to 69 percent. The length of stay and occupancy rate are projected to decline over the next decade. Most beds will be occupied by seriously ill patients.

The average length of stay is affected by the high acuity level of patients. The high acuity level of a patient determines the need for extended care after discharge. Home care is one type of extended care that can positively influence the cost of health care, allowing for shorter hospital stays while ensuring that a patient is cared for in a familiar setting. Furthermore, readmissions have been shown to decrease as a result of team-managed home care. Advances in technology allow more services to be performed in the home, including infusion therapy (such as total parenteral nutrition). Home care offers bigger challenges for home delivery of meals, as does the continuing decline in funding for meal programs for the elderly.

Ambulatory Care

Ambulatory care is expected to show significant growth throughout the next decade. The number of outpatient procedures continues to increase, resulting in a net increase in adjusted admissions. Surgical procedures in ambulatory care settings continue to increase nationwide. Technological advancements and reimbursement trends continue to support the shift from inpatient services to outpatient services. Emergency department visits increased due to a larger number of individuals without health insurance and the enforcement of the federal Emergency Medical Treatment and Labor Act. Outpatient visits will continue to increase by a rate of 15.7 percent per year.

Even though hospital foodservice departments continue to encounter declines in the number of meal demands for inpatients, the number of meals prepared for nonpatients is likely to increase. For example, as outpatient procedures increase, foodservice departments will serve more visitors and family members who accompany patients as well as employees associated with ambulatory care.

Case Management and Patient-Focused Care

The goals of *case management* and *patient focused* (or *patient centered*) care are to improve patient care and satisfaction, decrease the cost of delivery, and improve access to health care. Patient-centered care is a more advanced extension of case management, but both are designed to use critical pathways or standardized care paths that specify a "road map" for the care team and are specific to individual diagnoses. The standards of care or critical paths, developed with input from all team members, are based on the best-demonstrated practice within the facility. Comparing the standards and paths with those at other organizations can help further quality improvement efforts. The patient-focused care model uses a case manager or coordinator who is assigned to a patient on admission and is responsible for monitoring the patient's progress throughout the hospital stay.

Patient-centered care eliminates traditional departmental lines, opting instead for health care teams that focus on patients with related conditions. To realize this type of care, a change in employee attitudes and structural changes to patient care units are necessary. Changes in these units will affect the nutrition and foodservice department as well as clinical caregivers. In models across the nation, foodservice workers are cross-trained to deliver meals and assist patients with their other needs. Some models assimilate jobs previously done by foodservice staff, housekeeping staff, and nurses' aides into new positions, such as the multiskilled patient care employee.

Accountability and Ethics

Government intervention and regulation have placed new emphasis on institutional accountability as it relates to physician recruiting. Once able to recruit physicians with income guarantees and low-interest loans, hospitals now must use their physician workforce plans and development plans to access and document their requirements for additional physicians. Demand cannot be based on the institution's need alone but must be supported by hard evidence of community need. In addition to recruitment accountability, hospitals are confronted with questions related to joint ventures between physicians and hospitals, and that these joint ventures have been entered into for freestanding laboratories and diagnostic centers. A federal ban now prohibits physicians from referring patients to joint venture facilities where referral is a condition of investment. The Josephson Institute of Ethics states "*ethics* is about how we meet the challenges of doing right things when that will cost more than we want to pay."

Ethics play a role for nutrition and foodservice managers in their decisions regarding meal delivery and clinical care. For example, purchasers of food and supplies must avoid suppliers whose offer of favors or gifts would place them in a compromising purchasing position. Further discussion on ethics related to food procurement is presented in Chapter 18. As part of the health care team, registered dietitians must give input regarding the delivery of nutrition hydration services to terminally ill patients. Some ethical issues dealing with nutrition management are addressed by state-specific advance directives signed when patients are admitted to a facility. These advance directives, which reflect a patient's wishes, help physicians and other caregivers in their decisions about the course of treatment.

Environmental Trends

Despite inroads on the amount of waste sent to landfills, more effort is needed. Americans continue to generate more waste than ever before. Each individual generates about five tons of waste per year. If this rate of growth continues, many landfills will be closed and there will be a demand for new ones or for shipping the waste to offshore locations. Health care and foodservice, both separately and together, have been targets in the environmental controversy. The waste from foodservice operations is composed of 60 percent to 70 percent of solid waste that includes food, paper, and plastic supplies such as napkins and single-use plastic items. The remaining 30 to 40 percent is from food production and preparation. Waste management efforts in all areas of health care should consider four agendas: **reducing** the quantity of waste, **reusing** as many materials or items as possible, **recycling** used materials, and **rethinking** what we can do to protect the environment. The increase in environmental regulation and public concern is forcing health care institutions to take innovative measures in handling medical waste, which includes many hazardous products as well as infectious waste that usually is incinerated.

Many foodservice opportunities exist to decrease waste and to implement recycling systems. For example, using individual coffee mugs and soft drink cups and eliminating or limiting disposable tableware can reduce waste. Recycling office paper, glass, steel and aluminum cans, and corrugated paper is another waste-reduction effort.

Many health care organizations have found a way to simultaneously decrease landfill use and help those less fortunate. For example, programs designed to feed the hungry are operated in many metropolitan areas. Food products prepared by health care foodservice departments are picked up by volunteers and distributed to organizations that distribute the food to homeless or low-income individuals. These programs have an added advantage in that the foodservice manager can measure and monitor food waste to improve preparation forecasts. An in-depth look at the environ-

ment and the responsibility of health care foodservice managers is presented in Chapter 12.

Food Labeling and Nutrition Claims

In 1992, the Food and Drug Administration (FDA) announced food-labeling regulations in conjunction with the Nutrition Labeling and Education Act of 1990. Both the number of foods covered and the amount of information required on labels have increased. The purpose of this legislation and ensuing regulation is to provide consumers with more reliable and informative material. Since May 1994, all processed foods regulated by the FDA must be appropriately labeled, and labels must include standardized serving sizes, grams of saturated fat, and fiber content. The percentage of daily values provides the percentage of fat, saturated fat, cholesterol, sodium, carbohydrate, and fiber contributed by a single serving, based on a 2,000-calorie daily diet. The new guidelines allow seven nutrient or disease-specific relationship claims and provide more detailed ingredient listings. Labels that use free, lean, lite, or extra-lean must meet the established standards for these product descriptions.

In 2006, the Food Allergen Labeling and Consumer Protection Act of 2004 became effective. This law requires manufacturers to clearly identify on their food label if a food product has any ingredients that contain protein derived from any of the eight allergenic foods and food groups: milk, eggs, fish, Crustacean shellfish, tree nuts, peanuts, wheat, or soybeans. These eight foods and food groups account for 90 percent of all food allergies. Other allergens are not required to be listed. The type of tree nut, the type of fish, and the type of Crustacean must be listed.

An exemption to providing nutrition labels has been made for food served for immediate consumption, unless health claims are made. This exemption applies to restaurants and health care foodservice facilities. However, if health claims are made, these facilities have to meet the specific guidelines for the nutrient, and the claims must be verified by a minimum of three chemical analyses. For example, a claim that a product is low in cholesterol requires that the product have three verification analyses that prove it is at least 30 percent lower than the original product.

Foods that are *irradiated* must be labeled as such. Companies that wish to include genetically enhanced ingredients in their food products may label genetically enhanced ingredients and ingredients enhanced using biotechnology.

WORKFORCE ISSUES

Globalization, deregulation, and technology are changing the nature of jobs and work. Today more than two-thirds of the U.S. workforce is employed in producing services, not products. Of 21 million new jobs added through the 1990s, many will become part time, and virtually all will be in service industries such as foodservice, retailing, consulting, teaching, and legal work.

The past few years have seen a spike in the unemployment rate. The rate has been as high as 20 percent in some areas of car production, and on average has hovered around 10 percent nationwide. All races, ages, and sexes were involved in the unemployment, and some people have been unemployed for more than two years. There were more than 2.2 million people who wanted work, were available to work, and had looked for a job in the previous 12 months. Some jobs were added for seasonal work, a few factory jobs, and mining. In 2008 health care work employment had increased at the rate of 20,000 per month. Government was the area with the largest increase in employment. The census added 411,000 on a part-time basis.

The demand for institutional foodservice jobs such as chefs, cooks, and dietitians is expected to be the highest. Because of the increased number of dual-income families and women, who make up 48 percent of the workforce, and because of the aging of baby boomers, the demand for service workers has grown. Foodservice managers in health care will have to compete with other service industries for the dwindling labor resources. A reduction in skilled workers coupled with an increased need for foodservice workers will require higher pay scales, which will negatively affect budget and cost-control efforts.

Not only has the labor market diminished, the demographics have changed: the workforce of the next decade will be older, more culturally diverse, and will include more women, people with disabilities, and those with alternative sexual or affectional orientation. These trends will continue, especially with the increasing diversity of the population. The decrease in the number of teenage workers and the increase in the number of workers older than 50 changes the face of the average employee. Baby boomers will still be in the workforce before becoming eligible for Medicare. As a result, the largest pool of workers will also be the older labor force, with the number of workers aged 55 to 65 increasing to about 8.5 million. According to the Bureau of Labor Statistics (BLS; www.bls.gov/data), the median age of the labor force will continue to rise, even though the rate of growth in the youth labor force (16 to 24 years old) is expected to be larger than the growth rate for the overall labor force. The growth rate for the female labor force is expected to slow, but it will grow more rapidly than the male labor force. By 2010, the workforce will comprise 52 percent men and 48 percent women and for the first time in history the workforce will be composed of four generations:

Traditional (*Silent*), born before 1946, make up 7 percent of the workforce.
Baby boomers, born 1946–1964, make up 42 percent of the workforce.
Generation X, born from 1965 through 1979, make up 29 percent of the workforce.
Millennials, born 1980–2000, make up 22 percent of the workforce.
New Silent or Generation Z, born 2001—

In approximately 2017 Generation Z members will enter the workforce and most Traditional and a portion of baby boomers will be leaving the workforce. Generation Z members will bring completely new skills, attitudes, and needs to the workforce.

The full effects of the Americans with Disabilities Act have yet to be felt but are expected to be tied closely with the aging of the population, escalation of obesity, heart disease, and job shortage. The decreasing literacy rate among the nation's workers continues

to be an area of focus. A shrinking labor pool necessitates identifying employees as customers and focusing on their needs. Specifics on managing, recruiting, and retaining tomorrow's workforce are outlined in Chapters 2, 8, and 9.

Cultural Diversity of the Workforce

(See a philosophy statement in the Preface. This is a philosophy that my family and I have lived by for more than 40 years. This engraving hangs in our home as a reminder that we are all different.)

The following definition of *cultural diversity* is a collection of definitions and include "representation, in one social system of people with distinctly different group affiliations of cultural significance, any perceived differences among people; age, functional specialty, profession, sexual orientation, geographic origin, lifestyle, tenure, within an organization or position in an organized society. Refers to more than just skin color and gender—all kinds of differences—age, disabilities, status, military experiences, religion, education, plus gender, race, and nationally." The United States is a nation reflected by the growing number of minority workers. This trend will continue because racial and ethnic groups compose about 25 percent of the U.S. population. The total population in the United States is more than 305 million. According to the U.S. Census Bureau the white race alone makes up more than half of the population; Hispanic or Latino *ethnicity* is 15.4 percent; black or African American alone 12.4 percent; some other race alone 4.9 percent; Asian alone 4.4 percent; two or more races 2.3 percent; American Indian or Alaska Native alone 0.8 percent; and Native Hawaiian or Pacific Islander alone 0.14 percent.

Currently the Hispanic population is the fastest growing among minorities as a whole, and according to the Census Bureau in 2005, 45 percent of U.S. children under the age of five belonged to minority groups. Hispanics and Latino Americans accounted for almost half of the population from 2005 to 2006. Immigrants and their U.S. born descendants are expected to provide most of the U.S. population gains in the decades ahead. A report from Pew Research Center projects that by 2050, non-Hispanic whites will make up 47 percent and the Hispanic population will rise to 29 percent by 2050. The proportion of Asian Americans would double by 2050. The major increase in population is due to (illegal) immigration. Of the nation's children in 2050, 62 percent are expected to be nonwhite. Approximately 39 percent are projected to be Hispanic and 38 percent are projected to be single-race, non-Hispanic whites, of Hispanic origin, and it is expected that by the end of the decade, Hispanics will represent 11.1 percent of the labor pool.

Cultural diversity of the workforce is represented to some degree by managers nationwide but varies regionally. For instance, the African American population is primarily in the South and Southeast, whereas Hispanics are located in the Southwest, West, Florida, New York, and the Chicago metropolitan area. Native Americans are concentrated in Alaska, the Southwest, and the Plains states, but Asian Americans most likely live in the West, with concentrations in Hawaii, California, and Washington.

Along with gains in cultural diversity comes the necessity for managers to recognize opportunities to draw on differences that enhance quality and service. In addition, these differences must be understood to provide compatible leadership that can create career ladders and encourage minorities in entry-level health care positions to access the system for further development. Health care nutrition and foodservice departments represent entry points where training becomes more of a priority. Employee socialization and retention are specific concerns for foodservice directors.

The number of younger women (ages 25 to 29) entering the workforce continues to increase but at a substantially lower rate than before 1985. A slower economy and an escalation in the number of births for this age group are cited by the BLS as a reason for the slowdown. Incentives—benefits, flexible schedules, job sharing, maternity leave, and child-care centers—will need to be provided for them to return to work.

Age of the Workforce

Working teenagers (16 to 19 years old), a traditional foodservice complement, have declined in number due to the low birthrate. Despite the swell in this age group to a projected 8.8 million in 2005, their number in the labor pool will still be 1.2 million below the 1979 level.

The average age of the workforce today is 40-plus years. Workers aged 50 years and older are expected to remain the dominant age group during the remainder of the next decade. The aging of the workforce has been attributed to maturing of the baby boomers, lower birthrates, and increased life expectancy. The shrinking pool of available workers and the growing number of older workers has necessitated their selection as alternative labor. Today's older worker is healthier and can work longer than the same-age worker of a few decades ago.

Having knowledge of the average worker's age and the diversity of the labor force helps foodservice managers make the changes needed to attract and retain employees. The value system of most of the workforce will be based on worker individuality, maximum amount and control of free time away from work, and participation in deciding how work is accomplished. These values will require nutrition and foodservice managers to be flexible with schedules, including total hours worked, workdays, and responsibilities.

Infectious Disease in the Workplace

Closely tied to the Americans with Disabilities Act is the treatment of employees with AIDS in the workplace. In terms of knives and other tools and equipment that could cause cuts, certain risks are involved with kitchen employees who are HIV positive. Closely tied to AIDS—and perhaps more important to foodservice managers— is the near-epidemic number of cases of TB currently identified. Because TB is an airborne infection that is highly contagious, foodservice managers have to diligently ensure annual employee physical examinations.

Literacy and the Workforce

About 2.5 million or more Americans who are illiterate are expected to enter the workforce each year; many will be attracted to the service industry, specifically foodservice. Of Americans who finish high school, only two-thirds will have adequate skills for employment. With the predictions of future labor shortages, quality of education and on-the-job training are increasingly important employment considerations. *On-the-job-training* (OJT), once limited to specific job skills, has to go a step further to provide basic reading and writing skills as well as oral communication in English. Partnerships between educational institutions and health care organizations are in demand to improve the knowledge base of the fewer number of entry-level employees available for foodservice work. Some organizations now include basic literacy courses as part of the health care employee-training program intended to provide service areas with needed staff.

Employee as Customer

The leaders of today and tomorrow have to consider employees not only as a resource but also as a valuable asset to be empowered, trained, and properly motivated. Although expert predictions that the demands of tomorrow's workforce will be linked to autonomy, more time off, and their being included in decisions affecting their work may hold some truth, differing employee value systems must be considered as a factor in this scenario. Value systems vary from one individual to another based on age, culture, and past experiences.

Viewing the employee as a *customer* can be effectively demonstrated through scheduling. Flexible scheduling based on the desires and needs of the workforce is not necessarily new. However, not all foodservice managers have felt the need to be accommodating. Part-time and occasional staff can be used to provide adequate coverage while maintaining flexible scheduling for staff. Occasional staff may consist of full-time parents who wish to earn extra income, older workers who wish to remain active without jeopardizing their retirement income, or disabled workers who may be unable to work full-time hours. Over the past few years, 32-hour schedules have become commonplace in many health care institutions, allowing full-time benefits with an extra day off for personal activities. Foodservice managers might learn by observing schedule patterns from other health care departments. Over a number of years, a shortage of professionals has created the demand for flexible, imaginative scheduling to provide adequate coverage, and no method of coverage should be dismissed without being given adequate consideration.

The Obama health care plan may help employees with medical coverage—not only for low-income workers but for all workers. Benefits are not limited to health insurance and may even include paid time off, freedom to design work areas, on-site child care, elder care, maternity leave, and time off to care for an ailing family member, to name a few.

Compensation continues to be a priority concern for health care foodservice employees, traditionally among the lowest-paid positions. Compensation is a focus for employees deciding which jobs to pursue. Specifically, cooks and chefs can expect income gains due to higher demand for their technical expertise.

CUSTOMER-ORIENTED FOCUS

The views and demands of *customers* affect their choices and have a tremendous influence on the health care delivery system. To determine customer wants and needs, customers must first be identified. Seven customer groups can be identified: patients, family and visitors, physicians, employees, volunteers, vendors, and payers. Of these, in the immediate future seniors, their children—the baby boomers—and women will influence the purchase of health care services. The customer concept is relatively new to health care providers and may be somewhat disconcerting because it depicts the delivery of health care as a business, an outlook that many of today's health care leaders believe necessary for survival.

The trend of identifying and meeting customer needs will likely intensify. Added services intended to increase satisfaction eventually become expected, so that further service-expansion attempts must be made continually to ensure customer satisfaction. This phenomenon encourages the philosophies of continuous quality improvement and total quality management, discussed in Chapter 4. Frontline employees will become more important in providing customer satisfaction because they are the ones who represent the organization or department. Customers and their wants will be identified through market research and its application, discussed in Chapter 3.

Value in the Quality-Cost Equation

To provide *value*, quality must be delivered while keeping cost under control. Customers' demands for quality from their perspective have provided the stimulus for customer satisfaction programs in health care. These programs span the continuum from simple customer service guidelines to detailed continuous quality improvement programs. All have the essential objective of improving quality and customer satisfaction in an effort to improve outcomes and increase use. Whereas customer satisfaction programs emphasize service delivery, continuous quality improvement programs provide a mechanism for in-depth enhancement of systems, processes, and methods of delivery.

Nutrition and foodservice departments have many opportunities to provide full quality and satisfaction to customers. Three distinct opportunities related to the foodservice component are the product, the service or delivery of the product, and the nutritional value of the product. In addition to these foodservice opportunities, many more exist in the delivery of clinical nutrition care. Each of these opportunities for quality enhancement must be evaluated in the customer service or quality improvement process selected.

Programs and services have continued to evolve, with the purpose of generating revenue for nutrition and foodservice departments, but they are now developed with a dual focus on customer satisfaction. Approaches to patient meal service include menu enhancement, nontraditional offerings such as room service, and home meal delivery after discharge. Cafeterias continue to be the primary type of service in health care facilities, although many have added restaurants, 24-hour coffee shops, cooperative vending, and on- and off-site catering. Some hospitals, finding it necessary

to reduce costs, no longer offer 24-hour or weekend services. Many have installed vending operations that may be managed by hiring an outside contractor, by leasing machines and managing the operations in-house (cooperative vending), or by purchasing machines for independent operation. "Branding" is another concept adopted by some health care foodservice departments to improve satisfaction for a variety of customer groups, either by including products in the existing service areas or with fast-food franchises opening on-site. *Branding* is defined as the use of a nationally known labeled product for sale in the current foodservice area or the inclusion of an entire operation (for example, a McDonald's in a hospital lobby). More detailed discussion of quality and customer satisfaction is found in Chapter 4, and branding and catering information is presented in Chapter 3.

Nutrition Awareness

Today's consumers have an increased awareness of nutrition and the effect diet can have on their health. Nutrition information collected through research efforts is no longer the exclusive domain of professionals who pass this information to their patients. Consumers are bombarded at every turn with reports on the latest nutrition research through television, newspapers, magazines, and numerous books and pamphlets. Although intended to educate consumers, this information is often conflicting and not easily interpreted for application to daily dietary intake. Because informed consumers are not always wiser consumers, attempts must be made to meet their perceived needs if customer satisfaction is the goal.

Heightened nutrition awareness is closely linked with an increased emphasis on fitness. Yesterday's fitness fad is today's lifestyle for many consumers of health care and nutrition and foodservice. Even so, people continue to indulge their appetites, especially when dining out. The number one health problem is now obesity. Portions in fast-food outlets, restaurants, and other foodservice operations continue to be "supersize," adding additional unneeded calories.

Increased nutrition awareness and health education will prove beneficial for patients who desire to participate actively in their care. This trend may be one answer to lowering the cost of delivering health care while improving customer satisfaction. In contrast, the large number of less knowledgeable persons living at or below the poverty level will be further disadvantaged by the continued economic dual tiering of society and the growth of a minority immigrant population. The upward trend of poverty will negatively affect the number of individuals at nutritional risk in communities and further validate the role of nutrition awareness.

Demographic Changes

Three primary demographic changes will affect the delivery of nutrition and foodservice in health care: *aging population*, more *women as decision makers*, and *cultural diversity*. Today the median age is 36.7 years. Ages 0–14 years make up 20.2 percent of the population; 15–64 years, 67 percent; and 65 and over, 12.8 percent. The estimated birth rate is 13.83 births per 1,000 population and the death rate is estimated to be 8.3 deaths per 1,000 population. The health care needs of these three groups will continue to center on preventive medicine, fitness, nutrition, and well-child checkups. In addition, this age group will become the primary caregivers for the majority segment—the elderly. (The elderly are sometimes classified as either "young elderly," ages 65 to 74, or "older elderly," ages 75 and older.) Those from age 60 to 80 and older will be the largest segment of the population.

An Aging Population

The number of people older than 65 years of age in the United States will be 70 million by the year 2030. The average age of the old is increasing—the age over 85 is the fastest growing segment of the older population. At least 80 percent of the population over 65 years of age is diagnosed with one or more chronic illnesses, and is reflected in an increased acuity level of patients, an increased number of patients at nutritional risk and more older patients requiring health care than at any other time in history. However, it is important to remember that not all older people are going to be unhealthy or ill. Today's older adults are healthier and more independent than at any time in history. There is a trend for older adults to stay in their own homes rather than move in with their families or to long-term care facilities. These older adults are a diverse group. They know their bodies and what they can do. They are better educated and have more knowledge regarding health care issues and they want more input into their care.

The shift in longevity and poor health of some older adults fostering extensive growth in extended-care facilities, including nursing homes, adult day-care centers, retirement centers, and assisted living facilities. In addition to the increased growth in these freestanding facilities, a larger number of hospitals include skilled-nursing units and rehabilitation units. In addition to caring for the elderly once they become ill, health care organizations are proactively designing preventive care programs to evaluate the health needs of older persons and provide appropriate education. Evaluation includes individualized screens for nutritional risk and guidelines for improving nutrition status related to illness prevention and treatment.

Women as Primary Decision Makers

Women are the primary decision makers in health care delivery choices and want more involvement in matters dealing with their health and that of their families. Centers and specific departments that consider their unique needs continue to influence the delivery of care. Interest in women's health concerns also is evidenced by increased research in this area especially in heart disease and cancer. As the average life expectancy continues to increase, women are facing more responsibility in caring for parents and other extended family members as well as their immediate families. This fact, together with the expanding number of women entering the workforce, will further emphasize customer satisfaction from the perspective of women. As health care decision makers, women influence the balance between high-touch and high-tech aspects of care.

In addition to the nutrition and foodservice demands already mentioned—affordability, continuity of care, equal access, and so forth—the growing number of working women expect convenience. Food choices for this group are influenced by the makeup of the family unit, and many experts in nutrition and foodservice predict that children will become the new "gatekeepers" of the food supply. Convenient well-prepared nutritious food becomes a key element in this scenario as the demands of female consumers provide opportunities for health care foodservice managers. For example, the cafeteria can be extended to offer take-out services, bakery products, and prepackaged kids' meals.

Cultural Diversity in Menus

The effects of cultural diversity on foodservice are prominently reflected in menus enhanced with ethnic dishes. Some operators call for a return to more basic, home-style "American" food choices, but the question arises as to what that means. For example, one of the most popular foods in America is pizza, followed closely by Mexican and Asian food selections. These cuisines have become American menu staples. In planning menus, foodservice managers should consider the population to be served. Demographics vary by region in age and cultural diversity and should be evaluated before making menu selections. Although menus may return to basics in the coming decade and reflect lighter fare, the signature items of various cultures will find a place. Application of this and other information pertinent to menu planning is found in Chapter 16.

TECHNOLOGY TRENDS

The past several decades have been marked by a pronounced growth in technology. Information services underwent the most rapid growth. In general, health care has been slow to implement computerization, especially in foodservice. Many hospitals today, however, have chief information officers who coordinate computer systems planning and implementation. In addition to information technology, medical technology has significantly changed the delivery of health care. Both diagnostic advances and treatment technology have improved patient outcomes while placing extreme financial burdens on health care organizations. Because of heavy diagnostic and clinical advances, many nutrition and foodservice departments have been left out of the capital expenditure cycle or have spent more time justifying equipment needs. However, this does not mean that significant advances that are important to the delivery of cost-effective, high-quality foodservice have not been made in foodservice technology.

At a recent dialogue, conducted by the American Hospital Association, 10 panelists, who were CEOs or senior vice presidents, discussed "The future of care and the implications for hospitals and health systems." These high-level health care administrators came to the conclusion that "The next decade will bring a host of clinical and technological advances that promise to transform the way health care is delivered. Personalized medicine and genomics, the aging population, the implementation of reform and many other emerging trends will impact how hospitals and their leaders will operate." (For the full text see *H&HN Hospitals & Health Networks®*, October 2010, pp. 56–65.)

Information Systems

Information systems will continue to dominate the technological front in the coming decades. Information systems in health care organizations over the past decade have been primarily in the areas of financial, accounting, and human resource management. This emphasis will continue to become more refined in assisting management with making budget-related decisions and with reporting specific information for the new requirements established by Medicare and Medicaid.

Current emphasis is on the design and implementation of a universal electronic data interchange system for processing health care claims. This system necessitates the development of a common language for hospitals, the federal government, and insurers, along with standardization of core financial information. Most hospital billing departments do not find it easy to accommodate a common language or method because of the lack of integration of computer systems and the large volume of services billed. This type of common claims processing will make it increasingly necessary for hospitals to improve their current computer systems.

Medical professionals are including clinical information systems in their office practices. Much of this technology provides for more accurate diagnosis, improved customer care, and improved patient medical records. As the technology becomes more commonplace, future professionals will have greater access and comfort levels. Clinical information systems tie diagnostic testing results directly to nurses' stations or physicians' offices, a linkage that allows quick review and action on test results and facilitates improved patient care. *Bedside charting*, a term used more and more frequently in discussions of patient care, and the computerized medical record improve information flow, thereby assisting with reimbursement.

Information systems also are important in the foodservice department, where management control systems are numerous and their applications vary considerably. Systems may include software packages designed to manage information for clinical management and meal service; menu planning; forecasting and purchasing; inventory management; food safety; payroll; financial management; and in skilled-nursing facilities, material data sheets. Many vendors or distributors offer foodservice operators a direct computer link to warehouses for the purpose of placing orders and accessing information regarding purchase history. Foodservice inventory systems range from department-specific personal computers and software to mainframe systems designed for the organization. Information is entered into inventory either manually or through the use of a scanner.

Still other software programs include nutrition analysis and additional clinical applications. As it becomes increasingly important to evaluate past and current information to make the best decisions for tomorrow, advanced information systems will become more significant. The use of computer systems may not decrease staff needs, but in today's environment they are necessary to manage the increasing amount of information needed by managers to run their departments effectively. Computer software should be purchased based on individual needs. What works for a hospital department may not work for a nursing home. Detailed discussion on management information systems is covered in Chapter 10.

Medical Technology

The delivery of high-quality health care continues to rely on technology, the increased cost of which tends to affect health care faster than other businesses. This cost dynamic is due to rapid changes in technology that can be linked to equipment obsolescence over a short time period, acquisition or replacement costs, and the effects of competition among facilities. Some technological advances have been able to reduce labor needs, but more have required new or higher skill levels. A more demanding skill requirement has led to specialization within departments or fields, making it difficult to use staff for a variety of tasks. Technology also can be effective not only in diagnostics but also in treatment to lower costs and decrease the length of stay. Technology has been responsible for decreasing patient admissions and for increasing the use of outpatient services. More general surgery is being performed as laparoscopic surgery, which can be done in the outpatient setting.

Another type of *medical technology* with widespread effects on health care involves pharmaceuticals. The number of new medications entering the marketplace yearly is staggering. The rapid pace of development creates new problems for the FDA and for the public in that a number of medications have been recalled after their extended use was found to cause side effects not predicted in trials before FDA approval. In view of the AIDS crisis, for instance, demands for rapid approval and release of pharmaceuticals are not likely to decrease.

Food Technology

This section briefly describes developments in *food technology* that foodservice operators should become familiar with. They include *sous vide*, biotechnology, irradiation, and medical foods.

The sous vide ("under vacuum") process, developed and perfected in Europe, uses freshly prepared foods that are processed with low-temperature cooking and vacuum-sealed in individual pouches. That process presented some problems with bacterial growth during the 1980s, but perfection of the slow-cooking methods to achieve pasteurization and improved packaging has made it a safe, viable option for foodservice operators. This technology is proving to be the least controversial and most widely accepted by both foodservice professionals and customers. Because many of the products prepared and preserved with low-temperature cooking and vacuum sealing are considered gourmet in nature, foodservice managers can expand and improve menu options for patients and other customer groups. Sous vide products are excellent for room service when one portion may be needed.

Biotechnology is creating the taste of the future. In this form of *genetic engineering*, a gene foreign to a product is spliced or added to its DNA to enhance or inhibit qualities of the original product. This bioengineering technology is being used to improve the current food supply; for example, vegetables and fruits are engineered to resist spoilage, increase variety, improve nutritional content, enhance resistance to disease and freezing, and provide a longer shelf life. The major reason for pursuing these genetically altered products is to decrease the amount of chemicals used during growing; by altering certain genes, the plants can be made resistant to insects.

The FDA has developed a guidance document for companies that wish to declare genetically enhanced ingredients in their food products. The National Food Processors Association announced before the FDA ruling that, in its view, no new regulation was necessary for food produced through biotechnology. Groups opposing the FDA guidelines include the Center for Science in the Public Interest, the Environmental Defense Fund, and the National Wildlife Federation. Since the FDA decision, many—including a number of chefs—have publicly renounced bioengineered foods. It is not clear whether this disapproval mirrors sentiments of the general public or is limited to this group. Nutrition and foodservice managers should follow development on this topic so as to make informed buying decisions.

Although it has been approved for food since the 1960s, *irradiation* is a technological breakthrough affecting current food supplies. Irradiation refers to exposure of substances to gamma rays or radiant energy. Irradiation has been used since 1985 to control trichinella in pork and since 1992 to control pathogens and other bacteria in frozen chicken and in some vegetables and fruits, especially strawberries.

In the late 1990s, after extensive and thorough scientific reviews of studies conducted worldwide on the effects of irradiation on meat, the FDA approved irradiation of fresh and frozen red meats, including beef, lamb, and pork, to control disease-causing microorganisms.

Federal law requires that all irradiated foods be labeled with the international symbol identified as the "radura"—simple green petals (representing food) in a broken circle (representing the rays of the energy source)—and accompanied by the words "Treated by Irradiation" or "Treated with Radiation."

Cloned food is food that is an exact genetic copy of another. This means that every single bit of DNA is the same between the two. There are a number of types of cloning. There are strict rules/ guidelines on cloning, especially cloning humans. Cloning is used in hundreds of species, including goats, sheep, cows, mice, pigs, cats, dogs, and rabbits. Obviously not all cloned animals are used for food.

After years of research and development, fat replacers or substitutes are beginning to obtain FDA approval. Fat substitutes are classified by the core ingredient used in their production and are carbohydrate-, protein-, or fat-based. Carbohydrate-based fat substitutes are made from dextrins, modified food starches, polydextrose, and gums. Many generic forms of these fats have been approved for use in baking but are not heat stable enough for use in frying. The most common protein-based fat substitute is Simplesse®, produced by the NutraSweet Company and approved by the FDA in February 1990 for use in frozen desserts. Because protein is not an effective heat conductor, Simplesse cannot be used in frying but can be used at high temperatures, for example, in cheese melted on pizza. The most widely known fat-based replacement is Olestra®, produced by Procter & Gamble. The FDA has

spent 25 years studying Olestra. As of 2002, the product is moribund, if not totally dead. More than 18,000 people have submitted reports to the FDA of adverse reactions they attributed to the ingestion of Olestra. That is more reports than for all other food additives in history combined. Procter & Gamble has not sought FDA approval for the use of Olestra in products other than snack foods and has sold its factory. Sales of chips prepared with Olestra have steadily declined.

A new no-calorie fat substitute is being tested in the hope that it can eventually be used to slash calories in everything from cookies to burgers. Z-Trim™, the name of the new substitute, was invented by a government scientist and is an insoluble fiber (hulls of oats, soybeans, peas, and rice as well as bran from corn and wheat) that goes through the body without being digested. Z-Trim cannot be used for frying, but it can replace up to half the fat in many prepared foods. There is some concern that fat substitutes will not decrease the desire for fatty foods and may in fact increase overall fat consumption, similar to the effect sugar substitutes have had on sugar consumption.

Obesity is a growing national problem. Many calories could be eliminated by the use of nonsugar sweeteners. Many consumers are hesitant to reduce their sugar intake because of the many misconceptions about the products. Even with the hesitation and concern about the safety of nonsugar sweeteners, in April 2003 the World Health Organization stated that Americans' need for sugar substitutes is on the rise. The FDA has approved the use of saccharin (Sweet'N Low™, Sugar Twin™), aspartame (NutraSweet™, Equal™, Sugar Twin™ [blue box]), acesulfame-K (Ace-K™ or Sunett™, Sweet One™), sucralose (Splenda™) and sucalose (Splenda). Aspartame is found in more than 5,000 products, including Diet Coke®. Sucralose is found in many products, including Diet Rite Cola®. Saccharin is found in many products, including Sweet'N Low™ brand of cookies and candy. Foodservice personnel have a responsibility to continue to educate the public concerning the safety of the products.

Medical food is a food or a mixture of food components that is administered under the supervision of a physician and interdisciplinary team and is intended for specific dietary management of a disease for which the "food" was intended. Prebiotic and probiotics may be considered as medical foods. *Prebiotics* is a nondigestible food ingredient that beneficially affects the host by selectively stimulating the growth and activity of one or a limited number of bacteria in the colon. Probiotics are living organisms that, when administrated in adequate amounts, confer health benefits to the host.

Foodservice Equipment

Advantages in equipment should be considered annually when making capital equipment plans. Concerns for water, energy use and the environment must be considered when making capital purchases. Equipment needs vary from one institution to another and depend on the types of food purchased, the production methods used, staffing, the menu, and available space in the foodservice department. Under-the-counter storage equipment is available for more flexible storage. Equipment is also being designed to help operators to meet HACCP regulations. Most of the new equipment is designed to maximize storage. Recent advances in foodservice equipment include cook-and-chill units, microwaves, blast chillers, smaller versions of existing equipment, and equipment that can be used for multiproduction methods. Some of the newer equipment can be matched with other equipment to offer flexible operation. Energy efficiency is increasingly becoming imperative, resulting in higher demand for energy-efficient equipment.

Many smaller versions of ovens and other equipment on the market were developed in response to limitations on space and the desire of some operators to use equipment in the view of customers. Other operators have installed preparation equipment—for example, a pizza oven—in full view of their customers. Microwaves, once used for boiling water or reheating foods, are finding their way into preparation areas of many foodservice departments. Microwaves can be used to reheat the many frozen products on the market and are excellent for preparing vegetables.

Equipment that is water and energy intensive is being engineered to conserve water and sewage bills but also to heat that water. Proper ventilation equipment can provide saving on energy used to cool the kitchen and help ensure that cooking and ware-washing equipment work more efficiently.

Another equipment advance is use of robotics, computerized units that assist with repetitive motion, such as placing items on patients' trays and cooking hamburgers. Technology is available to fully automate many kitchen and service activities. Equipment designs no doubt will consider changes in tomorrow's labor force. Instructions must be clear and understandable to workers whose abilities to read English may be limited, and knobs or switches must be designed for physically challenged individuals.

Background of Foodservice Industry

Providing food in an institutional setting has evolved from the Middle Ages when large feudal groups were fed. Many large royal households fed as many as 250 people at each meal. Religious orders served quality food in abbeys to thousands of pilgrims on retreats. Florence Nightingale was the first "dietitian" when she insisted that the troops in field hospitals be provided nourishing food.

Today food is served in homes; restaurants; schools; colleges; universities; health care organizations; the military; corrections facilities; clubs and other social organizations; day-care centers; and industrial, business, and transportation enterprises. Each of the facilities plan, price their menus, and provide a variety of eating rooms, from elegant dining to tray service in health care to fast food that can be eaten in an automobile.

The foodservice industry is one of the world's largest businesses. Sale of processed food worldwide is approximately 3.2 trillion in U.S. currency. According to the Food Industry Overview, U.S. consumers spend approximately US$1 trillion annually on food, or nearly 10 percent of the gross domestic product (GDP). Worldwide foodservice is also the number one employer among all retail businesses, with more than 16.5 million persons employed, most being women and about 25 percent being teenagers. According to the BLS, foodservice and preparation jobs are the fastest-growing national occupation. It is predicted that it will continue to increase. The BLS also predicts a shortage of registered dietitians in the next decade.

There are approximately 1 million foodservice operations in the United States. Many U.S. households continuously rely on others for their food preparation. Before the economic downfall, more than half of every consumer food dollar will be spent on foodservice rather than groceries. Restaurants account for 62 percent of foodservice sales. Elder care is the fastest-growing market; correctional foodservice continues to grow and is expected to have a rapid growth in the next few years, with the greatest increase in federal prisons. More than 10 million meals per year come from correctional facilities.

Health care institutions, like many of the noncommercial foodservice operations, serve a captive audience. Their budgets for expense are included in the hospital room rate, and many health care foodservices are subsidized, which means they receive some funds from external sources.

Classifications of Foodservice

The *hospitality industry* is composed of three major segments: *lodging, food and beverage service,* and *travel and tourism. Lodging* includes hotels, motels, and so on and frequently offers foodservice to the customers. *Travel and tourism* includes retail stores, recreation sites, transportation, travel agencies, and so on. Foodservice may be available at some of the sites. The *food and beverage* services industry is made up of a broad scope of establishments. These establishments are classified as *commercial, noncommercial,* and *institutionals. Commercial foodservice* has as its primary activity the preparation and service of food. In noncommercial and institutional foodservice, the preparation and service of food is a secondary activity. The commercial segment includes fast-food, quick-service, or limited-menu restaurants; fine-dining restaurants; airport restaurants; convenience stores; buffet and self-serve restaurants; catering; supermarkets; food courts; and retail outlets such as department stores. These establishments set their own menu, price structure, and hours of service. Some, like airport restaurants, may serve the same customer only once or twice a year.

The *noncommercial segment,* where entities operate their own foodservice, includes hotel and motel restaurants, country club restaurants, cruise ships, trains, airlines, zoos, sporting events, and theme parks. Each of these establishments may depend on the economy. When the economy is good, customers tend to spend more money to indulge in eating in these restaurants. The *institutional segment* includes the military; correctional facilities; hospitals; child-care centers; senior-care facilities; extended-care facilities such as nursing homes and other health care centers; employee foodservice for offices, industrial complexes, and health care facilities; schools, colleges, and universities; and not-for-profit establishments. All of the institutional segments have several things in common: a captive audience; low cost per meal; many regulatory agencies' standards; and local, state, and federal government regulations that must be met.

In-house management of noncommercial institutional foodservice, referred to as *self-operated,* has remained steady over the past decade. Many noncommercial operations hire contract foodservice organizations that manage the foodservice department as well as other departments. *Contract foodservice management* is the provision of foodservice by a third-party company through a contract. The company meets the objectives of the department but is profit-oriented. The contract company provides management of the foodservice operation for the organization and in some instances may also provide clinical services. Some organizations may outsource some of their services, such as information services or purchasing. *Outsourcing* means that an outside company will provide a service that the organization may not have the staff or equipment to do on-site.

Self-operation is the opposite of contract management. *Self-operating foodservice* is defined as the organization or institution being responsible for the management and clinical components of foodservice. There is an ongoing discussion of the advantages and disadvantages of contract management versus self-operation. The advantages of using the contract companies include but are not limited to expertise, economy of scale, and service:

- *Expertise.* Provides the knowledge, skills, education, and resources that a company will use to operate the foodservice operation.
- *Economy of scale.* The work involved in developing resources for a foodservice operation is done economically, at a reduced cost per unit. The company offers buying power for food and equipment, expertise and in some instances money for renovation projects, computer technology, standardized recipes, and menus for a variety of diets.
- *Service.* Relieves the administration of worry about a department because the company will handle operational issues, quality control, customer satisfaction, and some staffing responsibilities, and the annual employee count is reduced because the employees are considered "management company" employees.

Disadvantages of the contract company versus self-operation include loss of control, expense, and divided loyalty:

- *Loss of control.* Hiring a contract company means relinquishing some control of the foodservice operation. Employees report to the manager of the contract company and are not part of the organization. Leadership roles are not clear unless they are clearly defined in the contract.
- *Expense.* The organization pays a management fee and also may pay the salaries and benefits of employees. The fees may be determined on a cost-per-day basis, plus a percentage of saving, or the revenue against expenses. Each contract may be different and must be carefully evaluated.
- *Divided loyalty.* Employees working for a contract company may have divided loyalties—the company or the organization. The contract should include a meeting between the organization's representative and the contract company's representative to plan and promote integrating loyalty. It is wise to be concerned over a power struggle.

Regardless of who operates the foodservice, it is vital that the needs of customers be the primary concern.

Role of Foodservice

The role of foodservice in a health care organization is to provide a variety of food that is nutritious and well prepared in a safe and sanitary environment that meets the financial obligation of the department while meeting the needs of customers and is served in a pleasing and attractive manner. The department will strive to meet the social, cultural, religious, and psychological needs of customers in meal planning and service. The staff provides education to its customers while they are patients in the health care facility, in outpatient consultations, in the community, and to the general public, as requested.

Employees in the foodservice department are leaders within the organization who adhere to the overall mission, vision, and values of the organization while dovetailing the department's mission, vision, and values and philosophy to those of the organization. The role of the foodservice is to develop goals and outcome objectives and to seek commitment to achieving the outcomes. The department works with other departments within the organization in a team effort to provide for customers. The largest challenge to face a foodservice department is to provide food to its customers while integrating the department's activities into the overall operation of the organization.

Managerial Ethics and Social Responsibility

Foodservice directors face *ethical challenges and social responsibility* as they balance the organization's need to know and the privacy requests of employees and cultural and ethical behaviors of a diverse workforce and customer base to ensure that the organization is working in a socially responsible manner. They also have a responsibility to the *stakeholders*. Stakeholders have a direct "stake" or interest in its performance as they are affected one way or another in what the organization does and how it performs. For health care the stakeholders include customers, vendors, competition, regulators (at all levels), owners, employees, labor unions, clients, and local community.

Ethics is defined as the principles of conduct governing an individual or business or the views, attitudes, and practices about what is right or wrong; it concerns moral standards and basic values. There are professional or business and personal ethics. *Business ethics* refers to principles of moral standard that business executives follow. *Personal ethics* is a code that is influenced by religion or philosophy of life as a moral code. Organizations such as the Academy of Nutrition and Dietetics (AND) and the Association of Nutrition and Foodservice Professionals (ANFP) have written codes of ethics that are guidelines for members of the organizations. (These codes may be found on the organizations' websites.) These codes are intended to promote and maintain the highest standards of food and nutrition services and personal contact among its members. Many codes of ethics are being replaced by standards. The term *standards* refers to some organizations' bills of rights for employees that assist managers in dealing with employees while ensuring those employees' rights.

All foodservice directors need to develop a personal code of ethics. The following should be included:

- Avoidance of conflict of interest
- Honesty and trustworthiness in all activities
- Respect for the rights of others, including cultural, ethnic, religious beliefs, and the right to privacy
- Loyalty to the employer
- Compliance with all applicable laws, regulations, rules, and policies
- Responsibility for one's own actions
- Honesty in credentials
- Adherence to a professional code of ethics
- Keeping confidential information confidential
- Protecting intellectual property

Social responsibility in organizations is changing. Organizations must operate to provide services to achieve the greatest good for the greatest number of people. This can be accomplished by an organization's support of charities or events of public interest or issues and time off for employees to participate in events such as health care fairs, wellness events, environmental, and other related community activities.

Social responsibility also includes the promotion of equal rights of all groups, a fair wage for work performed, and the avoidance of favoritism. Employees should be protected in freedom of speech and assembly. Employees should have the right to unionize. Employers should provide a safe and drug- and smoke-free work environment. Employees should be concerned about issues beyond business- or work-related issues including being proactive about ecology and environmental quality, the conservation of water and energy, pollution and the protection of patients' rights. As time and interest allow, employees should participate in community activities such as volunteering at health fairs, working with cancer-related and children's events.

STRESS

Job stress can affect all the systems of the body. *Stress* is a condition that can be physical or mental strain from situation(s) in the workplace. Foodservice is considered a high-stress occupation because of constant deadlines and demands, the objective of meeting the needs of customers, and in some instances the uneven distribution of the workload.

A foodservice director will need to be a buffer between staff and external stress. As an example, a customer in the cafeteria becomes angry over a perceived error in the amount of change received from a transaction. The foodservice director or cafeteria manager should intervene to deal with the problem, rather than leaving the cashier to fend for herself or himself because the relationship between the cashier and customer in the future could lead to additional stress.

To minimize the stress level in the workplace, foodservice directors should know their stress level and develop ways to cope.

Many books have been written on how to deal with stress. The following ideas may be helpful.

- Know what causes you the greatest stress. Accept your own mistakes as positive learning experiences. Do not constantly relive the experience and fret that it will happen again.
- Keep a positive outlook. See the big picture, focus on what you value, and do not let the little things destroy your attitude. Believe in yourself and your knowledge, skills, and abilities.
- Accept what you cannot change or control. If the administration tells you that you cannot change prices in the cafeteria, let it go. Do not worry about things that are beyond your scope of responsibility or control.
- Focus on one task at a time. Thinking about all the tasks you need to complete is a waste of energy and will not allow you to do your best with the task at hand.
- Use positive results from your work. While working hard and with lots of pressure, bask in the outcomes of your effort. For example, pleasing a customer, teaching a new employee a job task, or writing a well-received report to administration is a positive result.
- Eliminate as many stresses as possible.
- Clear your desk. Throw out clutter such as papers or materials that are no longer needed or used.
- Shut your door. Get rid of annoying or distracting background noises.
- Unclutter your life. Give up activities that cause stress and spend more time with yourself, nonstressful friends, or family members.

When the stress seems overwhelming, take a break. Get away from the situation. Take a walk, chat with a colleague, listen to music, do relaxation exercises that will help to loosen muscles, and release negative thoughts about the offending situation.

- Get a massage for overtired, overused muscles because this can relieve stress.
- Let others know you are stressed. Express your feelings without becoming overly angry.
- Be honest, be direct, and be definite. Learn to say no to something you do not want or need to do.
- Focus on the good things, and be grateful for what you have. Slow down; you can accomplish only one thing at a time. Keep your priorities in mind.
- Seek professional help if stress has increased your blood pressure, changed your life style, and changed your moods (depression)
- Be straightforward without being rude. Do not overreact. Take time out, review the situation, and try to discuss your feelings quietly.

Foodservice directors are better leaders and managers when they learn how to cope with stress and how to provide freedom from undue stress at work. When a work situation becomes over-stressful for the director, it usually affects the staff as well.

PERSONAL AND PROFESSIONAL DEVELOPMENT

Personal and professional involvement is an individual choice. Effective foodservice directors are responsible for maintaining and improving their knowledge and skills to be competent to carry out their duties. This can be accomplished in a number of ways. The following is a list of suggestions that other foodservices directors have found to be beneficial.

- The foodservice industry offers professional development and ongoing education and training.
- The AND, the ANFP, and many other professional organizations conduct annual education conventions where speakers provide information on the latest research on food and nutrition services that can be used to improve skills and continue professional growth.
- Most professional organizations on both the state and national level lobby for its members on issues of interest to the organization. A good example is reimbursement for medical nutrition therapy.
- Professional and trade organizations also publish magazines and journals that address the needs and interests of its members.
- Involvement in professional organizations at local, state, and national levels help improve the profession and assist younger persons entering the profession.
- Serving as a role model or mentor and sharing ideas with students and staff will help new members and will give a foodservice director a sense of "giving back" to the profession.
- Foodservice directors should use information gained in participating in professional activities to train staff and in providing written reports to administration of the facility to let them know how the involvement not only helps foodservice directors personally but is beneficial to the organization.
- Education is lifelong. To continue the education process, foodservice directors should enroll in courses at community colleges, universities, or off-site continuing education programs or attend seminars or workshops that will benefit them and their organization. Education can be obtained while sitting at home/office via webinars, e-learning, websites, videos related to the profession (such as food safety), teleconferences, and online courses through university flexible-learning programs.
- Read critically; read books, journals, trade magazines, and then read some more.
- Networking is building and maintaining positive relationships with people, typically outside current organizations or businesses. Networking with other professionals is an excellent source of support, ideas, and methods improvement. Networking on legislative issues with other professional organizations to lobby support for food and nutrition programs increases the awareness of these issues to the legislative body and the community.

Networking allows foodservice directors to know that their problems are not unique and that by sharing, problems may be solved. Networking can be accomplished by attending local, state, and national professional organization meetings and through websites, Internet chat rooms, telephone calls, and e-mail.

- At conferences offer your business card and collect cards from those you meet. Talk to other members, vendors, educators; ask questions without being intrusive or rude.
- Become involved in community affairs such as religious activities, schools, social and service organizations.
- If possible, participate in research within the organization or as a member of a focus group or a test site for evaluating a new piece of equipment or a new food product.
- Learn from suppliers. Suppliers have a wealth of information concerning new products or equipment. They are also available for hands-on demonstrations for incorporating new food items on menus, latest research reports, and in-service training on sanitation and proper equipment use. Many suppliers also sponsor trade shows where the newest equipment and food items are available, in addition to presentations by noted speakers in the field.
- Participation in professional organizations and networking provides many opportunities to continue on a career path or developing new skill set. It opens doors to what else is available within the profession or what is available if you desire to change professions. Building skills and experiences is lifelong learning. Using your interest and talents may lead to a unique new career. Networking and participation also can lead to lifelong friendships.

SUMMARY

This chapter analyzes the current and projected external environment for health care foodservices. The external environment includes trends and issues arising from the government, businesses and industries, health care institutions, workforce demographics, customer needs and demographics, and technology, the unknown effect the Obama health care plan will have on the delivery of health care. Many of these elements are evolving constantly and will continue to direct the operation of health care nutrition and foodservice departments.

As the environment changes, foodservice managers should modify the goals, objectives, and operation of their departments. Many trends discussed in this chapter will have a direct effect on how other information in the text should be applied to individual departments, and these will be noted in the relevant chapters.

By anticipating trends, successful managers will plan their departmental operations with a vision—both the department's and the facility's—of tomorrow. This is accomplished through conducting an internal and external environmental analysis and applying the information to organizing and planning functions, topics that are discussed fully in Chapter 5.

Clinical pathways
Cloned foods
Contract foodservice management
Cultural diversity
Empowering
Ethics
Genetically modified foods
Interdisciplinary health care providers
Irradiated foods
Medical foods

Medicare/Medicaid
Networking
Obama health care plan
Omnibus Budget Reconciliation Act (OBRA)
Organically grown foods
The Joint Commission
Self-operated
Sous vide foods
Stakeholders
Stress

DISCUSSION QUESTIONS

1. How will the Obama health care plan affect the delivery of health care, including foodservice?

2. How will trends and changes in regulatory agencies standards affect the foodservice operation?

3. What is the impact of having four generations working in the same department at the same time—the differences in how they process information and how they perform assigned tasks, and so on?

4. Name the methods to develop a cohesive workforce with the majority of the employees from different cultures, religions, and ethnicity.

5. What are the ways to be involved in networking and professional organizations?

6. State your own personal code of ethics and how this meshes with the organization's ethics.

7. Name some additional ways to reduce stress at work and in your personal life.

PART ONE

MANAGEMENT OF THE FOODSERVICE DEPARTMENT

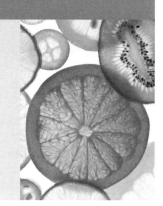

THE MANAGEMENT RESPONSIBILITIES of foodservice managers or directors are the same as those of other professional managers. All managers and directors plan, direct, control, and organize the tasks or activities of subordinates within their respective department or organization. These managers or directors may be classified as first-line or middle managers. Some managers or directors may have responsibilities for other departments besides foodservice. All managers or directors have the responsibility for planning, organizing, leading, controlling, communicating, making decisions, motivating subordinates, handling complaints, setting performance standards or outcomes, improving quality, satisfying customers, controlling the environment and its resources, marketing, and managing fiscal responsibilities. All managers must possess an array of skills in varying degrees, in particular: conceptual, interpersonal, technical, and political skills.

Part One provides information on the role of the manager or director as well as how to manage the foodservice operation. Following an overview in Chapter 1, Chapters 2 through 11 cover topics that managers can use to be more efficient and effective in an ever-changing climate and profession in which "doing more with less" has become the norm.

Chapter 3 outlines methods to market and promote the foodservice operation while increasing revenues. These functions continue to gain importance because of greater demands by surveying agencies and customers for quality food and service. This chapter also promotes "tooting the department's horn."

Chapter 4 gives information on how to develop a continuous quality improvement program and many of the tools that are used to set up and monitor the program. Many surveying and accreditation standards are based on continuous quality improve-

ment. Tools and data are provided to assist in meeting these standards.

Chapter 5 is an important chapter because it discusses planning. Planning is the first step in managing. Planning may include short- and long-term plans with the possible addition of strategic plans with measurable outcomes. Without planning, the efforts of the manager or director and the subordinates will fail. Using problem-solving and decision-making techniques, the manager or director is able to gather data, determine alternatives, and base decisions on facts and objectivity.

Chapter 6 discusses a variety of methods that can be used to organize a foodservice department and to use time wisely. Because of the ongoing reduction of staff and the introduction of new and sophisticated equipment and procedures, it becomes vital that the department(s) be organized in the most efficient manner to maintain a high level of productivity. Poor planning or organizing and time management—falling victim to overbooking, interruptions, missed deadlines, and myriad other problems—can cripple a foodservice department. Chapter 6 covers all these tasks.

The managers or directors must develop good communication skills to deal with individuals of diverse cultural and educational backgrounds. They will also need to communicate with personnel within the facility as well as persons from outside the facility who offer services to the organization. The ability to communicate in an understandable manner using written, verbal, and nonverbal skills is an essential skill that all managers or directors need to develop. Listening, sometimes a forgotten skill, is the most important communication skill of all. The art of communication is discussed in Chapter 7.

Managers or directors, to be successful, need to surround themselves with motivated subordinates. Human resource management is discussed in Chapter 8. The many rules, regulations, and laws that pertain to human resource management are provided. Hiring, orienting, training, job descriptions, and other personnel processes are also discussed.

Chapter 9 explains the importance of maintaining personnel records. The role of the director or manager in providing performance evaluations, disciplinary procedures, and union involvement is discussed.

Technology can be used to interface with other departments, vendors, and peers, to reduce paper, and to provide quick updates on materials and information. Chapter 10 shows how to manage information systems to enhance the foodservice operation by providing up-to-date information on the various systems and subsystems within the operation. A glossary of computer words is provided in the appendix.

Maintaining fiscal responsibility of the foodservice is important. Chapter 11 provides data on controls, budgets, and other financial information that can be used by managers or directors to follow and maintain a budget. They need to learn how to control the financial operation, labor hours, materials, personnel, and equipment as a business entity. Strict accounting and auditing procedures are necessary to ensure that controls are properly in place.

Throughout the chapters, words in italics indicate key terms that are defined.

CHAPTER 2
LEADERSHIP
Managing for Change

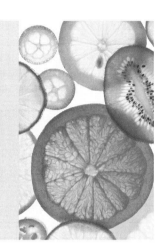

THE TRADITIONAL ROLE of nutrition and foodservice directors or managers has expanded into a more complex one, due in part to the trends described in Chapter 1. The political environment calls for a manager who is fiscally responsible, knows regulatory requirements, and understands how foodservice department functions affect the facility. Managers also must have a heightened awareness of workforce issues, customer needs, technological implications, and continuous quality improvement systems.

Management can be defined in a variety of ways. It is the process of reaching organizational goals by working with and through people and other organizational resources. The management process includes planning, organizing, leading, and controlling an organization's human, physical, and financial resources by influencing other people to get the job done, maintaining morale, and guiding the attitudes of an organization's members in an appropriate direction. The ultimate purpose of influencing is to increase productivity. Employee involvement is essential for improving service, whether employees participate as department team members or on cross-functional teams within the facility.

In this chapter, behaviors, traits, and skills that characterize an effective leader are explored, along with how they can be applied in various situations to guide employees and manage a foodservice department. The practical application of these three components is described within the context of creating a participative work environment that motivates and empowers employees. (Many of the concepts discussed in this chapter are further explained in other chapters.)

LEADERSHIP STYLE

Leadership style is defined by the behaviors, traits, and skills a manager exhibits over time in influencing the work of others to accomplish common goals for the department. Leadership style can be better understood by exploring certain theories on behavior and reviewing situational theories that link management behavior to work factors. In other words, an individual employee's unique level of job task development within the work environment may derive from or respond to a particular leadership style.

Behavior Theories of Effective Leadership

Theories on effective leadership styles have evolved from early research that focused on analyzing personality traits of individuals who demonstrated leadership ability. Studies conducted before World War II identified traits such as intelligence, self-confidence, and physical attractiveness as—not surprisingly—being desirable. These studies, however, were unable to isolate a single trait that could predict leadership ability. Research since World War II has focused more on behaviors as indicators for identifying what creates an effective leader.

Two recent studies, one by Rensis Likert in 1961 at Ohio State University (OSU) in Columbus and another by the University of Michigan in Ann Arbor in 1964, were conducted to identify leadership behaviors. The OSU studies concluded that leaders exhibit two main types of behavior, structural and consideration. *Structural* behavior is leadership activity that either delineates the relationship between the leader and the leader's followers or establishes well-defined procedures that the followers should adhere to in performing their jobs. *Consideration* behavior is leadership behavior that reflects friendship, mutual trust, respect, and warmth in relationships between a leader and followers. The conclusions of the studies showed that leaders who were both high in structural and consideration behaviors achieved high subordinate performance and satisfaction in most instances.

The Michigan studies, conducted by Rensis Likert (described by Dessler), defined two basic types of leader behavior: job-centered and employee-centered behavior. *Job-centered* behavior focuses primarily on the work or production a subordinate is doing as well as the job's technical aspects. *Employee-centered* behavior is leader behavior that focuses primarily on subordinates as people, on personality needs, and on building good interpersonal relationships. The conclusion of the study proved that employee-oriented leaders had high group productivity and higher job satisfaction

Using the behavioral approach, leadership styles have been defined or categorized using a variety of terms. Perhaps the most familiar categories (or terms) are *autocratic, democratic*, and *laissez-faire* approaches. Another classification uses terms such as *directive, supportive, participative*, and *achievement*. Work conducted by Robert R. Blake and Jane S. Mouton in the late 1970s grouped behaviors into five categories using a management grid to identify leadership styles:

1. *Task or authority-obedience management* describes a behavior that exhibits little concern for employees and emphasizes production activities. A task-management leader delegates little authority and is autocratic in dealings with subordinates.
2. *Country club management* is demonstrated by a manager whose primary interest is in keeping employees happy and satisfied in their work. The work environment is permissive, and pressure of any kind is avoided.
3. *Middle-of-the-road* characterizes the style of a manager who seems to focus on tasks and employees. However, decision making is marked by compromise and ambivalence, with constant fluctuation between opposing viewpoints.
4. *Improvised management* describes the management behavior of one who provides virtually no leadership to subordinates, with all productivity attributable to the employees' own initiative.
5. *Team management* is demonstrated by a manager who shows a high level of concern for both people and productivity. Unlike middle-of-the-road management, however, this behavior emphasizes the importance of mutual trust, understanding, and common objectives.

These leadership behaviors, and their variations, are revisited throughout this book as necessary.

Situational Leadership

The theories on situational leadership attempt to identify basic factors in the work environment that determine appropriate leadership behavior. One such theory, called the *contingency theory*, suggests that effective leadership behavior is based on three factors: the organization's task, the relationship between the leader and other members of the organization, and the leader's power base within the organization. The contingency theory assumes that a leader is either task-oriented or people-oriented and that he or she cannot change leadership styles to suit the work situation. Therefore, the work situation must be changed to suit the leader's style.

Numerous other theories dispute the contingency theory, saying that the leader, not the work environment, must be flexible in situational leadership. One such theory was proposed by Victor H. Vroom and Philip W. Yetton in 1973 and refined and updated in 1988 (described by Dessler and others), as the Vroom-Yetton-Jago model of leadership. This theory focuses on how much participation to allow subordinates in the decision-making process. The model is built on two principles: organizational decisions should have a beneficial effect on performance, and subordinates should accept and be committed to organizational decisions that are made. The Vroom-Yetton-Jago model suggests that there are five different decision styles or ways leaders make decisions, from the autocratic to consultative to group focused. Later Vroom-Jago developed another contingency leadership theory that focuses on how managers lead through their use of decision-making methods. The theory is that managers have three decision options and no one option is always superior to the other. The three choices are:

1. *Authority decision.* Leaders make the decision and then communicate the decision to the personnel.
2. *Consultative decision.* Leaders seek input from individual or group members and then make the decision.
3. *Group decision.* Leaders establish a group, tell them the problem, and then facilitate the group in making the decision.

A situational theory that assumes that a leader can be flexible in exhibiting the degree of control, concern for productivity and employees, structure provided, and risk taken in decision making is defined in *Effective Behavior in Organizations*, by Cohen, Fink, Gadon, Willits, and Josefowitz. The authors define leadership style using five distinct dimensions and argue that a leader may respond or exhibit behavior at various points along the dimensions, depending on the situation. These five dimensions (called the *five-dimension theory*) help describe how a leader might carry out various functions and can be applied directly to foodservice department functions.

1. *Retaining control versus sharing control.* The degree of control retained or shared is apparent based on who makes decisions (manager or employees), how decisions are made (with or without employee input), whether information is shared with staff, and the amount and nature of work delegated.

2. *High-task concern versus low-task concerns.* This dimension relates to the emphasis placed on the quality and quantity of production or output. A foodservice manager, for example, may place high or low emphasis on employee productivity. Although for financial reasons a high level of task concern may be desirable, it need not occur to the exclusion of concern for clients or workers.
3. *High-person concern versus low-person concern.* Concern for individuals—consumers or staff—considers the effect of actions or changes on department morale.
4. *Explicit versus implicit expectations (degree of structure provided).* This dimension is determined by how clearly and in how much detail tasks are identified; the number of written policies; and the form of communication, whether written or verbal.
5. *Cautious versus adventurous decision making.* The level of risk involved in decision making, a manager's level of visibility within the organization, and how willing the manager is to push the outer limits characterize this dimension of leadership style.

The situational leadership models discussed so far provide the basis for work presented by Paul Hersey and Kenneth Blanchard on situational leadership theory. Hersey and Blanchard defined *situational leadership theory* as "a model of leadership behavior that reflects how a leader should adjust his or her leadership style in accordance with the readiness of followers." Two important points in this theory are whether followers are ready to follow the leader and whether they do or do not accept the leader. Regardless of what the leader does, the group effectiveness depends on the action of the followers. Hersey and Blanchard define *readiness* as the extent to which people have the ability and willingness to accomplish a specific task. The four styles defined by Hersey and Blanchard, which are progressive and can be applied by management personnel at all levels, are *telling (high-task–low-relationship style)*, *selling (high-task–high-relationship styles)*, *participating (low-task–high-relationship style)*, and *delegating (low-task–low-relationship style)*. There are also four stages of employee readiness that states that they are people who are: (1) unable and unwilling to take responsibility for doing something, (2) unable but willing to do what the leaders wants, (3) are able or unwilling to do what the leaders wants, (4) are both unable and unwilling to do what is asked of them.

It is understood that managers will develop a leadership style that is preferable and most compatible with their individual makeup, but it is also desirable that the style be appropriate for dealing with a variety of employees and situations. Ultimately, complex situations or employees with mixed skill levels (or both) will necessitate the use of more than one leadership style.

The third style, *supportive leadership*, is exercised with employees who have knowledge concerning the tasks they are assigned but may still lack confidence in their abilities. A supportive leader shares responsibility for a task and decision making with employees while helping to accomplish it. The fourth leadership style recognizes employees who are highly motivated, knowledgeable about their job, and ready for full delegation from a manager. A delegating leadership style allows a manager to turn over responsibility for both decision making and problem solving to employees. Leaders whose employees are capable of taking on this responsibility should remember that delegation is not abdication but a sharing of responsibility. Employees will continue to need a leader's guidance to ensure task completion. Further discussion on delegation can be found in Chapter 5 on planning and decision making.

Depending on the employees' developmental level and the situation, more than one style can be used with the same employees. For example, an employee responsible for tray preparation, meal delivery, and cleanup may have varying levels of expertise in these areas. Whereas total delegation may be appropriate for meal preparation and cleanup, tasks related to meal service may require more of a directing or coaching role.

Gender and Leadership

Some leaders believe that gender differences in leadership is a non-issue. Leadership may have more to do with style than gender. Both females and males show some of the same qualities such as self-discipline, ambition, expertise in their field, and a strong visible presence. Women appear to be more successful in day-by-day leadership than men. Women leaders are significantly more participative than males. Women prefer to build consensus and use good interpersonal skills and be more democratic and participative by showing respect for others, caring for others, and sharing communication and information with others. Men tend to rely on directive and assertive behavior: "I am the boss, I am in control, and I am in command." Regardless of gender, an interactive leadership style is needed in today's ever-evolving health care organizations.

LEADERS AS MANAGERS

Leading and *managing* are two activities that take place in all organizations, and the two terms are often used interchangeably. The role of a *leader* is to create a vision for organizations or units, promote major changes in goals and procedures, set and communicate new directions, and inspire subordinates. *Managing* involves most of the kinds of activities that are included in a leader's role. A person can be a leader and a manager. Leadership is a component of management, but management involves more than just leadership.

Leadership style is defined by characteristic behaviors and traits in various situations, as well as the process of inspiring others to work hard to accomplish important tasks; then management applies these items in the planning, organizing, staffing, and controlling of resources to achieve goals. In this context, rather than being part of what defines management, leading dictates how management is carried out. In other words, good managers place more emphasis on leadership and apply what they know and learn to the daily and long-term management of their departments.

Leadership Characteristics for Effective Management

Based on the leadership theories discussed earlier, what attributes will a successful health care foodservice manager need in the future? Current literature and expert opinion lean toward two general categories: technical expertise and knowledge and interpersonal skills that promote a participative, enabling environment for employees. The common denominator between the two is flexibility, the essential ingredient for dealing with rapid changes that will permeate health care foodservice throughout the twenty-first century. As identified in Chapter 1, external environmental changes will alter both work methods and those who perform the work. Flexibility allows foodservice managers to plan, organize, and lead according to the dictates of the work situation and employee diversity. Flexibility in leadership style also helps employees deal with change. The effects of change are addressed in Chapter 5. The two key attributes, technical proficiency and interpersonal skills, are discussed next, followed by a brief statement on the qualities of a leader.

Technical Expertise and Knowledge

Technical proficiency uses the knowledge, tools, and techniques of a particular profession or job. A leader's technical skills include the ability to use administrative knowledge and tools to carry out basic management functions (described later in the chapter). They also include the ability to develop and implement standards and policies and procedures, to process paperwork in an orderly manner, to manage the work of the unit or department with the resources allocated, and to coordinate work and elicit the cooperation of employees and others within the organization. Administrative skills are used most often by top-level managers and least often by first-line supervisors. Managers on all levels are responsible for processing paperwork, whereas the responsibility for implementing standards falls primarily on first-line supervisors.

Technical skills are used frequently by first-line supervisors who have daily contact with employees and must spend a large portion of their time training, evaluating performance, and answering task-related questions. First-line supervisors in smaller organizations may be expected to perform tasks that in larger organizations are assigned to nonmanagerial employees, or they may be expected to act as lead workers on employee teams. Evaluation of technical skills should be one consideration given to employees who show supervisory potential. Although technical skills are important, an employee highly skilled in task performance but lacking the administrative and interpersonal skills required by the position may not be a good candidate for a supervisory position. At the same time, an otherwise competent manager who lacks technical skills may be less than successful if the position requires monitoring the performance of production-level employees. Put simply, both are needed. (See references for Standard of Professional Performance for the Management RD and Standards of Performance for Certified Dietary Managers.)

Effective leaders must view development for themselves, for their employees, and for the organization as a continuous process. *Technical knowledge* for foodservice managers, for example, may be enhanced through trade shows, which provide information on the latest equipment, supplies, and food items. Continuing or higher education classes and professional organization meetings also may provide an ongoing flow of information to manage a department effectively. Future demands will include technical expertise and knowledge in the following areas:

- Environmental protection rules
- The political environment—especially all the changes in the delivery of health care
- Marketing, revenue-generating programs and customer satisfaction
- Continuous quality improvement, surveying regulations changes
- Work redesign, productivity, and benchmarking
- Innovative cost-containment measures
- Food consumption patterns, sustainability, LEED, Green
- Food and equipment technology
- Human resource trends and changes in laws
- Food and water safety, waste management, protection of the environment
- Disaster and emergency planning
- Cultural diversity and generational difference in the workplace

This knowledge is important in establishing the strategic direction for a department that is in tune with the vision of the larger organization.

Interpersonal Skills

Effective leaders rely on basic *interpersonal skills*—communication, empathy, understanding, ethical conduct, motivation, mentoring, trustworthiness, intelligence, sharing the vision, goals, and objectives, self-confidence, and delegating—to influence the behavior of others in a positive manner to ensure peak performance. The higher the level of management, the less emphasis is placed on technical skills and the more emphasis is placed on interpersonal skills. Middle-level managers spend about 50 percent of their time applying their interpersonal skills. These skills also depend on a manager's awareness of the various beliefs, needs, and attitudes of group members and of their perceptions of themselves, their work, and the organization. Some would argue that these interpersonal skills make the difference between effective and ineffective leadership.

Interpersonal skills are important to managerial success in a foodservice department because they promote harmony among foodservice workers and try to fit the needs of individual workers into the operating requirements of the department. They also enable foodservice directors to develop a network of positive relationships with administrators and other hospital staff members (as well as with other health care workers, physicians, patients, and vendors). Without such relationships, few managers would meet their own professional goals or fulfill the organization's objectives.

Effective leaders have the ability to manage themselves, gaining rapport and building good relationships with others within and outside the organization. Leaders need to have a drive to succeed, to be energized, and to challenge employees to seek lifelong learning either by formal or informal education.

Successful leaders must prove their authenticity to employees; that is, that they are persons of character and integrity. Employees need to know that their manager can be trusted and that they consistently will be treated fairly. Managers who remain above reproach win their staff's respect and dedication. Department leaders must enforce rules that protect the safety and security of employees and customers. Employees come to know a leader's values through his or her actions and interactions with others. The behavior exhibited by managers when interacting with employees, peers, and vendors says more about their leadership style than does any verbal rhetoric.

Effective leaders consistently follow two practices: promoting an environment or culture that fosters learning, innovation, and risk taking, and believing that employees are the most important resource in the department and treating them accordingly. In this nurturing environment, a manager has an open-door policy to ensure that employee needs are met, and that he or she most likely will find employees doing things right and will offer praise accordingly.

Successful leaders also have these characteristics: they are visible and approachable to employees; they seek feedback on decisions, procedures, and so on; they give clear directions to **all** staff members. The leader also provides a degree of freedom in assignments (empowering), balancing the positive and negative aspects of the job. It is important for the successful leader to keep a perspective, to learn from all situations and decisions, either good or bad, trust their own instincts, and above all be true to themselves and find a happy medium between work and outside of work.

Effective *communication* is perhaps one of the most important interpersonal skills, helping to instill in employees a department's vision and departmental objectives as well as being attuned to their needs and providing performance feedback. Identifying how a department fits into an organization's vision—and clearly articulating this to employees—is a necessary characteristic of an effective leader. Chapter 7 identifies effective communication skills.

Formal Versus Informal Leaders

In every organization there is a *formal leader*, one who has the legal authority and responsibility to operate the department, make decisions, control finances, and other functions granted by the organization/position. There is also an *informal leader* who has no legal authority but has a great deal of influence and power within the department and in some instances the total operation. The informal leader does not have an "official" title as a leader, but may hold any position within the department/organization. The informal leader is frequently contacted by other employees for additional information and is a spokesperson for a group. The contacts will depend on the issues. It is important for the "legal" leader to know who the informal leader is and when a change is made that the informal leader accepts it and persuades others to cooperate.

Managers' Roles

Current and future managers must view their roles in light of changes and trends that dictate the need for strong leadership. The application of leadership can be seen in the traditional roles of management, as described in the theory developed by Henry Mintzberg. The three roles identified in the Mintzberg model are interpersonal, informational, and decisional.

The *interpersonal* role involves building and maintaining contacts and relationships with a variety of people inside and outside the department. This role requires the manager to act as a symbol representing the department; to function as a liaison with others outside the department; and to provide supervision in hiring, training, and motivating employees. The importance of interpersonal skills for a leader-manager was discussed in the subsection on leadership characteristics for effective management. As the demands for quality, customer satisfaction, and employee empowerment continue to evolve, a manager's interpersonal skills take on added importance.

The *informational* role requires a manager to monitor operations through data collection and analysis, to disseminate information to employees and others, and to act as a spokesperson outside the department. The manager's informational role can be defined in terms of *effective communication*, as outlined in Chapter 7. A manager must keep up to date on events by attending organizational and professional meetings, reading current literature, and networking. The manager must then disseminate relevant information to other department members, acting as the department spokesperson, information conduit, and negotiator who "sells" or persuades others to buy into plans for additional resources or policy changes that affect patients and coworkers. In this spokesperson role, a manager keeps others up to date on changes within the department.

The *decisional* role requires a manager to be innovative, to handle conflict and problem resolution, and to allocate resources. An innovative manager must identify and interpret trends so as to anticipate and plan for future service opportunities and improvements. He or she must proactively seek new business or program possibilities and discover new approaches to effective problem solving. Conflict management occurs at all levels of management, and frontline supervisors are required to deal decisively with disruptions that can arise daily in a health care environment. In general, the higher the level of management, the less time is spent in dealing with conflict.

Because the decision-making role also involves the allocation of resources, a manager must set priorities for departmental functions and how resources—from department personnel to food and equipment, time, information, and money—are used. Decision-making responsibilities can be closely controlled by a manager or shared with supervisors and frontline employees, depending on the matter being decided and on the leadership style. Decision making is discussed as it relates to individuals, teams, and a participative work environment later in this chapter and in Chapter 5.

These three management roles are interdependent. For example, a manager can gather outside information by using interpersonal skills and then use decision-making skills in applying the information to determine how work is planned and executed within the department. The roles of management as outlined in this section need not be the sole responsibility of a manager. In fact, it is through sharing of these roles and responsibility that a participative work environment is created and fostered.

Managers of health care foodservice departments must fulfill their roles within the context of providing food and nutrition services to the organization's customers. To accomplish this goal, they must use specific functions of management—planning, organizing, staffing, leading, and controlling—to ensure that a department's resources are used efficiently and effectively.

Levels of Management

The number of management levels in a foodservice department depends on many factors, including the number of employees, hours of operation, the complexity and scope of service, and the department's organizational structure. In smaller organizations where there are fewer employees and limited hours of operation, only two levels of management—department director and supervisors or lead employees—may be needed. Most medium to large foodservice departments have at least three levels of management: top level (director), middle level (managers), and first-line (supervisors).

The scope of service can influence the number of both management positions and levels. A department responsible only for feeding patients or residents will have fewer management personnel and levels than one responsible for feeding patients and nonpatients. If additional services are provided (for example, catering, vending service, coffee shops, child care, extended care, bakery operations, physician dining facilities), more management levels may be needed, such as a director, assistant directors, managers, and supervisors. Added meals mean additional preparation and service requirements and, consequently, more employees.

Traditionally, levels of management have been differentiated using the functional-hierarchical organizational structure shown in Figure 2.1. This structure, developed in the late nineteenth century and supported by the "scientific management" theory of Frederick Taylor, is based on a rigid chain of command and layers of management with varying levels of authority and responsibility. Total authority and control in this model rest with management. Using the functional-hierarchical structure, organizations assign different levels of management according to the responsibilities and authority needed to fulfill them. In this context, *responsibility* is a manager's obligation to perform certain tasks or duties, and *authority* is his or her power to allocate specific resources in the performance of those tasks or duties. For example, a hospital's CEO has more responsibility for the overall operation of the hospital and therefore more authority to direct the use of hospital resources than does the foodservice director.

Other management structures used by health care organizations to foster teamwork and employee empowerment are *matrix design, product-line management*, and *team-based organization organizational design*. These models create an organizational structure that shares responsibility and authority to move decision making to the lowest possible level in the organization. They also make it possible to have fewer layers of management by virtue of shared responsibility and authority. Organizational structure is discussed in more detail in Chapter 6.

All levels of management have one thing in common: all managers must use leadership skills to plan, organize, coordinate, and control the resources for which they are responsible. Foodservice directors must develop departmental plans that are based on the goals, vision, mission, and objectives of the institution. Middle managers also must guide and monitor the performance of their departments.

The scope of first-line managers is narrower, but they, too, must plan, coordinate, and control the daily activities (for example, efficient operation of the tray line in the food preparation area) of employees they supervise. Again, the more participative the work environment, the more the functions of management are shared among various levels of management.

Basic Functions of Management

Coordinating the work of individuals, teams, or a department requires managers in any organization and at any level to perform four basic managerial functions: *planning, organizing, leading*, and

FIGURE 2.1 Levels of Health Care Management

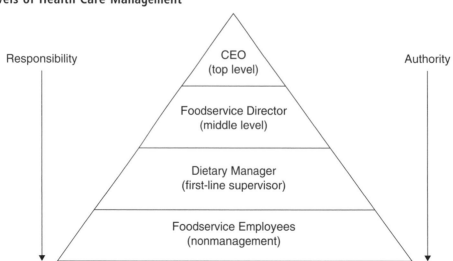

controlling. These four functions are interrelated, and the extent to which a manager exercises them depends on the complexity of the problems or issues in question and on the manager's level within the organization. For example, although top- and middle-level managers typically spend more time on planning and control functions, participative work environments bid managers at all levels to provide input and be accountable for carrying out the work of the organization. All management levels contribute to the organizing function, which defines the scope of jobs and determines staffing requirements. As mentioned earlier in this chapter, the function of leading places increased demands on all levels of managers in influencing work completion by employees. The next four subsections take a closer look at each of these basic functions of management.

Planning

Through *planning*, the future course of an organization or group is determined. The *planning function* helps set goals and objectives and define policies and procedures to achieve them. Planning is a continuous process of reviewing information, weighing alternatives, making decisions about those alternatives, and devising strategies to make the best use of available resources. Information reviewed includes trends and issues in the external environment and long-range plans for the organization.

Most organizations engage in two types of planning, *operational* and *strategic*, each of which is defined by the time span covered by the plan. For example, when developing short-range plans for day-to-day operations, a foodservice manager engages in *operational planning*. These short-range plans generally are based on existing facilities and markets. *Strategic planning*, on the other hand, emphasizes long-range issues and new opportunities related to the organization's mission and objectives. A third type of planning, called *performance planning*, is built on individual employee potential, contribution, and achievement. Planning is discussed further in Chapter 5.

Planning occurs at every level of management. Top-level management in a hospital—for instance, the CEO—must work with other decision makers within the organization and the board of directors to develop the hospital's vision and strategic plan, which will guide overall activities and changes in the institution for a long period—five years or more. One element in the strategic plan might be to add a skilled-nursing unit. In turn, a foodservice director would need to develop specific policies and operating plans for cooperating with other departments to deliver meals and nutrition services, taking into consideration regulations of the surveying and accreditation agencies. First-line foodservice managers also would need to participate in this process, for example, if it appears necessary to restructure meal delivery times to ensure that meals are delivered within the guidelines established for the unit. The planning function establishes the general picture of what is to be done and how it is to be accomplished.

Organizing

The *organizing* function involves defining fine points of job specifications and determining how work is to be grouped, who is to do the work, what authority is needed, how much staff is needed, and how work will be accomplished by using what resources, and how to coordinate activities of individuals and groups. Whether they are responsible for the whole department or for a smaller unit such as the cafeteria, all foodservice managers must consider how their objectives can be broken down into specific tasks and assignments and how these assignments can best relate to one another in authority, responsibility, and communication of information. Managers must then decide which tasks to accomplish personally and which ones to delegate. It is vital that the authority needed to make use of appropriate resources be delegated along with the responsibility. Finally, the organizing function also includes the task of staffing the positions identified. Recruiting, interviewing, hiring, orienting, training, and developing new employees are major parts of most managers' responsibilities. The human resource, or personnel, department may assist managers in some or all of these staffing responsibilities.

Influencing

Influencing is a function that has been titled *motivating, leading*, and *direction*. *Influencing* is the process of guiding the activities of an organization's members by enthusiasm, hard work, and inspiration, in an appropriate direction to help the organization move toward goal attainment. The ultimate purpose is to increase productivity. Influencing requires managers to use their interpersonal skills to influence individuals and teams and to communicate information and instructions. Individuals and teams must be motivated to accept and strive to meet departmental and organizational objectives as established through the planning and organizing functions. Effective influencing requires a manager to understand how to motivate employees to achieve individual goals and how to coordinate the work and interactions of employee groups.

Controlling

Controlling is the process of measuring work performance to actual outcomes that are consistent with the planned outcomes specified by the goals and objectives. Because goals and objectives should be accomplished with the most effective and efficient use of resources, control is essential. It is the medium by which accountability—for instance, adherence to timelines, resource use, and quality of outcomes—is ensured. Ensuring control involves several actions:

- Establishing standards of performance or outcome and communicating them to the persons who must meet those standards
- Devising systems for measuring performance, either by monitoring the work process or by examining the work product
- Evaluating performance measures with the standards set
- Adjusting performance as necessary by first determining why it does not meet established standards

TABLE 2.1. Types of Power

Source of Power	Description of Power Source
1. Position or legal power	The power to control others because of position or title held
2. Expert power	The power to control others because of expert knowledge, experience, or information that one possesses
3. Interpersonal or referent power	The power to control others because of personal charisma or personality
4. Reward power	The power to control others by giving rewards; power based on control of resources to compensate individuals for good performance
5. Coercive or punitive power	The power to control others by punishing those who make mistakes or perform poorly
6. Personal power	The power to influence, power received from a manager's relationship with others

MANAGERIAL POWER

Managerial power is the ability to influence someone or something to change the course of events or overcome resistance and to get people to do something they would not otherwise do. Just because managers have power does not ensure that they will use it or even use it wisely. Power may originate from the leader, the subordinate, the position, or the leader's ability to dispense reward and punishment.

There are basically five types of power: expert, referent, legitimate, reward, and coercive. Table 2.1 describes each of the types.

The two major types of power based on their sources are *position* and *personal*. *Position power* is based on the rank of a manager in an organization, and the power of the position is given by the manager's superior. It encompasses legitimate, reward, and coercive power. *Personal power* is based on a person's individual characteristics and is given in part by subordinates. Personal power encompasses expert and referent power.

Legitimate power is the power granted to the position or formal authority to carry out the responsibilities of the position. Some managers believe that this power can be used to tell employees what to do by virtue of the position and authority over the person. This power can be ambiguous. A manager and subordinate can disagree on the directive and leave room for open conflict. The subordinate may do the job as directed but will do only "what has to be done."

Reward or *punitive power* is the strongest source of power because of the authority to give rewards or the threat of punishment to subordinates. Not all employees will receive the best assignments or receive the largest reward. This power must be handled carefully and objectively. This power has the potential to increase motivation in those who receive rewards, but it can also decrease motivation for those who do not receive them or if the reward is insufficient.

Coercive power is the ability to administer punishment by either withholding a reward (salary increase) or giving out punishment (letter of reprimand). A major problem with the use of coercive power is that subordinates can devise methods to disguise their objectionable behavior or they can retaliate. Coercing employees by reducing pay, reducing work hours, or refusing requested days off can result in work slowdown, absenteeism, or union complaints or grievances. All personnel within an organization can use coercive power, from the subordinate who withholds needed information, making a situation worse, or uses subtle effective methods to fail to meet time commitments to the CEO who uses this power as a threat to the manager.

Expert power is based on specialized knowledge in a specific field that others do not possess. The power comes when others need this expertise. An example is the physician-patient relationship. Expert power is held by all in an organization: the secretary who knows where certain information is filed, the plumber who can repair a leak, and the computer expert who can repair the computer and retrieve data.

Interpersonal or *referent power* is the power to control others through charisma, respect, and interpersonal relationships. It is also a power of subtle occurrence. Subordinates may emulate the superior by mimicking the superior's gestures or other mannerisms. This power has great potential due to relationships with department staff and others within an organization where the manager has no legal power.

Power should be used to achieve the objectives, but care should be taken to avoid using excessive power. The right type of power to use depends on the situation and circumstances surrounding it. Power can be used to influence specific behaviors and to affect the behavior and attitudes of other people. Power should be shared by empowering others (discussed later in this chapter).

MANAGERS' RESPONSIBILITIES

Managers are responsible for management functions, resource management, and production of a service or a product. In the above discussion, the management functions of managers—planning, organizing, influencing, and controlling—were explained. In later chapters, directing, staffing, communicating, and representing will be discussed. *Resource management* is the authority and responsibility to manage the resources allocated to a department. These resources are made up of "8Ms":

1. Men: The number of personnel allocated in the budget
2. Minutes: The number of productive and nonproductive hours/minutes for each worker
3. Machines: Equipment available to meet outcomes
4. Money: To purchase supplies, pay personnel, and maintain and renovate area
5. Methods: Policies, procedures, goals, and objectives that define what to do and how to do it
6. Materials: Needed to prepare food and maintain a safe and sanitary environment
7. Markets: Regular customers and potential customers through promotion and advertising
8. Motivator: To produce the best-quality products to meet expected outcomes

Managers also have the responsibility for meeting the outcomes or organizational goals. These goals include providing a safe place for employment, providing a quality product, adhering to the mission, vision, and values of the organization, and providing for the wants and needs of customers.

Managers will be more likely to succeed in their responsibilities if they possess: integrity, credibility, consistency in values, and moral leadership as shown by the manager's actions and personal example, and if they have set high ethical standard for others to follow.

PARTICIPATIVE MANAGEMENT

Creating a work environment in which employees are not only allowed but openly encouraged to participate in job-related decisions takes dedication and persistence on the part of all management levels. The reason for creating such an environment is to be positioned to respond to changing demographics and demands of the workforce, increased emphasis on customer satisfaction, and the demands for continuous quality improvement.

Participative management has positive effects for both the organization and employees. Because employees are closer to the customers, they can more readily identify and meet customers' needs. Employees empowered to act instantly to satisfy customers win customer dedication and return business for the organization and gain a feeling of self-worth and further incentive to complete their jobs. These feelings motivate employees, improve the quality of their work life, and increase their level of commitment to the department and to the organization. Another benefit to promoting employee autonomy is that the organization gains from employees' knowledge and experience, in turn giving them a sense of ownership in the work process.

Managers may act *proactively* or *reactively* to a situation. A proactive manager will take actions to prevent a disaster. For example, the proactive manager will have plans for various situations and will react calmly to the crisis. The manager will take action to intervene to prevent or contain a situation.

Using the reactive management style the manager *reacts* to a crisis immediately because no plans were in place, employees had not been trained, and policies and procedures were not followed. It may take days to solve the crisis. Managers who act in a proactive manner know and practice good management techniques and train their employees how to act in a crisis.

Creating a Participative Culture

Organizational culture (and therefore departmental culture) is identified by how things get done. As is true for other social units, a facility's cultural climate (or personality) is determined by the accepted norms, values, and beliefs demonstrated through the behaviors and relationships of its management and employees in various situations. It influences how employees view and perform their jobs, how they work with colleagues, and how they look at their institution's future. The internal culture is a blend of the following components:

- The external environment (that is, the larger community) in which the organization exists
- The employee selection process
- Execution of managerial functions
- Accepted behaviors within the organization
- Organizational structure and processes
- The removal of deviate members (unsatisfactory workers)

Creating a participative environment requires a change in the views, beliefs, and behaviors of managers and employees. These changes influence how things get done and, eventually, the culture (or "feel") of the organization.

A *culture inventory*, or *audit* (often conducted by consultants), may help an organization assess its current culture by asking employees to define their ideal culture. For example, questioning employees about how they feel about their jobs, whether they feel comfortable approaching their supervisors, to what extent they regard customers as being important to the organization, whether they feel that reward and recognition are linked to satisfying customers, and so on can disclose much about an organizational climate. Once audit results have been tabulated, analysis of the information can uncover areas in which change is needed to support continuous quality improvement. Audit results should be shared with staff and an action plan created to define how the ideal continuous quality improvement culture can be promoted. More on culture as it relates to quality is detailed in Chapter 4.

Management Responsibilities in a Participative Culture

To establish a participative work culture setting that enables employees and strengthens their commitment, managers must assume a number of responsibilities. Some key tasks are listed below as well as other employee development techniques:

- Training and developing employees to their highest potential
- Sharing decision-making authority
- Building a team mind-set
- Compensating and rewarding employee achievement
- Removing obstacles to employee advancement
- Communicating effectively

Other development techniques such as:

- *On-the-job training* (OJT) is training developed to assist the employees to learn and apply the principles and procedures to complete a job. This type of development is used for all employees at all levels of the organization.
- *Job rotation* is a method used to move trainees or seasoned employees from a job or department to other areas within the organization to broaden their experience and to identify the employee's strong and weak points. This type of training may be used for new college graduates who need to discover the jobs they prefer, or are best qualified for, as well as broaden their knowledge of the organization.

- *Apprenticeship* is a method that has been used for centuries. Apprenticeship is a structural process where individuals may become skilled workers. The training involves assigning a nonskilled person to the guidance/teaching of a master craftsperson, for example, assigning a cook's helper to a chef.

Training and Development

Managers must assess employee development levels to appropriately match capabilities to work situations. One key to ensuring a participative culture is to provide the right mix of information, power, and incentive that will positively influence departmental performance.

A positive work environment is fueled by the development of employee potential. This is accomplished through new employee *orientation, continuing education, in-service training, cross-functional training* across jobs and across department lines, *skill enhancement programs* both inside and outside the organization, and *daily coaching* from managers. This also includes lifelong learning. Lifelong learning includes many variances such as the organization paying for tuition to a deserving employee(s) to complete a GED, or to attend a local community college or a specialized training program where certification may be earned. Another method of lifelong learning includes paid time off to attend job-related training that is held on a consistent basis that relates to skills that are specific to the job, such as technology training. *Management development training* is specialized training to improve current or future management performance, knowledge, skills, attitude, communication, and other skills that may be taught. In addition, successful empowerment ensures that roles, relationships, job duties, and performance expectations are clearly defined up front for new employees.

Employees and especially managers can become more proactive and productive when a *mentoring program* is available. Mentoring is where a "seasoned" employee acts as a counselor/trainer to a new member of the organization. The *mentor* provides support, guidance, and assistance as the new employee goes through difficult times and challenges to help the employee overcome problems. The mentor is a volunteer committed to helping the employee learn new ways. The mentor is an adviser who introduces the employee to others in the profession or workplace. Mentors provide answers concerning foodservice basics, and they help the employee assimilate into the organization.

A mentor needs to have these qualities and character:

- A reputation for honesty and effectiveness within the organization
- Respect for senior management as well as all levels of employee positions
- Excellent communication skills, especially the ability to listen
- A willingness to invest the time needed
- A personal stake in seeing that the employee succeeds
- A good sense of humor
- A pleasant nonjudgmental personality

Further discussion on the manager's training responsibility can be found in Chapter 8.

Shared Decision Making

As mentioned earlier, shared power and *decision-making* authority between managers and employees enables employees to influence their day-to-day work life, which enhances job ownership and commitment. Therefore, when job descriptions are written or revised, when work processes are designed or reviewed, or when procedures are changed, employees should be polled for their input. This can be done by using questionnaires that disclose how the work is done, seeking suggestions on how the job should be done, or group meetings in which managers and employees brainstorm new methods. *Brainstorming* is an idea- and information-sharing session at which everyone is allowed to give input without being judged. Authority can be shared in employee performance appraisals, at which employees can participate in rating the quality and quantity of their work and in setting goals to improve or enhance their performance. Empowerment is discussed further in a later subsection.

Team Building

Participative management appreciates the benefits of having employees work in *teams* to influence quality improvement, customer satisfaction, and job performance. Managers must be part of the team, not above it, providing the information and training needed to foster team success. Once employees become accustomed to working in groups to influence job design or to solve problems, they will be capable of meeting with less input or guidance from the manager. This does not mean that a manager should abdicate responsibility for ensuring that meeting time is scheduled, recommendations are considered fully, and resources are available to implement team recommendations.

Compensation and Rewards

Employee incentives, either formal (*compensation*) or informal (*rewards*), are key to nurturing a participative work environment. *Formal rewards* encompass pay policies, employee benefits, and career paths, all of which usually are set up and administered by the human resource department. Some organizations have implemented formal employee profit-sharing and gain-sharing programs. *Informal rewards* can include anything from verbal praise and positive feedback for a job well done to outside training programs or celebrations (at the work site or elsewhere) on reaching a specific goal or goals. Team and group performance as well as individual performance should be rewarded. It should be remembered that in a participative environment, improvement and innovation cannot take place without mistakes. Employees should be rewarded for effort and initiative even if the desired outcome is not reached. Tolerance of minor "failures" and mistakes encourages employees to try again without fear of being punished or losing their job.

Obstacle Removal

In a participative environment, the department manager must anticipate potential *obstacles* to employee advancement and seek to remove them. For example, policies and procedures that prevent employees from making appropriate decisions to satisfy customers may jeopardize employee morale, the customer base, and productivity. Appropriate decisions are those that fall within an employee's job scope and capabilities. Although policies and procedures provide adequate structure, efficiency, and safety of operations, procedure overload can result in avoidable delay while stifling employee spirit. Another obstacle is an employee who refuses to participate or support team efforts. It is the manager's responsibility to identify such persons, coach them toward involvement, or apply the established disciplinary steps to remove them. Other obstacles include budget constraints, productivity and labor demands, unrealistic demands and expectations from other departments, lack of understanding or cooperation (or both) from other organization members, insufficient employee knowledge or expertise, and time constraints for meetings and problem solving.

Communication

Effective *communication* in a participative work climate includes (among other methods) conducting meetings for the purposes of identifying strategic plans for the organization and updating employees on the status of organizational goals. Employees also should be informed of how department goals fit into the larger organization's vision, how the employees contribute to accomplishing department goals, and what future planning efforts will include. Good communication in a participative setting moves in two directions—"downward" from managers and "upward" from employees—which means that managers must sharpen their listening skills. Chapter 7 is devoted to the skillful use of communication techniques.

By bridging communication gaps with other departments, managers become more aware of conditions faced by others in the organization. Thus, they can sensitize their staff and improve relations throughout the facility. By opening communication across departmental lines, managers learn what is considered politically correct in an organization's cultural climate, thereby better protecting their staff against uncomfortable situations.

Employee Involvement

A participative or high-involvement manager understands the values and beliefs that motivate employee *involvement* through empowerment. This section explores theories on motivation and their application in a collaborative work environment. Also, the levels of empowerment and its application to health care foodservice are described.

Motivating Employees

Motivation is the process by which individuals are stimulated to act on their innermost needs, desires, and drives. *Needs* are unfulfilled physical or psychological desires of an individual. Motivation is a repetitive, circular process: an individual's needs cause him or her to behave in a way that fulfills, or promises to fulfill, those needs. Once needs have been met (either partially or fully), the individual feels satisfaction. The feeling of satisfaction reinforces the need, and the need-fulfillment-satisfaction cycle of motivation is repeated.

One of the most important managerial responsibilities is to motivate employees to work toward organizational and departmental goals and objectives. To accomplish this task, the manager must find a way to make those aims fit each employee's needs. Motivation is only part of work performance; individual ability and the work environment also bear on performance level. In other words, employees need to know how to do their work well (ability); they need to want to do their work well (motivation); and they need adequate equipment, supplies, facilities, and authority to do their work well (environment). The absence of any one of these three factors jeopardizes performance. The way employees are treated and the workplace atmosphere are also important factors. Everyone wants to feel a part of the team and to be recognized as special and unique individuals. Managers need to recognize the diversity among employees and respect cultural differences in the workplace. Demographic characteristics can be an issue if staff members do not believe or they question if they are "one of us." If a manager's socioeconomic, ethnic, nationality, sex, or religious backgrounds are different from those of a subordinate, the manager must create a climate of understanding acceptance and "togetherness." The leader must be sensitive to the cultures and social values of the workforce.

Compensation (money) and benefits programs are the most tangible means for motivating and rewarding employees for their work. (Compensation and benefits are discussed in more detail in Chapter 9.) However, how well money and benefits alone motivate employees to performance levels beyond the minimum required to accomplish the work at hand is questionable. Compensation and benefits are extrinsic motivators, having limited long-term effect. In fact, employees generally rate four things above salary: appreciation for work done, a sense of "being in on things," help with personal problems, and job security.

More theories about worker motivation have been proposed than can be described within the scope of this manual on foodservice management. It may be useful, however, to explain basic theories that have influenced modern management practices. The flagship theories can be divided into three categories: content theories, process theories, and reinforcement theory.

Content Theories of Motivation

Content theories of motivation focus on specific factors that influence an individual to behave in a certain way. These factors are related to the individual's basic biological needs and immediate environment.

One proponent of content theory was Abraham H. Maslow, a psychologist who developed a theory known as the *hierarchy of needs*, discussed in his book *Motivation and Personality* (1954). As shown in Figure 2.2, Maslow believed that certain needs (for

FIGURE 2.2   Maslow's Hierarchy of Needs

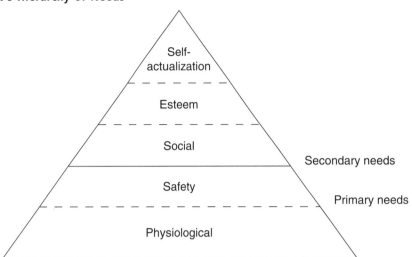

example, physiological and safety needs) are more basic (or primary) than other higher (or secondary) needs (for example, esteem). Maslow concluded that a person's primary needs will affect his or her behavior before any secondary needs have a chance to affect that person's actions. Once the primary needs have been fulfilled, however, they no longer operate as strong motivators, and the drive to fulfill needs farther up in the hierarchy begins to dominate the person's behavior.

According to Maslow, a work environment that allows employees to meet their physiological and safety needs will succeed, for employees will be motivated to better performance than in an environment that ignores their basic needs. The influence of Maslow's theory on modern management practices partially explains the reasoning behind the fair wage and salary practices in most of today's organizations. Maslow's influence also can be seen in medical and life insurance benefits, safety standards, and retirement plans.

Most foodservice directors do not directly control the compensation and benefits offered to their employees (see Chapter 9). Foodservice directors, however, can reward good performance with promotions and regular salary increases. They also can make sure that their departments are pleasant and safe places in which to work and, by exercising fair and professional management, can ensure employees of reasonably secure prospects for future employment.

Another content theory that is influential in the development of modern management practices is psychologist Frederick Herzberg's *two-factor theory* of motivation, or the *maintenance motivation theory*, based on studies he conducted during the 1950s. He concluded that two sets of factors—which he called *hygiene factors* and *motivation factors*—influence employee attitudes and behavior. *Hygiene* factors include such things as personnel policies, job security, salary and benefits, seniority benefits, the ability to interact with one's peers, and adequate working conditions. Herzberg believed that hygiene factors can prevent job dissatisfaction if employees perceive them to be adequate and fair but that these factors cannot increase motivation levels or job satisfaction. *Motivation factors* include responsibility, recognition, achievement, advancement, work that is challenging, feeling of personal accomplishment, and

other elements related to job content. Herzberg believed that these motivation factors are the conditions under which employee performance is motivated. In other words, giving additional responsibility or recognition for a job provides motivation.

Herzberg emphasized that managers need to work simultaneously on hygiene and motivation factors to foster a positively motivated workforce. Two major ideas advocated by Herzberg and his colleagues were that *intrinsic motivation*—motivation that comes from within the person—is important for keeping employees motivated and that the nature of the job, such as whether it was sufficiently engaging and challenging, was also extremely important. The *extrinsic factors* are associated with dissatisfaction and include such factors as company policy, salary, supervision, working conditions, and relationships with peers. This theory has important application in the operation of foodservice departments and should be considered during the process of job design, job enrichment, or job enlargement because motivation factors may influence the level of employee productivity in new positions.

Process Theories of Motivation

Another theory about motivation was developed by David McClelland and John Atkinson (described by Dessler and other writers on management). They agree with Herzberg that higher-level needs are most important at work. They developed a theory called *McClelland's achievement, power and affiliation theory*. This theory focuses on the needs that people acquire through their life experiences. The theory emphasizes three of the many needs developed in a lifetime.

1. *Need for achievement.* The desire to do something better or more efficiently than it has ever been done before. Individuals with a high need to achieve prefer to:
   - Set achievable goals for themselves.
   - Work on tasks of moderate difficulty.
   - Take moderate risks.
   - Take personal responsibility for their actions.

- Receive specific and concrete feedback on their performance.

   McClelland claims that "in some businesses people's needs to achieve are so strong that it is more motivating than the quest for profits."

2. *Need for power.* The desire to control, influence, or be responsible for others. Managers with a high need for power are likely to seek advancement and take on increasing work activities to earn advancement. They enjoy decision-making roles and competitive situations.

3. *Need for affiliation.* The desire to maintain close, friendly personal relationships. Managers with a high need for affiliation have a cooperative, team-centered management style. They prefer to influence subordinates to complete tasks through team efforts. This type of manager must beware that his or her need for social approval and friendship does not interfere with a willingness to make managerial decisions.

Whereas content theories focus on the *why* of behavior, process theories focus on *how* motivation occurs. *Process theories* look at motivation from the point at which individual behavior is energized through the behavior choices that person makes to the quality of the effort.

Among the body of process theories, *expectancy theory* proposes that motivation begins with a desire for something, such as more recognition on the job, higher pay, or a stronger feeling of accomplishment. In this theory, individuals would then consider whether the effort to do a certain job (performance) could be expected to achieve their goals.

Expectancy theory can help managers understand motivation on an employee-by-employee basis because it takes individual differences among employees into account in a way that content theories do not. For example, Herzberg's theory suggests that job enlargement would increase the level of motivation in all individuals. Expectancy theory admits that not everyone is willing or even able to accept job enlargement as a likely means for achieving what they want.

Reinforcement Theory of Motivation

Originally, *reinforcement theory* was based on the behavior of animals under experimental conditions. Rat performance in mazes, for example, tested the psychological theory of reinforcement. B. F. Skinner and other psychologists have demonstrated how the theory can be applied to human behavior. Basically, reinforcement theory assumes that behavior that brings positive results probably will be repeated, whereas behavior that has negative results probably will not.

Four basic elements are at work in the theory: *Positive reinforcement* strengthens a specific behavior because the result of the behavior is desirable to the individual. *Avoidance* strengthens a specific behavior because the result allows the individual to escape an undesirable result. *Punishment* weakens a specific behavior because the result is undesirable to the individual. *Extinction* weakens a specific behavior because no desirable result is provided by the behavior.

For example, a foodservice director who praises an employee for preparing an especially attractive casserole provides positive reinforcement, and the employee is likely to repeat the work behavior. But for employees who are careful to wash their hands after handling uncooked meat because of past counseling for violating hand-washing procedures, avoidance is at work; that is, the employees behave in a certain way to avoid another counseling session.

Managers often use punishment to reduce the likelihood that employees will repeat inappropriate behavior. However, this approach (for example, punishing foodservice employees for breaking rules or missing work) can lead to anger and resentment among employees. When practical, reinforcing proper behavior through praise and reward should be used in place of punishment.

A foodservice director might use extinction to discourage inappropriate behavior that was rewarded in the past. Suppose that an employee who habitually engages in horseplay in the department was rewarded in the past when a previous director or other managers joined in the laughter at the employee's antics. The director could discourage the behavior by ignoring it instead of rewarding or punishing it.

Application of Motivational Theories

No one theory of motivation is completely relevant to every work situation or to every employee. Managers with effective leadership qualities are sensitive to employee differences, but they also recognize that each of the theories has some application to their ability to motivate employees. General motivation guidelines suggested by these theories are summarized below.

- Reinforce desired performance or achievement by providing formal rewards (fair salaries, benefits, and opportunities for advancement).
- Design jobs that are interesting and challenging as defined by each employee's skills.
- When an employee's performance falls short of expectations, praise positive aspects of the performance and suggest specific improvements without threats or punishment.
- Recognize and reinforce improvements through praise and other rewards.
- Make employees feel important by encouraging, helping, and supporting them in their work.
- Provide for advancement and growth in position by additional training or education.
- Allow employees to set their own goals within the limits of the department's objectives and the organization's goals.
- Provide a work environment that is responsive to employees' needs.
- Treat employees as the unique individuals they are by learning their names, interests, and concerns.
- Show trust in employees by delegating responsibilities to them and by emphasizing their contribution to the organization.

- Keep employees fully informed about policies, procedures, and organizational changes that affect their jobs.
- Protect employee privacy and confidential information as prescribed by law.
- Encourage employees to participate in planning department activities and solving work-related problems.

Motivating employees is a challenging responsibility because each employee is unique, bringing different needs, desires, and perceptions to the work situation. Good managers help pave the way for employees to realize their full potential and to become satisfied and proud contributors to their organization. To help all employees reach this state, managers must provide them with opportunities to participate, to gain self-esteem through greater responsibility, and to achieve a real sense of accomplishment.

Empowering Employees

Employee empowerment is best defined as employees organized into self-divided teams and empowered to do their jobs and even to change work processes if that will improve product quality. This is accomplished through intrinsic motivation and is a positive outcome of a participative work environment created by a flexible situational leadership style. Employees are trained, retrained, and cross-trained in a variety of jobs. Facilitators (supervisors) work with the employees to provide the resources necessary to meet the customers' needs. Empowerment simply means the sharing of power with those who have less. For empowerment to be successful, managers must delegate more formal authority to make specific decisions and avoid the sudden withdrawal of shared power at the first sign of trouble. Subordinates must be allowed to learn to use their increased power. Managers need to carefully consider how much power to share and how to enable others to share that power. To make empowerment successful, managers also need to:

- Communicate information.
- Train subordinates in how to use the "new" power.
- Define objectives clearly.
- Clarify any policy that will need to be used to enable subordinates to have a solid framework for decisions to be made.
- Define limits of what situations employees will be supported to handle and when the managers need to be involved.
- Share decision-making power.
- Provide rewards and recognition.
- Delegate meaningful work.
- Be accessible to coach, answer questions, discuss action, and provide support.

When employees choose responsibility for becoming involved and managers commit to encouraging that involvement, employee empowerment is under way.

The remainder of this subsection focuses on the varying levels of empowerment and when it is appropriate to apply these levels.

Levels of Empowerment

David Bowen and Edward Lawler define three levels of employee empowerment: *suggestion, job,* and *high involvement*. Each level has a place in foodservice operations where employee empowerment is a priority. All three can provide a road map for managers seeking to change a tightly controlled work environment into a highly participative one.

With *suggestion involvement*, employees are encouraged to contribute ideas through formal suggestion systems, but there is little change in how day-to-day work is accomplished. Or employees are encouraged to make recommendations for change, but management usually retains power to decide whether the recommendations are implemented. Suggestion involvement, then, is closely related to a control model of management. Managers may use suggestion involvement as the first step to leading employees to high (or full) involvement, or they may decide that this level is appropriate for their department based on the organizational culture. Suggestion involvement may be appropriate to certain tasks or situations, whereas job involvement or high involvement is better suited to others.

Job involvement takes a large step up from the typical control model. At this level, employees are involved in job design (how to do their work), they exercise a larger variety of skills, get more feedback on how the work is proceeding, and are responsible for an identifiable piece of work. This level of involvement offers more employee enrichment, which leads to higher motivation, commitment, and quality of work. The job involvement level is where many organizations begin emphasizing a team approach. Teams are especially important in health care foodservice because no one individual is responsible for customer contact from beginning to end. The complex nature of the work and service delivery make it necessary to increase emphasis on job completion through teamwork. Also at this level of involvement in employee empowerment, training becomes more important. With more demand for employee involvement, managers must ensure that workers have the knowledge and skills to make decisions effectively. Finally, managers at the job involvement level become more supportive and less directive in their situational leadership approach.

High involvement derives from employees' keen sense of how they do their jobs, how their group or team performs, and how successfully the organization performs as a whole. This level of involvement thrives in a culture that promotes employee empowerment and participative management, where information on the organization's business performance is shared; skill development in teamwork, problem solving, and business operations is offered; and employee participation in job-related decisions is promoted. Managers at this level must be highly competent in participatory management and team building, coaching, training, and delegation skills. Strategies of high-involvement empowerment also can be more costly in terms of additional time taken in hiring employees and in their training and development.

Application of Empowerment to Foodservice

Is it appropriate in every situation to empower foodservice employees to make decisions? Probably not. Recall that policies and procedures are established to provide consistent and safe service. For example, it is unwise to authorize employees on a patient tray line to make substitutions, which might compromise patients' nutrition needs or food preferences. Using another example, a standard greeting for answering the phone or addressing customers in cafeteria lines promotes an image of continuity and corporate identity. Management judgment and discretion come into play when the application of empowerment versus strict procedural adherence is at issue.

Individual differences in value systems and belief systems must be taken into account when making empowerment application decisions. For those employees whose cultural comfort zone is more amenable to structure and management-based decisions, tasks requiring strict adherence to procedural protocol are more readily completed. Regardless of whether employees require more control than autonomy (or vice versa), they should be selected for positions that allow them to use their skills to maximum potential.

Image

The image a foodservice department presents is crucial to customer satisfaction. *Image* is the perception customers form of the product and service provided. The organizational image is often found in an organization's values and culture. It also includes the building, grounds, personnel, logo, stationery, and above all, whether customers' needs and wants are met.

An organization's image must also be presented by all units within the organization. Because all patients are served food while customers in the facility, the image a foodservice department presents helps form the image customers have of the facility and the foodservice department. To enhance this image, a foodservice department should ensure that:

- Employees are dressed in clean, well-fitting uniforms with visible name tags that identify them as foodservice personnel.
- Materials for patients' trays—tray covers, napkins, glassware, and china—are color coordinated, clean, and pleasing to the eye. No cracked or chipped china, no spotted flatware.
- Dining facilities post menus that offer a variety of nutritious foods that meet the ethnic and cultural needs of customers, prices, and nutrition information for each menu item.
- Service is personalized, and employees are courteous to all customers.
- Dining facilities are accessible to customers with handicaps.
- Dining areas present a pleasant ambience.
- Surveys and focus groups are used to determine the needs of customers; outcomes are implemented as appropriate, and the results are shared and used as a marketing tool.
- Current customer needs are met while potential new customers are sought.
- Hours of service are posted; the operation opens and closes as stated.

- Employees are hired and trained to focus on service to customers.

Chapter 3 also discusses image.

Roadblocks to Participative Management

Participative management and employee empowerment are not always accomplished easily, and *roadblocks* lie ahead if the organization is unsupportive of an empowered workforce. Although it can be difficult for managers or employees to exert influence outside their department without commitment to participative management from the top, managers can begin with suggestion involvement, encouraging employee input on how things are done within their department.

Employee skepticism may present another roadblock to participative management if employees doubt management's sincerity to welcome their input in decision making and job completion. Skepticism can be due to employees' past experiences with the current organization or a previous one. For example, employees whose participation and input were solicited in the past but consistently overruled may doubt a manager's seriousness. Long-time employees who have seen programs, processes, and managers come and go may feel that this is just another empty effort. For employees who view the manager as being lazy or abdicating responsibilities, this may be the thought at first glance, but a manager who continues to encourage and support them eventually wins their allegiance.

A third obstacle to participative management may be the employees' level of development. Without adequate training and information, employees are incapable of providing input. Managers must be responsible for employee education to ensure success while providing constant feedback and praise. Again, not all employees desire autonomy on the job or opportunity for input.

If cultural differences provide a stumbling block to empowerment, managers must recognize this opportunity and find a way to use the differences. Chapter 8 further discusses the issue of cultural differences.

Fear of failure or job insecurity can hamper employee involvement. Fear that the manager is "setting me up to fail so I can be fired" may be unfounded, but it is up to the manager to reassure employees. This can be done by starting at the basic level and allowing the employees to offer suggestions but taking the ultimate responsibility for the decision until employees are trusting enough to move beyond this level.

Managers themselves can be obstacles to a participative work environment. Those who "grew up" (that is, developed their management styles) in nonparticipative environments may face some of the same fears their employees do in trying to change to participatory management. They may not be willing to give up the power and authority that come with their position, feeling that they worked hard for it and that by sharing it, they somehow admit their inadequacy. It may also appear to some managers that by sharing their power and authority, they—and therefore their jobs—become devalued. It may be difficult for some managers to give up responsibility and authority because they need to be in control and to know what is going on. Being responsible and knowledgeable is possible in a participative environment if the manager is a member of the overall team. Managers who simply may not have the skills and information necessary to be participative leaders will have to defer to the organization's responsibility for making this knowledge available.

SUMMARY

An emphasis on customer satisfaction, continuous quality improvement, and increased demands from employees for participation places more demand on managers to become effective leaders. A practical approach to leadership can be established using the styles identified by Kenneth Blanchard and colleagues—directing, coaching, supporting, and delegating. Each style requires leaders to be flexible in the application of their style based on employees' developmental level and the task's complexity.

An effective leader is flexible and possesses both technical expertise and interpersonal skills. The application of these skills is important to accomplishing the management functions of planning, organizing, leading, and controlling. Interpersonal skills are extremely important to creating and nurturing a participative work environment that enables employees and allows them to be active in decision making. Managers who advocate a participative setting possess skills for communicating effectively, training, coaching, sharing decision making, team building, providing rewards and recognition, delegating work, removing obstacles, and bridging gaps with other departments.

Providing a collaborative environment for employees stimulates their feelings of self-worth and inspires a commitment to the organization. Empowerment can be simplistic and allow only suggestion involvement or be more complex and allow for involvement with job design and completion and decision making. Creating a participative work environment takes time and requires change on the part of managers and employees. It is an evolutionary process that can suffer setbacks due to obstacles. These roadblocks can be overcome with understanding and persistence on the part of employees and managers.

Benefits of a participative work environment accrue to employees and organization alike. When allowed to influence their work life, employees develop a higher level of self-esteem and job satisfaction. Organizations gain from employee loyalty and enhancements in customer service, productivity, and quality.

KEY TERMS

Behavior theories on leadership
Compensation/reward
Empowerment
Formal versus informal leaders
Herzberg's two-factor theory
Interpersonal skills
Leaders
Leadership style
Levels of management
Managers

Maslow's hierarchy of needs
McClelland's achievement, power, and affiliation theory
Mentor
Motivation
Participative culture
Participative management and culture
Power
Rewards
Situational leadership
Training and development

DISCUSSION QUESTIONS

1. How does leadership style impact a foodservice operation?
2. What is the difference in leadership and management?
3. Explain the importance of understanding the role of behavioral theories and how they affect the manager and the employees.

4. Name the characteristics needed to be an effective leader and or manager.
5. Describe the functions and responsibilities of a manager and a leader.
6. What are the various theories of motivation?

CHAPTER 3

MARKETING AND REVENUE-GENERATING SERVICES

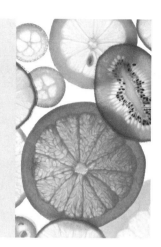

LEARNING OBJECTIVES

- Differentiate between service and goods.
- Plan revenue-generating services, such as a catered event.
- Compute the cost for the catered event.
- Compare the difference between promotion, advertising, and marketing.
- List examples of promotional techniques used in foodservice.
- Explain the role of image in a foodservice department.

N THE PAST, health care providers managed operations with little concern for environmental pressures and changes in the marketplace. However, given that health care technology has expanded and that the percentage of the gross national product spent on health care has increased, the health care system now must change its approach to be more consistent with other sectors. It is no longer immune to the complexities and uncertainties of its environment.

A number of uncontrollable pressures within the health care environment (discussed in Chapter 1) make health care delivery today increasingly more turbulent and stressful. These pressures have forced providers to learn and implement new skills to make their operations more cost-effective and revenue-producing while maintaining quality standards. Primary among these responses has been the implementation of marketing, which has long been used in other consumer-oriented fields.

Marketing is often confused with sales, advertising, and public relations. In fact, these activities are part of marketing. To produce targeted results, not only must marketing become a way of doing

business in the health care operation, it must become a function of management. In the health care context, marketing is oriented to consumers, as opposed to sales or a product.

When applied to the health care field, *marketing* is defined as a tool that strives to meet the needs, wants, and demands of the customers to obtain products and service of quality and value while the organization ensures the ethics and philosophy of the organization are good and sound and as a result revenue is produced. It is an activity that produces sales, and therefore revenue that can be added to the bottom line for the department/organization. The American Marketing Association defines marketing as "the performance of business activities that direct the flow of goods and service from the producer to the customer." Because many different health care options currently exist and because changes in health care delivery will continue, providers must design services with the opinions and perceptions of their customers in mind. Therefore, health care nutrition and foodservice departments are becoming increasingly—and more overtly—important in facilities' overall marketing strategies and revenue producing.

This chapter introduces key marketing concepts, including services management, the difference between goods and services, types of markets, market and basis for segmentation, target markets, marketing mix, and advertising and promotion revenue-generating methods. These concepts then are applied to devising a cyclical, five-phase marketing management model based on the following elements:

- *Information*: Maintaining records; collecting, analyzing, and interpreting data
- *Planning*: Operational and strategic planning, the planning process, documentation and components of the marketing plan

- *Implementation*: Dealing with change, employee training, advertising and promotion
- *Evaluation*: Monitoring and measuring marketing outcome
- *Feedback*: Reporting successes, failures, or both, and returning to the information phase

KEY MARKETING CONCEPTS

Although relatively new to the health care field, marketing is a discipline of sophisticated and proven theories, techniques, and concepts. Although a complete discussion of these areas is beyond the scope of this book, it is critical that managers in health care foodservice be familiar with at least three of the concepts: *service marketing, markets and segmentation*, and *marketing mix*.

Services Marketing

Since the early 1980s, the *service sector* of the nation's economy has grown at an astounding rate. According to the Bureau of the Census, this sector, of which the health care field is a member, accounts for more than 50 percent of both the gross domestic product and consumer expenditures. Despite the importance of the service sector, only recently has services marketing been differentiated from goods marketing. Marketing techniques—originally developed to sell *goods*—are not always appropriate for selling *services*.

Goods Versus Services

Before services marketing is examined, the distinction between goods and services must be understood. *Goods* may be objects, devices, or things; when goods are purchased, something tangible such as revenue (money) is acquired for possession. *Services*, on the other hand, are mostly intangible; a service is an activity performed for the benefit of a purchaser. A service often is transacted on a personal basis and usually does not result in ownership (possession) of a physical (or tangible) item. A service is created by its provider; for example, a facility that employs a meal hostess to deliver patient trays or a chef to carve roasted meat on a cafeteria line is a service provider.

Most health care foodservice operations probably deliver a combination of goods and services. In such operations, acquisition of goods and supplies, preparation and service of meals, and cleanup afterward are performed for patients and other customers by foodservice employees. Hence, health care foodservice is considered an industry—a service industry—even though tangibles (food and equipment) are involved.

Characteristics of Services

Although service industries themselves are heterogeneous (ranging from barber shops to health care operations), certain generalizations can be made about the characteristics of services. The most important of these characteristics are intangibility, simultaneous production and consumption, less uniformity and standardization, and absence of inventories.

Intangibility

Services provided by health care foodservice operations are consumed but not possessed. What is being bought is a performance of an activity rendered by a foodservice employee or group of employees for the benefit of a customer. Generally, the provision of services is a people-intensive process. To the patient, the meal hostess's delivery of the breakfast tray is as much a part of the meal as the tangible portion, the food.

Simultaneous Production and Consumption

Goods are generally produced, sold, and then consumed, with much emphasis placed on distributing goods at the "right place" and at the "right time." Services are produced and consumed simultaneously, meaning that the service provider is often physically present while consumption takes place: the clinical dietitian produces an educational service while (at the same time) the patient consumes it. Because the dialogue occurs between customer and service provider, the manner in which services are delivered becomes important. How foodservice employees conduct themselves in the presence of a customer can influence future business. Figure 3.1 shows production and consumption of goods versus services over time.

Less Uniformity and Standardization

Because people are involved on both the production and consumption sides, services are less uniform and standardized than are goods. With extensive involvement of people, a degree of variability in the outcome is introduced. Whereas a patient may expect his or her favorite breakfast cereal always to taste the same, two different meal hostesses could do an effective but different job in delivering the breakfast tray to the patient.

Absence of Inventories

In most service settings, some levels of inventory must be maintained, which is the case with food and supplies in foodservice departments. However, some resources cannot be stored for future sale and thus are considered *perishable*. A sale is lost (perished) when a hospital guest finds the wait time in the hospital restaurant to be too long, and the sale cannot be recovered. Along with surges in demand, service organizations also experience slack periods. Because of this variability in demand, service operations are often concerned with how to manage demand. For example, the above-described hospital restaurant with long wait times might feature special offers during low periods of demand in an attempt to manage demand more effectively.

Markets and Segmentation

To maximize the success of a health care foodservice operation, its manager must be able to identify the potential market for the operation's goods and services. A *market* is simply a group of individuals or organizations that might want or need the good or service being offered for sale.

FIGURE 3.1 Production and Consumption of Goods Versus Services

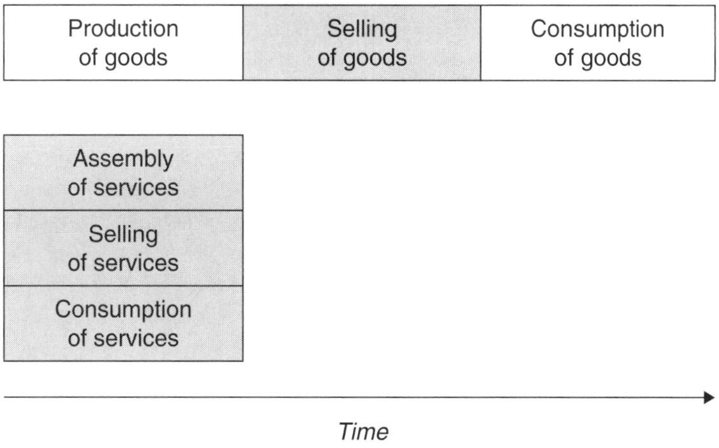

Production of goods	Selling of goods	Consumption of goods

Assembly of services
Selling of services
Consumption of services

Time

Shaded boxes indicate the points at which buyers and sellers interact. For services, each point can influence buyer satisfaction and must be addressed by the operation's marketing program.

Types of Markets

If a buyer is the one who will use the product to satisfy personal needs, the buyer is part of the consumer market. When a product is purchased for business purposes, the buyer is part of the organizational market. Different marketing strategies must be used when dealing with consumer versus organizational markets. Clearly, many health care foodservice operations market not only to individual consumers but also to organizations. Marketing nutrition counseling services to an individual on an outpatient basis, then, probably would require a different approach from that used to market the same services on a contract basis to a nearby nursing home.

Segmentation

Most managers find it necessary to further divide consumer and organizational markets into smaller, more homogeneous "submarkets" that are likely to purchase a specific product. This process, referred to as *market segmentation*, recognizes that buyers are not all alike. Appropriately implemented, market segmentation can be one of the health care foodservice manager's most powerful marketing tools.

Basis for Segmentation

Almost any buyer characteristic may be used as a basis for segmenting markets into submarkets. Common characteristics used to define segments of consumer markets include *geographical, demographical, psychographic*, and *behavioral* dimensions of buyers.

Geographical Dimension (Where the Customers Live) *Geographical segmentation* is a logical segmentation characteristic because it is based on the assumption that consumers' wants and needs vary depending on where they live. Most health care operations provide services in a specific geographical area, called a *service area*, such as cafeteria service. Basic statistics about a service area's

population and health care needs should be analyzed by an operation's management staff, including foodservice. This could prove beneficial when reviewing existing services and when considering new ventures. For instance, when menus are developed or revised, the menu planner must consider the regional food and beverage preferences of potential customers.

Demographical Dimension (Statistical Data or Customer Profile) Most health care operations segment their markets according to the diagnosis of a patient, such as pediatrics and oncology. Other demographic characteristics, such as age, gender, family size, income, occupation, stage in the family, life cycle, ethnicity, religion, and nationality, are segmentation variables that have long been popular bases for determining market segments in the health care industry. The health care services, including food and nutrition services, used by an individual are highly associated with demographical variables. These variables have a major effect on most of the functional units of a foodservice operation. When a health care operation serves certain diagnostic segments, patient menus must be developed for those segments (for example, fat-controlled menus for patients with heart disease and diabetic menus for patients with diabetes). Likewise, the age of the patients served must be considered. The specific effects of selected demographical variables on menu planning and meal service are described in Chapters 16 and 21, respectively.

Psychographical Dimension (Different Groups Based on Social Class, Lifestyle, or Personality Characteristics) Because individuals within the same demographical group do not always exhibit the same buying behaviors, other dimensions must be considered. One of these, *psychographical* segmentation, divides buyers into groups based on social class, lifestyle, or personality characteristics. Lifestyle is an important factor because it is a strong predictor of future health care consumption. Likewise, it has an effect on the types of food and beverages desired by a foodservice operation's customers, both patients and nonpatients. In the lifestyle category, health-conscious consumer segments typically select menu choices with lower fat, sugar, and sodium than regular menu items.

Behavioral Dimension (Groups Based on Consumer Knowledge, Attitude, Use, or Response to a Product) *Behavioral segmentation* based on the knowledge, attitude, use, or response of consumers to actual services is another dimension. A number of factors can be analyzed when attempting to segment a market according to this dimension. Factors applicable to a health care foodservice operation include the benefit sought by consumers in terms of quality, service, and value; consumer usage rate (that is, how often a consumer will use the operation's services); and the consumers' general attitudes toward an operation's products.

Target Markets

Based on the dimensions described above, a number of market segments could be created from the consumer market of a health care foodservice operation. It might be tempting to create a large collection of goods and services to meet the wants and needs of each segment. However, most marketers agree that to market to everyone is to market to no one. Therefore, foodservice managers need to choose a few meaningful segments and concentrate efforts on satisfying those selected submarkets. A market segment toward which the organization directs its marketing efforts is called a *target market*. Target markets may be a *local market* where brands are tailored for the local customer and the promotion to the needs and wants and needs of a local market. *Niche market* is a subgroup usually defined as a group with a distinctive set of traits that may want special combination of benefits. Most often in a health care operation, this selection process is not left entirely to the discretion of foodservice managers. They may be involved in identifying target markets, but the final decision as to where efforts are concentrated will be made by the facility as a whole.

The *marketing cycle* identifies the customers who make up the market and is illustrated in Figure 3.2. The marketing cycle is complete if a customer's behavior was changed to produce a profit for product(s) that were identified to meet the identified needs or wants; feedback from customers and staff was obtained; and there was a profit that could be reinvested for additional research and development.

Marketing Mix

A successful health care foodservice operation focuses on the wants and needs of its customers and markets the operation's products efficiently. To accomplish this objective, foodservice management must adjust specific elements of its operation as necessary so that its products will appeal to potential customers. Elements over which an operation has control to influence the salability of its products are called the marketing mix (see Figure 3.3).

Traditionally, elements of the marketing mix considered common among all businesses and industries include product, place, promotion, and price. A fifth element that must be included for most service sector businesses, including health care foodservice, is public image. When considering a specific type of business or industry, this list can be customized. Each element is essential to ensuring that a health care foodservice positions its products optimally to meet the wants and needs of its customers.

Product

A health care foodservice's *product* is a combination of goods, services, place, ideas, activities, organizations, and people that are unique to foodservice and that meet the wants and needs of targeted customers. Of several factors that influence how acceptable a product is to customers, quality is a key measure. Quality is discussed in Chapter 4, but the main point here is that foodservice managers can adjust quality to meet customer expectations. Other adjustable product characteristics include labeling (such as naming the employee cafeteria or cafeteria products in inviting and interesting ways) and packaging (how goods and services are combined to affect sales). Closely related to packaging is accommodation. For instance, when a foodservice operation joins forces (combines) with a health care operation as a whole to provide an elegant dinner for new parents, the product has been qualitatively adjusted, resulting in a special accommodation.

Place

Health care foodservice products are offered for sale in a specific *place*. The location and method of distribution must be convenient and attractive to customers. Because the typical operation serves a variety of patients and nonpatients, multiple locations for foodser-

FIGURE 3.2   Determining the Market Cycle

Identify customer needs and wants (survey, past records, and the like)

↓

Develop product(s), pricing, and distribution method

↓

Customer purchases product(s)

↓

Determine if product met needs or wants (sales records, feedback from staff)

FIGURE 3.3 Health Care Foodservice Marketing Mix

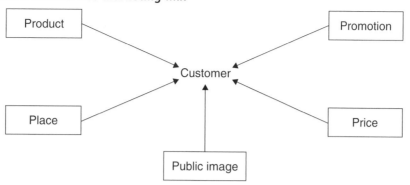

vice facilities may be a major marketing consideration. Sales may be enhanced by implementing new methods of distribution, such as offering take-out services. Physical characteristics of place—shape, size, and certainly the facility's decor—are important to a marketing effort.

Promotion

Promotion includes those methods by which an operation makes potential customers aware of its products. Many forms of communication take place between an operation and its potential customers. Promotion is focused toward short-term results. The major goal is to build sales for a short period of time. A good method to use in promotion is discount coupons (see Figure 3.6 and 3.7), two-for-one special promotions, and free samples. Promotions are cost-effective. *Advertising* is market-centered communications that includes advertising, sales, promotion, publicity, public relations, and personal selling. Advertising needs more time for results and can produce greater profits than a promotion. The goal of advertising is to strengthen a brand and the building of long-term sales and loyalty of customers. Advertising is nonpersonal communication from an identified sponsor using mass media such as television for the promotion of ideas, goods, or services. *Promotion* is the coordination of a marketer's communication efforts to influence attitude or behavior; it is used to publicize products or services and generates revenue. Advertising and sales promotion facilitates customization of the message and image conveyed to groups identified as potential customers (for example, visitors). As an example, table tents can be used in hospital coffee shops to describe a new food item and therefore promote its sale to coffee shop patrons who might not normally purchase such an item. Most foodservice managers know that word-of-mouth communication by satisfied customers can have a positive effect on sales. For example, the popularity of a Sunday brunch for hospital visitors could increase significantly from the endorsement of satisfied customers and increase revenue.

The following methods can be used to enhance *advertising, promotion, image,* and *increase revenues* for the department:

- Design menus that use a simple format, familiar menu terms or explanations of product, photos of a finished product, contrasting colors for paper, and print and typeface large enough to be read easily. Provide items that promote a healthy lifestyle and include a breakdown of nutrients.
- Post menus in the cafeteria or send out on the Internet; include them in the organization's newsletter.
- Distribute menus to customers. In health care, menus can be kept and used by customers as educational tools. Attach any daily special item to the menu. Include hours of service, location, telephone numbers, and payment options.
- Carefully name menu items. Use a name that will portray an image of the food and be clear and descriptive. Use a name to convey information to avoid confusion or surprises. In health care, a brief description of a product will tell patients something about the food.
- Add new items. Use fliers or the Internet to promote the item, explain how it is prepared, its nutritive value, the recipe, the name of the person who prepared the item, and a short acceptance survey for patrons to fill out and give to the cashier for possible incorporation into the menu system.
- Institute theme meals or weeks or months. Make theme meals and holiday meals special. Vendors and the Internet list special days, weeks, and months. Food for a theme day is important, but it takes more than just food. Advertise, promote, reduce prices (if there is an employee dining area where other notable events may be scheduled), and involve an interdisciplinary team in the event, as well as customers. Have employees dress in costumes as appropriate, and decorate the dining area and patient trays (as appropriate). Change the ambience and the sound (music, special entertainment, games, or activities), if appropriate, and use theme-day napkins, placements, and other decorations as appropriate and that meet budgetary constraints.
- Promote nutrition and foodservice, develop special events for National Nutrition Month, Pride in Foodservice Week, Registered Dietitian Week, and other health care–related weeks such as Nursing Week (see Figures 3.4 and 3.5).
- Meal deals. As appropriate, use discounts, coupons, and meal deals as another form of advertising and promotion. Any discounts may need budgetary approval from the administration. Discounts may be used for specials, such as

"buy one, get the second one at half-price," the introduction of a new product, or for the delivery of multiple meals to a patient unit. Coupons for discounts could be included in payroll envelopes and an in-house newsletter. Meal deals usually constitute an entire meal, without substitution, usually at a reduced price. *Bundling* of a group of products under one price encourages increased sales and offers faster service. Bundled meals usually are given special names such as "blue plate special," "chef's choice," and the like (see Figures 3.6 and 3.7).

- Use a departmental or organization newsletter to highlight the foodservice department. A newsletter is a simple tool for informing customers about the foodservice operation, a new menu item or recipe, or nutritional facts. These newsletters are usually one page (front and back) with foodservice news such as a new service. Newsletters are an excellent way to tell customers more about what, how, and why certain services and products are offered. Copies should be placed in lobbies, on patients' trays, and in the cafeteria. When applicable menus, daily specials, and other happenings in the department may be sent via e-mail blast. (Be sure this is approved by administration.) Include a special phone number that contains a prerecording of the day's menu selections, specials, and a short nutrition tip.
- Use *self-branding*, defined as creating a special product line and creating a unique name for the product. Develop a line of products that are unique to the department and label as "XYZ health care cookies" or "Chef Laurie's fried chicken." Advertise and promote the product. (Be aware of product names and your right to use them, ways to protect them; be aware of intellectual property, copyrights, and trademarks, and so on.)
- Stage an open house as a way to inform clients, families, physicians, and other health care providers of the department's efforts. Holidays, the organization's anniversary day, and renovation completion are all good opportunities for an open house.
- Develop friendships with writers in local media. The media can be a friend or an enemy. In using outside media, it is always best to check with the administration and public relations for assistance and permission for publication. When applicable, provide accurate information and a press release with photos, contact names, e-mail addresses, and telephone numbers. Give enough description to avoid delay or misinformation. Where photos of individuals are used, a signed released form may be necessary.

FIGURE 3.4   A Gift Certificate Used in a Promotion

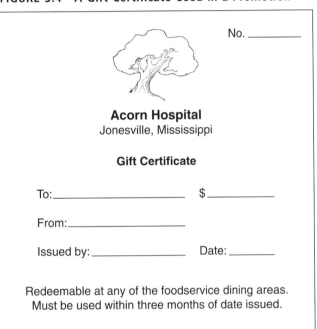

No. _____

Acorn Hospital
Jonesville, Mississippi

Gift Certificate

To:_____ $_____

From:_____

Issued by: _____   Date: _____

Redeemable at any of the foodservice dining areas.
Must be used within three months of date issued.

Figure 3.5   A Menu Used for a Special Event or Theme-Day Promotion

1950s Party
Roll Back the Price Day
June 3rd

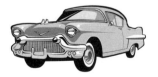

Enter the Best Dressed Costume of the 1950s
Win a Prize

MUSIC, GAMES, FUN
(Elvis may appear.)

1950s Menu
June 3rd — 11:30 A.M. – 2:00 P.M.

All beef hot dogs	15¢
Hamburgers	25¢
Additional tomatoes and lettuce	5¢
French fries	10¢
Chicken baskets	75¢
(Chicken, fries and drink)	
Fountain drinks	
Cherry Coke	5¢
Chocolate root beer	5¢
Regular fountain drinks	5¢
Sundaes (choice of toppings)	25¢
Sodas (choice of flavors)	20¢
*Other items available at regular price	

Remember: Bring canned food for
City Food Cabinet.

FIGURE 3.6 A Reduced-Price Coupon Used in a Promotion

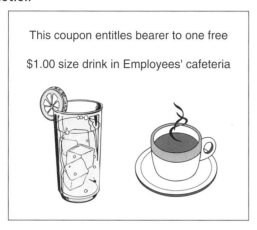

This coupon entitles bearer to one free

$1.00 size drink in Employees' cafeteria

FIGURE 3.7 Another Example of a Reduced-Price Coupon Used in a Promotion

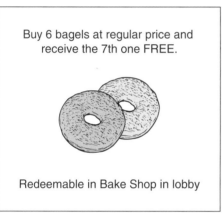

Buy 6 bagels at regular price and receive the 7th one FREE.

Redeemable in Bake Shop in lobby

- Make use of the ever-evolving Internet technology. Websites are an excellent way to communicate with the public concerning products and service. Websites can be used to promote new products, menus, nutrition information, food safety tips, recipes, culinary tips, and special offerings. Include contact information such as address, telephone and fax numbers, and e-mail addresses. Websites must be kept up to date, and all information must be current and accurate.
- Use brochures and fliers to advertise and promote a special foodservice project for such things as daily specials, hours of operation, catering, nutritional counseling, and food safety information. This is an excellent way to let customers know about the happenings. All brochures must contain accurate information, be easy to read and attractive, and include descriptions of how the product(s) and service(s) will help customers.
- Catering is a good method to use to market the foodservice to both in-facility customers and the community. Catering places the foodservice in a different light and provides an

opportunity to enhance the image of foodservice and to generate revenue.

- Use payroll stuffers to promote upcoming events, changes, and so forth that are "stuffed" into employees' paycheck envelopes.
- Package and merchandise items to be sold in an appealing and attractive manner. A *packaged product* that offers a visual appeal is more likely to be purchased. For example, when packaging sandwiches and other "grab and go" items package the food in an attractive manner that allows the customer to visualize the product. *Merchandising* is the most effective method of selecting, displaying, pricing, and advertising.
- Install vending (preferably self-operated, except for canned sodas) in high-traffic areas.
- Provide a take-out/pick-up service. Facility employees order meals, using telephone or Internet, for meal delivery/ pick-up between certain hours. Set aside a pick-up area in café or main kitchen area where employees pay and pick up meals or deliver meals to employees in their work area. These ideas would need a business plan and justification and approval of administration.
- Provide for home meals or bakery items for sale for employees to pick up on their way home.
- Day before a major holiday (Thanksgiving and Christmas) offer "Special Holiday Takeouts" such as pies, cookies, relish or deli trays. Do not offer cooked turkeys or ham because this could strain the production staff. Work with administration and the foodservice staff to develop a program.
- Establish *point-of-sale* items that are located near the take-out service or near the cash register. These point-of-sale items could include chips, fruit, candy, gums, mints (both with sugar and sugar-free as well as low fat), and so forth. When space and equipment are available some of the following ideas will increase revenue: microwave oven and bags of popcorn; freezer that is stocked with ice cream or other frozen confectionaries; specialty coffees, including a special insulated container with special blended coffees such as hazelnut, or special flavored creamers; pretzels with a pretzel machine. There are other point-of-sale items that may produce revenue. Appoint a committee to brainstorm various ideas. Before beginning a point-of-sales program determine if space, equipment, and personnel are available and if the idea will produce revenue after the cost of equipment, space, and labor have been defined.
- Justify the installation of a variety of kiosks for specialty coffee service and snacks; hand-dipped or bought ice-cream sandwiches a variety of flavors of cones, take-out pizza and sub sandwiches.
- Institute a meal ticket system via payroll deduction (increases meal count and increases revenue).
- Provide meals for sale for family members who are staying at the facility. Provide gourmet meal service to family members in celebration of a birthday, anniversary, or birth of a new baby.

Most of these revenue-producing ideas will require a business plan with a justification. The business plan can be simple or complex as described in Chapter 4. A simple plan would include:

- Description of the service to be implemented.
- The product or service to be offered.
- The target market (internal—staff; external—physicians, visitors, community who will purchase the product or service).
- Check the competition providing the same or equal service and product within a five-mile range of the facility.
- A written justification for the request will need to be written and discussed with upper administration (include a profit/loss statement pricing, sales volume, expense [labor and supplies] gross/net income).
- A marketing plan, which includes how and to whom the product or service will be sold.
- Catered event as a source of revenue.

Foodservice *catering* is a specialized service where food, beverages, and services are provided for special events, usually a onetime event such as a wedding, or routine staff meetings. Catering services cost extra but can enhance the revenue for the department. Catered events may be held in the health care facility (conference room, dining room, foyer, or auditorium) that has been set up for the occasion. Catering may also be held off-site in such places as a park, lodge, or home of a facility manager. Catering is hard work and requires excellent management skills and creativity.

To have a successful catered event at least the following must be followed. The caterer must:

- Meet with the client to determine type of catering, date, time, place, and approximate budget for the event.
- Visit the site where the event is to be held.
- Determine whether kitchen facilities are available at the site and whether they can be used by the caterer.
- Ask if there are provisions for cleanup and garbage disposal.
- Ask if wine or other alcoholic beverages may be served on the site.
- Determine the menu (with the group requesting the catered event). Review the standard menus with the client and provide cost for each menu type. Decide if standard catering menu will need to be modified if so, provide the cost for changes.
- Write a contract that confirms the order, date, time, and location of the event method of payment, who owns leftover food and supplies and a guaranteed number of expected guest (provisions for either under or over guaranteed number) and other needed details. (Give a copy to the group requesting the catering and keep a copy for the department records.)
- Determine the number of persons to be served. Will an RSVP be requested? Provide the exact time for any changes from the original or contract or menu. Explain additional costs for changes.

- Outline the service requirements—fine dining with silver, china, glassware, linens, or casual using disposals. What type of service—waiters or self-serve, such as a buffet?
- Is there a theme? If so, coordinate the flowers, linens, food presentation table setup, employee uniforms, and any equipment that may need to be rented (tables, chairs, linens, uniforms, and so on). Other requests might include ice carvings or an on-site music group.
- Prepare schedules for each separate unit of service, determine staff needs, supervision, needed supplies, and if off-site, the mode of transportation of equipment, personnel, and supplies to the site. Determine staffing (include overtime and fringe benefits if applicable) for prepreparation, on-site service, and after the event cleanup. (Cleanup may include the on-site and the facility kitchen for dishwashing, and so on.)
- Hire qualified persons needed to accomplish a successful catered event.
- Check with purchasing and others who may order supplies to determine if all special beverages and other items have been ordered and will be delivered to the off-site and at the specified time.
- Conduct a special training program for all personnel from production to cleanup.

All catered events must be priced. This includes:

- Raw food and beverage cost per person multiplied by the number of guests
- Labor cost (number of people (non-facility personnel) including X number of hours $\times$ rate of pay $+$ benefits (and as applicable overtime)
- Rental cost (tables, chairs, delivery, setup and breakdown, uniforms, specialized equipment)
- Determine markup (facility policy from 30 to 100 percent, depending on all overhead expenses that have to be paid, and supervisors' time)

Example of the cost for a seated luncheon for 50 people.

1. Raw food and beverage (1) $4/person $\times$ 50 guest = $200.
2. Labor cost 4 employees $\times$ 20 hours $\times$ $15/hours $+$ 20% benefits = $(4 \times 20 \times \$15 + 20\%)[2]$.
3. Rental and service cost.
4. 30% markup (this is low but food, labor, and supplies have already been included in the cost).
5. 18% gratuity for staff (this is not always included but is most often for events for more than 100).
6. Add $1 + 2 + 3 + 4 + 5$ to secure the cost of the event.

[(1) if wine or other alcoholic beverages are served this cost should appear as a separate item on the invoice and the contract will need to include who has ownership of the unused beverages and food.]

[(2) Labor is the most expensive cost in catering.]

A *profitability analysis* must be made for all catering events. A *profitability analysis* is a financial calculation that compares cost with revenue to determine whether the event is profitable or whether the event lost money. Determine what caused the loss of a profit.

Feedback

For promotion and advertising to be successful the foodservice director must seek *feedback*. This can be accomplished by oral interviews with customers during the meal period, informal and formal written surveys. Once the results of the survey have been tabulated the foodservice director and staff will need to carefully evaluate the results and make changes that are feasible, economical, and in the best interest of the department and organization. If customers seek results of the survey the foodservice director will need to be honest and provide information; information can be general or specific.

Price (the Amount of Money to Charge for a Product)

Price must be established that reconciles the value of the product to customers with the value of the exchange to the foodservice operation. Before purchase, price is one of the few indicators of quality. Unfortunately, it also may be one of the least reliable quality indicators because a variety of variables, some related to quality and some not, are used to establish prices. Accurate cost information is critical to effective pricing. When establishing product prices, foodservice managers must consider not only their costs but other factors, key among which are the demand of consumers for products and the prices charged by competitors for comparable products. Because the cost, demand, and competition variables differ from one geographical region to another, price variations for similar products are often noted.

Public Image

Public image is the way current and potential customers evaluate their views and perceptions of the products (food) and service or how service is presented in the market place. Every organization creates an image (e.g., McDonald's). Some images are easily recognized for quality of products and services. Boards of directors and upper management create the image for the organization. A foodservice facility's image and reputation is tied to the overall image of the organization as well as continuing to enhance this image through quality products and service among customers and potential customers, peers, community, and the public at large. Some ways this image can be portrayed includes participating in nutrition-related interviews in print or broadcast media. Another might be participating in annual tasting events sponsored by a local restaurant association. Both could influence the public's perception of food quality at the facility. Responding to community needs by donating unused prepared foods to congregate feeding programs, such as soup kitchens, could be viewed positively. Each organization must clearly define its own image specific to that organization.

Other ideas include:

- Walking around to observe if the employees' dress code is being followed.
- Checking all dining areas for cleanliness, attractiveness, pleasant ambience, no loud music or television, the area meets temperature needs of customers, and is a place where someone may want to visit/eat again.
- Serving fresh-quality nutritious food, garnished, rendered with quick service by courteous employees.
- Observing patient meal service to determine if the meals meet the medical therapy needs of the patient. The trays are attractive—no chipped china or glassware, placemats and napkins are color coordinated; food items on trays are placed where patients can easily reach them, cartons of beverages, and other items on the tray are easy to open. Meal servers greet the patient by name and offer assistance within their job description.
- Observing the image in extended-care facilities—are clients given a choice of meal service, either tray or dining room? The entire area presents a home environment. The dining environment is pleasant with flowers, artwork, table cloths, and reusable napkins. The food is prepared in a nutritious manner served by clean-uniformed waitstaff who are helpful and courteous, a variety of food selections are available to meet the medical nutrition therapy of the customers.
- Observing in a school or college—are there healthy food choices available? Flexible hours of service for college students, students have input into food choices/menus.

It is important that the image portrayed by foodservice reflects positively on the whole organization. The initial evaluation of the revenue of the foodservice products could serve as the foundation of a comprehensive, structural marketing plan.

MARKETING MANAGEMENT MODEL

Successful marketing of health care foodservice products (food) is a challenging task, unachievable without managerial involvement and a systematic approach. The *marketing management process* is a sequence of steps designed to ensure that the right decisions are made to effectively sell an organization's goods and services. In many health care organizations, the coordination of this process is centralized in marketing/customer service department. Foodservice managers, along with other operational managers, should be actively involved in this process. Their level of participation depends on the complexity of the marketing unit. Although market research may be conducted by an organization's marketing department, foodservice managers should use this information to develop new ventures and services.

Numerous models depict the marketing management process, and the following discussion lists those minimum essential elements that make up a tried-and-true marketing management process. A review of marketing management models reveals that they differ primarily in the number of elements around which they are organized. Elements may range from as few as three to as many as ten in a marketing management model that is more appropriate for large or multiunit foodservice operations. However, on a smaller scale, many points of this model can be used in smaller health care facilities. The model in this discussion uses five: *information, planning, implementation, evaluation*, and *feedback*. These elements are best described as cyclical, with each element—or phase—evolving from the previous one. *Feedback* is composed of the processes that enable information to flow from the evaluation element back to the information element.

Phase 1: Information

Sound *information* makes for sound decision making. Thus, marketing information, provided either by routine record keeping or as a result of market research, is extremely valuable to the marketing management process. Especially in light of today's health care environment, it is imperative that organizational and departmental managers, including foodservice, develop effective and efficient marketing information systems to get the precise information required for sound and timely decision making.

A *marketing information system* is a set of ongoing organized procedures, personnel, and equipment that collects, sorts, analyzes, stores, and retrieves information for use by marketing decision makers. According to Philip Kotler and Roberta N. Clarke, the marketing information system is composed of four subsystems: internal records, marketing intelligence, research, and analytical marketing. (This information would be used by both small and large organizations.)

Internal Records

Probably the most well-established subsystem of the information element is made up of *internal records*, routine data sources generated many times during the course of day-to-day operations. The data generally focus on issues of cost, inventory, dollar sales, volume of services, and other recurrent data that are routinely collected. From these records, a foodservice manager can develop basic statistics such as number of meals by diet type, average customer check in the employee cafeteria, and restaurant seat turnover.

The internal records should be *evaluated* routinely to determine where problems might exist. The goal is to design a resource network that is most effective that meets the foodservice manager's information needs cost-effectively. The ability to use these statistics to support future decision making can be greatly enhanced if the data are computerized, as detailed in Chapter 11.

Marketing Intelligence

Environmental intelligence describes a network of procedures and sources that provide managers with information about the organization's external marketing environment. This subsystem yields valuable information from a routine scan of relevant articles from magazines and journals and from outside parties, such as suppliers. A particularly effective method for gathering this type of information is to hire "mystery shoppers" for the purpose of purchasing and

evaluating services from the operation and to compare them with those purchased from competing foodservice operations. This provides information about the types of service offered, prices charged by competitors, and staff performance in the manager's own and similar operations.

Research

Market research, the systematic assembly of data that uses statistical technology to analyze the potential sales success of a good or service, is a highly developed field of study. Because market research provides information on the basis of which business decisions are made, it must be conducted carefully to ensure that the results reflect the situation accurately. It also can be costly. Unless a foodservice manager has the training to carry out market research, it is wise to enlist the services of the facility's marketing department or hire a consultant. Regardless of who conducts the research, the foodservice manager should monitor its progress to ensure that appropriate methods are carried out in the proper sequence. A recommended sequence is to define the problem, collect the data, analyze the data, and interpret the research findings.

Step 1: Define the Problem The problem must be defined in enough detail that subsequent steps in the research process can be planned and carried out based on reality of the purpose. Problems that might be defined include:

- Whether opportunities exist for off-premises catering services
- Why competitors are gaining a bigger share of the outpatient weight loss business
- Whether implementation of a take-out bakery counter would be profitable
- What promotional activities would have a positive effect on demand in a hospital's restaurant during slack periods
- Whether to outsource some of the duties of the department, such as housekeeping

Step 2: Collect the Data *Data collection* involves determining what data are needed, what collection method(s) will be used, and the actual collection of data. After the problem has been defined clearly, researchers/foodservice directors must review already-existing departmental and hospital data. Because the implementation of new promotional activities in the hospital restaurant might require expenditures for equipment, supplies, and training, the foodservice manager will need to investigate the cost-effectiveness of various techniques. In this case, past sales records (including average check amount) and seat turnover would be reviewed in terms of previous promotions. Interviews with the restaurant waitstaff might provide additional insight into customer reactions to promotions.

The next step is to review secondary or previously published data. A number of governmental and public agencies can provide valuable data, however, the best sources of secondary data most likely are found in the publications of trade and professional associations.

If secondary data fail to provide the documentation required, researchers/foodservice directors must turn to primary data. Each design involves standardized techniques so that data will be valid and reliable. In considering which promotional techniques to implement in a hospital restaurant, for example, researchers might use an observational method by recording reactions of customers to various promotional techniques. As an alternative, a customer survey questionnaire could be used to determine what techniques to consider. The effectiveness of the techniques could be evaluated by experimental design by determining the effect of each technique on sales in the hospital restaurant.

Step 3: Analyze the Data   Once data have been collected, they must be *analyzed*. The data need to be valid and reliable, and be tested statistically to measure relationships among the data. There measurements would help the foodservice manager determine the relative effectiveness of two or more promotional techniques—for example, in the introduction of new menus items, whether a table tent or cafeteria signage would bring better results.

Step 4: Interpret the Research Findings   Following data analysis, study results should be *interpreted* and *recommendations* made. At this point, the foodservice manager would decide which promotional technique(s) to implement in the restaurant. Study results should be documented in report form for the benefit of future studies.

Market research techniques can be highly technical and, if not conducted carefully, could result in flawed information on which decisions are made. A less formal technique includes development and completion of a marketing mix checklist, discussed earlier in the chapter. Other informal, qualitative market research tools that can provide valuable information about an operation's products, customers, and competition are focus groups and analyses of strengths, weaknesses, opportunities, and threats of the department to develop a strategic plan for the department.

Analytical Marketing

The fourth subsystem, called *analytical marketing*, comprises a set of advanced techniques for analyzing data. Usually it incorporates statistical, spreadsheet, and database software systems. Large organizations use analytical marketing extensively because it focuses on diagnosing relationships within a set of data, determining statistical reliability, and using mathematical models to predict outcome. Because it is highly technical, this technique generally is not used in smaller organizations or at the departmental level. The information generated from this subsystem flows into Phase 2, planning, and is used for decision-making purposes.

Phase 2: Planning

Planning, the second phase in the marketing management cycle, usually occurs at two levels in a health care organization. Planning at the organizational level, called *corporate marketing*, focuses on organizational objectives, upper management's view of the organizational mission, and resource allocation for the organization as a whole. At the departmental level, the planning process may be focused on the implementation of promotional activities in the restaurant or as broad as developing a three-year departmental marketing plan. Regardless of its scope, the planning process should be driven by the information collected in phase 1 of the cycle. The planning process results in marketing goals and programs to be implemented.

Planning Process

Each phase (and all its components) of the marketing management cycle must be aimed at *satisfying customers'* wants and needs in an ethical manner. Therefore, most health care operations satisfy three requirements before adopting a specific model for their planning process. These requirements are discussed in the following subsections.

Identify and Evaluate Opportunities and Threats   At the outset of the planning process, the health care operation's mission statement and established objectives that include a time for completion need to be reviewed. Next, the foodservice manager should review the market information system to identify marketplace opportunities that are consistent with the organization's objectives. This activity, called a *marketing opportunity analysis*, apprises managers not only of benefits associated with specific opportunities but also potential problems. Marketing opportunity analysis pays close attention to the environment in which the health care organization and foodservice facility operate. It identifies competitor facilities and compares their strengths and weaknesses with those of the foodservice operation. Such analysis allows the foodservice manager to select opportunities that are best suited to the operation. At the same time, effort should be made to correct weaknesses disclosed by the analysis.

Marketing opportunity analysis should be conducted by the foodservice manager when considering projects such as expanding existing catering services to off-premises events. Even though the market information system may indicate that this is a likely opportunity, careful analysis should be made before further action.

Analyze Market Segments and Select Target Markets   The results of opportunity analysis lead to decisions about where marketing efforts will be directed. It is important to stress that the health care foodservice manager must identify specific markets from all the possible market segments. To accomplish this, the market segments should be analyzed carefully to determine which ones are likely to have heavy users of the services and which hold little potential or present unreasonable risk. Specific targeting can improve revenue and may help control costs.

Referring back to the catering expansion example, based on the principles of segmenting and targeting markets, the foodservice manager must determine the focus for the proposed project. Operational characteristics necessary to support the venture for each segment under consideration must be explored. Examples of operational characteristics include hours of operation, the number of employees to consider, the addition of new employees, and cost-effectiveness of the venture. If the most promising market appears to be current hospital employees, a possible outcome of this analysis would be to design the off-premises business primarily for this segment.

Plan and Develop a Marketing Mix The third requirement in the planning process is to construct the marketing mix, discussed earlier in this chapter. The main objective is to determine the characteristics of product, place, promotion, price, and public image so that the wants and needs of target markets (customers) can be satisfied and the desired outcome of the marketing project can be achieved.

For the off-premises catering project, the existing marketing mix of the on-premises catering program can serve as the basis. For example, the product (food) must be analyzed to determine how the product can be offered by the off-premises facility. Specifically, menu offerings, hours of service, and methods of service would be considered. Simply offering the services off-premises changes the place element of the mix. The remaining elements of promotion, price, and the public image would require analysis and revision as well.

Marketing Plan All details resulting from the planning process should be documented in a working document called a *marketing plan*. The marketing plan identifies a systematic, structured program of action to be undertaken over a specified period (for example, one year) to achieve targeted financial results. Simply stated, the marketing plan provides the details necessary to achieve the stated goals.

Many health care operations specify a format for the marketing plan and justification for the proposed service. Otherwise, the foodservice manager should adopt a format similar to that suggested in *Marketing for Health Care Organizations*, by Kotler and Armstrong. Format components for the plan are as follows:

- *Executive summary.* The plan's main goals and recommendations are summarized so that readers can determine areas of major emphasis. The summary also facilitates plan evaluation.

- *Marketing opportunity analysis.* Results of the marketing opportunity analysis are provided, along with background information, forecasts, and assumptions. This section also should include a comparison of the operation's strengths and weaknesses with those of its competitors.
- *Current marketing situation.* Is the market overcrowded? What is the competition? A description of the product, the competition, and the distribution process should be included.
- *Threats and opportunity analysis.* What will be the ramification if this product is introduced? Will it bring positive or negative reactions? Will it generate revenue, improve image?
- *Goals and objectives.* Measurable goals and objectives for the foodservice department and its projects must be specified. Generally, these must be related to overall organizational goals for the specified time period.
- *Marketing strategy.* The foodservice marketing strategy consists of a coordinated set of decisions about target markets and the marketing mix that will be developed to appeal to these markets.
- *Actions plans.* Action plans turn the marketing strategy into a specific set of actions required to achieve the operation's goals and objectives. A table is an appropriate format for an action plan because it can include a timeline, which enables management and employees to determine when various activities will be initiated and completed (Figure 3.8).
- *Budgets.* Resources must support the proposals recommended in the marketing plan. A budget that shows projected revenues and expenses related to marketing activities must be provided.
- *Controls.* This section describes controls that will be used to monitor the plan's progress. For example, by arranging goals and budgets by appropriate time periods (usually monthly or quarterly), the health care operation's management can review results periodically.

FIGURE 3.8 Sample Action Plan

Action Plan

Topic:	Off-Premises Catering	
Strategy: Distribute brochure promoting off-premise catering to supervisory and managerial staff		
		Person Responsible
Action	**Completion Date**	(Coordinated by)
Establish format for brochure	September 15	M. Bloom
Identify possible photographs and topics for copy	September 22	T. Warren
Take photographs	September 30	Contracted out (T. Warren)
Write copy	October 5	T. Hardy
Design layout of brochure	October 12	T. Warren
Approve layout, copy, and photographs	October 19	M. Bloom
Obtain mailing labels	October 26	L. Williams
Print brochures	October 26	Contracted out (T. Warren)
Mail brochures	November 6	L. Williams

Phase 3: Implementation

Implementation of the marketing management process begins once actions are taken to initiate the marketing plan. These actions include organizing and coordinating procedures, people, tasks, and the development of a marketing budget. This budget needs to include allocation of money for each activity in the market plan. The budget must be realistic, incorporating research data. For instance, before a new menu is introduced, a number of operational procedures must be developed or changed, or both. To ensure that all necessary ingredients are available for the proposed menu items, new vendors may need to be located, and new purchasing contracts may need to be signed. The food storage, inventory, and requisition systems will require revision to incorporate new ingredients. Production records such as recipes and production schedules will have to be developed to support the new menu.

In preparation for the introduction of new products, the responsibilities for preparing and serving food items on the new menu must be assigned. As a result, employee training may be required. Physical facilities, such as equipment or storage facilities, may need to be modified. Advertising and promoting the new menu by means of signage, merchandising, and personal selling are important implementation activities that the manager will need to oversee both before and during the actual introduction of a new menu.

Although it may sound simple, implementation is only the beginning. Managers must *monitor* the process continually using techniques such as sales analysis, operating ratios (food cost to revenue), and customer comments. All procedures specified in the marketing plan must be reviewed and operations altered as necessary to ensure success. Without the proper implementation and effective monitoring procedures, even the best marketing plan will fail.

Phase 4: Evaluation

Results of the marketing effort must be *measured* and *evaluated* to determine whether the plan objectives have been achieved. A variety of qualitative, quantitative, and financial analysis methods can help make this determination. For example, recall the promotional technique of special offers during low-demand periods in the hospital restaurant (discussed under "Absence of Inventories" earlier in this chapter). Sales analyses should be conducted to show whether dollar sales increased during those slack periods. If sales did increase, the foodservice manager would then compare the actual increase with the increase forecast. Customer counts during hours of operation must also be monitored to see whether volume objectives were reached.

Sometimes a comprehensive review and appraisal of the marketing effort can be beneficial. Called a *marketing audit*, this activity evaluates an operation's marketing environment within the frame-work of operations organization-wide. The marketing audit must be conducted systematically and impartially to produce valid results, so it may be necessary to contract an outside consultant to perform it to ensure an unbiased analysis of the operation's strengths and weaknesses.

Phase 5: Feedback

The marketing management process is not linear but cyclical in nature. Therefore, at the end of the evaluation phase, information about the programs presented in the marketing plan should flow back to the information phase. *Feedback* is composed of a wide variety of techniques designed to facilitate this process. For instance, a status report could be discussed in a management staff meeting where the actual performance against the proposal is discussed Feedback information on successes and failures identified by this process could provide valuable input and create new marketing opportunities. This feature of cyclicity acknowledges the dynamic nature of health care foodservice operations and allows for adjustments in response to ongoing competitive and environmental changes. Implementing new strategies and ventures can be both frightening and exciting for a foodservice manager. Using this five-phase model can help managers design programs for almost any situation that may arise.

SUMMARY

All too often, health care foodservice managers try to advertise, promote, and sell goods and services without giving adequate thought to marketing. In times of intense competition and rapid change in this environment, a thorough understanding of marketing principles and techniques is needed to maximize service to customers and revenues for the operation and its parent organization.

This chapter covered several key marketing concepts that foodservice managers must grasp to design, plan, and implement effective marketing programs. Ideally, these concepts should be implemented within the context of the five-phase marketing management model presented.

Managers should assess their operations continuously for opportunities to apply marketing principles and techniques. The marketing orientation is critical in these times because of the pressure to satisfy increasingly complex and sophisticated wants and needs of health care foodservice customers.

To enhance revenue a list of ideas are offered as well as a method to determine pricing of an off-site catered event.

Image of foodservice operation must relate to the overall organization image. A positive image of the foodservice operation is vital. A good image will invite customers to return for a meal. Suggestions are offered to enhance the image of the operation.

KEY TERMS

Advertising

Behavioral dimension

Bundling

Customers

Demographical dimension

Feedback

Geographical dimension

Market management model

Market mix

Market plan

Market segmentation

Marketing audit

Merchandising

Packing

Promotion

Psychographic dimension

Self-branding

Target markets

DISCUSSION QUESTIONS

1. Determine the differences between promotion, advertising, and marketing.
2. Discuss the market segment that could be found in your locale.
3. How would you develop a marketing plan for a health care foodservice?
4. Explain the method you would use to develop a promotion plan to introduce a new service.
5. How would you plan an off-site breakfast buffet for 100 people? Refer to the model in the text.
6. Elaborate on methods to improve the image of a foodservice operation.

CHAPTER 4

QUALITY MANAGEMENT

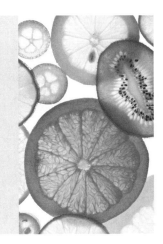

LEARNING OBJECTIVES

- Follow all surveying agencies regulation.
- Develop a continuous quality improvement program.
- Establish procedures to empower employees to work with internal and external department teams.
- Implement team management as it relates to quality management.
- Define benchmarking as it relates to quality management.

A PRIMARY RESPONSIBILITY of nutrition and foodservice managers is to help ensure the highest quality of patient care through the provision of high-quality food products and service to all consumers. The trends mentioned in Chapter 1 have caused renewed interest in health care quality management—in particular, health care reform issues, an expanding body of regulations, a shrinking and changing labor force, increased customer demands, and computer technology.

Health care organizations have become value-driven, stressing both quality and cost containment. *Value* is defined here as the relationship between quality and cost, or a focus on delivering the highest quality at the lowest possible cost. A value-driven approach requires more emphasis on quality of care and service, with cost containment becoming the added benefit of delivering high quality.

This chapter provides a brief background of quality in general industry and health care, with The Joint Commission (TJC) information that relates to quality and patient service. Specific characteristics of organizational culture that are supportive of continuous quality improvement (CQI) are presented, with description of the infrastructure necessary for implementing a CQI program.

The chapter also gives guidelines for developing a CQI plan that ensures service quality, quality control, and quality assessment related to clinical care. Quality of service and products are discussed throughout the book.

DEVELOPMENT OF QUALITY IN HEALTH CARE

Health care reform has forced administrators to transform their view of quality as an intangible to one that recognizes quality as an identifiable, measurable, and improvable entity. Although responsibility for quality was once delegated to a single department, managers now recognize quality improvement as the responsibility of each individual in an organization. *Quality improvement* is seen as a long-term proactive (rather than retrospective) strategy to improve patient care and satisfaction, increase utilization, strengthen productivity, and enhance cost-effectiveness throughout the organization. It has as its purpose to provide a continuous assessment of the department to meet the needs of customers. When developing continuous quality initiatives the director will need to focus on the plans for the facility and department as well as cost measures. The first step is to evaluate the goals of the organization and the department.

General History of Quality Management

In the 1930s, Walter A. Shewhart provided a scientific foundation for quality control measurement in industry and manufacturing. He believed that efforts should focus on identifying and correcting problems during the manufacture of products rather than on correcting the final product. Shewhart is credited with designing the plan-do-check-act (PDCA) cycle shown in Figure 4.1.

W. Edwards Deming, who was originally trained as a statistician, began teaching statistical quality control in Japan shortly after

FIGURE 4.1 Shewhart's PDCA Cycle for Process Improvement

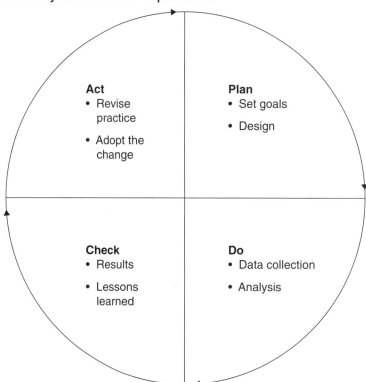

World War II. He is recognized internationally as a primary contributor to the Japanese quality improvement program. Deming advocated that the way to achieve product quality is to continuously improve the design of a product and the process used to manufacture it by reducing waste. He expanded the PDCA cycle, defining each of the four quadrants in Shewhart's model and providing specific suggestions to foster improvement (Figure 4.2). He was a prominent pioneer in the quality movement, maintaining that 90 percent of variations in quality are due to systemic factors such as procedures, suppliers, and equipment not under employees' control. He thought that it was management's responsibility to reduce variation and to involve employees in the continuous improvement of system processes.

Deming also is credited with the use of statistical process control tools that are the foundation of total quality management (TQM). In Causey's handbook *An Executive's Pocket Guide to QI/TQM Terminology* (1992), TQM is defined as "a continuous quality improvement management system, directed from the top, empowering employees and focused on systemic, not individual employee problems, and continually strives to make improvements and satisfy customers."

In 1951, in his *Quality Control Handbook*, Joseph Juran introduced the dimension of economics to quality by categorizing the costs of quality as "avoidable" and "unavoidable." According to Juran, avoidable costs are associated with defects and product failures, scrapped materials, labor hours for rework and repair, complaint processing, and losses resulting from unhappy customers. Unavoidable costs, he explains, are associated with prevention, inspection, sampling, sorting, and other quality-control initiatives.

Juran's work provided managers with objective measures for deciding how much to invest in quality improvement.

According to Garvin (1988), Armand Feigenbaum expanded manufacturing quality control in 1956 by proposing a *total quality control system*, adding product development, vendor selection, and customer service to the existing quality system. Feigenbaum supported reliability engineering designed to prevent defects and to emphasize attention to quality throughout the design process.

Another well-known name in the quality movement is Philip Crosby, who focused on management expectations and human relations. Crosby believed in getting the job done correctly the first time—or *zero defects,* achieved through training, communicating quality results, goal setting, and personal feedback.

The Joint Commission's Influence on Health Care Quality

The Joint Commission is a private, not-for-profit organization dedicated to improving the quality of patient care for all types of hospitals, home care organizations, nursing homes, and other long-term care facilities; behavioral health care and managed behavior health care organizations; ambulatory care providers, including outpatient surgery facilities, rehabilitation centers, infusion centers, physician group practices, and clinical laboratories; and health care networks, including health plans, integrated delivery networks, and preferred provider organizations.

Health care organizations voluntarily seek TJC accreditation because it raises community confidence and provides educational

FIGURE 4.2 Deming's PDCA Cycle

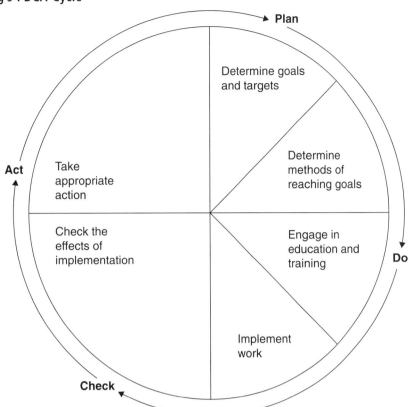

tools to improve care, service, and programs. When "accredited," an organization has proved its commitment to patient focus as measured against the highest and most rigorous standards of performance.

Standards of performance vary according to the classification of the health care environment. These standards are developed by TJC and its board, which includes administrators, nurses, physicians, and consumers, with input from individuals as well as professional organizations such as the Academy of Nutrition and Dietetics (AND). This group of people sets the standards by which health care is measured.

To earn and maintain accreditation, at least once every 18 months to three years, an organization undergoes an unannounced on-site survey by a select team that has been trained externally by TJC. The team usually is composed of a physician, an administrator, and a nurse. In large complex organizations, a survey may include a clinical laboratory person, a behavioral health care provider, and an outpatient surveyor. These surveyors make firsthand observations, visit patients and staff, and review paperwork. The survey team helps identify the organization's strengths and weaknesses in such areas as patient care, patient rights, organizational ethics, ongoing improvement procedures, and organizational leadership. The emphasis of the survey is on validation of performance improvement through a continuous quality improvement; and positive health outcomes as measured against the standards that were designed from patients' point of view that focus on the delivery of care and not on policies and procedures. The survey is

flexible and customized for the type of organization being evaluated. It is more consultative and educational in its approach. TJC assists organizations to provide quality by the implementation of *continuous quality improvement* (CQI). CQI is a process that emphasizes quality management through a proactive process. It further stresses the relationship of interdisciplinary team cooperation in making the process work.

Surveyors provide a preliminary report at the conclusion of the survey. The accreditation may be awarded on several levels based on the organization's compliance with TJC standards. Organizations receiving recommendation for improvement are required to bring the areas cited into compliance within a specific time.

In 1997 TJC developed an adjunct to the accreditation process: *ORYX—The Next Evaluation in Accreditation*. (ORYX is a proprietary term; the letters do not stand for anything.) ORYX requires organizations to provide TJC with data regarding their "outcomes" (actual patient care results) that show patterns and trends leading to improvements in patient care.

The ORYX includes performance measures: "quantitative tools that provide an indication of an organization's performance in relation to a specified process or outcome." Another component of ORYX is the identification by TJC of care performance measures to eventually permit comparisons to performance across hospitals. Data derived from care measures are used to monitor a health care organization's performance on a continuous basis, focus surveys on areas that need the most clinical improvements, and help to identify best practices to facilitate benchmarking.

Until the late 1980s, the quality process in health care institutions was designed to meet the demands of outside regulations or guidelines. For nutrition and foodservice departments, reviews have come from the Health Care Financing Administration, now called the Center for Medicare and Medicaid Services (CMS), and TJC. The CMS is responsible for reviewing organizations that serve patients who receive Medicare funds. TJC reviews are educational and must be requested by the facility being surveyed.

Move to CQI in Health Care

The term *continuous quality improvement*, or CQI, has been selected by many to identify their quality initiatives. For the purposes of this text, CQI is defined as "the base theory that quality can be improved on a continuous, or never-ending basis," a definition taken from *An Executive's Pocket Guide to QI/TQM Terminology*. The concept of CQI is based on the principle that poor quality is the result of poorly functioning or poorly structured processes that can be improved. To further define CQI provides a method of *continually* assessing the performance of a department to meet the needs of the customer. The CQI concept was first introduced in the *JCHO Accreditation Manual for Healthcare* in 1992. TJC's position is that 95 percent of an organization's problems can be solved through process improvement, and the JC encouraged all hospitals to have some type of CQI process in place. The remaining 5 percent of problems should be handled through traditional quality assessment and peer review.

TJC had renamed the "Quality Assessment and Improvement" chapter as "Organizational Performance Improvement." Representatives for TJC advise hospitals to learn the concepts of CQI without abandoning traditional monitoring and evaluation of quality assurance. This advice means that traditional quality assurance will continue to play a major role in accreditation standards with TJC.

TJC concedes that many different approaches lead to CQI and that it endorses no one method. However, elements of CQI have been incorporated into the standards for accreditation as:

- The key role that leaders (individually and collectively) play in enabling the assessment and improvement of performance
- The fact that most problems or opportunities for improvement derive from process weaknesses, not from individual incompetence
- The need for careful coordination of work across departments and professional groups
- The importance of seeking judgments about quality from patients and other "customers" and using such judgments to identify areas for improvement
- The importance of carefully setting priorities for improvement
- The need for both systematic improvement of the performance of important functions and maintenance of the stability of these functions

Another standard addresses the education of health care executives about quality improvement. The standard requires facilities to demonstrate that the executive team has acquired education in the approaches and methods of quality improvement. A plan must be in place to demonstrate how the organization will meet quality improvement standards for:

- Setting priorities for quality improvement activities
- Allocating resources for improvement activities
- Training staff members regarding quality improvement
- Fostering better communication and coordination of quality improvement activities
- Determining how the effectiveness of their contributions to quality improvement is analyzed

CREATING A CQI CULTURE

To create a *culture* that fosters CQI, an organization or department must adhere to the principles for creating a participative culture as described in Chapter 2. *Culture*, identified as the way things get done in an organization, influences not only how employees view and perform their jobs and how they work with colleagues but also how they view their customers and how they view quality.

Principles That Drive a CQI Culture

CQI requires the integration of quality and change management methods, practices, concepts, and beliefs into an organization's current culture. Adopting any CQI process means integrating a focus on quality into all aspects of the organization, making it everyone's priority. Three principles are essential to establishing a CQI culture:

1. Customer satisfaction
2. Scientific approach (evidence based)
3. Involvement of the total organization in improving quality for customer satisfaction (team approach)

For the CQI program to be effective it will need the endorsement, support, leadership, and communication from the board and other management staff. Creating a CQI environment takes structure, planning, trust, patience, positive change, and time to develop; that is, to monitor and make appropriate changes for continuous quality improvements. The CQI program must be organization-wide. This is accomplished through training programs, management support, teamwork, and tools of quality improvement. CQI will need to be included in job descriptions as general duties and responsibilities, Performance appraisal criteria can be set that rewards employees for concentrating on customer satisfaction, working teams, and improving process. Health care organizations that embrace CQI have been found to have certain cultural characteristics in common. Table 4.1 lists these characteristics.

Customer Satisfaction

A customer-focused organization recognizes the need to identify and exceed customers' expectations. An organization focused on quality improvement recognizes that the purpose of improvement is to provide the best service at the lowest possible cost and that without this value-driven goal, customer orientation is futile. Potential customers—individual patients, physicians, managed care

TABLE 4.1   Cultural Traits Shared by CQI Organizations

Characteristic	Summary
Quality definition	Knowing what quality "looks like" in an organization (for example, a statement on how to greet customers)
Business strategy	Business plan incorporating strategies for quality goals and objectives, along with written plans for meeting them
Communication	Two-way flow between employees and leaders
Supplier partnerships	Organization-vendor commitment to provide best value at lowest possible cost
Error-free attitude	Mind-set to "do it right the first time—every time"
Fact-based versus result-based management	Process versus outcome (quantity) orientation; long-term versus short-term results
Employee empowerment	Employee autonomy, involvement, ownership of work process
Physician involvement	Improved quality of practice patterns through multidisciplinary teamwork, critical paths, physician liaisons
Training and retraining	Continuing education through hands-on learning, cross-functional training, development of in-house expertise, for example
Problem solving through teamwork	Inter- and intradepartmental evaluation, decision making, prioritizing; some accountability to quality council
Work process focus	Realization that processes account for 85 to 95 percent of problems and that individuals may or may not account for remaining 5 to 15 percent
Innovation and risk taking	Employee freedom to be creative and experiment without fear of reprisal or job loss
Reward and recognition	Social (verbal congratulations), tangible (success celebrations), or symbolic (plaques or pins) acknowledgment for effort and accomplishment

organizations, payers, colleagues, someone from other departments, families and visitors—have choices when it comes to selecting health care. Often, these choices may conflict. For example, patients may want some say in the health care facility they use and the physician they see. To remain competitive, organizations must seek to be the provider of choice for all of these customer groups that meet their wants and needs.

Customers are more likely to take their business elsewhere because of poor service than for any other reason, and secondly for the lack of the organization meeting the needs of patients. Changing patronage due to unsatisfactory service is more common than changing due to unsatisfactory quality or cost of the product. Research has shown that customers will even pay more for products if they *perceive* the service to be of excellent quality.

In health care, *customer satisfaction* often has focused only on external customers (patients, for example). However, internal customers include nurses, physicians, laboratory technicians, nurses' aides, and other health care professionals. This is especially important to foodservice managers, who must understand the needs of internal customers and balance them with those of external customers. For example, nurses can influence how patients and their families perceive product service and quality. If nurses are dissatisfied when calling for patient tray service or if they find the cafeteria service to be inferior, they can affect how to monitor quality indicators and to work with the director to assist in developing tools and reports on the effectiveness of the program. Another effective technique for helping employees develop a customer focus is to have them meet as a group to identify their customers. The group defines the customers and makes posters for "customer-focused," which are displayed throughout the department as a reminder to new and veteran employees.

Scientific Approach—Evidence-Based

Customer satisfaction and patronage need to be carefully managed through the use of informal and formal surveys. These surveys may be conducted by the health care facility patient service resident, by various departments as well as outside consulting firms who specialize in surveying patients on a nationwide basis. Patients with major concerns about their treatment may be interviewed by the patient representative while they are still in the health care facility, with a follow-up telephone call or printed survey after discharge. Information gathered from these interviews must be shared with any department that patients perceived to present a problem or praise. The director of any department mentioned will need to evaluate the problem and make improvements/changes as merited.

An example of a department survey may occur while making meal rounds; a foodservice representative may ask pertinent questions that relate to the food, the service, and the personnel. Foodservice personnel need to consistently ask customers what they want and whether their expectations are being met. Cafeteria customers may be given a written survey or asked by frontline employees to participate in a focus group to gauge their acceptance of meal items and the quality of service provided. If problems are mentioned the supervisor will need to alert the director or dietitian. Results will need to be tabulated and analyzed, and additional data gathered to problem solve. Actions taken may include retraining, change in policies/procedures, or corrective action. Ongoing surveys provide feedback to determine if the action plans were effective. The problem will need to be documented and the outcomes recorded as part of an ongoing CQI program.

Health care facilities may also send out written questionnaires to discharge patients concerning the care they received while they were a patient. This information is carefully evaluated as part of the organization's CQI program. Changes may be made as needed. Outside consultants may be employed to randomly select discharged patients to complete a written survey. The answers from the surveys are sent to the organization along with a comparison of how well its competition is doing. Health care facilities take the information from the surveys seriously. All departments that are surveyed receive the information and are expected to review the information and compare it to the standards as established by the administration and the department. When standards are not met a written report is developed to include methods of how the department standards can be made to meet the organization's standards.

Teams

Health care organizations that embrace CQI have been found to have certain cultural characteristics in common. There are 13 different characteristics, as noted in Table 4.1. The main feature of CQI is a *team* approach with support from higher management and the removal of artificial work barriers. Through training programs and management support, organization-wide involvement on the part of each employee can be enhanced. Once employees are trained in teamwork and in the tools of quality improvement, they should be encouraged to participate in teams. With this training and support comes accountability. Often employees are reluctant to participate without understanding the importance of their roles. Accountability and employees' value to the organization are conveyed by including guidelines in general duties and responsibilities in job descriptions. Performance-appraisal criteria can be set that reward employees for concentrating on customer satisfaction, working in teams, and improving processes.

Problem Solving Through Teamwork

One of the principles of CQI is involving the entire organization in improving quality. This is best accomplished through intradepartmental or interdepartmental teams. *Intradepartmental teams* usually focus on processes or service areas within one department (sometimes as related to one other department, which acts as a "customer"). *Interdepartmental teams*, or cross-functional teams, are formed when a process needs to be evaluated and spans two or more departments.

Intradepartmental teams usually identify the project or process to be worked on. This may be done during an initial meeting of a team created to identify customer needs, or it may be done as a department task. As mentioned earlier, processes and problems can be listed, prioritized, and then posted so that employees can volunteer. Accountability for actions of intradepartmental teams lies with the department manager and the team leader, although team members should have some understanding and "ownership" of the process being studied. The team leader is generally selected by the team or may be appointed by a manager based on the knowledge of an individual. An intradepartmental team can have up to 10 members and usually will include a supervisor. Once they become experienced with CQI, employees can form teams and meet without a supervisor. However, it should be made clear that the progress,

actions, and outcomes of the team must be shared with the department manager. Team meetings can take from 30 minutes up to one hour per week. The life span of intradepartmental teams can vary from short term to indefinite, depending on how productive they are in identifying and addressing CQI issues. Implementation of team recommendations will be department-based and occur based on complexity. For example, if a team's goal was to decrease the amount of time it takes for a patient to receive a late tray, the action plan may include steps to shorten the time between receiving the order and preparing the tray. All of these steps would occur inside the department.

Interdepartmental (cross-functional) *teams* are selected based on input and priority level established by the quality council, to which they are accountable. Membership (commonly limited to eight members) should be representative of each functional area involved in the process under investigation and should include department managers and supervisors. The team's life span depends on the complexity of the process under investigation and of the recommendations to be implemented. Generally, the team will have to meet for more than one hour per week. The quality council should monitor the performance of cross-functional teams to determine whether politics or turf battles might compromise final recommendations. As a rule, the "owners" of the process under study are accountable for implementation of recommendations, with assistance from team members and the quality council.

Generally speaking, CQI teams, whether intradepartmental or cross-functional, consist of a team facilitator, team leader, and team members. The facilitator is responsible for providing training and information about the process under study, suggesting tools for problem solving or measurement, providing feedback and support, ensuring equal participation, and if necessary, mediating and resolving conflicts. A facilitator may not be necessary for every process improvement. For example, an intradepartmental team whose leader has had experience in teamwork and understands the fundamentals of process improvement may not need a facilitator.

The leader of a CQI team is responsible for guiding the team to resolution through achieving the desired objectives or problem resolution. Conducting team meetings, providing direction and focus to the team, and keeping the group on track and on time are some of the leader's responsibilities. (It may be necessary to appoint a team member to be a timekeeper to ensure efficient use of time.) The leader also is responsible for conveying the team's need for resources, recommendations, and other concerns to the quality council or to management. Documentation and reporting of team activity and progress is an important function of the team leader. A sample team documentation form is shown in Exhibit 4.1.

Team members should be vested with some sense of ownership in, and knowledge of, the process or problem being investigated. Members provide ideas and different perspectives through their active participation. They must agree to adhere to meeting ground rules, to support the leader, and to support implementation of the recommendations agreed on by the team. Assignments must be performed on time to ensure smooth progress during team meetings. More information for conducting team meetings is provided in Chapter 7.

EXHIBIT 4.1   Team Documentation Form

Name of project/issue: _____

Date: _____ Assigned by (title) _____

Team leader: _____

Team members: (inter- or intradepartmental) [9 members maximum]

_____

_____

List who the customers are: _____

What is the proposed outcome? _____

Tools and resources to be used: _____

Action plan: _____ Who is responsible? _____

How will outcomes be measured? _____

Meeting dates: _____ Finish date: _____

Report outcomes to: _____

_____

_____

_____

Source: Developed by Ruby P. Puckett, 2011. Used by permission.

Work Process Focus

Organizations successful in creating a CQI culture understand that processes, not individuals, create inefficiencies or problems. A *process* is a sequence of events or tasks performed to reach a desired outcome. For example, a patient's receiving his or her tray late is the outcome of a late-tray process, which comprises several steps from receipt of an order by the foodservice department to delivery of the tray to the patient. Productivity is improved when unnecessary steps in a process are eliminated or when steps can be combined. Although some processes can be improved by making minor adjustments, others must be replaced or redesigned entirely. Quality management experts estimate that 85 to 95 percent of all problems within an organization are caused by work processes and systems, leaving only 5 to 15 percent that are controlled (not necessarily caused) by individuals. Viewing related tasks as processes provides employees with a broader view of how work is accomplished. This type of thinking allows them to understand that quality of output (outcome) is affected by quality of input (process or system).

Innovation and Risk Taking

Testing the unknown and trying unproven solutions and ideas is another characteristic of a CQI culture. An environment that encourages innovation and experimentation leads to creative thinking on the part of all workers. Once employees are assured that they can take reasonable chances to improve care or service without fear of punishment for failure, more ideas will be tested. Thus, creativity

among all department members can be nurtured, rather than depending on the experiences and ideas of a few.

Reward and Recognition

Without properly recognizing and rewarding employees and managers who are successful with CQI initiatives, it will be difficult to sustain their long-term commitment. Rewards and recognition may be social, tangible, or symbolic. Congratulations to a team from the manager or upper leadership is a type of social reward. Celebrations, such as fairs where teams are encouraged to display the work and results of their efforts, are more tangible. Plaques, pins, or ribbons are examples of symbolic reward and recognition for involvement as well as for success. Positive reinforcement is crucial to sustaining long-term empowerment and assisting with success. It is important that the reward and recognition be genuine. Some CQI proponents caution that team-of-the-month awards or other such distinctions may prove counterproductive to the CQI process because they honor only one group among many and create negative competition and possible resentment among those who did not "win." However, these types of programs have also been advocated to establish friendly competition, which leads to more staff members becoming involved in the organizational culture.

Components of the Foodservice CQI Plan

A CQI plan for health care nutrition and foodservices has three components: quality control to ensure safe and wholesome products, customer service, and clinical quality assessment. The following sections describe each component.

Quality Control

Quality assessment measures the overall quality of care delivered to patients, whereas *quality control* as it relates to foodservice management measures systems for handling, preparing, and serving food. Customer satisfaction is gauged by addressing quality from the customer's point of view—for example, food temperature, appearance, palatability, and nutrition content. The handling, preparation, and service of food also are measured against standards for infection control, aesthetic appeal, and safety. Feedback tools in a quality-control program may include:

- Sanitation reports (internal, external)
- Safety reports
- Temperatures of refrigerators, walk-in refrigeration units, and dish machines
- Downtime on the tray line
- Cart delivery time
- Trays per labor minute
- Portion control
- Food temperatures
- Patient questionnaires or surveys
- Verbal compliments and complaints
- Comment cards
- Observation of customer service as measured against preestablished guidelines
- Timeliness of cafeteria service and other meal service

The *quality control program* must be adhered to in every food and nutrition service department. If the program is carefully developed, monitored, and evaluated, and if it has built-in routine follow-up procedures, CQI and customer satisfaction are enhanced.

A comprehensive quality control program includes:

- Defining objectives and standards for foodservice
- Monitoring quality procedure

- Making necessary procedural changes
- Making reports to the designated person
- Implementing audit procedures to determine the effectiveness of the quality indicators
- Written policies and procedures with established standards that help identify strengths and weaknesses in food and service quality

Once standards or guidelines are in place, appropriate training must be completed to convey responsibility and expectations to staff and supervisors. The standards are then used to measure compliance to ensure consistent and safe operations.

Quality Control of Food Products

The sampling of food products, measurement of food temperatures, and sensory appraisal of product characteristics allow comparison of observed quality with the standard established for each item. Inspection criteria for food production and service include food appearance, taste, texture, and safety and tray appearance. Through evaluation and analysis, foodservice directors can identify what went wrong, how often, and why. For example, evaluating a patient tray would include making sure that an attractive garnish is present, that the meat is adequately browned, that the vegetables complement the meal in color and are not overcooked, and that everything is at appropriate serving temperature. Then corrective action can eliminate or reduce quality deficiencies.

Success of a quality control program depends on the commitment of all employees to the provision of high-quality food. Quality control activities should be incorporated into regular job routines and duties for each position. For example, each position on the tray line can be responsible for checking temperatures and ensuring that each menu item is attractively served on the plate. Failure of staff members to follow established criteria for food product safety should be documented and addressed. The director should prepare a foodservice quality checklist as a routine evaluation tool. Exhibit 4.2 is an example of quality checklist inspection criteria.

EXHIBIT 4.2 Inspection Criteria for Food Production and Service

Food appearance

☐ Satisfactory and appropriate color and texture

☐ Pleasing and varied food color-texture combinations

☐ Attractive garnishes

☐ Variety in shape and size of food items

☐ Adequate portion size

Food taste

☐ Pleasant flavor combinations

☐ Taste integrity of each item

☐ Adequate seasoning

☐ No undesirable or odd flavors

☐ Pleasing aroma

☐ Proper temperature

Food texture

☐ No item overcooked or undercooked

☐ Variety of textures

☐ Suitable moisture content

☐ No toughness or stringiness

☐ Suitable for consumers being served

Food safety

☐ Proper hot serving temperatures: for liquids, 185°F (85°C); for cooked cereals, 175°F (79°C); for soups, 180°F (82°C); for meats, 150°F (65°C); for eggs, 145°F (63°C); for vegetables, 160°F (71°C). (Temperatures requirements vary among foodservice organizations.)

☐ Proper cold serving temperatures: for liquids, 35°F (2°C); for solid foods, 45°F (7°C)

☐ Foods prepared and portioned using utensils or disposable gloves to avoid contamination by employees' hands

☐ Two clean spoons used for tasting food products

☐ Special care used in handling clean dishes and flatware to prevent contamination

☐ Unused raw ingredients or cooked leftover foods labeled, refrigerated promptly, and used within 24 to 48 hours, frozen immediately, or discarded

☐ No reuse of single-use utensils and containers

☐ Employees' clothing and personal hygiene at established standards

☐ Tray appearance

☐ Adequate tray size, no overcrowding

☐ Specified setup used

☐ Each item placed on tray correctly and arranged for eating convenience

☐ Dishes and flatware in good condition

☐ Food neatly served

☐ Separate dishes for foods that contain liquid

☐ Neat overall appearance, no spills

☐ Tray accuracy

☐ All food items specified on menu present on tray

☐ Food on tray allowed on patient diet

☐ No unnecessary utensils on tray

Source: Developed by Ruby P. Puckett © 2011.

Customer Service and Satisfaction

Whether it is called *guest relations, customer service*, or customer relations, the concept is the same. It is estimated that more than 60 percent of the nation's hospitals have introduced some type of customer relations training for their employees. The purpose of these programs is to improve customer satisfaction to obtain repeat business and to increase market share through word-of-mouth referrals.

Often customer satisfaction is based on the interaction between the customer and service personnel and occurs at the time service is delivered. In this respect, customer satisfaction depends on employee performance. Research conducted on the results of meeting customer needs has shown measurable benefits in profits, cost savings, and market share. Customers often do not complain when they have received less-than-satisfactory service; however, they do tell 9 or 10 other people about the problem. It is estimated that it costs an organization five to six times as much to gain a new customer as it does to keep a current one. To retain current customers while attracting new ones, health care foodservice managers must strive toward two goals. First, they must instill in employees the fact that customer orientation drives customer satisfaction. Next, they must design and launch a strategic quality service plan.

From Customer Orientation to Customer Satisfaction

To embrace the concept of customer relations, employees must first recognize that they have customers. Customers include patients, residents, their families and significant others, physicians, and other staff members. The thought of identifying a patient as a customer has been disconcerting for some health care professionals, but without viewing patients as end users of their services, providers do nothing more than develop systems and processes for their own convenience. Although these systems and processes may be based on the best medical practice and perceived need, they often are created at the expense of customer satisfaction. Referring to patients as customers recognizes their autonomy and capability of demanding high-quality care and information about the services they buy.

The nutrition and foodservice department can play a key role in developing a positive image for patients and their caregivers. Although much of what customer-patients come in contact within the hospital setting is technical and beyond their general understanding, food is the one thing they do know. They know whether the food is prepared to their satisfaction, whether it is delivered when they are hungry, whether it is at the right temperature, and whether the person delivering the meal is polite and attentive to their needs. Therefore, it is vitally important for the foodservice manager to ensure that staff members understand their role in customer satisfaction.

Although the customer-patient is certainly a key focus, this is not the only type of customer encountered by foodservice employees. Physicians, family members, and other hospital staff are served in the cafeteria, physician dining rooms, coffee shops, and so on. Service quality can be compromised not only because it may be difficult to persuade foodservice staff to accept other hospital employees as customers but also because satisfaction is based on customer expectations and perceptions. By comparing their expectations of service quality with actual service delivery, they judge whether satisfaction has been attained.

From Service Plan to Customer Satisfaction

In the book *Service America*, Karl Albrecht and Ron Zemke identify three features of outstanding service organizations: a defined, customer-focused service strategy; customer-oriented frontline employees; and customer-friendly systems.

It is impossible to expect employees to provide exemplary service if no quality service plan or strategy is in place. A *service strategy* is based on feedback from the customer and also the organization's strategy and mission. The plan should include a written statement or mission that all employees can understand and support. A health care foodservice strategy may include the following elements:

- Greeting customers by name according to organization policy, making eye contact
- Extending extra effort to be helpful
- Providing timely and prompt service
- Listening to customers' needs and responding to them
- Maintaining appropriate appearance according to departmental policy
- Maintaining a safe and pleasant environment
- Providing what was promised

Once the departmental strategy is written, employees must be trained to deliver the service as outlined. Training may be done through modeling behavior, scripting phrases for greeting customers, or practical examples of ways to handle specific customer issues or requests. This strategy and training are useful in developing customer-oriented frontline employees.

Used consistently as monitoring and measuring devices for service performance, these feedback mechanisms keep managers up to date regarding customer perception of timeliness of meal service, temperature of food items, and staff courtesy. Once surveys are tabulated, they should be analyzed for potential problem areas so that action plans can be created and implemented for improvement. Ongoing surveys provide feedback to determine in turn whether the action plans were effective.

Customer-friendly systems are based on understanding what the customer wants, and in a quality-oriented and participative work environment, feedback is encouraged so as to get this information. Employees are best positioned to know which systems or processes are not customer-friendly and in some instances can work around these systems to offer better service. Policies and procedures are developed to ensure safe, consistent service, but before being implemented, they should be evaluated from both the customer and employee points of view. Management can then evaluate how relevant these guidelines are to promoting customer satisfaction. Once a system or process is identified as not being customer-friendly, customers' input must be obtained to correct the situation.

Clinical Quality Assessment

The quality assessment program, according to TJC, "is an ongoing, planned, and systematic process to monitor and evaluate the quality and appropriateness of patient care." It is used to improve clinical patient care and to identify problems. The minimum requirements of the quality assessment plan include:

- The use of evidence-based indicators or performance measures
- Ongoing monitoring (that is, a process that tracks quality assessment system components to determine the system's level of compliance to the indicators)
- Analysis of performance data against reference databases (benchmarking)
- The use of multidisciplinary teams when processes and systems are being evaluated across departmental lines

- The use of individual peer review when the performance of an individual practitioner is being evaluated
- Annual review and revision of the plan to ensure effectiveness

Although TJC appears to be moving away from thresholds to standards, monitoring against established standards is applicable. CQI, on the other hand, emphasizes changing the target as improvement occurs. However, ongoing monitoring is compatible with the quality control aspects of CQI. TJC is looking for sustained improvement over time, and if the threshold is met consistently, monitoring can be deferred until a later date but must occur again to ensure sustained improvement or compliance.

TJC still emphasizes the concept of individual competency—that good results occur when competent people work in effective systems. TJC also recognizes that ineffective systems can hinder good performance and results. Thus, when individual weaknesses do occur, the organization is expected to identify them and provide guidance or training for improvement.

Peer review continues to be a part of TJC's standards, indicating the persistent need for professional judgments in the review of process and of individual performance. The best judgments must be made based on the latest information available. In TJC's view, those best qualified to determine whether the best judgment was made are peers. (Check the latest edition of TJC standards for changes.)

Quality Programs

Quality programs continually change and have evolved from quality control → quality assurance → continuous quality improvement → total quality management of satisfying the customer → ISO 9000 (described in detail later in this chapter).

Quality control is a method or process to ensure that what is produced meets some preestablished standards. Quality control monitors quality at all steps of the operation to the finished product. Quality control ensures early detection of a defective part, procedure, and process and can save the cost of further work on the item. Measures need to be developed before implementing the program if less than 100 percent acceptable.

Quality assurance is the next step in the evolution of quality. Quality assurance is a process of identifying and solving problems within a department or area of an organization. TQM tools can be used to monitor quality assurance within a foodservice department.

Continuous quality improvement, CQI, is the process of evaluating and always searching for which things within an organization can be improved and what can be done to achieve the improvement. A patient questionnaire not only indicates what is acceptable but also evaluates what category of food or service needs to be targeted to achieve improvement. It requires integration of quality and change targeted to achieve improved management methods, practices, concepts, and beliefs into the organization's culture.

Even with these three processes, problems seem to occur that do not have a solution. CQI uses the tools of *total quality management* (TQM), which seeks to achieve continuous process improvement so that variability is reduced. TQM commits to quality objectives, continuous improvement, and doing it "right the first time." TQM is a management system that has six components:

1. Change the processes, not the people.
2. Focus on the customer.
3. Empower employees.
4. Use a team approach to accomplish change.
5. Control processes through sequential steps.
6. Expect a long-term organizational commitment.

TQM was designed to look at problems and improvements that could be made across departmental boundaries. An example would be an interdisciplinary approach to the education of a patient. TQM puts the focus on the problem or product to be improved. The process is interdepartmental, and administration usually assigns it to a committee composed of representatives of departments affected by the problem. The committee should focus on a workable positive outcome for all departments. The committee may be a self-managed group assigned to work on a specific problem or process, and when the task is completed, it is disbanded. Ideally, administration assigns a leader who is disinterested, has no vested interest in the outcome, is able to be objective, and is a good negotiator. A group works best when it can reach an agreeable solution; the solution is implemented, evaluated, and monitored; and necessary adjustments are made.

When a TQM team follows a "standard guide," consistency and group acceptance seem to improve. A guide may suggest the following:

- Choose the product or process that needs to be improved. This may be a management decision or a regulatory problem. For a foodservice department, this may include:
  Late tray service
  Height or weight of patients
  Use of floor stock
  Weekend coverage
  Adherence to all regulatory agency standards
- Organize the team and appoint a facilitator and a recorder. Depending on the product or process to be improved, members could include:
  Personnel from the area of problem
  Member of management
  Members of departments that are affected by the process or problem
- Use benchmarking data to determine the best performance. Use other data that will provide needed information.
- Perform an analysis to determine how performance standards can be met, improved, or beat. For example, XYZ hospital can serve nine trays per minute; your facility serves only seven. What makes the difference: equipment, menu, personnel, materials available, work methods, or physical conditions? Who serves patients' trays, foodservice or cross-functional trained personnel?
- Devise and perform a pilot study and analyze data: can time be improved; what is the cost of improvement; should schedules or personnel change (or both)?

FIGURE 4.3   Flowchart for Patient Late Tray Process

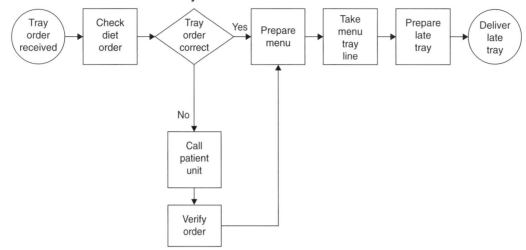

■ Implement and monitor improvements. Will improvements enhance patient services and meet the needs, wants, and perceptions of patients?

Total Quality Management

TQM provides the techniques, concepts, and tools to analyze data for application in CQI. The tools of TQM help identify and analyze current processes either within or across departmental lines. Once data are collected and analyzed, steps can be taken to improve a complex process. Unnecessary or nonvalue-added steps can be eliminated and the process streamlined to provide better care or service.

TQM Tools

Statistics-based process control is the foundation of TQM. Tools of TQM, such as flowcharts, Pareto charts, and cause-and-effect diagrams, provide a common statistical language and visual aids for analyzing a process or problem. Not all TQM tools are required to evaluate any one process or problem, and only those that clearly will facilitate decision making should be selected for the issue in question. Quality improvement tools can be divided into two general categories: those used for *problem identification* and those used for *problem analysis*. However, some tools can be used for problem identification and analysis.

Tools used for problem identification include *flowcharts* and *brainstorming*. Recall from Chapter 2 that brainstorming is a group session devoted to sharing ideas and information without judging their value. A top-down flowchart is explained in Chapter 5. Another type of flowchart is a detailed flowchart that is used to identify steps or tasks in a process. This flowchart may identify the current path or establish a new road map or direction. Flowcharts are usually drawn using squares, rectangles, diamonds, and circles, with circles specifying the beginning and final steps in the process. Squares or rectangles represent the in-between steps, and diamonds represent decision points and questions. Flowcharts are beneficial

in that they disclose duplicate steps and steps that can be combined or performed in a different order to prevent unnecessary feedback loops. *Feedback loops* are steps or events that require a product or customer to return to a previous step in the process. An example of a flowchart for the late tray process is shown in Figure 4.3.

Tools used for problem identification or analysis include Pareto charts, cause-and-effect diagrams, and run charts. A *Pareto chart* is simply a bar graph used to prioritize problems and determine which should be solved first. In constructing a Pareto chart, categories must be designed and the unit of measure (for example, hour, error, dollar, or job category) selected. After data are gathered, they must be broken down, or aggregated, by category; items should be ranked in descending order from left to right. Efforts can then focus on the categories with the greatest effect or frequency. An example of a Pareto chart reflecting the problems associated with late tray delivery is provided in Figure 4.4.

Cause-and-effect diagrams, also called *fishbone* or *Ishikawa* diagrams, are used to represent the relationship between an effect and all the possible causes contributing to it. Team brainstorming may be used to create a fishbone diagram. Causes are generally divided into four categories: materials, methods, equipment, and employees. An example of a cause-and-effect diagram related to late tray delivery is provided in Figure 4.5.

A *run chart* can be used to identify trends or shifts over several observation periods. Run charts provide information regarding long-range averages to determine whether changes are occurring. This allows for an investigation of increases and decreases in averages. For example, a run chart can disclose the number of patients over a 12-month period who waited longer than 15 minutes to receive a late tray. Figure 4.6 charts this scenario.

Another common tool used for problem analysis is a control chart. *Process control charts* are run charts that allow the use of probability and statistics to set upper and lower control limits for tasks to study those above or below the norm. A control chart assists in determining which variations are acceptable and to be expected versus those that are unacceptable. Unacceptable variations are usually unpredictable and are related to a special cause. Correction

FIGURE 4.4   Pareto Chart of Problems Associated with Patient Late Tray

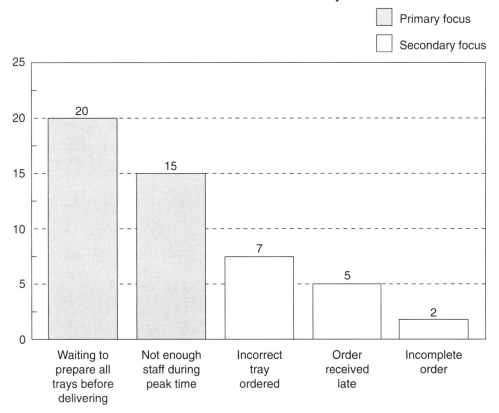

FIGURE 4.5   Cause-and-Effect Diagram for Patients Not Receiving Late Trays

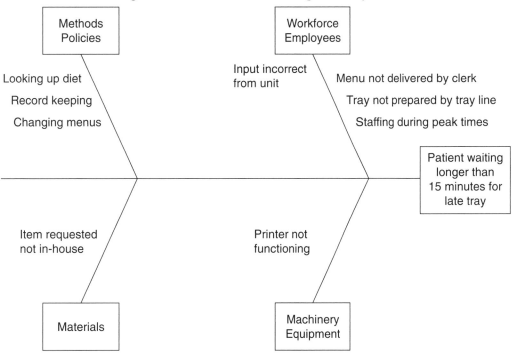

FIGURE 4.6 Run Chart for Late Trays Longer than 15 Minutes

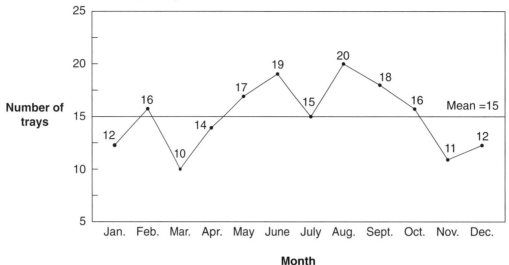

of the variation requires removal of the special cause. Acceptable or expected variations are usually caused by the process itself, and the only way to correct these variations is to change the process. Special causes must be eliminated before the control chart can be used as a monitoring tool because as a monitoring tool, chart measurements are expected to stay between the upper and lower limits established. For example, the start of a tray line may be within plus or minus 10 minutes of the preestablished time. If a time occurs outside this control, investigation should occur (Figure 4.7).

Some foodservice employees may require training in the proper use of improvement process tools of TQM. A manager or supervisor should work with these individuals to model the behavior of conducting a meeting, using the tools, and making decisions for improvement based on the results.

Other Regulatory Agencies

There are at least six national organizations that survey and certify that standards are being met in health care organizations. There are also local (county health departments) and state agencies (public health). The surveys include a number of standards that directly relate to food and nutrition service, while other food- and nutrition-related standards can be found in human resources, pharmacy, nursing, emergency preparedness, pharmacy, safety, and leadership standards. These standards all have one thing in common: to ensure that health care organizations are providing safe environments, quality, efficient, and effective service to the customers while improving the accreditation process by making the standards clear, relevant, and applicable to the specific health care setting.

The six survey agencies include:

1. The Joint Commission (TJC)
2. Center for Medicaid and State/Survey and Certification Group (CMS)
3. Omnibus Budget Reconciliation Act (OBRA)

4. Occupational Safety & Health Administration (OSHA)
5. National Patient Safety Goals (NPSGs)
6. Health Insurance Portability and Accountability Act (HIPPA)

The *CMS* requires an ongoing quality assurance and assessment program that monitors client care and outcomes. The *National Social Security Act* mandates that facilities participating in Medicare and Medicaid programs meet minimum health and safety standards. *Medicare* is a federal insurance program with payments for service made by the federal government through intermediaries. *Medicaid* is a state program that provides medical service to people receiving public assistance under the Social Security program as well as needy people. The requirements pertain to hospitals, skilled-nursing facilities, and a wide range of other providers and suppliers of health services. State-level officials are generally responsible for conducting on-site surveys for Medicare and Medicaid requirements, which is referred to as the *certification process*. The federal government has the following responsibilities:

- Review survey and certification reports submitted by state agencies.
- Evaluate fiscal, administrative, and procedural aspects of its agreements with the state.
- Conduct some on-site inspections.
- Review and approve state budgets and expense reports dealing with survey and certification activities.

Foodservice professionals have the responsibility to be familiar with the regulations established by the federal government and state regulations for the facility in which they are employed.

Coordination of state licensing requirements and TJC and other regulations require interdisciplinary cooperation and exchange of information. CMS will accept TJC findings. TJC standards generally meet many of the federal standards. All of these guidelines, recom-

Figure 4.7   Control Chart of Tray-Line Start Times

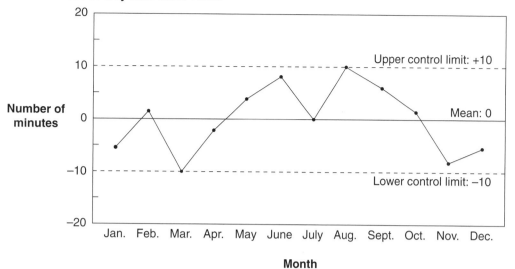

mendations, standards, and interpretations of each regulatory or professional organization intersect to provide guidelines for quality of care to clients.

Center for Medicare and Medicaid Services

CMS views the Medicare Quality Improvement Organization (QIO) programs as a cornerstone in its efforts to improve quality and efficiency of care for Medicare beneficiaries. CMS is undertaking activities to ensure that the program is focused, structured, and managed to maximize its ability for creating value. The program is supporting partnerships that engage a broad set of stakeholders for the purpose of improving the quality of care for all patients based on common goals and measures.

Improvements have recently occurred on clinical quality measures; however, there is still a need for improvement for higher levels of quality. CMS has expanded its emphasis on demonstrable, systematic quality improvement. In 2005 a Quality Improvement Roadmap was issued that emphasized "the right care for every person every time." The road map described five activities that CMS uses to achieve this goal:

- Work through partnerships, including HHS, with other federal and state agencies, and with nongovernmental partners including health professionals.
- Publish quality measurements and information.
- Improve quality and avoid unnecessary cost.
- Assist practitioners and providers in taking the necessary steps to make the care effective and less costly, in particular greater use of effective electronic health systems.
- Become an active partner in driving the creation and set of evidence about the effectiveness of health care technologies, bring effective innovations to patients more rapidly and help doctors and patients use treatments we pay for more effectively. (More information can be found by reading

Michael O. Leavitt, Secretary of Health and Human Services, *Report to Congress: Improving the Medicare Improvement Program* 2006; reports are routinely made to Congress. A Standard of Work, SOW, has been issued for care perimeters for 2012. More information is available on the web.)

CMS as an agency of the U.S. Department of Health and Human Services administers the Medicare program. CMS issues standards that must be honored by institutions such as nursing facilities that receive Medicare funds. CMS and TJC standards are similar, but they are not identical. CMS standards vary in their administration from state to state. Many standards in CMS address dietetic and foodservices and are too numerous to detail in this book.

CMS also manages reimbursement through the prospective payment system. This system dictates that reimbursement for care be based on certain clinical factors that have been defined and documented.

Standards for documentation are required to help ensure that a facility can receive all reimbursement to which it is entitled. The documentation system uses minimum data sets that identify all the data that feed into the prospective payment system and defines reimbursement. Minimum data sets must be provided to CMS in an electronic format.

All of the standards deal with reimbursement; however, if quality of service is not geared to each client's need, reimbursement may be limited. CMS uses quality indicators for tracking and benchmarking care, and these may be found in the standards.

The Omnibus Budget Reconciliation Act (OBRA) is an act that was passed by Congress in 1987. The Act mandates that residents in nursing homes need a suitable home where they can live their lives as individuals. The act requires choice, dignity, and self-determination; each home is required by law to provide services and activities to attain the highest practicable physical, mental, and psychosocial well-being of each resident.

The Office of Regulatory Services (ORS) is the agency that enforces state and federal requirements. There is a survey of deficiencies as well as a survey due to a complaint. During a complaint survey, ORS can survey the entire facility if it is considered necessary. The written survey reports are a matter of public record and the last five years of reports are available for public inspection,

Surveys are unannounced and are conducted simultaneously with the state licensing survey. The surveys can occur between 9 and 15 months unless a complaint is made that requires a survey.

The survey is oriented to reviewing care outcomes for residents. OBRA has developed guidelines to cover all areas of the facility. In the *Survey Protocol for Long-Term Care Facilities* a section for dietetic services is included. These protocols are found under Sub-Task 5B-Kitchen/Foodservice Observation and under Sub-Task 5C Resident Review. The following are surveyed: Investigated Protocol; hydration, unintended weight loss, and dining and foodservice.

The *State OBRA Operational Manual for Surveyors* lists the standards to be used for long-term care surveys. (Copies of these standards are available from the web or the state surveyor's office.) The standards are listed as **F Tags** and outline the required guidelines that **must** be met. The **F** Tag numbers for foodservice include F310–312 Activities of daily living; F314 Pressure ulcers; F322 Nasogastric tubes; **F325–328 Nutrition; F360–371 Dietary Services and F464 Dining and Resident Activities**. Other Tag numbers that relate to other departments within the facility and also include food and nutrition services include F 441 Infection control; F454 Life Safety: F517 Fire safety; F518 Disaster and Emergency preparedness; and F520 Quality assessment and assurance.

Other Governmental Agencies

The Food and Drug Administration (FDA), U.S. Department of Agriculture (USDA), and other governmental agencies ensure that businesses and organizations are accountable to the public. The Centers for Disease Control and Prevention (CDC) also evaluate an organization and its procedures in case of food-borne illness. The Commission on the Accreditation for Dietetic Education oversees dietetic education for both a written review of the programs and a site visit. The Certifying Board, a separate entity of the Dietary Managers Association, also reviews all of its programs.

ISO 9000 Series In the 1980s, global corporations began pushing for standards that measure quality management. To compete in a global market, many companies had to offer assurance to purchasers of their products and services that what they were buying was what was expected. If a company wants to be able to convey to its customers that its products meet the highest quality, they can obtain ISO 9000 certification. ISO is designed by the International Organization for Standardization that uses stringent international quality standards. **ISO 9000** is a certificate attesting that an organization's factor, laboratory, or office has met quality management requirements determined by the International Organization for Standardization in Geneva. It permits entry into some markets not otherwise accessible. It demonstrates process quality and consistency but does **not** focus on end products. The standards, once met, assure customers that a company uses specific steps to test products it sells; con-

tinuously trains its employees to ensure they have up-to-date skills, knowledge, and abilities; maintains satisfactory records of operations; and corrects problems when they occur. In 1997 ISO 14000 implemented standards to demonstrate they are environmentally responsible. Companies achieving this certification must have demonstrated that they are environmentally responsible. The certification is costly (may be several hundreds of thousands of dollars) and may take a year or more to meet the goal.

TJC Dietetic Standards TJC has established specific standards for food and nutrition services. Other standards that relate to dietetic services have been integrated into other unit standards such as leadership, infection control, engineering, emergency planning, safety, and patient rights. These standards are universal throughout the organization.

TJC issues its *Accreditation Manual for Healthcare* once a year. Annual reviews of these standards ensure continued compliance. Scoring categories include:

- Category A—Yes (satisfactory compliance: score 2), no (insufficient compliance: score 0)
- Category C—Multiple observations of noncompliance
  — 0–1 observation, satisfactory compliance: score 2
  — 2 observations, partial compliance: score 1
  — 3 or more observations, insufficient compliance: score 0
- Category B (qualitative and quantitative components) discontinues
- "Bulleted" (multiconcepts) EPs—Reduced EPs based on "criticality"—immediacy of impact on quality of care and patient safety as result of noncompliance

Important changes for 2011 will become a major part of future standards. Perhaps the most important new standard refers to the National Patient Safety Goals, which is a program that provides a significant focus on patient safety within health care and is designed to stimulate organizational improvement activities for the more pressing safety issues that all organizations are struggling to manage effectively. Three National Patient Safety Goals for foodservice are: "Do not use abbreviations," hand hygiene, and universal protocol. (To learn more check out www.jointcommission.org/PatientSafety/NationalPatientSafetyGoals/.)

The following standards are important for the foodservice and director to know and implement procedures/processes/rules to be in compliance.

- **PC 01.02.01** Hospital Assesses and Reassesses Patients
- PC **01.03.01** Hospital Plans the Patient Care
- PC **02.01.05** Hospital Provides Interdisciplinary, Collaborative Care
- PC **02.03.01** Hospital Provides Patient Education and Training, Discharge Education Plans and Referrals
- HR **01.04.01** Hospital Provides Orientation to Staff, Orientation to Departments, Patient Population
- HR **01.05.03** Staff Participates in Ongoing Education and Training, Dietetic Service Staff Training (Departmental and Interdepartmental)

There are other standards where foodservice must meet the standards; these are found in Emergency Preparedness, Safety, Infection Control, and Leadership. Each foodservice director has a responsibility to know **all** standards that are applicable to food and nutrition services and to develop a policy, procedure, process, or rule to show compliance.

An organization that is routinely surveyed by TJC must obtain a new *Accreditation Manual for Healthcare* annually to ensure continued compliance. Some of the recent changes have specific effects on nutrition and foodservice departments.

The specific standards for nutrition service are discussed in this book other than those that have been standards for many years (see earlier). Standards should be reviewed annually and, as applicable, processes should be implemented to focus on patient care. An organization's quality control or quality assurances educator should be consulted for input. The TJC website (www.jcaho.org) is updated frequently. It contains information on preparing for a hospital survey, changes in standards, and the latest information relating to TJC.

Critical Paths

TJC defines *critical paths* as a "descriptive tool or standardized specification(s) for care of the typical patient in the typical situation; developed by a formal process that incorporates the best scientific evidence of effectiveness with expert opinion. Synonyms or near-synonyms include clinical policy, clinical standard, parameter (or practice parameter), protocol, algorithm, review criteria, and preferred practice pattern." Interdisciplinary standards of care for particular patient types can be used to establish quality criteria for measurement. If databases that include a large number of facilities are used, practice patterns can be developed and tracked for improved patient outcomes. Dietitians should be involved in developing critical paths to ensure that the appropriate nutritional intervention is included.

These types of protocols or practice guidelines provide a means of bringing physicians into CQI. Independent of the TQM movement, for many years the American Medical Association has been a proponent of practice guidelines. These guidelines become critical paths and help to define when there are variations in care. Once the critical paths have been used for long periods, it is possible to identify expected variations versus unexpected variations in care and outcome. Critical paths are used to reduce variations in treatment from a clinical standpoint. However, these variations should concentrate not just on variations of practitioners but also on the hospital systems that may contribute to the variations. Health care institutions must pay attention to operational systems as well as to clinical systems to affect a true picture of CQI.

Comparative Outcome Measures

As stressed throughout this chapter, information and data are of primary importance in quality improvement. Data provide the information necessary to determine where efforts should be concentrated. Severity-adjusted databases have become more common over the past few years and are being used by a number of businesses to provide comparisons on physicians and hospitals during provider contract negotiations. Health care institutions, through cooperative partnerships, have established comparative databases to assess variations in practice patterns that are used as indicators of quality. Through the use of these databases, hospitals can determine which diagnosis-related groups should receive special emphasis and will have the greatest return in improving patient care and reducing associated costs.

Standards established by databases with many contributing hospitals can provide information on length of stay, charge or cost of care, and mortality. This information can be used to focus quality initiatives within a facility. Morbidity can be indirectly assessed by length of stay. No outcome data currently in use can define absolute medical quality, but measurements of these aspects of quality can be useful for physicians and health care organizations to use their time and other resources more wisely and begin problem solving. Such comparisons must be adjusted for severity against an established norm. There is no consensus among health care practitioners regarding the use of severity-adjusted databases because of fear that not every variation between facilities can be taken into consideration and boiled down for a simple comparison. However, these types of comparisons seem inevitable, and at least 12 states currently have established severity-adjusted databases.

The federal government uses a similar database, called MEDPAR, with Medicare patient information. Although proponents recognize that only practitioners with the patient and medical record in front of them can truly define the quality of care, they think that some aspects of care are measurable.

Case Management

Closely related to critical paths is the concept of *case management*, which furthers continuous quality initiatives by allowing a coordinated prospective review of patient care, that is, review **before** admission. A case manager participates in planning for a patient's admission, monitoring the concurrent stay using critical paths, and retrospectively evaluating the stay after discharge. A nurse or other health care professional is responsible for coordinating all aspects of care during the patient's stay. This may also be referred to as outcome management.

Case management is seen as a method to improve inpatient care; decrease length of stay; reduce rate of readmission, negative outcome, or both; and provide cost-effective care. Discharge planning begins at the time of admission to ensure a smooth transition to home with no additional care, to home with home care services, or to a long-term care facility.

Process Reengineering

TQM stresses the use of statistical tools to identify and modify work processes on a continuous basis. These modifications are generally incremental and implemented over short time frames. *Process reengineering*, on the other hand, makes radical changes by creating new processes to replace inefficient ones. Accomplished through team effort in a concentrated time frame and generally taking longer than the time needed to make minor quality improvements, process reengineering is most useful when the scope of the project is cross-functional and complex. Reengineering may require a structural change as well as a cultural change in the organization. Rather than using statistical tools, a modeling process involving computer technology is used.

Process reengineering is an analytical approach to quality improvement, with analysis occurring from the top down. For example, the late tray process diagrammed in Figure 4.5 would begin with providing a patient with a late tray. From this point, the various steps would be charted with second-level steps and possibly even substeps to the process. This breakdown allows each activity to be subcategorized to the lowest level necessary to facilitate transformation or improvement. Process reengineering also provides information regarding the inputs to the process, outputs of the process, controls affecting the process, and mechanisms used to complete the process.

Benchmarking

Benchmarking is the practice of comparing the performance of key indicators of an organization or company's operation in-house with similar operations in other organizations producing the same type of products using a measurable scale. Benchmarking is also the process of identifying *best practice* internally as well as externally, against competitors using benchmarking and best practice to help achieve best practice/superior performance. Benchmarking not only determines who is the very best, but who sets the standards for comparison and what standards are being measured. Benchmarking also measures performance and quantitative productivity against standards. Benchmarking helps to identify best practices internally as well as externally, against competitors. Using benchmarking and best practices can help achieve not best practices but superior performance. Benchmarking is a TQM tool that allows an organization or company to set attainable goals based on what other organizations or companies are achieving. Benchmarking can also identify trends that need to be monitored. Benchmarking foodservice is easier to quantify than clinical (patient care) productivity; however, clinical productivity can also be measured using different tools to monitor quality, quantity, and outcomes.

Benchmarking may be internal and external. Internal benchmarking compares current data with records of past data (performances or standards) to determine if its own standards are met or surpassed. External benchmarking compares an organization or department's performance and productivity with that of other organizations of comparable size or service to determine whether the organization is performing at, above, or below the established industry standards. Internal benchmarking allows a manager to compare data, note variation, identify why something occurred, and justify the reason. If there is a pattern developing, the manager can use the data to change schedules or production methods or revise standards. Whatever the reason for a change in quantity, quality, or outcomes, it must be evaluated for positive or negative effects on the organization. When changes are made, they will need to be monitored and evaluated for effectiveness and for meeting outcome goals.

External benchmarking is more difficult because it involves comparing organizations within an industry. Comparing the performance of a small community hospital with that of a large university hospital is difficult and perhaps invalid. To obtain data that is valid and useful, the comparisons should be made using standards that are similar to each other in size, governing authority, self-operation, management, services provided, or the ability to share meaningful information.

Many professional organizations offer benchmarking services. These benchmarking companies collect data on a nationwide scale and compare one organization against another. These companies set standards and costs for their services.

SUMMARY

In the past, health care institutions measured the quality of clinical care with an emphasis on quality assessment. Quality assessment focused on reactive or retrospective monitoring of individual variance and performance. The recent emphasis on CQI views quality in terms of both process improvement and customer perspective.

Continuous quality improvement is influenced by regulatory agencies, but a quality-committed organization will practice it with or without outside influence. Benefits of CQI include customer satisfaction, employee morale through involvement and ownership, and a cost-effective business approach that offers better value to the customer. The best reason for an organization to adopt a CQI agenda is to compete at a higher level, improve quality, and reduce cost.

An organization can expect to generate from 20 to 30 percent in cost savings by implementing a CQI process. The costs of implementing a CQI process include the labor for training and conducting team meetings, training materials, and possibly the use of a consultant. These costs are more than offset by the savings generated when processes are improved to decrease nonvalue-added steps. Occasionally the solution to a process or system problem will cost more in the short term to correct than to leave it as is. But when the cost of the solution is considered over the long term, with the customer in mind and in regard to savings from process improvement, it may be determined to be the best solution.

Private and governmental agencies help health care organizations to maintain a high degree of quality services through surveys using a preset group of standards and through benchmarking internally and externally to determine who is "the best."

Benchmarking
Cause-and-effect diagram
CMS
Continuous Quality Improvement (CQI)
Customers
Deming
Fish diagram
Flowchart
Ishikawa diagrams

ISO 9000 Series
Joint Commission Standards
OBRA
Pareto chart
Quality assurance
Quality control
Run chart
Shewhart
Total Quality Management (TQM)

ADDITIONAL RESOURCES

Changes in State Operations Manual, Chapter 7: Survey and Enforcement Process for Skilled Nursing Facilities and Nursing Facilities (Rev. 63-09-10-10) https://www.cms.gov/manuals/downloads/som107c07.pdf

Survey Reports for MSD 3.0 the CMS 802 and 672: www.cms.gov/cmsforms/downloads.cms802.pdf, www.cms.gov/cmsforms/downloads.cms672.pdf

Joint Commission, January 2011: www.jointcommission.org/assests.1/18/2011_sag.pdf

Changes effective July 01, 2011: EP.28, and 29, RI.01.01.01 (patients' rights). Revised Fire Alarm and Fire Protection Systems Required for Hospitals Check Environmental Standards: revised EP.2 new EP.25, EC.02.03.05. In July 2012 Changes in National Safety Goals for Hospitals and Long Term Care Organizations will become effective.

DISCUSSION QUESTIONS

1. Explain methods/tools needed to establish a quality improvement program.
2. Discuss how to use the various TQM charts and diagrams to solve problems.
3. What is the importance of surveying patient and cafeteria services (that is, developing a survey form, implementing it, evaluating the results, and determining methods for follow-up)?
4. Describe role of customers in the quality improvement program.
5. Discuss the importance of internal and external benchmarking.
6. Explain procedures needed to meet TJC, CMS, and OBRA standards.

CHAPTER 5

PLANNING AND DECISION MAKING

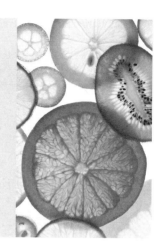

LEARNING OBJECTIVES

- Apply the planning process for short- and long-term activities.
- Show how a strategic planning process can improve the effectiveness and efficiency of a foodservice operation.
- Choose basic skills in problem solving and decision making.
- Write policies and procedures for a foodservice operation.
- Create a simple business plan.
- Define operational objectives for performance expectations.

PLANNING HAS BEEN identified as the first function or step in management and is applicable at all levels of management. It also defines an organization's goals and establishes a process of determining how the management system will achieve its goals, how it will get where it wants to go. The purpose of planning is to help organizations reach their objectives. Generally speaking, the higher the level of management, the more time is spent in formal planning activities. Formal planning is performed on a regular time cycle by a group of people working together. Formal planning involves the use of systematic procedures and comprehensive data and is recorded in writing. Upper management may spend as much as 50 percent of the time planning, compared with less than 10 percent by first-line managers. *Planning* can be defined as the process of identifying expected outcomes and determining possible courses of action using appropriate resources to achieve the desired outcome.

Planning involves establishing core values, developing mission and vision statements, setting goals and objectives for the organiza-

tion and its various units. *Core values* are broad beliefs about what an organization is and is not. A *goal* is a broad term used to describe what an organization hopes to accomplish over a relatively long period. *Objectives* are more concrete and specific statements of how an organization or a unit in the organization intends to accomplish a goal. In addition to setting goals and objectives, planning involves developing strategies. *Strategies* are precise action plans for achieving the organization's goals and objectives while making the best use of available resources.

Health care foodservice planning is designed to support organizational goals or mission, meet customers' needs, and provide for efficient and effective use of departmental resources. To accomplish this, planning must respond to the demands of the external and internal environmental trends and issues addressed in Chapter 1. Knowledge of these trends allows a manager to be proactive in establishing future objectives and strategies or action plans that take advantage of projected shifts in the business environment. Planning sets the framework within which the other management functions—decision making, organizing, staffing, leading, and controlling—can be accomplished.

Planning applies to diverse activities in the foodservice department and varies in complexity from writing an annual business plan to preparing daily menus or work schedules. Foodservice managers may be required to plan or help plan any number of organizational agendas. Some of these are:

- Annual objectives as part of the institution's business plan
- Policies and procedures for the foodservice operation
- Projects or new business opportunities
- Human resource recruitment and retention
- New or remodeled facilities
- Departmental safety

- Continuous quality improvement and customer satisfaction activities
- Strategies for support of a new product line
- Patient-centered care strategies
- Employee performance planning

In this chapter, steps in the planning process are discussed, including key types of planning and how they apply to nutrition and foodservice department operations. A model and steps are provided for writing a department business plan based on the organization's strategic focus. An approach to writing up departmental policies and procedures is presented, as are tools for monitoring planning efforts and specific suggestions for writing effective objectives. Finally, the decision-making process, including group decision making, and planning for change, are reviewed.

PLANNING PROCESS

The planning process in a participative organization is characterized by involvement of managers and employees at as many levels as is feasible. In Chapter 2, three levels of employee empowerment (participation) were identified as suggestion involvement, job involvement, and high involvement. The extent of involvement by various levels of management and employees depends on the type of planning and the level of participation with which the organization or department is comfortable. In most organizations, top managers set the organization's overall goals, middle managers set their departments' objectives for meeting those goals, and first-line managers make everyday strategy decisions in fulfilling their departments' objectives.

Kinds of Planning

There are three basic kinds of organizational planning: strategic planning, operational planning, and individual performance planning. *Strategic planning* assists management in making nonrecurring, significant decisions that affect the culture and direction of the organization. It also assists the organization in adapting to the external business environment. Strategic planning is based on the values and purpose of the organization, in addition to the expectations of customers and the community at large.

Operational planning deals with the process by which the organization's larger mission and long-range goals are broken down into shorter-range objectives and activities. This type of planning is accomplished by members of a particular department or unit.

As they develop operational plans, managers prepare standing plans, periodic plans, or single-use plans. *Standing plans* guide activities that tend to be repeated frequently in the organization over long periods. Standing plans include policies and procedures and standards of operation. *Periodic plans* identify a specific course of action for a designated period and are rewritten at the end of that period. Annual department business plans and budgets are examples of periodic plans. *Single-use plans* define a course of action that is not likely to be repeated, such as program or project plans (for example, remodeling the cafeteria). Standing plans, periodic plans, and single-use plans represent the major outcomes of operational planning.

The third kind of planning, *performance planning* with individuals within the department, is often overlooked by managers but is essential in setting goals for individual performance. Performance planning attempts to elicit maximum motivation and commitment from individual employees to contribute to departmental and organizational goal achievement. Individual performance planning as it relates to coaching is discussed in Chapter 9. The remainder of this chapter focuses on strategic and operational planning.

Steps in the Planning Process

Integral to the planning process is to know what you, the team and department, want to accomplish and how best to attain these goals. To plan effectively, it is important to know the organization's current status; what factors influence its future; and how the organization, department, or employees must be positioned to attain success in that future. Although the following seven basic steps apply more directly to strategic planning than to operational planning, they have applicability in all levels of organizational planning.

1. *State organizational objectives* in a clear, concise method before beginning to plan.
2. *Collect data.* Gathering information such as forecasts, benchmarking, and competition to identify the current status and strategies of the organization or department and to predict future implications will yield details of internal strengths and weaknesses and external opportunities and threats.
3. *Analyze the collected data.* Analyzing the information assesses what effect it has on current organizational strategies and identifies alternative or new strategies.
4. *Develop goals and objectives.* Based on the information gathered and the strategic focus established long- and short-term desired outcomes can be identified. This step also includes assigning specific timelines for meeting objectives.
5. *Develop action plans.* These delineate specific assigned responsibilities, contingency plans, and time frames for task completion.
6. *Implement the action plans.* This step begins movement toward the established objectives.
7. *Monitor or evaluate the effectiveness of the plan.* Was the action plan appropriate to the objectives set and to the degree of goal attainment accomplished? If not, the action plans and objectives should be reevaluated. Feedback is necessary at every process.

The seven steps of the planning process can be examined by grouping similar activities into three phases: first, data gathering and analysis, including current status, strengths and weaknesses, and opportunities and threats (SWOT); second, development of goals and objectives with appropriate strategies or action plans; and third, implementation, evaluation, and modification of the goals and action plans.

Time and the Planning Process

The dimension of time is a major element in all planning activities. Timelines serve to enforce operational controls, structure, a sense of focus, and direction for everyone charged with carrying out plan objectives. The terms, *long-range planning* and *short-range planning*, are sometimes used to describe strategic planning and operational planning, respectively. As mentioned, long-range planning involves the major activities or strategic changes an organization will undertake during the next two to five years, sometimes even as far as 10 or more years into the future. Long-range planning, such as deciding on the organization's core values, mission, and goals, rests in the hands of top-level managers and the board of trustees. *Intermediate-range planning* is a type of operational planning that covers shorter periods, perhaps one to three years. Responsibility for intermediate-range planning is shared by top- and middle-level managers. Short-range planning covers operational activities that are to take place in the near future, for example, the next week or the next fiscal year. Such planning usually involves the participation of first-line managers and employees.

The time frame for long-range planning depends on the degree of uncertainty in forecasts and predictions. The further into the future planning efforts extend, the more they are based on speculation and guesswork and, therefore, the less valid the predictions and subsequent planning become. For this reason, careful research is conducted to validate forecasts and predictions before long-range planning is undertaken.

Planning time frames also are influenced by need. This is especially true for short-range planning. For example, in planning departmental involvement in implementation of a new organization-wide safety program, dates for implementation may be set by upper management based on immediacy of need for the program to control injuries. Department managers would then be required to develop and implement the necessary objectives and action plan within the established time frame. Timelines may be influenced by the item being planned, such as the development and implementation of a particular product line. The organization may wish to have the new product line available in six months to meet the demands of the market and customers. However, the influence of technology, need for infrastructure changes, or difficulty in attracting the appropriate human resources may prevent meeting the established timeline. In this case, the nature and complexity of the planning event set the time frame.

STRATEGIC PLANNING

In health care organizations, the CEO usually is responsible for strategic planning, together with the board of directors (also referred to as the board of trustees, the governing board, or the board of commissioners). Most of the time, the board has ultimate responsibility for how the institution is run, with the CEO representing the board in his or her management capacity.

Depending on the size of the organization and the complexity of its structure, there may be a planning committee or a department responsible for planning activities. Commonly, a planning department led by a vice president or director is responsible for gathering and disseminating information for individuals at various levels who assist in planning activities. Large organizations often use outside consultants to conduct an internal analysis and make suggestions for areas that need attention. *Strategic planning* is long-range planning that focuses on the organization as a whole and that matches an organization's resources and capabilities to its market opportunity for long-term growth and survival. It involves defining a clear organizational mission, setting appropriate objectives, designing a sound business plan, and coordinating functional strategies. The following sections describe the three phases of strategic planning.

Phase 1: Data Gathering and Analysis

Collecting and analyzing data are the basis of long-term strategic planning for the organization. Organizations with planning departments have the capacity to gather and analyze data on an ongoing basis. Others may assign this responsibility to individuals in the organization or rely entirely on consultants. Either way, a number of activities must be carried out continuously to ensure availability of adequate information for long-range planning. These include:

- An analysis of the environment
  - Conducting market research and analysis to identify current and potential customers; this includes collecting data on consumer markets
  - Gathering information on customers' profiles, including average age, which services they use, their sources of payment for these services, how long they stay in the institution, why they choose to use the services, and what other services they may want
  - Monitoring current market share and forecasting future market share activity; market share is defined as the percentage of patients using the institution compared with the total number of possible patients in a designated area
  - Conducting an internal analysis of the services offered, number of admissions (inpatient and outpatient), emergency department visits, length of stay, patient days, surgical procedures, meals served, and other specific departmental activity and financial reports that may help guide strategy
  - Gathering information on physician referral patterns to other hospitals and physicians; other physician-related information includes average physician age, specialties, number of admissions, and level of satisfaction with the services offered by the institution
  - Studying the market for new business opportunities or product lines and making feasibility, pricing, and promotion recommendations
  - Collecting information on the external environment (competition, business environment, political and economic trends); information about other health care organizations may include their past growth and performance, their current position and image in their service areas, and their current services and future plans

- Collecting information on new technology developments and their effects on the future of health care delivery
- Collecting and analyzing data on workforce issues to predict labor requirements
- Monitoring and collecting information on the facility's financial operation; for example, data on expenditures for personnel and equipment and supplies
- Analyze the operations resources

Designing systems and methods for gathering the above information may fall to the planning department or committee or be handled by the institution's marketing department. The methods for acquiring this information are reviewed in detail in Chapter 3.

Once the appropriate data have been gathered, the organization's current business position must be evaluated using a systematic evaluation of resources and capabilities and to identify core competences. *Core competencies* define what the organization does best—expertise in room service, cutting technology, outstanding cancer research, and so on. This evaluation is conducted by the board, the CEO, top-level managers, and possibly a consultant. Analysis of the internal environment includes identifying the organization's current *strengths* and *weakness* as well as *opportunities* and *threats* (SWOTs) posed by the external environment. *Strengths* are internal resources that are available, unique skills of personnel, good market share, and outstanding reputation. *Weaknesses* are the lack of resources needed to carry out the mission, outdated equipment and facilities, weak management, and poor planning.

Opportunities can mean gaining new market share, resources available, new facilities with emerging technologies, superior research labs in the field of brain and cancer research, and exploiting in a positive manner the threats they must face, whether negative, external, and or environmental factors. *Threats* can be the new health care bill, increased competition from emergency care facilities, customer demands and reduced funding, and the environment. The external environment is influenced by events and circumstances beyond the organization's control. In contrast, the internal environment, although based on external pressures, is within the organization's control. Analysis is taken a step further to predict what probable effect environmental pressures will have on the organization's operation in the foreseeable future. Based on the information collected, the strategic planning team prepares strategies for responding to the projected environmental influences. For example, the shift from inpatients to outpatients is an external factor that affects the organization's future plans for delivery of service. The SWOT evaluation is an analysis of the organizations' existing strengths, weakness, opportunities, and threats in order to identify a *strategic niche* that the organization can exploit. *Niche* is the organization's product or service that has some competitive edge.

As part of the strategic planning process, managers and the board may reconsider the institution's mission as represented in its mission statement. Typically, the *mission statement* is a written document developed by management—with input from managers and nonmanagers—that describes and explains the organization's mission and what it intends to achieve in terms of its customers, products, and resources. Simply, it is a statement that defines the purpose and answers the question "What business are we in?" The mission forces management to identify the scope of products and services. The organizational mission is the purpose for which, or the reason why, an organization exists. For example, the statement may include a description of the hospital's primary functions, its philosophy and values, the levels of care and types of service it offers, the population or special groups it intends to serve, and its special relationship with other organizations. A *mission* is defined by what organizations stand for and how they perceive their function in the community and to their customer base.

In addition to a mission statement, an organization may write a *vision statement*. The vision statement is designed to denote where the organization would like to be positioned in the future. Without a vision of where the organization is going, it is impossible to devise a plan to get there.

A *value statement* may be included in the mission statement but more frequently is a stand-alone statement of beliefs about what is right or wrong or what the organization values. Values shape the way an organization and individual behaves. Values must be accepted by the organization, be clearly written, and be carried out by top management on a daily basis. *Core values* are the organizations broad beliefs about what is and is not appropriate.

Phase 2: Establishing Goals, Objectives, Strategies, and Plans

Based on evaluation of the data, goals and strategies are set for the entire organization and are the basis of the departmental business plan and objectives. *Strategic plans* focus on the future of the organization and incorporate both internal and external environmental demands and resources needed to achieve these plans. *Tactical plans* are plans that translate the strategic plans into specific goals for specific units within the organization, plans that departments will carry out in the short term. Once goals and strategies are written, they are evaluated to determine whether and how they best fit the organization and their potential for leading the organization to success. Selection of strategies should reflect a balance between the organization's potential for taking advantage of opportunities or overcoming threats and the values of its management and established mission.

In addition to forming the basis for department planning, the identification of goals and strategies for the entire organization requires upper management to form and be responsible for specific action plans at their level. An example of an objective and action plan is the development of the organization's long-term capital expenditure plan. This budget is based on the need for resources identified in both the long-range strategic planning and the departmental planning process. The long-term capital budget must be approved by the governing body or board. The capital budget is the organization's action plan for fiscal and other resource allocation.

Action plans focus on how the goal and objectives of the strategic planning process are to be accomplished. Department directors can expect to become involved in this phase when the chosen strategic alternatives affect their departments or are relevant to all managers throughout the organization. For example, the planning committee may decide that the institution must improve its management competence at all levels and, therefore, establishes a plan for organization-wide management training.

Action plans include designating the person (or group) responsible for completing the activities, along with specific statements of the measurements used to identify when the objective has been met. Timelines are specified for each step in the action plan to ensure that objectives are met according to the established strategic plan.

Phase 3: Implementing, Evaluating, and Modifying Goals and Action Plans

Once an organization knows its mission, vision, values, and strategic direction, it has a strong foundation for implementing operational planning and setting objectives. However, an organization concerned with long-term success will not stop at implementation but will continue to gather information, evaluate its mission in light of that information, and adjust its strategic plan as necessary, including corrective action.

Strategic thinking moves with the environment; as the environment changes, the organization must respond and adapt accordingly. An example is a change in an organization's financial status, a real issue for many institutions across the country. Even organizations that were once in financial trouble but managed to recover have to modify their strategic focus for future advancement, not just recovery. Once implemented there must be follow-up using an evaluation that answers the question "How effective was the plan, are changes still needed; if yes, what adjustments need to be made; will corrective action be necessary if there is failure?"

Middle Manager's Role in Strategic Planning

Although information collection is important to strategic planning, much of it also is valuable to operational planning. Department managers must be aware of what is being monitored or surveyed in their organizations and use these data in operations planning. Upper management must communicate to department managers and staff the organization's future direction and provide regular updates on goal accomplishment. Providing communication on these issues is important to having a highly committed and motivated workforce. To accomplish this, the director needs to conduct staff meetings to discuss and review the strategic plan and organizational goals.

During the early phases of strategic planning, middle managers are often a source of data, reports, and knowledge for strategic planners. If appropriate for the alternatives being considered, department directors also may be asked to respond, for example, the foodservice director might be called on to find outreach contracts for the delivery of nutrition services in physicians' offices, wellness centers, and extended-care facilities. A foodservice director might need to answer any number of questions about suggested alternatives. For example:

- How would the new strategy fit the established objectives of the department as well as the values and beliefs of its staff?

- Would the department be able to implement the new strategy with its current resources, or would new resources be needed?
- How much would it cost the department—in human resources, time, money, equipment, training for new methods, and other support systems—to implement the strategy?
- How would the department need to change its structure or its relationship with other departments to ensure that the strategy would be implemented most effectively?
- Would this strategy be relevant to the market the department currently serves?
- Would the strategy represent a risk that the department is ready to assume?

These questions would be addressed in the department's business plan, and objectives would be written to meet the challenges identified. The department director needs to have a considerable amount of information before responding to such questions and making recommendations to strategic planners. In addition to increased commitment, motivation, and involvement of others in the department, gathering this information and evaluating the suggested changes offer two other advantages for the director: having access to more comprehensive information and being equipped to inform and prepare department employees for major changes that might take place over the long term.

STANDING OPERATIONAL PLANNING

Primary responsibility for operational planning rests with the manager or director of the foodservice department. *Standing operational planning* is the basis for daily recurring departmental functions and assists in establishing structure and accountability for all members of the department. The largest portion of this planning is policies and procedures, in addition to which are departmental reports that monitor financial success and provide information to others within the organization. These reports also form the foundation for information necessary for periodic planning, such as budgets or business plans. Examples of various reports include productivity reports; continuous quality improvement (CQI) monitoring; cash register reports; turnover, overtime, and other payroll reports; and meal equivalent information (that is, the number of meals served).

Policies and Procedures

Policies are general guidelines—usually written—that tell "what to do" when carrying out essential and frequently repeated activities. Policies give direction for action and therefore are helpful in reducing the need to make operating decisions each time an activity takes place. *Procedures* can be defined as prescribed ways to accomplish an objective or "how to do it." Procedures specify how to do something; who will do it using what skills, materials, equipment, and other resources; and what the time frame will be for accomplishing the task. In contrast to policies, procedures list in chronological order the steps required to achieve an objective or to carry out a policy. *Rules* are written statements of what is to be done. An example of a rule is that the employee dining room will open at the stated times.

Although the policies of the foodservice department must be relevant to its activities, the policies also must be consistent with policies of the institution and reflect the requirements of standard-setting organizations (for example, The Joint Commission [TJC], discussed in more detail in Chapter 4). TJC's standards for dietetic services mandate that policies and procedures be in written form. The standards must be reviewed annually to ensure departmental compliance.

Department Policies and Procedures Manual

Writing a policies and procedures manual is the final phase in a long process of planning departmental activities. The manual must be written specifically for the facility foodservice department. A well-written manual depends on input from a number of sources:

- Managers, professionals, and employees in the department
- The department's records
- Relevant standard-setting organizations and regulatory agencies
- Manuals written for other facility foodservice departments
- The foodservice director's own experience

The policy and procedures manual should be written for the unique operation of the department. Other materials may be useful as guidelines and references. All policies and procedures in the manual must be consistent with the organization's policies and accrediting agents surveying standards.

Although each department's manual is based on input from many sources and can be written by different individuals, the foodservice director completes the final editing and approval of each policy and procedure. Having only one editor will ensure that the writing style and format are consistent throughout the manual. Exhibit 5.1 illustrates the basic format for a policy and procedure statement. Exhibit 5.2 shows an example of a foodservice policy. Only policies that are actually used by the department should be included in the manual.

Once policies have been established, procedures can be developed for carrying them out. Like policies, procedures should be written for every area of the foodservice department's activities—purchasing, production, service, clinical care, sanitation, and personal hygiene, among others.

Procedures are usually specific, step-by-step descriptions of a particular technique and often include illustrations that enhance the description. Each procedure should be described in a separate entry in the manual.

In addition to a written policies and procedures manual, the accrediting agents also require the foodservice department to review and update the manual annually. The department director is responsible for this process but may enlist the help of the foodservice staff. Policies and procedures no longer relevant or now obsolete must be revised or deleted. Once revisions have been approved by appropriate administrative and medical staff in accordance with the organization's policy, their signatures must appear on the relevant pages of the manual or on a cover page. Such changes include, for example, price increases in the cafeteria, changes in nutrition care policies, and changes in the services offered that would affect staffing levels and budgets. When policies and procedures involve another department, the two departments should meet and jointly agree on them. Copies of the joint policies and procedures should be signed by both department heads and placed in each department's manual. An example of a joint policy would be between engineering and foodservice for the maintenance of the foodservice equipment. Finally, the director must communicate changes to department employees to ensure that everyone involved in implementing the changes knows how they are to be carried out. Copies of the revised or deleted materials should be destroyed.

The manual is a tool for routine decision making, new employee training, and veteran employee retraining. Regular updating of the policies and procedures manual also is important to ensuring smooth departmental operations. Finally, the manual serves as documentation of the standards against which employees' performance will be evaluated.

Periodic Operational Planning

Periodic operational planning is conducted for specific purposes and within designated time frames. Examples of this type of planning include development of the department budgets (including operating budget, capital budget, and cash budget, for example) and the annual department business plan. Annual department business planning is similar to *strategic* planning where the same seven steps are applied in the three phases previously identified. Information affecting the department must be gathered and analyzed, objectives and action plans must be developed and implemented, and goals and action plans must be evaluated and modified as deemed necessary.

EXHIBIT 5.1   Policy and Procedure Format for the Foodservice Department

Department of Food and Nutrition Services, Community Hospital	
POLICY MANUAL	Policy number: _____
	Effective date: _____

Subject: _____

Area of responsibility: _____

Classification:_____

Approved by: _____

Primary responsibility: _____

Distribution: _____

Review date: _____

Revise date: _____

Person responsible: _____

Purpose:

Policy:

Procedure:

Special instructions or illustrations:

Source: Developed by Ruby P. Puckett ©.

EXHIBIT 5.2 Sample Policy and Procedure for the Foodservice Department's Policies and Procedures Manual

Department of Food and	
Nutrition Services,	
Community Hospital	Policy number: 1306
	Effective date: March xxxxx
POLICY MANUAL	Page 1 of 2

Subject: Taste Panels

Area of responsibility: General administration

Classification: Purchasing

Approved by: Director, Food and Nutrition Services

Primary responsibility: Assistant Director,
            Procurement and Production, and
            Food Stores Manager

Distribution: Standard

Review date:					
Revise date:					
Person responsible:					

Purpose: To determine the acceptability of a product before purchase and service.

Policy: Taste panels will be conducted at least monthly, more often if deemed necessary, to objectively evaluate products.

Procedure:

1. Taste panels will be regularly scheduled on the third Friday of each month at 1:30 p.m.

2. A group of no more than 10 and no fewer than 5 people will be selected prior to the date of the panel by the Food Stores Manager and as appointed by the Director.

3. The panel will include representatives from Purchasing, Nursing Services, Food and Nutrition Services, Administration, and other interested personnel.

4. Tabulation of the results of the panel will be completed by the Food Stores Manager and kept on file for future reference.

5. Results of the panel will be discussed with the Director, Assistant Director, Clinical Dietitians, and/or Production Manager.

6. The MN dietitian, Production Manager, Assistant Directors, and Director may recommend products for testing. This should be done at least a month prior to scheduled panel.

7. Procedure outlined in policy for taste panels dated 10/04/xx is still applicable (attached).

EXHIBIT 5.2 (*Continued*)

Department of Food and

Nutrition Services,

Community Hospital

Policy number: 1306

Effective date: March xxxxx

POLICY MANUAL

Page 2 of 2

Before a new product is to be used on the menu, it will be tested for acceptance.

Procedure:

1. Except on approved occasions, the taste panel will be conducted on the third Friday of each month at 1:30 p.m.

2. The Assistant Director for Production and Service will have the overall responsibility of the panel.

3. Assistance will be given by the Food Stores Manager (that is, he or she will invite participants, tabulate forms, and so on).

4. Water, cups, plates, napkins, and utensils will be made available for each participant.

5. There will be no talking, except to ask questions, during the taste panel.

6. Each product is to be individually evaluated by each participant.

7. Each individual is to independently score the results.

8. There will be no joking, horseplay, and so forth allowed during the meeting.

9. Answering pages and telephone calls will be kept to a minimum.

10. There will be no more than 12 people at each panel (including the Production Manager and the Assistant Director, Procurement and Production).

11. No food is to be taken out of the conference room by the participants.

12. The panel will be made up of:
    Director
    Assistant Director, Procurement and Production
    Assistant Director, Nutrition Services or Clinical Dietitian
    Food Stores Manager
    Production Manager
    Other foodservice personnel as invited
    Nursing Services representative
    Purchasing representative
    Administration representative

The Assistant Director, Procurement and Production, will invite persons from the preceding list to participate. Invitations will be issued a week in advance. Those unable to attend should notify the Assistant Director as soon as possible. After participants have tasted products and finished the evaluation phase, they are to return to their work area.

Everyone should be honest and objective in the evaluation.

Department Budget

The budget, a planning tool, is a good means of forecasting long-range expenditures for personnel, equipment, supplies, and other resources. Therefore, it is important that managers learn to use department budgets to ensure that necessary resources are available to meet department objectives.

The department budget actually is a composite of different types of budgets. The *operational budget*, for example, projects the number, types, and levels of service to be offered over the defined period and the resources needed to support service delivery. The *capital budget* forecasts major purchases in plant and equipment, new construction or facilities renovation (or both), and furnishings. The *cash budget* estimates cash income and expenditures over the budget period to ensure sufficient cash availability to meet the department's and the organization's financial obligations. The operating and capital budgets are primary components of the department's financial plan and become part of its business plan.

Because the overall department budget also is a tool for controlling departmental performance, each of these components will be discussed in greater detail in Chapter 11.

Department Business Plan

The purpose of a business plan is to develop an organized written plan that contains elements of a business venture. A department business plan is a tool or process that can be used to organize department-specific operational planning. As mentioned earlier, the strategic direction is set by upper management and the board of directors and is the foundation for departmental operational planning. During the strategic planning process, specific areas are targeted for development or concentration of effort. Based on the direction set and the specific goals the organization wishes to accomplish, the department must assess how its role fits in the larger picture and plan accordingly. Once the strategic focus has been determined, the foodservice director must evaluate his or her current ability to assist in accomplishing the organizational goals and then set the necessary objectives to assist in goal attainment.

Depending on an organization's size, structure, and level of service offered, departmental business planning may or may not be part of the organization's process and may or may not be required of managers. However, many benefits are to be gained by developing a business plan. One benefit is improved performance by clearly identifying and understanding the strengths and weaknesses of the department, which allows management to plan proactively for potential problems instead of becoming embroiled in crisis management. Clarity of objectives as delineated in a business plan in turn sets clear performance, priority, and accountability expectations by providing standards against which to measure. The instrument coordinates the planning effort throughout the department and provides a framework for making key decisions. As an educational tool, the business plan can present an opportunity to promote staff involvement and ownership in the department's future.

The department business plan can be utilized externally. For example, in a business expansion effort to provide meal service to a smaller organization, a well-written business plan could help "sell" the idea to the potential client. The complexity of the business plan is directly related to the size and makeup of the organization and department.

Lessons from Other Industries

To better understand business plans, it is helpful to look at their use in other industries. Generally, business plans are composed of five components: market strategy, production or service strategy, research and development strategy, organization and management strategy, and financial strategy.

Each of these areas can be applied to health care foodservice and included in the planning process. The *market strategy* (or plan) identifies who customers are; what products or services will be sold to them; and the policies regarding pricing, promotions, and distribution as explained in Chapter 3. Marketing strategy information applies to both the data gathering and analysis phase and the objective and action plan phase.

As in other planning activities, *production strategy* begins with gathering and analyzing data to identify current capabilities of meal production and service and to predict future needs based on the objectives. The foodservice director must learn whether changes are needed in the department's infrastructure, whether additional capital equipment or technology is needed, or whether changes in the marketing mix are needed. For example, if a department was using a hot pellet system for meal delivery and determined there was a need to change to a cook-chill system, changes would be necessary in the production strategy to modify preparation, storage, tray assembly, and service.

The third strategy in the general industry model is *research and development*. This applies to foodservice departments that wish to develop new programs for clinical services or new revenue-producing ventures. New development may include expanding catering to the outside, implementing a vending program, opening a coffee shop, or opening a branded chain operation within the facility. The research and development portion of the business plan is based on market analysis of who customers are and what they want. Often this portion of the business plan is completed by managers as a single-use program plan. However, for its effectiveness to be monitored, it must be an ongoing element of the overall business plan.

The *organization* and *management strategy* of the business plan includes an explanation of the functions that must be performed and who will perform them. This portion includes staffing needs, training and skill development needs, procedures and control measures necessary to support the department or new programs, and the level of employee involvement. The organization and management strategy may include an explanation of how things currently are done in the department and what procedural changes will be necessary to support new objectives. This portion of the business plan may include training programs that will be needed or will assist in translating customer needs into continuous quality improvement.

The last strategy of the model used by business and industry is the *financial strategy*. As mentioned above, both the operating and capital budgets become a part of the annual business plan. Further-

FIGURE 5.1   Top-Down Flowchart of the Major Steps in a Business Planning Process

Before beginning the planning process	During the business planning process	After the business planning process

	Phase 1	Phase 2		Phase 3
#1 Organize the process	**#2** Gather and analyze data	**#3** Write objectives and action plans	**#4** Write the business plan	**#5** Implement, evaluate, and modify
1. Who is to be involved? 2. Decide roles. 3. Method of involvement. 4. Establish deadline.	1. Organization's strategic plan. 2. Existing business plan. 3. Gather reports and data. 4. Internal strengths. 5. Internal weaknesses. 6. External opportunities. 7. External threats.	1. Write objectives. 2. Write action plans. 3. Set timelines and dates. 4. Assign responsibility. 5. Develop contingency plans.	1. Decide on format. 2. Develop cover page. 3. Write executive summary.	1. Follow steps in action plan. 2. Evaluate effectiveness. 3. Modify objectives or action plans. 4. Implement contingency plans.

more, when new programs or products are proposed, the financial plan must address revenues and cost of the investment. It may be necessary to establish a pro forma or projected profit-and-loss statement. The pro forma is usually based on one budget year and on the projections made from the marketing, production, research and development, and organization and management strategies.

Business Planning Phases

Although the five components mentioned above should be addressed in the department business plan, the three phases used for strategic planning discussed earlier in this chapter should be used to develop the business plan. Figure 5.1 illustrates a top-down flowchart of the business planning process for the department. A top-down flow-chart is another tool that can be used by the manager, especially for project planning.

Before the process can begin, deadlines must be set, and the manager must determine who is to be involved, when, and in what capacity. Staff may be involved through small group meetings, employee meetings, management meetings, or one-on-one sessions with the director. The director in a high-involvement department may ask employees to participate in the data-gathering and analysis phase or wait and include input on the writing of the objective and action plan.

Either way, providing opportunity for involvement ensures commitment from the staff who will have to assist in carrying out the action plan. Once the method and time for employee involvement have been established, the director needs to provide the necessary information regarding the organization's strategic plan, without which managers and employees will be unable to contribute informed suggestions.

Once deadlines are set and staff involvement has been identified, Phase 1 of the planning process begins. A *situational diagnosis* is conducted to determine internal strengths and weaknesses and external opportunities and threats, or SWOTs. This portion of the situational analysis might be conducted through staff brainstorming. A list of SWOTs may look like the one in Figure 5.2. This portion of the analysis and the next portion, defining the current business definition, form the foundation of objectives needed for the coming year for improvement and those needed to support the organizational strategy.

The internal analysis will include the business definition—what is being done now—and the number of meals served, customer groups served, where services are being provided, and the clinical services provided. Analysis also will include the number of employees, hours of operation, and service. Internal environment will include the strategic plans made by the organization. An example of a strategic goal for the organization that affects departmental planning is focusing on the customer while implementing continuous quality improvement. The department is then responsible for making its contribution and setting specific objectives for how its members will contribute. Questions to be asked may include:

- What does the strategic direction mean in relation to what is going on in the department now and the forces in the external environment?
- What objectives must be set to assist in accomplishing the organizational goal?

Another example of building on strategic plans is the organization's decision to undertake a major building project. The

FIGURE 5.2   Foodservice Department SWOT Analysis

Strengths
- Highly qualified and concerned staff
- Low employee turnover
- High employee morale
- Positive internal image, especially in catering and cafeteria
- Ability to function within operating budget
- Strong inventory control and purchasing procedures
- High department productivity

Weaknesses
- Timeliness of patient late trays
- Timeliness of food production
- Constraints of the physical plant in relationship to meal delivery
- Aging equipment
- Limited computer access

Opportunities
- Train employees for enhanced quality of service
- Replace current patient tray line
- Improve patient satisfaction with a new patient tray delivery system
- Convert production to a cook-chill system

Threats
- Shortage of qualified service employees due to changes in the workforce
- Difficulty of serving patient meals if tray assembly and delivery systems are not updated

department director would have to assess whether adequate facilities and staff are available to provide the needed meal service. If not, necessary data would be gathered and analyzed to determine needs. Objectives for the department would be based on the information gathered.

In *Phase 2*, specific departmental objectives are written to assist in accomplishing the organizational goal. The objectives must be measurable and include time frames for accomplishment as well as specific action plans. Action plans are then developed to support the objectives. The action plan must be specific about time frame for accomplishment, who is responsible, and how success will be measured. Also included are contingency plans in the event the initial plan was either ineffective or the objective needed to be modified. If the objective involves capital expenditures, the appropriate financial information is included in the action plan. Details for writing appropriate, measurable objectives are covered later in this chapter.

Phase 3 of the business plan, like the strategic organizational plan, requires the manager to provide leadership for implementing the agreed-on action plans. The steps of the implementation process are delegated by the manager. The foodservice director's responsibility does not end with implementation of the action plan, the effectiveness of which in meeting established objectives must be monitored and changes made as necessary. As mentioned, the validity of the objectives must be continuously evaluated in relationship to the changing environment. For example, if the foodservice department based one of its objectives on providing meal service to a long-term care facility to be acquired by the institution, but upper management decided to forgo the purchase, the objective and action plan would need modification.

Business Plan Format

A written plan should be made even if only for inside use. This will help solidify the importance of the planning process and provide documentation for coordination of efforts. The format for the business plan may vary by organization, but the fundamentals are similar across organizations. The first thing the manager needs to do is determine whether the organization has adopted a format. If not, guidelines built on the five components mentioned previously—market plan, production plan, research and development plan, organization and management plan, and financial plan—may be used. Another approach, used by Rotanz Associates and specific to health care, is represented in Figure 5.3. Not used in the Rotanz model but added by the author are a table of contents and an executive summary briefly highlighting each major section.

The executive summary is the most important component of a business plan and must be written in a positive tone. It must be short and concise. If it is too long, the executive may put it aside, throw it out, or read it at a later date.

The summary should avoid threats—implied by words such as "shall" and "will"—but choose words that show action as if the project was in existence. Use short sentences and paragraphs, and do not use boldface type or highlighted text except as absolutely necessary. Do not be trite or whine. Be sure all pertinent and essential information is included.

Scheduling Techniques

Managers often find that a visual representation of work over time is helpful in scheduling routine activities. The *Gantt chart*, a

FIGURE 5.3 Sample Business Plan Outline for the Foodservice Department

I.   Title page
    A. Name of the institution
    B. Name of department or functional areas
    C. Date of preparation and time period covered by the plan
    D. Name(s) of person(s) preparing the report
II. Table of contents
    A. Major headings with page numbers
    B. Appendix of figures, charts, graphs, tables, or other supporting documentation
III. Executive summary
    A. Brief description of the department (mission, purpose and goals, products and services (major functions)
    B. Current position or changes, or how plan is consistent with current status
    C. Significant strengths, weaknesses, opportunities, and threats that directly affect goals
    D. Financial and other resource requirements
    E. Main objectives, strategies, or plans
IV. Development process
    A. Details how the information was gathered
    B. Identifies sources used to develop the plan
V.   Business definition
    A. Overview of current department status
    B. Resources
        1. Technologies that affect services
        2. Facilities that affect services
        3. Human resources
            a. Department-based employees
            b. Common interfaces with other departments
        4. Current budget
            a. Capital. Are funds available? How will the project be financed: Bonds? Loans? Grants?
            b. Operating; industry analysis, business and economic trends, legal or regulatory issues, risk
    C. Principal customers
        1. Identify various groups (patients, physicians, employees, and so on)
        2. Identify characteristics (age, needs, changing environment, and so on)
    D. Sustainable competitive advantage
        1. Strengths that have long-term effects
VI. Strategic focus of the department
    A. Brief statement of major emphasis for department
VII. Key results areas (identify those areas important to department—may come from strategic plan or department environmental analysis). Examples:
    A. Human resources (attraction, retention, or training, staffing competencies, compensation)
    B. New products or business opportunities
    C. Financial performance/risk, cash flow, source of funds, capital equipment needs and break-even analysis, justifications
    D. Facilities development, any renovations needed, sustainability, waste management
    E. Quality and customer satisfaction, survey results, benchmarking
    F. Market segment, description, and strategy
VIII. Environmental assessment
    A. Business or health care environment
    B. Market segmentation
        1. Specific breakdown of groups served
        2. Brief details that identify differences
        3. Description of strategy
    C. Market needs assessment
        1. How were needs of the specific markets determined? Competition, 5-year goals
        2. Do these needs vary? Promotion, advertising, surveying?

FIGURE 5.3 (*Continued*)

     D. Customer concentration
       1. Location of customer groups—will it change in 5 years?
       2. Demographics: cultural, economic, and social
       3. Common disease entity—cardio, cancer, obesity
       4. Age category specialty such as pediatrics
       5. Professional category
     E. Competitive (SWOT) analysis
       1. Strengths
       2. Weaknesses
       3. Opportunities
       4. Threats
IX.   Business objectives
     A. Action steps
     B. Person(s) responsible
     D. Completion dates
     E. Measurement of success
X.   Appendix

Source: Adapted from Rotanz, 1990, revised by Ruby Puckett 2010.

nonmathematical graphic method of coordinating and organizing multiple tasks to complete a project on time, is one such device. It can help a manager plan a variety of related tasks or schedule the work of a group of employees who perform the same task. The chart in Exhibit 5.3 is an example of a schedule for a catering service. The Gantt technique is useful for relatively simple planning tasks. More sophisticated methods must be applied as a project grows more complex.

A planning technique used for short-term projects is the *planning grid*, shown in Exhibit 5.4, which provides the planning team with an organized format for reaching a goal. The first step in completing a planning grid is to identify the objective or outcome of the planning effort. The achievement of the outcome with the final action step is the measurement that determines when the planning is complete. The first action step might simply be to schedule the first planning session with the relevant team. The rest of the planning grid is completed by the team using various techniques of teamwork participation.

Another tool, the *program evaluation and review evaluation* (PERT), can be used for planning as well as for controlling more complex departmental activities. Much more quantitative than the Gantt chart, PERT is best used by managers who are skilled in using mathematical methods for planning complex projects. Briefly, PERT helps to define a network of relationships among activities and events that occur in the course of a project and then to calculate the time needed for each event and the time lapse between one event and another. PERT is often used to reduce the total time needed to complete a project and to keep the project on schedule by making adjustments in the network of relationships. A similar quantitative planning tool for sophisticated, nonrepetitive technical projects is the *critical plan method*. Both the critical plan method and PERT are used by industrial and management engineers to plan and schedule activities for a one-time project (such as a major renovation of a department) and can, therefore, be considered methods for single-use planning.

EXHIBIT 5.3   Sample Gantt Chart for Planning a Catered Dinner

	Week 1	Week 2	Week 3	Week 4	Week 5	Week 6
Activity A	xxxxxx					
Activity B		xxxxxx				
Activity C			xxxxxx			
Activity D				xxxxxx		
Activity E					xxxxxx	
Activity F						xxxxxx

Activity A: Plan menu.
Activity B: Order supplies (including tables, linens, chairs, and flowers).
Activity C: Order food (after checking recipes).
Activity D: Make arrangements for security (including parking facilities and coatroom).
Activity E: Hire and train additional workers.
Activity F: Set tables and make general arrangements.

EXHIBIT 5.4   Planning Grid Format for Short-Term or Project Planning

Objective or outcome:								
Team members:								
Item #	Action Step	Product Outcome	Responsibility	Due Date	Whom to Involve/Contact	Budget or Cost	Other Resources	Other Categories
1								
	Final step	Objective achieved						

Objectives

Although the use of a business plan can assist the department manager in determining which areas need attention and what specific objectives should be, a business plan is not necessary to establish operational objectives. *Operational objectives* are the foundation for directing performance expectations. Writing and executing clear objectives avoid crisis management and allow managers time to further develop employees (Figure 5.4). Objectives also assist in bringing the department together, with everyone moving in the same direction.

Characteristics of Well-Written Goals and Objectives

Goals are developed before objectives and are closely related. *Goals* are more global and general, are also broad, are long term from 5 to 10 years, and most important, they are what the organization wants to achieve. Goals keep the organization on track in an efficient and effective manner by looking into the future to predict what is necessary for success. There are many things that need to be studied for this predication such as:

FIGURE 5.4   Steps in the Development of Department Objectives

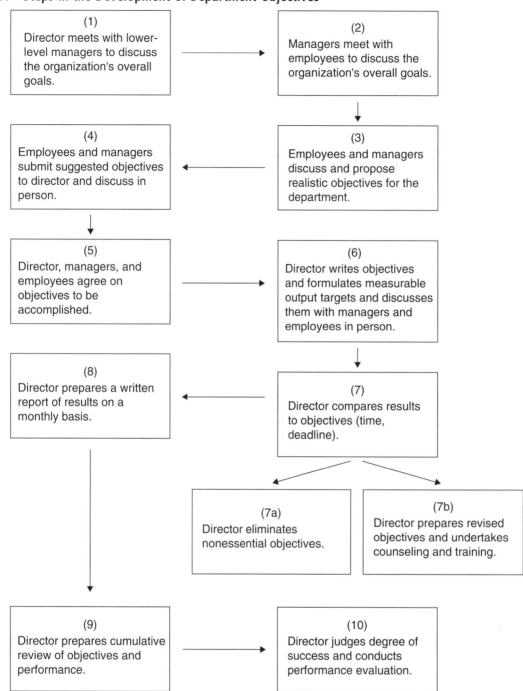

(1)
Director meets with lower-level managers to discuss the organization's overall goals.

(2)
Managers meet with employees to discuss the organization's overall goals.

(4)
Employees and managers submit suggested objectives to director and discuss in person.

(3)
Employees and managers discuss and propose realistic objectives for the department.

(5)
Director, managers, and employees agree on objectives to be accomplished.

(6)
Director writes objectives and formulates measurable output targets and discusses them with managers and employees in person.

(8)
Director prepares a written report of results on a monthly basis.

(7)
Director compares results to objectives (time, deadline).

(7a)
Director eliminates nonessential objectives.

(7b)
Director prepares revised objectives and undertakes counseling and training.

(9)
Director prepares cumulative review of objectives and performance.

(10)
Director judges degree of success and conducts performance evaluation.

Source: Ruby P. Puckett; used by permission.

- Technology
- Regulations, laws, standards
- Revenues/sales
- Employee development/staffing needs
- Productivity
- Quality control/assurance
- Cross-functional integration
- Customer satisfaction and relations.

- Cost controls/management
- Financial restraints/available resources
- New opportunities objective

Goals need to be reviewed annually to determine if they mesh with the organization's vision and mission; as appropriate, goals may need to be changed when there is a change in the environment (financial, standards, regulations, and so forth).

Goals need to describe the outcomes of the goal topics listed earlier; do they meet the vision and mission of the organization, are there enough resources available to meet the goal, is this goal affordable, are they realistic and reasonable (who, what, when, how, why, where, will need to be answered), and finally there must be a time limit as to when the goal is to be accomplished.

Once goals are set *objectives* must be developed. Objectives must be specific statements that explain how the broader goals of the organization are to be accomplished. The more specific an objective is, the more efficiently it can be reached. In addition, specific objectives are essential as tools for adequately evaluating and controlling the performance of the organization as a whole. As a director you may have input in the overall objectives of the organization, specific departments, and individual employees. You will be responsible for developing objectives for the department. Share ideas and plans with your supervisor, talk to the staff, and others who may have suggestion that may enhance the foodservice operation, for example customers and staff may want more healthy foods served In the cafeteria.

A well-written objective has the following characteristics:

- *Specificity.* The objective identifies the specific outcome of an activity. The results of quantitative objectives (that is, those whose results can be measured mathematically) are easier to determine than the results of qualitative objectives. For example, the objective of increasing the productivity of the tray preparation line by 2 percent is a quantitative objective. The objective of improving employee morale is qualitative and is, therefore, harder to measure. However, a manager should not be discouraged from setting qualitative objectives because other factors can be measured that are good evidence of employee morale, such as the number of employee grievances filed or the rate of absenteeism.
- *Conciseness.* The objective is succinct, uncluttered by identification of the method for accomplishing a task, for example; that is, it contains no extra information.
- *Time dimension.* The objective is time-related in that everyone involved understands by what point a task must be accomplished.
- *Reality.* The objective is achievable and within the work group's capabilities and available resources. On the other hand, an objective should not be so easily achieved that the work group does not feel challenged to give its best performance.
- *Method.* Each objective is accomplished by an action plan that outlines the steps for achieving the objective.
- *Value dimension.* Objectives should have value to the department and to those responsible for carrying them out.

In the following example, a foodservice department objective reflects one of the hospital's overall goals: to provide service in a cost-effective manner. The department implements this goal by stating its own objective:

To reduce the overall cost of each patient meal by 1 percent by the end of the current fiscal year, thereby reducing the overall cost per patient meal per patient day.

This objective is specific, and its achievement can be measured (quantified) against the financial information from department records. The objective is stated concisely, clearly, and within a designated time frame. Objectives must *RUMBA:*

R, realistic. Is it logical, can it be accomplished?
U, understandable. Does the staff understand the change (what is to be accomplished)?
M, measurable. Does it contain a method of how the objective will be measured (reduce by 1 percent, cut staff by 4.0 FTEs)?
B, behavioral. Will a change be accomplished?
A, acceptable. Is it possible to achieve?

Objectives also need to be specific, simple (one action for each objective), observable (can the manager observe a change), and is the objective too easy or is it challenging.

To decide whether the objective is realistic, the foodservice director would need to assess the costs involved in current meal preparation and delivery and decide whether a 1 percent reduction is feasible and, if so, through what means—reductions in staff, changes in methods of preparation, or some other adjustment. Devising or amending production methods involves the creation of action plans. It also incorporates a value element in that it must be worthwhile to those who must perform the tasks that lead to attainment of the objective.

To implement departmental objectives effectively, each one must be prioritized in relation to the others. In addition, each objective must be broken down into its component tasks in an action plan. The resources available for accomplishing each task should be assigned according to the objective's relative priority.

Steps for Writing Objectives with Outcome Measures

A manager who uses a department business plan will have a clear idea of what areas would benefit from having objectives established. Otherwise, the first step is to determine which areas need objectives. Experts estimate that about 20 percent of the activities in any business necessitate having specific objectives in place. Setting objectives for everything in the department is extremely time-consuming and can frustrate the monitoring process. Once the determination is made as to which areas need objectives, five steps can be used to establish clear ones:

1. State the problem or opportunity clearly.
2. Decide what the expected outcome is to be.
3. State the end product—what will be achieved by the outcome.
4. Establish possible action steps, including the measurement to be used.
5. Refine the possible action steps into a concrete plan.

After the target areas for objectives have been identified, the next step is to identify the challenge or opportunity at issue. A general statement is then written to identify what the desired outcome or change would look like. The next activity is to refine the general statement, keeping in mind how the outcome will be tracked and measured. Once the objective is clearly written, all possible actions are listed. From this list, an organized sequential list is formed. The action steps to be followed to accomplish each task should be described in specific procedures (discussed in the previous section). A time frame for completing each task also must be established. Scheduling becomes a more complex process as tasks require more steps and more people to perform them. Action plans that lead to attaining objectives identify who is responsible for each step and provide timelines for completion.

Assigning responsibility for fulfilling each objective and completing its component tasks is the foodservice director's role. One person may be involved in a task, or the whole department may work to fulfill the overall objective. It is vital that the person assigned primary responsibility for completing the task be given sufficient authority and resources. As mentioned earlier in this chapter, once the action steps have been outlined with responsibilities and timelines, monitoring must occur to ensure success. *Progress reports* should also be kept as records of the department's objective setting and fulfillment process so as to document for top-level managers the department's progress in fulfilling institutional goals. The reports can also be used as part of the institution's evaluation and control system. The objective and action plan should be put in writing and shared with everyone who will be affected either directly or indirectly.

Management by Objectives

Peter Drucker is usually credited with developing the systematic technique of goal setting and implementation called *management by objectives* (MBO). This tool is best applied by a department director as part of an organization-wide program for meeting the organization's goals. Briefly, *MBO* is a method by which a manager and a subordinate (a person directly supervised by that manager) cooperate in setting objectives that the subordinate intends to accomplish in his or her position. Usually, both agree to document in the subordinate's personnel file the objectives to be reached by a certain date, at which time the manager evaluates the subordinate's success in achieving the objectives. If performance has been satisfactory, the manager can reward the subordinate according to the personnel policies established by the organization for salary increases, benefits, promotions, and so forth. If performance has not been successful, both must reach agreement about the problem and identify ways to solve it. That is, they must define a new set of objectives.

The MBO tool has several advantages when used carefully and cooperatively. First, it is a powerful morale booster and motivator of employee productivity. By involving employees in defining objectives, MBO fosters a greater commitment to the organization by demonstrating how the employees' objectives are intertwined with the organization's goals and strategies. Furthermore, MBO makes a clear connection between performance and reward, thus ensuring for both employee and manager that evaluation is an objective and fair process rather than a subjective one. Finally, MBO provides a systematic tool for planning employee activities as well as for controlling them and keeping them on the same course as the department and the organization.

DECISION MAKING

Decision making can be defined as the process of assessing a situation or objective, considering options or alternatives, and selecting the one most likely to provide the best possible outcome for those involved. As discussed in Chapter 2, decision making is a key managerial activity and a significant part of the four basic management functions of planning, organizing, leading, and controlling. The purpose of decision making in health care foodservice is to coordinate objectives and activities of the department so that its members deliver optimal nutrition care and meal service to designated customers.

Managers are required to make decisions for problem or conflict resolution and for identifying objectives. Throughout the planning process, managers make decisions in determining which objectives the department should pursue in the future. They also make decisions during implementation of the objectives. Additional decisions are made regarding effectiveness of the objectives, appropriateness of the action plans, and alternatives in the event neither is determined to be appropriate.

Planning drives much of the daily work in health care foodservice by establishing appropriate written policies and procedures. However, problems may occur that require decisions and changes in these policies and procedures. Even with problem resolution, decision making is more effective when based on information-gathering procedures that contribute to developing appropriate actions.

Three Elements Essential to Effective Decision Making

Three elements are critical to making decisions effectively and in a timely manner. These are the *authority or freedom to take action, knowledge of the situation or issue under consideration*, and *motivation to make a decision*. Having authority to act is especially important if employees are to participate in the decision-making process. For instance, unless authorized to do so as part of his or her job description or as defined under a specific policy or procedure, a tray line worker cannot make menu substitutions for patients receiving a diabetic diet. Even if so authorized, the employee cannot do so without knowledge and expertise in diabetic diets and in the nutritive value of foods and food equivalents. Even if authorized and properly trained, without sufficient motivation—for example, a line employee being evaluated for promotion to a supervisory position requiring more of a decision-making role—there is little or no will to make the decision.

Obstacles to Effective Decision Making

Unfortunately, more obstacles can preclude good decision making than there are factors that promote it. This section identifies four such roadblocks:

1. *Individual bias* locks a decision maker into a perspective that can sabotage the best choice for a given situation or even eliminate other alternatives from consideration.
2. *Lack of knowledge or ability.*
3. The *lack of clear objectives* can inhibit the decision-making process.
4. Without *availability of crucial resources* (for example, finances, time, or staff), less-than-satisfactory decisions can result.

One barrier that should be avoided, especially by new managers or new line employees, is fear of taking risks or making mistakes. Resistance to change can bottleneck even the simplest decisions. (Planning and managing for change are covered later in this chapter.)

Influences on Decision Making

When making decisions that will affect the entire organization, the manager must be able to identify elements that may influence the decision-making process and understand how their influence plays a part. For example, decisions are often made based on past experiences of the decision maker; a manager who tried an approach that proved to be ineffective may be reluctant to make that choice again (even if the situation is different). Although learning from the past is desirable, it is also important to ensure that logical choices are not precluded because of limited failures. The same is true for experimentation: A manager who tries a decision in a limited setting and finds it to prove effective may fear applying it in a larger context. Each person brings to the decision-making process his or her own personal and social views and values that will have an effect on the outcome. In addition, decisions are influenced by the departmental or organizational values. The final influence on the decision-making process comes from other managers or people whose judgment the decision maker trusts.

Decision-Making Process

The decision-making process follows the same steps whether a first-line manager is solving a minor production problem or a top-level manager is deciding what the objectives are to be for the coming year. The following are six steps to any decision-making process that should be followed to provide for an optimal outcome:

1. Establish objectives or define the problem.
2. Gather data.
3. Identify alternative solutions or outcomes.
4. Evaluate relative values of alternatives.
5. Activate action plan to implement best choice.
6. Follow up and evaluate the decision.

Establish Objectives or Define the Problem

Decisions are made based on a clearly defined expectation of the outcome. This is true whether the decisions are being made in con-

nection with solving a problem, resolving a conflict, or allocating resources. To make the best possible decision, it is necessary to establish clear objectives that will lead to the optimal outcome or resolution. Defining the problem allows the manager to understand the full implication of his or her decisions. What may appear to be a small, simple problem can turn out to be much larger and involve multiple processes or systems. For example, on noticing a rise in employee complaints about work conditions, higher-than-average absenteeism, an increase in the number of kitchen accidents, or a falling off of employee dependability in timely task completion, a manager might easily jump to the conclusion that "today's employees are unreliable and careless." In fact, such symptoms may signal an operational crisis on the horizon.

An alert manager thoroughly explores a problem to find its possible causes. For instance, rumors of layoffs, a wage freeze, or employee perception of supervisory apathy could explain any one of the observations cited above. Whatever the cause of disruptions or negative changes in the department's operations, investigating beyond the first impression is worth the time and effort. The manager avoids wasting time on treating symptoms while the real problem may remain undetected. It also avoids time spent in crisis management once the problem erupts. Clarity in defining the problem simplifies the rest of the decision-making process and, indeed, may make the rest of the process unnecessary.

Gather Data

The second step in decision making is to gather data that have a bearing on the decision. A manager should not settle for an assumption that involves any reasonable doubt on any point.

Two major points should be considered when gathering data. First, how can the facts be gathered and, second, how much data should be gathered. Facts may be gathered by:

- Reviewing existing policies and procedures and mission and value statements
- Reviewing past events when a similar problem was encountered
- Observing employees, equipment, and so forth. Write down the facts observed, and accurately describe what was found. List all facts and any related conditions that have a bearing on the decision. Take the time to be thorough.
- Interviewing anyone who will be affected by the decision. Listen to what is being said. Observe behavior. Do not rush, do not criticize. Be objective and nonjudgmental.

Once all the facts have been gathered, organize and evaluate them. Decide what are facts and what are opinions. Are these facts reliable? Additional observations and interviews may be necessary.

Identify Alternative Solutions or Outcomes

With the problem clearly defined, the manager can move on to the third step in the decision-making process, developing alternative courses of action to deal with the problem. In some situations, alternatives may already have been defined by the organization's policies and procedures, and the manager must simply carry them out. For example, if an employee repeatedly ignored a work schedule by arriving late and had received first an unofficial reprimand and later a written warning about the consequences of repeated tardiness, the manager usually has only one choice in dealing with the problem, according to the organization's personnel policies.

With other scenarios, however, the manager will have to collect information to arrive at relevant and valid alternatives. Depending on how quickly the decision must be made, the manager may involve employees or other managers to brainstorm ideas and possible alternatives. When making decisions about nonroutine problems or conflicts, all possible outcomes of the alternatives outlined must be considered to ensure a winning situation.

Evaluate Relative Values of Alternatives

Each alternative must be carefully examined for its strong and weak points. To do this, the manager must gather all information pertinent to each alternative and then answer these questions:

- Is the alternative feasible? For example, does it violate any departmental policy or procedure? Does it conform to legal, regulatory, or code restrictions? Does the alternative risk overstepping firmly established bounds of authority?
- Is the alternative satisfactory? Even when an option is feasible—that is, even if no strict organizational barriers are in its way—the option may not suit the unofficial social norms of the work group. Implementing changes that are socially unacceptable to the staff would meet with stiff resistance.
- If the alternative is both feasible and satisfactory, will its consequences be acceptable to the manager, the department, and the organization?

Information gathering for each option may require a review of policies and procedures, an examination of previous memos or other documentation on the same or a similar problem, or an analysis of job descriptions. Additional information may be gained from personal experience and observation and from discussions with other managers in the organization.

Activate Action Plan to Implement Best Choice

Answering the above questions will help eliminate all but a few options. The best of these probably will be the one that allows the most positive answers to the questions of feasibility, satisfaction, and potential consequences. However, not all options are mutually exclusive. If two seem to be equally good solutions to a problem, perhaps they can be used in tandem or sequentially. For example, offering a new special diet menu to patients might require them to make choices that are somewhat more complicated than what they are accustomed to. Should the nutrition staff show the staff nurses how to help patients fill out their menus, or should the nutrition staff urge patients to call the foodservice department with questions or problems? The staff may be able to implement both alternatives and, in doing so, provide two options that will ensure that patient menus are filled out properly.

Implementing the most appropriate solution may in turn require another set of decisions. The manager may need to choose the most efficient and effective method for carrying out the solution from several possible alternatives. On learning that standing plans have already been developed that would be workable for the proposed activity, the manager may need to prepare a single-use plan for a brand-new effort. For example, the existing policy on the delivery of meal carts would need revision if the number of personnel assigned to cart delivery was reduced because of a low patient census.

Follow Up and Evaluate the Decision

The final step in the decision-making process is to evaluate the option(s) chosen. Do the chosen actions have the desired effect? If not, why? At this point, the decision-making process may have to begin again from Step 1, and the problem may need to be reanalyzed in light of the failed attempt to solve it. If the chosen actions fail to meet expectations, the manager should not assume that the problem was incorrectly identified. Indeed, the action may have been well chosen and well planned but may have lacked good implementation. In any case, timely follow-up is essential to the decision-making process because it keeps poor decisions from wasting department resources and derailing its efforts.

TEAM DECISION MAKING

All steps in the decision-making process can be taken by an individual manager or by a team. For the sake of time and efficiency, a manager can and should make certain decisions independently. However, research studies and management experience have shown that managers who involve subordinates significantly in the decision-making process have a more satisfied, committed, and productive staff. Research has further demonstrated that team efforts make for more sound decisions than does an individual effort to resolve the same problem.

Team decision making can offer other advantages as well. For one thing, individuals working together bring their cumulative knowledge and experience to the decision-making process. Therefore, a group is likely to generate not only more but better alternatives and be better able to evaluate them. Once a decision is made, group members are likely more motivated to implement it because of their ownership in formulating it. Also, routinely sharing decision making makes a stronger working team.

Team decision making has its limitations, however. A significant drawback is that it can be time-consuming and therefore not the best approach if a decision must be made quickly. Other problems arise if the decision-making process is not carefully carried out. For example, if decision makers fail to assign responsibility for specific tasks in the action plan, no one assumes responsibility, even though the manager's superiors will hold the manager responsible. Furthermore, fear of suggesting what may be workable but radical alternatives could discourage creativity in suggesting options. Therefore, the team may generate a decision that appears to be endorsed by most members but is really a less-than-satisfactory compromise. Often this is a problem when a manager or other group member resistant to suggestions tries to dominate the decision-making process.

As a decision-making technique, brainstorming (discussed earlier) is applied most often to solving problems that are unusual and especially challenging. To generate the most creative alternatives for the group to consider, brainstorming encourages participants to suggest novel, even radical, ideas. Everyone in the group must agree in advance to conform to an important ground rule of brainstorming: criticizing the ideas of other participants is not permitted. Instead, participants must try to build on the ideas advanced until a solution is found that is feasible and satisfactory and that has the fewest negative consequences.

Another technique that engages a work group in participative decision making is *quality circles*. Quality circles are made up of small groups of usually 5 to 10 people who perform the same type of work and who voluntarily meet on a regular basis while on duty to discuss work-related problems. The group strives to improve quality of products, service, or work processes while seeking solutions that can be sent to management for approval and to be implemented by the quality circle group. In a wider sense, however, a quality circle is an environment in which a team decision-making process takes place. Various decision-making techniques, including brainstorming, can be used by a quality circle to arrive at decisions, depending on what kind of problem the group is attempting to solve.

Whatever techniques are used, according to Megginson and others, effective team decision making is characterized by the following:

- It is fair to all members of the group.
- It provides an opportunity to gather together people with different attitudes.
- It permits members of the group to explain what they think should be done to solve the problem.
- It fosters group discipline through social pressure and persuasion.
- It permits the cooperative solution of problems.

In contrast, team decision making is ineffective when any of the following conditions result:

- It tries to give each member what he or she wants.
- The manager or some other group member tries to manipulate participants to reach his or her "right" decision.
- The manager considers the team decision-making process as only a forum to sell his or her idea to the group and does not listen to alternative ideas.

- Discipline is ignored in the process of exchanging ideas.
- The manager only appears to seek the advice of the group, without actually planning to implement it.

PLANNING, DECISION MAKING, AND RESISTANCE TO CHANGE

Most decisions, whether made by top-level managers, department heads, or groups within departments, require some change in the way things work. As in other aspects of everyday life, change is a constant in the work setting. Therefore, resistance to change, no matter how insignificant it is, might seem a curious phenomenon. The major reasons for resistance to change are listed below:

- Ignorance—Do not understand the reason for the change
- Comparison—Old methods versus new methods, inconvenience
- Disbelief–New system will not work
- Loss of power—I already know the system—the new system will mean I have to learn a new way
- Mistrust—Why is there a need for change, insecurity
- Frustration—Reduced political power and career opportunities
- Fear—Of losing status or economic well-being
- Fear—Of the unknown
- Change in relationships

Managers must contend with this resistance, both in employees and in themselves. A positive attitude toward change is critical to an effective management and leadership style. Change in products, equipment, methods, and clientele is a fact of life and a necessity for survival in health care institutions. Effective managers not only accept change but strive to be instrumental in bringing it about by constantly searching for ways to improve their departments.

Managing change begins with a self-examination of the manager's own attitudes toward impending change and his or her sensitivity to the reasons why employees resist change. When the manager is open, honest, and has a concern for the employee, the employee is more likely to accept the change. The manager will need to seek input from the employees and honestly explain how the change will impact them such as change in schedules, standards for work, and so forth. The manager must be able to describe the results of the change to calm employee concerns and unwarranted fears. In many cases these results are due to a manager's failure to explain the changes adequately. Fear is a major resistance to change. Fear of losing status or economic well-being and a general fear of the unknown is further exacerbated when employees are not allowed to participate in making decisions that affect them. For this reason, group decision making is becoming an important element of effective management.

Change involves principles of managing—goals and objective setting, decision making, formal and informal groups, participation, teams, communications and training. To help overcome resistance employees must be provided the opportunity, through training, to learn new procedures, new skills, methods, and to gain confidence in conquering new skills.

Attempts to change the way a group works often imply criticism of the status quo. Suggested changes in procedures or products may cause employees to feel that their past performance has been less than satisfactory and that their work is being criticized. Unfortunately, many employees have previous experience with poorly implemented procedural changes and tend to be suspicious, even angry, when new methods are proposed. An alert manager anticipates this problem and makes every effort to prepare employees for changes in procedures, products, or services. Extra effort should be made to assure employees that suggested changes are not a criticism of their past performance but merely represent more efficient procedures.

Because change almost always causes some negative reaction among employees, managing change well also means managing employee emotions so that sensitivity to the emotional connotations of change helps a manager effect change smoothly. Setting the stage by creating a positive work environment within the foodservice department is the first step in the right direction.

The next step is for managers to cultivate employee awareness of, and interest in, the change process. This will make the trial and adoption stages easier for everyone involved.

Apprising employees of possible changes can help lessen their anxiety and distrust. Generating employee interest and their suggestions for ways to try out new plans can result in a more cohesive work group and in helping employees develop their own management skills.

Employees must feel that the change will be good for them. Therefore, changes that are well planned and well executed enhance growth and positive development toward the goals and objectives of the organization. In contrast, hasty or poorly planned changes may lead to problems and lack of productivity. A manager's effectiveness can be measured in part by his or her skill in initiating and leading constructive planning for change.

Once the change has been implemented it will need to be evaluated. Was this the correct change, was it beneficial to the department, are additional changes necessary for a more efficient operation? Were the criteria the best ones? What was the change necessary and did it meet the reason for the change? What were the benefits, disadvantages? What was the overall impact on employees, the department, and the department resources? Was the training program sufficient or too long; did it cover enough material? Did others provide enough information concerning the change to remove fears of the employees? Did I, as the manager, do my best to remove fears of the employees? Did I involve others in decision making? What could I have done to reduce the resistance to the change?

SUMMARY

Planning is the most basic of all management functions. It determines the purpose of an organization and its many parts. It forms the basis for controlling the numerous activities that help the organization achieve its purpose. Long-term planning often involves a consideration of the organization's business environment and ways the organization intends to respond to change in the environment.

Effective business plans rely on upper management's commitment and involvement. Objectives and action plans should address all significant factors that affect the department's short- and long-term performance. The business plan must be forward looking and based on a realistic analysis of the situation. Key management and staff members charged with implementing plans should be involved in plan development. Plans should foresee contingencies and outline courses of action in the event that organizational plans or direction change. For example, if a decision is made to remodel an existing part of the department and then a decision is made to build a new kitchen, contingency plans would be needed

When developing goals and objectives a review of the resources available needed to implement the goal must be made. If resources are not available the goal may need to be revised to meet the needed resources or be considered for a later date. Resources include staff, space equipment, time, and money. Employee input for all short-term or long-term goals or plans empowers and motivates the staff. The final goals and plans need to be discussed with the staff and copies of the final product need to be posted.

KEY TERMS

Business plan	Objectives
Core values, rules	Planning
Decision making	Policies and procedures
Gantt chart	Program evaluation and review technique (PERT)
Goals	Resistance to change
Long-range planning	Short-range planning
Management by objectives (MBO)	Strategic planning
Mission	Strategies
Vision	SWOT (strengths, weaknesses, opportunities, threats)

1. Explain the steps needed for the development of a business plan for opening a coffee shop in the lobby of the facility.
2. How would you design methods, such as goals, objectives, and strategies, for the serving of late trays?
3. Define a common problem, using the decision-making process to solve.
4. Explain the importance of strategic planning. Include SWOT.
5. Discuss the best format for writing an operational objective for reducing overtime.
6. Develop a program to help employees accept a change to room service from the traditional delivery system.

CHAPTER 6

ORGANIZATION AND TIME MANAGEMENT

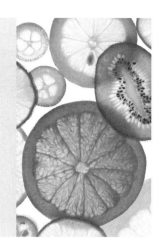

LEARNING OBJECTIVES

- Explain the difference between committees, task forces, and teams and the role each plays in an organization.
- Apply the systems approach to a foodservice operation.
- Identify the advantages and disadvantages of various organizational structures.
- Write a competency-based job description.
- Incorporate job analysis, job descriptions, work division, and job enrichment to develop staffing needs.
- Calculate the number of full-time equivalents (FTEs) needed to operate a foodservice organization.
- Determine ways to effectively use time, prepare a time schedule.

ORGANIZING IS THE process of dividing the work done in an organization (or a unit within the organization) into smaller parts and assigning responsibility for those parts to specific positions. Historically, organizations believed work was accomplished most efficiently when divided into specialized tasks and given to specialists of those tasks. More recently, the idea of specialization is being questioned in light of job diversity that creates multiskilled workers, a more desirable approach. The change from a specialized skills approach to a multiple-skills approach is attributed to a number of trends. These include demands for a customer-orientation and patient-centered care, the movement toward continuous quality improvement, changes in workforce demographics, and the demand for participative management.

This chapter answers the question of how health care facilities should be organized to meet their goals efficiently and effectively, and explores various organizational structures. Each structure is explained in terms of the extent and type of departmentalization within an institution, the degree to which decentralization of tasks and decision making is a prominent feature of an institution, and job design factors in a specific corporate climate. Organizational structure is determined by how the role of a foodservice department is defined in a larger organization (for example, through teams). In addition, foodservice department organization is determined by including the proper exercise of authority, staffing, and scheduling. Time management is viewed as a resource whose function is to maximize productivity.

DETERMINING ORGANIZATIONAL STRUCTURE

The system a facility chooses as most appropriate for conducting its work is called the *organizational structure*. It is a formal system of task, workflow, reporting relationships and communication channels that link the various parts of an organization to one another. Health care facilities continue to explore various organizational structures to determine the one best suited to meet quality demands within limitations imposed by cost constraints. It is important that decisions be made quickly, that employees participate in decision making, and that customer demands (especially those of patients) be met to ensure a health care institution's long-term viability. With these considerations in mind, the following sections discuss three common entities in health care organizational structure: departments, committees, and teams.

Departments

The formation of departments, or *departmentalization*, can fall into any of several categories: functional, product, geographical, customer, process or equipment, and time. It is also the process of

FIGURE 6.1 Functional Organization of a Foodservice Department

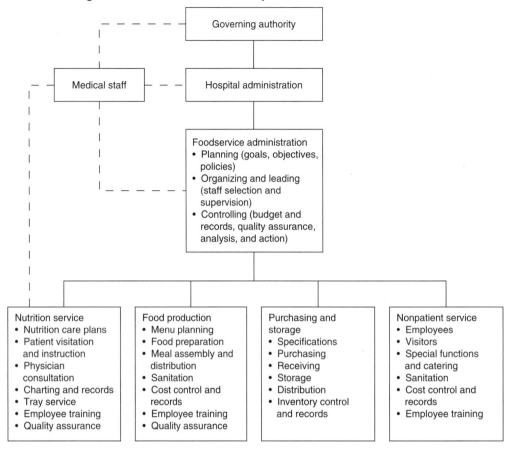

grouping together people and jobs into a work unit. In the past, only functional and time departmentalization were relevant to foodservice departments in health care institutions. However, changes in health care focus have made product, customer, and process departmentalization pertinent components of a facility's structure. For departmentalization to be effective, the concept of separation and reintegration must be taken into account when deciding how to form an organization. *Separation* represents division of labor by pulling the organization apart and making it more complex. The value of separation becomes evident when groups are reintegrated, forming the support structure for operations. *Reintegration* refers to the degree of coordination, cooperation, and communication that flow among units in the organization.

Usually top-level managers determine which department structure is appropriate for their institutions. Most likely, a combination of categories will be the best choice. Six departmentalization types are briefly described.

Functional Departmentalization

Functional departmentalization groups jobs into departments or units in which employees perform the same or similar activities. Most units within hospital foodservice departments are organized according to function, such as nutrition services, food production,

purchasing and storage, and nonpatient services (Figure 6.1). A manager or supervisor is usually in charge of each unit's activities. Functional departmentalization makes sense from the standpoint of having like functions centralized. For example, although decentralizing meal service may be desirable, it does not make sense to decentralize food preparation.

Functional departmentalization can cause conflicts between departments in meeting customer demands. Those closest to patients (for example, nurses) have a unique perspective of patients' requirements and may fault another department, such as foodservice, whenever patients' needs go unmet. Because foodservice staff are removed from the patients, they may not comprehend the urgency of nurses' requests. For example, interrupting a work activity to get an item requested by a nurse interferes with getting items ready for the tray line. This type of functional cross-purpose does not allow employees to engage in the full cycle of their work. In this example, a conflict occurs between nursing and foodservice. However, if the foodservice employee is involved in the full cycle of fulfilling a patient's dietary needs, he or she would understand that both tasks are of equal importance. The employee could then understand that the choice is not between completing a department task versus a nursing request but a choice of meeting an immediate patient need and scheduling or postponing a task for a future need. With the patient in clear focus, the foodservice staff could see that the positive consequences of meeting the patient's need would outweigh the negative consequences of not having all items ready for the tray line to start.

Product Departmentalization

Product departmentalization creates work units based on the product or service the unit delivers. This form of departmentalization is used most often in large manufacturing companies and financial institutions. In recent years, health care institutions have experimented with product-line departmentalization, defined by body system units or by the traditional nursing care units. Therefore, product lines may include cardiac care, obstetrics, oncology, or orthopedics.

The idea of product-line departmentalization is to coordinate the efforts of all health professionals involved in caring for a particular patient type. This coordination enhances the quality of care and improves costs associated with that care. Product-line management is further enhanced by critical paths that standardize the intervention at various stages of a patient's stay. (Critical paths are covered in detail in Chapter 4 on quality management.) Dietitians are among the practitioners who will have a role in product-line management and interdisciplinary care of patients. Although most product lines will likely be managed by a nurse, other professionals may lead. An example of this type of product line is an orthopedic or rehabilitation unit where a physical therapist may be the manager. Product-line departmentalization may or may not require that dietitians and others from foodservice report to the manager of the product line. If, for example, 100 percent of a dietitian's time is devoted to a particular unit, he or she conceivably could report to the product-line manager.

Geographical Departmentalization

Geographical departmentalization groups an organization's activities according to the places in which the activities are performed. This type of departmentalization is used in fast-food operations, contract feeding services, and large school districts. For example, food may be purchased, delivered, and stored in a central warehouse. The food may be prepared at a single second location or be disseminated to individual sites for preparation and service. Geographical departmentalization allows concentrated effort around fewer tasks.

Customer Departmentalization

Customer departmentalization focuses each department's or unit's work on the customer to be served. For example, a contract feeding company might service hotels, health care institutions, and schools. Therefore, it would structure its departments according to the different needs of these three customer types.

Customer departmentalization can be seen in large hospitals in which professionals and nonprofessionals work as a team in a patient-focused or patient-centered care unit. The traditional term, *nursing unit*, is being replaced with *patient care unit*, which attests to the influence patients have on how care is delivered. During a typical hospital stay, the average patient will come in contact with more than 25 individuals a day. It is estimated that nursing personnel spend more than 52 percent of their time in nonprofessional tasks such as paperwork, ordering supplies, handling communication, housekeeping, and performing personal service duties. Services related to patient support take about 22 percent of their time, leaving only 26 percent available for direct patient care. This revelation has led many organizations to patient-focused care units.

Patient-focused care units are designed to rely on a highly cross-trained staff that functions as a team. During a patient's stay, treatment is given by the same team members; this reduces the number of caregivers they have to see. This care allows a high level of comfort for patients and their families. Many organizations have dissolved the nursing station and provided bedside terminals and decentralized supplies, which allow staff to "float," thereby leaving them available to meet patients' needs. Frequently, with customer departmentalization, a clerical person in the unit handles patient admission at the bedside. Support generalists may be responsible for housekeeping, foodservice, and stocking and ordering supplies.

In addition to providing better care, patient-centered care acts to improve staff's work environment. Everyone has an equal place on the team and in patient care. This can be especially rewarding to foodservice employees who have traditionally felt left out of caring for patients. Rewards are based on team effort and quality of care. To ensure high-quality care, measurements must include clinical outcomes as well as patient satisfaction. Cross-functional or cross-trained employees are an effective means of allowing people from diverse areas within an organization to exchange information, solve problems, reduce duplication, and coordinate projects. In the beginning, it takes time for members to learn to work with diversity. It takes time to build trust and teamwork, especially among people from different professional backgrounds, experiences, and perspectives. A good example of this type of a team is the interdisciplinary team for "special diseases" such as the parenteral-enteral nutrition team.

For foodservice departments, this means that some of their work may also be decentralized to these units, which also means that the staff may be decentralized, as in the case of dietitians who specialize in diabetes, pediatrics, and dialysis. As team members, they will contribute to the care of patients while increasing their skills and the number of tasks they are capable of completing.

In recent reports, this type of decentralization has not been successful. Many foodservice departments are again serving and retrieving trays. Dietitians and dietetic technicians are still employees of foodservice departments but serve as members of interdisciplinary teams with the same rights of input as any other member. Because of the critical shortage of nurses, various methods are being tested to enable nurses to provide more direct patient care.

Process or Equipment Departmentalization

Process departmentalization divides work groups according to their different production processes or the specialized equipment their work requires. Foodservice departments are exploring this type of departmentalization. Employee involvement and teamwork have placed new emphasis on process departmentalization, and employees are grouped together to manage a process from beginning to end, rather than seeing only one specialized piece of the process. For example, a process team established for patient feeding would include not only servers on the tray line but also cooks, dietitians, hostesses, purchasing personnel, and a supervisor or manager. Process departmentalization requires the manager of the process to have a broad knowledge base and understanding of the interactions of various parts of the process. Process focus has been shown to improve not only the quality of work produced but also employee commitment to work. Teams and self-managed teams are discussed later in this chapter.

Process departmentalization allows employees to cross-train and gain information about all steps of the process. This way, they no longer place blame on one step in the process; instead, they see how everyone working together can enhance the overall process to improve outcome. This type of work unit division can go further than foodservice department units and can include nurses or other professionals on the patient unit. If an organization is using customer departmentalization and patient care units, a person on this work team may be a service generalist from the patient unit.

Time Departmentalization

Time departmentalization is often used along with another form of departmentalization when the work to be done fills more than a standard eight-hour workday. Hospitals use time departmentalization in grouping work according to shifts. In most foodservice departments, two shifts are needed to cover the 12- to 14-hour period of meal service for patients and nonpatients.

Committees

Although most work in health care organizations continues to be accomplished in departments and intradepartmental units, some activities require that individuals from different departments (or from different units within a department) work together on a common task. In this case, a work team such as a committee, task force, or project team is formed. Historically, team members come from about the same level in the organization. However, with participative management and continuous quality improvement, this no longer may be the case. For example, a task force whose assignment is to explore a new process for preparing department budgets might consist of persons from the same level. Members of the work team would include all department directors and a representative from the finance department. A different type of work team might review the patient admission process for improvement. This team would include clerks who actually complete the process as well as managers, directors, and perhaps administrators. To build a team that works in harmony requires substantial effort; teams must be given high priority and attention. Some good employees do not make good team players. Usually a team can achieve more than an individual. Teams contribute significant achievements in all phases of life. The military would never win a battle if it did not work as a team with the same objective of winning with as few casualties as possible.

Work teams can take several forms, some of which are listed here:

• *Ad hoc committees* are created for a short period to perform a specific task (for example, evaluating new computer training packages).

• *Standing committees* work together for a longer period than do ad hoc committees to deal with an ongoing subject of relevance to all committee members. For example, several departments might send representatives to a multidisciplinary patient education committee whose task is to develop materials and programs to teach patients about topics that draw from the department's knowledge. For example, a program on diabetic patient education might require help from the medical staff, nursing staff, pharmacy, laboratory, and a dietitian.

• *Task forces* are similar to ad hoc committees in that they are short term and have a narrow purpose. Usually, however, task forces are formal teams charged with solving or reporting on specific problems. Another difference is that a task force always has representatives from various departments, whereas committee members may be from the same department. The purpose of a task force is to integrate the work of discrete departments that on a daily basis work independently. Another difference is that the task force membership may change as the team works through a project. For example, a task force whose purpose is to evaluate a hospital's eating disorders program might be composed of nutritionists, psychologists, and physicians initially, with marketing specialists brought in later to suggest ways the program could improve to better fulfill the community's needs.

• *Project teams* are similar to task forces and ad hoc committees in that their purpose and duration are limited. However, the task that a project team is to accomplish may take as much as a third or half of members' work time. For example, the development of an eating disorders program might be assigned to a project team so that the program can get under way as quickly as possible. A project team manager coordinates the work of the different specialists. These specialists must report to the project manager as well as to their regular department or unit directors until their work on the project is completed.

• *Cross-functional teams* are made up of employees from about the same hierarchical level (dietitians, nurses, pharmacists, and the like) but different work areas who work together to accomplish a task or job. These employees work in the same organization and blend their knowledge, experience, and talents to meet outcome objectives and goals.

• *Virtual teams* are an extension of electronic meetings. Virtual teams allow groups to meet without concern for space or time. This is accomplished through communication links such as conference calls, video conferencing, e-mail, and chat rooms. The members may be geographically distant and in various time zones.

• *Problem-solving teams* are specialized teams appointed to solve a specific problem. Teams are composed of members that may be involved in the problem. These teams strive to improve quality (usually throughout the organization), to provide more efficient processes, and to improve the overall work environment. Once the problem has been solved the team is disbanded. A new team will be appointed to solve another problem.

- *Self-managed teams* are groups of employees that self-regulate their abilities and behaviors. A self-managed team is the highest level of employee involvement.

- *Self-managed work teams* are groups of interdependent individuals who select their own teams and can self-regulate their behavior to complete a whole task. These employees can control their own work schedules and performance goals. Team members interact with employees at all levels of the organization. The team manages a budget and takes responsibility for productivity, cost, and quality. Members are empowered to make major changes in their work process without going through management.

Self-managed teams benefit the organization because people are taking more responsibility. Reduction in the work force and economic conditions in organizations has caused a decrease in the number of middle managers and employees, making self-managed teams more important. Self-managed teams may work in some areas of the foodservice department. For example, dietitians, technicians, patient host, and clerical support personnel can form a self-managed team with responsibility for making decisions that relate to the tasks they perform for patient care and supporting meal service to customers.

Self-managed teams foster effective communications among departments that share common goals and objectives. Self-managed teams permit integration of departments with similar goals and objectives.

- They offer a medium for coordinating the opinions and experience of specialists from several different functional areas.
- They provide a forum for team decision making.
- They create broad-based support for projects that demand the involvement of several different departments or units within departments.

Generally speaking, foodservice directors are required to serve on various hospital committees, among them the emergency preparedness planning committee, continuous quality improvement committee, safety committee, and infection control committee. (The advantages of team decision making are discussed in Chapter 5.)

Teams

The importance of teamwork in a participative management structure is emphasized throughout this segment of the manual. Teamwork is important at the job-involvement level of empowerment to help employees make decisions that affect their work group. Teamwork is valuable in health care foodservice because of department complexity and job interrelationships; the more complex the organization or department, the greater will be the return on an investment in teamwork. For example, because many individuals are involved in providing a patient with a meal tray, collaborating on the task provides a clear goal to be accomplished. In a complex department like health care foodservice, the various sections of the department have a variety of goals. For instance, those purchasing food see their goal as obtaining and providing raw materials to the cooks. The cooks see their goal as preparing food for the tray line. The tray line server's goal is to complete the tray for a hostess to deliver. When all of these members act as a team, the goal becomes serving patients. In addition, an organization with a focus on customers and continuous quality improvement can benefit from the ideas and accomplishments created by teams. *Risk taking* is a positive outcome of teamwork, and research has shown that team workers are more likely to take risks than are individuals. These statements, while supported by the author, are based on the information presented by various leaders in business and specifically in health care and foodservice.

Characteristics of High-Performance Teams

Much time and research have been devoted to singling out competencies or characteristics of high-performance teams. Stellar teams exhibit the following characteristics:

- *Clear definition of roles and purposes.* The team has clear goals and strategies for goal accomplishment.
- *Interpersonal relationships.* Interactions among team members and with key people outside the team are ruled by trust, collaboration, responsiveness, and support.
- *Member empowerment.* Team workers have access to necessary skills and resources. Policies and practices support team objectives.
- *Open and honest communication.* Members express understanding and acceptance of others, practice active listening, and value different opinions and perspectives.
- *Member participation.* Members perform roles and functions as needed, share responsibility for leadership and team development, are adaptable, and explore various ideas and approaches.
- *High performance.* High output, excellent quality, effective decisions, and an efficient problem-solving process are apparent.
- *Exemplary individual contributions.* Workers' efforts are recognized by everyone. Team accomplishments are recognized, and members feel respected and recognized by the organization.
- *Individual motivation.* Workers feel good about their membership, are confident and motivated, have a sense of pride and satisfaction, and have a strong sense of cohesion and team spirit.
- *Mutual accountability.* Each member is accountable for the success of the goals of the project or task.
- *Commitment.* Members are committed to the goals of the team, a meaningful purpose.
- *Specific outcomes.* Performance goals.
- *Complementary skills.* Members have complementary skills (technical or functional)—problem solving, decision making, communication, and interpersonal.

Leader or Manager Responsibility to Teams

An environment that fosters teamwork is created through participative management and employee empowerment. The manager is responsible for communicating a clear vision or purpose for the team. (Communication related to teams is detailed in Chapter 7.) The working environment culture must support team members and efforts for goal accomplishment. Many of the necessities for a participative work environment also are critical to effective teamwork. These include providing flexibility by eliminating unnecessary procedures and allowing employees freedom to develop new ideas, permitting people to take risks and make mistakes, setting challenging goals with clear standards for accomplishment, providing recognition and praise, clearly communicating expectations and plans, and being committed to provide whatever is necessary for goal accomplishment.

The manager is responsible for providing employee training so that employees have the skills needed for problem solving and team interaction. Education and reeducation are based on the demands and needs of the team members and individual levels of competency. It is the manager's responsibility to assess level of competency and, if needed, to provide individual coaching for employees. The manager must ensure that everyone is given ample opportunity to participate and that outspoken members do not make all decisions and dominate the group. Before employees are asked to work in a team, they must be trained in how to conduct team meetings, how to participate, how to make decisions, and how to follow the ground rules for team meetings (see Chapter 7). Once everyone has been trained, individual abilities can be addressed. The competency of team members can be assessed through observation by a manager and frequently can be measured by the output or lack of output by the team.

The manager may have to assist with resolving conflict and with providing problem-solving tools. Statistical tools used to measure and analyze problems (reviewed in Chapter 4) and situational leadership (see Chapter 2) should be kept in mind with teams.

Group Development or Team Stages

Blanchard and associates identify four distinct stages of team or group development: orientation, dissatisfaction, resolution, and production. (Other writers refer to these four stages as forming, storming, norming, and performing.) Orientation, or Stage 1, characterizes a newly formed group whose members have high expectations and some enthusiasm but may experience anxiety about their role and feel a need to find their place. They test the leader but at the same time are dependent on authority and the hierarchy to provide guidance. During this stage, the group will have a low productivity level but a high commitment level. The leader will have to provide specific directions and a clear vision with desired outcomes to decrease anxiety and allow members to understand what is expected.

At Stage 2, dissatisfaction, teams are somewhat disillusioned about team accomplishment. They may feel dissatisfaction with authority; be frustrated with goals, tasks, or action plans; feel confused and incompetent; compete for power or attention, or both; and experience dependence and counter-dependence. Although their morale and commitment may be waning, their level of productivity is on the upswing. The manager or leader will have to create a supportive environment that allows members to explore their feelings of discontent while providing enough coaching to move the group forward. Understanding that this stage of team growth is normal will allow members to stay focused and committed.

At Stage 3, resolution, teams have moved toward some resolution of what dissatisfied them at Stage 2. Members begin to develop harmony, trust, support, and respect for one another. Self-esteem and confidence are strong, leading to more open communication and feedback. A team language begins to develop as responsibility and control are shared by group members. The manager or leader must continue to provide support but from a distance as team members begin to take active roles and become responsible for the outcome of the group.

Production, the final stage, is represented by a high level of productivity and morale. Team members are excited about their team and collaborate and work interdependently within the group and subgroups and as a whole in the team. There is a feeling of team strength, leadership is shared, tasks are being accomplished, and the team members have a high level of confidence. The team leader will have to further remove himself or herself from the leadership role and move toward delegation, allowing team members to accomplish desired outcomes.

Team Building

Team building is important to producing a desired outcome or high performance. Otherwise, both loyalty and performance will be jeopardized. Trust is developed through team building, which allows open discussion and feedback among members. The first step to building high-performance teams is to nurture a collaborative relationship between managers and team members. Managers must share their power and authority in an effort to reinforce the responsibility given to teams. A commitment from the manager means giving the time necessary for team development and always attending scheduled meetings.

To form a high-performance team, members must understand and believe in the purpose of the team and in their ability to influence work. Team members must trust one another, the leader, and the reason for the team. Team building can provide enjoyment and allow personal growth of members. For department members to begin functioning in teams, the manager will have to ensure commitment from them to join in. For the best results, participation in teamwork should be voluntary because some individuals feel uncomfortable functioning in teams, just as they feel uncomfortable giving opinions. These employees should be given other individual tasks to complete. It is also possible that individuals who are reluctant to join teams will come around after they see there is nothing to fear and after team members provide positive feedback.

Team-building efforts must focus on the task or content of the meeting and the process. Teamwork is effective when team members are chosen for their knowledge, and the task portion of teamwork. Team building must address how members relate, go about the task, and communicate to build a functional team. The team process can affect the outcome. Team building should concentrate on how things are going, encourage full participation, and emphasize listening and building consensus rather than majority rule. Byron Lane has suggested two ways to increase awareness of process:

1. When process problems develop in which people are dropping out, forming subgroups, or not listening, stop the meeting. Ask members to discuss how they feel about what is happening. They may be apprehensive at first, but as teams develop, they will be more willing to share their concerns.
2. At the end of each meeting, allow 10 to 15 minutes to discuss the process. Ask the team members, "How did we do today?" Once they realize that process is important enough to discuss, they will pay closer attention.

Team building should be fun and produce synergy. *Synergy* is the creation of a whole greater than the sums of individual parts. If possible, off-site training and development sessions should be held with team members. If this is not possible, time should be set aside for the department to celebrate and reward team participation. Effective team building requires as much interaction time as possible for team members. Early meetings should focus on how they can work together, what they think they can accomplish, and what issues are important to them in terms of decision making. (Team decision making is discussed in Chapter 5.) Feedback to the director and the department is virtual or employees may resent the team and its authority.

SYSTEMS APPROACH TO FOODSERVICE ORGANIZATIONS

M. C. Spears, R. P. Puckett, and other management foodservice professionals advocate the use of a systems approach in foodservice organizations. A *system* is a collection of interrelated parts, facts, principles, rules, or subsystems unified by design to obtain stated objectives or outcomes. A system that interacts with external environments is an *open system*. A system that does not interact with its environment is a *closed system*. The systems approach to management involves keeping the objectives or outcomes in mind throughout the performance of all activities. This approach requires communication and coordination among all parts of the organization. The basic systems model of an organization is depicted in Figure 6.2.

A system is composed of subsystems. A subsystem depends on the whole system. That is, it is not independent but is a complete

FIGURE 6.2   Making Coleslaw Using a Systems Approach

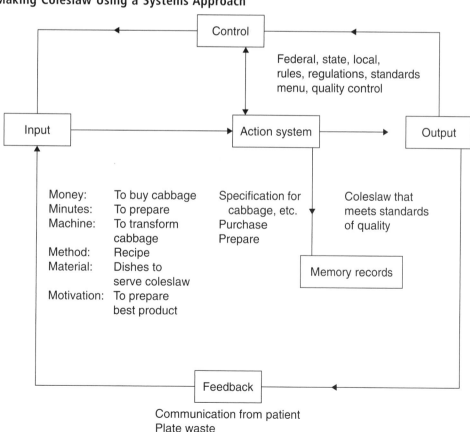

system within itself. The system also has controls, records, feedback, decision making, linking processes, and balance. The linking process is necessary to coordinate the functional *subsystems* from resources to goals or outcomes. Decisions may be made by management at any point to alter the action. Communication is vital. It includes all types of information: oral, written, computer forms, or data throughout the system. The system must be kept in balance by the manager's ability to maintain organizational stability during changes in technology, economics, and political and social conditions.

A foodservice department usually has at least the following major systems: management system, action system, control system, and output system. Each of these systems contains smaller systems with rules and regulations that must be followed.

The *input* is made up of management systems and basically defines the resources available. The *management system* is made up of the seven Ms: man (personnel), machines (equipment and physical resources), money (budget), motivation, materials, methods, and minutes. The *action or transformation system* transforms the raw materials into finished products and services. This action must use the seven Ms of other functional subsystems and the linking processes. These systems work together to produce the outputs, which are the finished products and services of the department. (Linking or interlocking is made up of *procurement, production, distribution, service and sanitation, security,* and *maintenance,* which are functional subsystems working in harmony to produce the output.)

Records are important, used to forecast, to meet budget requirements and personnel needs. These records are used for the action or transformation systems.

The *control system* refers to the plans, goals, and objectives of the organization and to outside influences (such as local, state, and federal laws and regulations). The control system is necessary to assure that foodservice personnel use the management system in concert with the action system to have an efficient and effective output system. The menu is the most important aspect of the control system. The menu also relates to the management and action systems.

The output system is the result of the other systems working together to produce a finished product that meets quality and quantity, customer satisfaction, and financial accountability. For example, a patient is not served whole raw cabbage, but coleslaw is an acceptable product. Coleslaw is served to a patient as a result of the output system. Feedback gives the manager the opportunity to make necessary changes at all steps of the system, to refine the action or transformation process.

The system must know the environment in which it exists. It must comply with all local and state rules and regulations as well as internal policies and procedures.

ORGANIZING THE FOODSERVICE DEPARTMENT

The division of work and its efficient coordination are important in every health care institution, and The Joint Commission (TJC) recognizes this importance in its standards. TJC and Center for Medicare and Medicaid Services (CMS) standards require that all departments or services be organized, directed and staffed, and integrated with other units and departments or services of the organization. For foodservice, the standards stress organization in a manner designed to ensure provision of optimal nutrition care and high-quality foodservices.

All health care employees must be aware of their place in the organization—who their supervisor is and who their peers are. This is called *organization structure* because it divides labor into distinct tasks and coordinates them. An organizational chart for the foodservice department is posted within the department. An *organizational chart* is a visual representation of the division and coordination of work within an organization or department within an organization. It illustrates relationships among units and lines of authority through the use of boxes and connecting lines. The chart is an unbroken line of authority that extends from the top of the organization to the lowest subordinate and clarifies to whom and how information and discussions should flow. The foodservice department's organizational chart is to be reviewed and revised at least once a year or whenever changes are made in the department's structure.

An organizational chart is a useful tool because it shows the characteristics of the larger organization and its units. For example, the organizational chart in Figure 6.3 shows how the various positions in one type of foodservice department relate to each other and to the administration of the hospital. However, no chart can show the dynamic interconnections and interactions among members of the organization. The following items are depicted on an organizational chart:

• *Chain of command.* The solid lines in Figure 6.3 demonstrate that the upper levels of the organization are linked to each of the lower levels through a defined set of relationships. Flattening of organization structure allows problems to be answered more quickly and efficiently as one or more layers of supervision have been removed. *Authority* is the right to perform or command. Managers are given authority to direct the operation of the foodservice department, and with this authority, the manager can give orders or directions and expect them to be obeyed or followed.

• *Unity of command.* Each employee is linked by a vertical line to only **one** supervisor. This ensures that each employee reports to, and is accountable only to, his or her immediate superior, an unbroken line of authority. When the unity of command is broken, the employee usually has to cope with conflicting demands from several supervisors.

• *Departmentalization.* The organizational chart also shows how jobs are grouped into those that have common tasks that can be coordinated by a supervisor. For example, Figure 6.3 shows that the foodservice department is split into three units: nutrition care services, food procurement and production, and nonpatient operations. Each unit is further divided into areas of specialization.

• *Divisional structure.* This structure groups together people working on the same product, in the same area or with similar customers. Divisional structure works well in today's unemployment and economic downfall. It brings everyone together, under one boss rather than several bosses. It helps the employees and bosses see the entire picture (product) and to reduce or eliminate redundancy.

• *Lines of communication.* In addition to showing the chain of command, organizational charts show how information should flow through the organization. Solid lines in all the flowcharts shown (Figure 6.1 and Figures 6.3 through 6.9) indicate both the flow of authority and the flow of formal communication among different positions in the chart. Broken lines show that information must also flow outside the chain of command. For example, in Figure 6.3, although the assistant directors of nutrition care services, food procurement and production, and nonpatient operations do not supervise each other, they must communicate and coordinate their efforts to ensure efficient operation of the whole department. In addition, the broken line in Figure 6.3 between the medical staff and the foodservice director indicates that the medical staff advises the foodservice department on the most appropriate service for particular patients but does not have direct authority over the department.

• *Span of control.* Span of control refers to the number of employees each manager must supervise directly. In a large organizational structure (see Figure 6.3), each manager tends to have a narrow span of control, whereas in a less complex structure (see Figure 6.6), each manager's span of control is wider.

- A tall organizational structure (Figure 6.3) consists of multi-reporting layers within the organization, giving span of control to three assistant directors.
- A flat organizational structure (Figure 6.5) has fewer layers of supervisors and subordinates.
- The wider or larger the span, the more efficient the organization.
- The wide span of control speeds up decision making, increases flexibility, empowers employees, and allows employees to get closer to customers. Employee training is necessary in an organization with a wide span of control.

• *Reduced staff.* To save expense or the use of specialized services or skills these services can be contracted out. In some instances,

FIGURE 6.4 Organization of a Small Institution's Top-Level Management

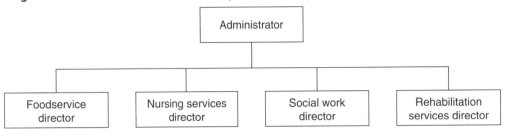

FIGURE 6.5 One Management Level in a Small Foodservice Department

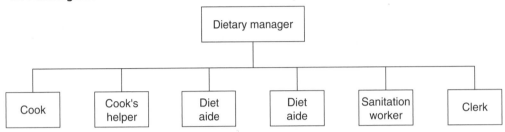

this will reduce the number of FTEs or reduce the number of hours. Full-time employees on the afternoon shift may be replaced with part-time employees, thereby reducing hours and types of service. Purchasing may be delegated to the purchasing department and information service may be contracted to an information service company specializing in foodservice operation.

Functional-Hierarchical Structure

Most health care organizations and foodservice departments continue to use the functional-hierarchical structure. The functional-hierarchical structure is present in organizations that group similar tasks (functions) together (for example, food production), with the chain of command and span of control increasing as one moves to the top of the pyramid (hierarchy). The more management levels there are in an organization, the more complex the organization is. For example, Figure 6.3 represents five management levels: CEO, vice president of operations, foodservice director, foodservice assistant directors, and managers. A large organization such as this has a *tall organizational chart*. Smaller organizations tend to have a *flat structure* because they have fewer levels of management.

Figure 6.4 is an example of an organizational chart for a small health care institution. Small hospitals and extended-care facilities, particularly those in small communities or rural settings, frequently do not have the services of a full-time registered dietitian. Therefore, to meet TJC, Omnibus Budget Reconciliation Act (OBRA), and Medicare-Medicaid requirements (CMS) for supervision of patient nutritional care, such institutions hire a dietetic consultant or part-time registered dietitian. A dietary manager has responsibility for the day-to-day supervision of the foodservice department in such institutions. The certified dietary manager is an experienced foodservice operations manager recognized as a professional. Certified dietary managers are educated, competent professional employed by

both health care and non–health care organizations. They are certified by the Certifying Board for Dietary Managers (CBDM). To maintain certification, members must secure additional safety and sanitation credential and continuing education credit every three years. The organizational chart for a small foodservice department is shown in Figure 6.5. Figure 6.6 illustrates two levels of management within a much larger foodservice department.

During the past hundred years the functional-hierarchical structure has contributed to the large economic growth of the U.S. economy; it now appears to have outlived its usefulness. Its limitations include turf orientation around departments or functions; limited information to employees, rendering them incapable of contributing to the big picture; communication difficulties due to the number of layers employees must go through; limited career growth; and rewards based on competitive individual or departmental progress, which limits contributions to the organization as a whole.

Alternative Organizational Structures

Changes in health care have required organizations to revisit the traditional functional-hierarchical structure to look for alternative structures. Options considered by some organizations have included removing a level of management by phasing out middle managers or reducing the number of managers at all levels, supposedly to improve communication with less vertical and horizontal boundaries. Still other attempts have been to invert the pyramid, putting employees at the top and the CEO at the bottom. However, this latter attempt did nothing with the direction of the power and authority. A new structure needs to be developed for managers to empower employees, one that is not designed to direct and control.

One possibility, the *matrix model*, consists of two organizational structures superimposed on each other (see Figure 6.7) such as

FIGURE 6.6 Two Management Levels in a Large Foodservice Department

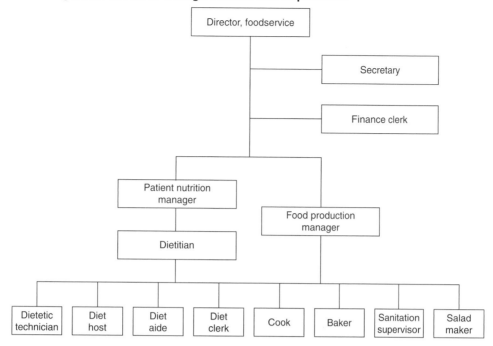

FIGURE 6.7 Matrix Structure for a Health Care Institution Showing Project Management

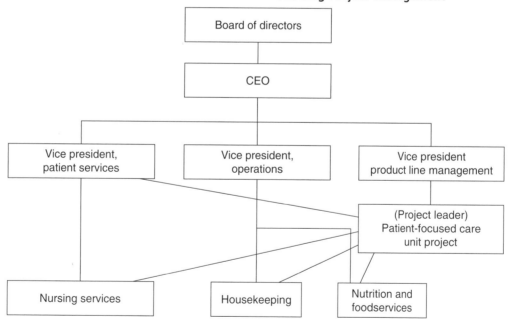

functional and divisional structure. This structure uses cross-functional teams to integrate functional expertise with divisional focus. This type of organizational chart allows for the continuation of the functional-hierarchical structure with the addition of project leaders. Top levels of the organization are still preeminent in regard to the chain of command and span of control in these two models. These two models differ in that the matrix structure in Figure 6.7 shows individuals or teams reporting to two different supervisors.

Many of the relationships depicted in the matrix model occur in the traditional hierarchical structure without being "legitimized" on the organizational chart.

This type of structure is felt to be effective at cutting the time for decision making and is flexible enough to accommodate temporary teams such as committees, task forces, and project teams. It allows for changes in the informal structure without creating problems for the fixed hierarchical structure. It also allows a clear picture

FIGURE 6.8 **Nutrition and Foodservices Process Structure**

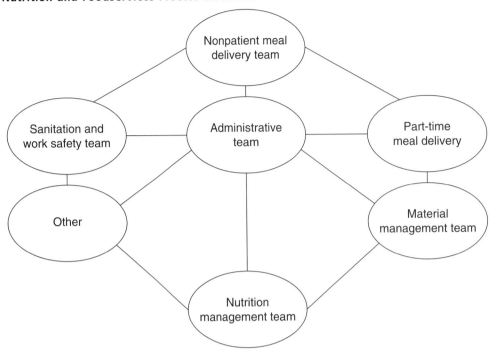

Note. The lines in this figure represent communication that may occur between any of the teams.

of product lines and customer or service units. Although the matrix model is more accommodating to organizational teams, there are problems associated with it. Problems include power struggle and ambiguity regarding the reporting structure (Who is the boss?). This structure can send conflicting messages: prioritizing tasks may cause focus on the team rather than the organization; it could increase personnel cost. For this reason, the appropriateness of such a structure for frontline employees is questionable. The matrix model may prove more beneficial at the supervisory or professional staff level, where ambiguity regarding reporting structure is more comfortable. Good interpersonal skills and conflict-management skills are essential for managers and employees if a matrix structure is used. These skills are helpful in improving communication and building relationships that facilitate dealing with ambiguity. For example, a dietitian may be asked to join a project team for developing a skilled-nursing unit in the hospital. Conflict may arise if the team decides that meals should be delivered at a specific time. Good interpersonal skills will allow the dietitian to communicate the needs of the unit and the limitations of the department in meeting these needs.

Functioning in teams requires an organizational structure that is designed to depict cross-functional processes rather than functional departmentalization. It is difficult to assign a specific chain of command because process management functions tend to intersect. The organizational chart in Figure 6.8 shows a *bubble diagram* for a nutrition and foodservice department. This structure represents different teams focused on the major core process of delivering patient care and foodservices. Comparing this diagram with the functional–hierarchical diagrams in Figures 6.3 through 6.6 uncovers the following innovations afforded by a bubble structure:

- Management layers have been replaced with team leaders and facilitators who coach and facilitate rather than control.
- Team members are responsible for decision making. Consensus building becomes important in this type of decision making, requiring a coordinated communication process as discussed in Chapter 7.
- Team empowerment allows communication with other teams, customers, suppliers, executive teams, and so on.
- Teams have a broader view of the organization and their contribution to its vision.
- Turf protection is replaced with cooperation within and across teams.
- Mobility of team members is increased through cross-functional participation on other teams within the department and organization.
- Team rewards can be provided in addition to rewards for individual development.

Organizational Culture

Organizational culture is the mechanism for guiding employee behavior; it is the personality of the organization. Organizational culture determines how employees view their jobs, how they act toward fellow employees and customers, and what style of leadership the manager uses. It also means the values they and the organization possess and the manner in which they behave.

The organizational culture usually reflects the mission, vision, shared beliefs, and values that guide behavior of the organization.

An organization's culture may have an effect on its structure, depending on how weak the culture.

Characteristics of Organizational Culture

Robbins and Coulter, in the tenth edition of their book, *Management* (2009), define *organizational culture* as being strong or weak. Strong cultures—those in which the key values are deeply held and widely shared—have a greater influence than do a weaker culture. Strong cultures include values that are widely shared, the culture is consistent in conveying what is important, most employees know and can tell stories about the company history or its heroes, employees identify with the company culture, and there is a connection between values and behavior. The company helps new employees learn the company core values, its belief about the right way to behave. From core values organizational culture can be observed by the way it does things (ethical or unethical), the company philosophy, rituals and rites, special language, and how it meets its mission.

On entering an organization, one can get a feel of the culture by the way employees behave. Employees communicate and represent the culture by their actions, the camaraderie of the personnel, the way customers are treated, and the values they display.

There is a *workplace spirituality culture*. Workplace spirituality is a practice that encourages members to integrate spiritual life and work life. Workplace spirituality has its foundation in strong ethics, recognizes the value of each person, respects diversity, and focuses on developing meaningful work and jobs. In this management environment, employees can become more creative and productive. Without this type of environment employees may become disenchanted, frustrated, and leave the job. This is a major move for most organizations and it behooves managers to learn more and perhaps implement this culture.

Factors That Influence Department Structure

Although health care foodservice departments typically perform the same basic functions, several factors influence how these functions are organized and staffed. Different types of health care institution (acute care hospital, nursing home, for example), its size (the number of beds it contains or the number of residents it cares for), and the type of services it offers (patient meal service, nutrition care service, cafeteria service, and so on) play a major role in the organizational structure.

In addition, an organization's philosophy and leadership style will affect the department structure selected. For example, an organization that promotes process development, teamwork, and employee involvement will seek a structure that depicts a dynamic, cross-functional approach.

Department Members and Responsibilities

As the sample organizational charts for foodservice departments demonstrate, the manager, staff members, and foodservice workers in various organizations have different titles and cultures. In addition, directors and managers have various levels of skill and responsibility and different levels of formal training and education. The foodservice director in Figure 6.3 heads a large and complex department in a large acute care hospital. Two levels of management below the level of director manage numerous department services and employees. In contrast, a consultant (a part-time registered dietitian) advises the manager of a foodservice department in a small hospital or extended-care facility like the one shown in Figure 6.9. The consultant might work only 8 to 40 hours per month in such a facility.

The titles, responsibilities, and educational backgrounds of foodservice managers in various health care institutions can be described as follows:

- *Foodservice director.* In most large health care institutions and in many medium and small ones, the foodservice director is responsible for the overall operation of the nutrition and foodservice department. The director usually holds a bachelor of science degree. In large organizations, advanced education in business management, health science education, institutional administration, or other related fields may be required. The foodservice director may or may not be a registered dietitian (RD). The director may belong to a number of professional organizations such as Association for Healthcare Foodservice, RD, LD, DTR, the Academy of Nutrition and Dietetics (formerly American Dietetic Association [ADA]), and the management practice group or, if a certified dietary manager, the Association of Nutrition and Foodservice Professionals (ANFP, formerly Dietary Managers Association [DMA]). Other titles that correspond to this position include director of dietetics, director of nutrition and foodservice, and foodservice administrator.

- *Certified dietary manager.* The certified dietary manager (CDM) has satisfactorily completed a course of study approved by the Certifying Board of the ANFP. The approved course usually requires 120 or more classroom hours and 150 hours of on-the-job training (field experience). The dietary manager (DM) is certified by passing a national credentialing examination and earning 45 continuing education clock hours in each of the three years during the certification period.

CDMs belong to the ANFP. Other titles that correspond to this position include foodservice director or manager and dietetic assistant (see earlier definition).

- *Dietetic technician registered.* A dietetic technician has successfully completed an associate's degree program that meets the educational standards established by the AND and has 450 hours of supervised field experience. A dietetic technician may become registered (DTR) by successfully passing a national certifying examination and maintaining 50 clock hours of AND-approved continuing education over a five-year period. The dietetic technician can work in food systems management under the supervision of, or in consultation with, an RD. The dietetic technician may also work as a member of a health care team under the supervision of an RD. Dietetic technicians may belong to the AND under the category of technician members. In addition, graduates of dietetic technician programs approved by the ANFP may also become CDMs through the ANFP credentialing process.

- *Registered dietitian.* An RD has earned a bachelor of science degree in dietetics, nutrition, or food systems management

FIGURE 6.9 Organization of a Foodservice Department with a Dietary Consultant in a Small Hospital or Extended-Care Facility

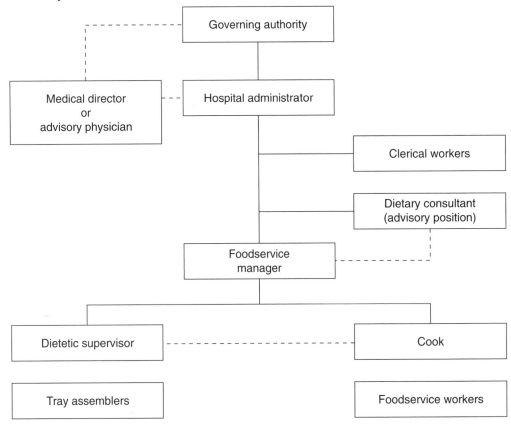

from a college or university, the program being approved by the Commission on the Accreditation of Dietetic Education (CADE). On successful completion of the academic and on-the-job training components (internship) of the program, students become eligible to take the national registration examination for dietitians. The successful applicant becomes an RD. To maintain the RD status, 75 hours of approved continuing education must be accrued in five years. RDs work as medical nutrition therapy dietitians in a variety of health care institutions. Some medical nutrition dietitians are certified in diabetes care, weight management, and other special areas of practice. Community dietitians work as counselors and coordinators of nutrition awareness and disease prevention programs. Management dietitians specialize in food systems, clinical management, or other areas of management and work in health care institutions, schools, colleges, cafeterias, and restaurants, and as consultant and advisers to the foodservice industry. Business dietitians work in related business areas such as sales, marketing, and public relations. Education dietitians teach nutrition and food systems in colleges, universities, and hospitals; conduct research; and write books and articles on foodservice. Consultant dietitians, who practice independently, may advise business and industry, and counsel patients in a variety of settings. These consulting dietitians are entrepreneurs, many owning companies and employing other dietitians.

In some states, RDs are also licensed by the state and are entitled to use the LD (licensed dietitian) designation or other titles following their names. All dietitians are eligible for AND membership. Many RDs also belong to the Association for Healthcare Foodservice and other related associations.

Shared Services

Given the high cost of food and substantial increases in labor costs, it is difficult for a foodservice manager to stay within a budget and to forecast realistically for the following year. The pressure to contain costs and at the same time improve the quality of foodservice is unrelenting. As a result, more and more foodservice managers are looking at shared foodservice systems as a means of providing high-quality food for patients and staff at a reasonable cost.

Shared service systems are categorized according to the degree of control and responsibility exercised by the participating institutions. Thus, a shared service can be classified as a referred service, a purchased service, a multiple-sponsor service, or a regional service. Usually shared foodservice systems are either a purchased service or a multiple-sponsor service. Purchased service is a payment paid for directly by the institution. The purchasing institution acts as an intermediary between the patient and the provider and therefore assumes some responsibility for quality of service. In a multiple-control and operate the service. Control can be established through an agreement among the institutions or through a separate corporation or cooperative. Although the nature and extent of shared food-services vary, the major types of sharing are in professional and managerial expertise, food purchasing, and food production systems.

Shared Professional and Managerial Expertise

The sharing of professional and managerial expertise is of major importance to small and rural hospitals and extended-care facilities. The opportunity to use the services of highly trained personnel on a part-time basis allows a health care institution to provide patient services that it otherwise could not afford to offer. Although large hospitals seldom share dietetic and other professional foodservice personnel among themselves, these institutions sometimes do so with small institutions. Usually, fees for this service are paid directly to the large hospital, which pays the shared personnel their salary, with additional compensation for travel when necessary. The shared personnel usually are required to submit reports to the administrators of both institutions, to meet accreditation requirements, and to evaluate the shared program.

Shared managerial services are similar to shared professional personnel services. Management services that can be shared include meal planning, financial record keeping, data processing for foodservice functions, payroll operations, in-service training and education, and policies and procedures planning.

Shared Food Purchasing and Production

Shared food-purchasing systems are the most common of the shared services. Standardized and least-perishable items are most often purchased through shared systems, but dairy products, frozen meat, poultry, fish, frozen entrées, and nonfood supplies are also frequently available. Agreement on product specifications among participating institutions is essential in attaining the greatest cost savings in shared purchasing arrangements. Shared food purchasing also implies sharing ideas about food quality, processing techniques, consumer acceptance data, and reliable information on new products. Management time is saved in shared purchasing arrangements because the buyer in the participating institution does not have to negotiate prices or see as many vendors, a benefit discussed further in Chapter 18.

Shared food production systems are feasible, provided a comprehensive planning and evaluation procedure is used in the developmental stages. Foodservice managers and CEOs of the institutions involved must agree on long-range goals in level of service, quality, nutrition counseling, bacteriological control, menu variety, and flexibility of the system in the face of changing circumstances.

The decision of whether to enter a shared production system or to maintain independent status needs documentation. One method of documentation is to survey patients, medical staff, employees, and outpatients about availability, quality, and level of service currently being provided or desired. Opportunities for sharing often involve a shift to different systems of food production and service. Careful consideration of the foodservice systems will help identify the strengths and weaknesses of the present or proposed system. Data to be collected include capital investment requirements, operating costs, quality and comprehensiveness of services, acceptability of services to client groups, and legal considerations such as taxes and contracts.

Multidepartments and Multifacilities

In an effort to flatten organizations, a facility may opt for multidepartment management, which has foodservice directors responsible for the management of more than one department within an organization, such as housekeeping, grounds, laundry, or other service departments. Another possibility is that foodservice directors may be required to provide management services to more than one facility within a corporation. For example, separate departments for dietetic education programs, wellness, weight management, or community education could be incorporated into a foodservice director's responsibilities in a large facility. A multifacility corporation that has a number of hospitals or extended-care institutions may require a foodservice director to oversee more than one of the corporation's units. These services may include the shared management services mentioned earlier.

DISTRIBUTING AUTHORITY

Authority, the legitimate power an organization grants to some of its members, is used to direct and manage the actions of employees of the organization in achieving its goals. *Line of authority* is the authority that entitles a manager to direct the work of employees. (Authority and leadership are discussed in Chapter 2.) Just as there are patterns for grouping work in organizations, there are also patterns for the way authority is shared among managers at various levels, depending on the structure selected. Along with authority comes accountability. *Accountability* is where an individual is held accountable for how well they use their authority and *responsibility* for performing their assigned task. Accountability may be two-pronged—punishment and reward. If an employee does not perform to standards there will be a penalty and if predetermined responsibilities are met a reward will follow.

Two terms are commonly used to describe the degree to which power is distributed in an organization: centralization and decentralization. *Centralization* refers to the concentration of authority at the top levels of management, where a high proportion of power to make important decisions lies. In contrast, *decentralization* refers to a more widespread sharing of decision-making power throughout the various management levels. Decentralization of authority is evident in organizations that promote teamwork, employee empowerment, and creative decision making and is effective for complex organizations that experience constant change (such as health care facilities). The process by which managers allocate authority to workers who report to them is called *delegation*.

Delegation

By allowing another person (for example, a line employee) to act for him or her in the workings of an organization, a manager is sharing authority and responsibility. A manager can share power through *delegation* but does not give power away. Delegation enables managers to accomplish more than they could if they attempted to do every task themselves. By delegating tasks, managers can spend time on the functions of planning and staff development. Delegation of responsibility and authority is especially important during a manager's absence, when an assistant (or understudy) can assume interim responsibility for the unit's performance and has the authority to carry out the responsibility. In large departments, a manager may need to train more than one assistant to assume certain portions of the manager's work.

Another advantage of delegation is that it permits the manager to share responsibility for a task with an employee who has more skill or training to perform that task. Delegation is important as a training device, providing employees with additional skills and knowledge. If poorly managed, however, the process of delegation can have some negative side effects. The most obvious problem is that some essential task may not be accomplished or it may be performed badly or late.

To work well, the process of delegation should follow these four steps:

1. The manager must assign a clear objective or a well-defined task to the employee.
2. The manager must grant the employee the necessary authority to accomplish the task and must ensure that everyone involved in the activity understands that the employee has been given this authority.
3. The employee in turn must understand the objective and accept the authority and responsibility for accomplishing it. This acceptance creates an obligation on the part of the employee to accomplish the task.
4. The manager must hold the employee accountable for accomplishing the task satisfactorily.

In addition to these basic elements of delegation, managers should consider several other factors when deciding to share their responsibility. For example:

- Managers must select employees who have the skills to accomplish the task or are willing to learn the required skills.
- Although managers should allow employees to assume responsibility for the whole task, they should monitor the employees' progress (especially if an employee is new to the assignment) to ensure success.
- Managers should anticipate some mistakes and be prepared to guide employees in correcting them.
- Managers should be certain that the lines of communication with employees are always open and that employees can rely on the managers' advice and support when needed and on praise when it is deserved.

Delegation becomes increasingly important as a manager rises to higher levels of management in the organization. How well the manager can accomplish the work of the organization is reflected by how well the manager leads the work of employees who report to him or her. Some management duties do not lend themselves to delegation and are better shared or left to the manager. They include:

- Establishing missions, goals, and objectives for the entire unit under the manager's responsibility
- Making policy decisions
- Defining standards of performance for the entire unit
- Monitoring the unit's achievement of these standards
- Taking corrective action when the standards are not met

Line and Staff Responsibilities

When managers delegate authority, they must consider the difference between employees in line positions and employees in staff positions. A *line employee* is part of the direct chain of command that has been established to accomplish the primary work of the organization. *Staff employees* support the line positions with their advice and special knowledge. In health care institutions, staff positions are found in departments of finance, human resources, marketing, legal affairs, planning, infection control, safety, management engineering, and data processing, among others. Staff positions usually do not have authority over line positions except when application of staff advice is crucial to the effective performance of line responsibilities. For example, the human resources director usually has no direct authority over tray line workers. However, because he or she has special knowledge about Occupational Safety and Health Administration (OSHA) safety standards, the human resources director knows that a worker without proper hair covering poses a risk and so apprises the foodservice director, who has authority in this case.

STAFFING THE FOODSERVICE DEPARTMENT

Before a foodservice department is organized a *work simplification plan* will need to be developed. *Work simplification* is the breakdown of the jobs into simple repetitive task to maximize efficiency, which is good for a stable environment such as serving patient trays but is less effective in a changing environment such as delivering medical nutrition therapy. Organizing the work of a department presumes that a competent staff is in place to accomplish the tasks that have been assigned. Building an effective staff involves making decisions about the tasks that need to be performed, the skills required to perform those tasks, the time needed to complete performance, and the number of employees needed to perform the work of the department.

Determination of Employee Staffing Needs

In a health care institution, several variables affect the type and number of job tasks to be performed by the foodservice department. In determining department workload, managers should ask the following questions:

- What types of service does the department offer? Is the department responsible for an employee cafeteria, a coffee shop, a patient dining room, patient tray service, outpatient clinics, or multidepartment management?
- What type of meal plan is required for the institution's patient population? Are patients offered three, four, or five meals per day, room services, tray service?

- How varied are the menu items (for example, limited, spoken, on demand, or extensive variation)? How complex are the recipes (simple, average, involved)?
- In what form are foods purchased—mostly frozen, fresh, or canned? Do prepared foods require less processing than fresh or whole ingredients?
- How many and what types of modified diets will the department need to accommodate?
- Which type of service system is used, centralized or decentralized?
- Who determines the division of labor between foodservice and nursing?
- What percentage of convenience food is used?
- Are disposable or china tableware used?
- How much time is available for meal preparation and service?
- How efficient are the department's physical facilities and equipment?
- What type of washing system is used for service ware and dishware?
- How extensively are the department's information systems automated? What are the computer links with hospital information systems?

Determining workload, type, and number of meals, service location, and so on provides information used to determine staff numbers. For example, a department that provides meal service to patients only will need less staff than a department that must staff a cafeteria. An organization using convenience food items needs fewer skilled cooks than one choosing to cook everything from scratch. All of the preceding questions assist in determining the number and skill level of employees needed by the department. To determine or forecast future needs for staff review current staff (number and positions), and update job analysis. This is a good predictor to use if new services or building additions are added.

Job Analysis

When the workload for the department and individual has been identified, a job analysis is made. *Job analysis* is a procedure to determine the duties of a particular job and the kinds of skills, experience, knowledge, and abilities needed for performing various job tasks successfully—the type of person to be hired for the job. Each foodservice task must be evaluated according to the mental and physical effort it requires, the equipment it uses, and the time and work conditions it demands. Job analysis is a tool for identifying the standard operating procedures, tools and equipment needed, and orientation and training programs. Accurate job analysis can be used to determine pay scale. A manager can gather this information by observing foodservice workers as they perform each task and by discussing their work with them. A manager should ask all relevant questions about the job:

- Who is responsible for performing the task?
- What supplies are needed, and what equipment is required?
- Why is the task performed, and why is it performed this way?
- When must the task be started, and when must it be completed?
- Where is the task performed?
- How exactly is the task performed?

Job analysis and recording of the information gathered during the analysis often benefit from the use of a questionnaire (Exhibit 6.1). Organizing the information in this way helps ensure that all tasks are analyzed on the basis of comparable observations.

EXHIBIT 6.1   Food and Medical Nutrition Therapy Job Questionnaire

Name _____

Many employees see their job and its duties differently from the way their supervisors do. Before writing job descriptions and work schedules, it is a good idea to have each employee fill out a job study questionnaire. The following questionnaire can be used to determine if you and your employees see the duties and other facets of the job in the same way. This form can also be used as an evaluation and management tool to determine if the quality and quantity of work performed meet the expectations in the work standards.

Date _____

Name _____   Job title _____

Department   Food and Nutrition Services   Hours on duty _____

Your immediate supervisor _____

Length of employment in present position _____

List your duties in order of importance as you think they are. List the most important duty as no. 1, the next as no. 2, and so forth.

_____

_____

_____

_____

_____

What do you think is the least important duty (or duties) of your job?

_____

_____

Could this work be done by people who are less trained? ___ If so, and considering the task was taken by another person, how much more time would you have available per week? ___

Does your job require you to operate any equipment? Yes ___ No ___

If so, list the kinds of equipment you use.

_____

_____

Were you trained to use the equipment properly? Yes _____ No _____

In your opinion, how much education should be required for your job? _____

What training was necessary to do your job? _____

If you failed to complete your duties or do your work properly, would anyone know? Yes _____ No _____ Who? _____

What would be the results? _____

Would the error be connected directly to you? _____

If not, what job (or position) would assume the responsibility? _____

Under the present organizational system, do you clearly understand:

A. Who your supervisor is?   Yes _____ No _____

B. Who directs the work of your supervisor?   Yes _____ No _____

Does your position give you authority over other employees in the department?

Yes _____ No _____ If yes, what positions?

Do other departments in the hospital have control over your job duties (medical, nursing, ward clerks)? Yes _____ No _____

Considering all the duties required of you, which is most pleasant? _____

_____

Why? _____

Which duty is most unpleasant to you? _____

Why? _____

To be discussed by employee and immediate supervisor:

    A. Quality of work   D. Job satisfaction

    B. Quantity of work   E. Suggestions to make job more pleasant

    C. Safety and sanitary standards

Source: Puckett© 2010 (revised). Used by permission.

Job Descriptions and Specifications

The results of job analyses are documented and used to develop job descriptions. A *job description* consists of written statements detailing the duties and responsibilities of the person holding that position. It may also contain personal competencies, equipment use, and qualifications. (See Exhibit 6.2.) Standards of performance are beneficial in developing job descriptions as they can distinguish between various levels of jobs. Job descriptions state the task to be accomplished and how the job is to be accomplished. Job descriptions should clearly define the functions of the job without jargon. Job descriptions can be used in performance evaluations and training for a specific job. A *job specification* describes the qualifications required of the person responsible for performing those tasks and applies to all candidates who apply for that job. In most organizations, the job description and job specification are combined on one standard form.

In recent years, TJC has placed increased emphasis on staff competency. Professionals are being forced to be accountable to the public to ensure competency. Professional and continuing education plus licensure or certification are several ways to determine competency. Job descriptions and performance evaluations written in competency terms is another method that can be used to ensure competency. *Competency* is multidimensional and includes "knowledge, psychomotor skills, critical thinking abilities, and interpersonal attributes." These traits need to be incorporated into the professional food and nutrition job description. Competencies for clinical RDs need to be for age-specific populations of customers (infants, adolescents, adults, or elderly). TJC human resources standards define the key processes that should be carried out by leaders of the organization to ensure competent staff.

An up-to-date job description and specification form must be kept for every job in the foodservice department. The form must be closely followed when a new employee is hired for a position, when a current employee and his or her supervisor develop objectives for the employee's performance, and when the employee's performance is evaluated by the supervisor. Exhibit 6.2 is an example of a combined job description and job specification for a position in the foodservice department.

EXHIBIT 6.2 Sample Job Description and Job Specification

Job Title: Tray Line Server—Room Service   Job Code: 99999

Department   Nutrition/Foodservices

Reports to: Medical Nutrition Specialist

Shift:

Position Summary: Responsible for foodservice to patients and other related duties including sanitation for patient foodservice areas. Has a working knowledge of foodservice procedures and delivery. There are five tray line positions as well as room service, which may rotate either monthly or bimonthly.

Minimum Qualifications: Ability to read and write English (other language may be a plus), to communicate with staff, patients, and other customers; a basic understanding of weights and measures. Experience is not required, on-the-job training will be offered in customer service, safety, and sanitation for handling food. Must be able to relate directly to customers and nursing personnel and work as a team member.

Licenses, Certificates, or Similar Qualifications: None required

Essential Functions:

1. Checks daily assignment sheet for shift duties.
2. Prepares station for serving food from tray line or for room service. Physical requirements include:
   - Transporting 22.5-inch-by-16-inch trays of food weighing up to 25 pounds. Trays are stored in carts at heights from 4 to 6 feet.
   - Stocking food on steam tables. Requires lifting food pans weighing up to 20 pounds from heights of 11 to 62 inches and loading them onto a food bar 35 inches in height.
   - Stocking beverage/ice-cream cooling units. Requires reaching over edge of cooling unit 35 inches in height with a forward reach up to 28 inches.
   - Starter position responsible for placing hot pellets or other heat-keeping devices on the tray using caution in handling hot materials.
   - When assigned to room service may be responsible for setting up as many as five separate tray requests and delivering them to patients in the time allotted for this duty.
3. Checks quality, temperature, and appearance of food, relaying any problems to supervisor. Physical requirements include corrected visual acuity of 20/20 and good sense of smell.
4. Serves food from station on tray line. Requires using appropriate utensils, such as large spoodles, ladles, and knives, for proper portion control. Beverages are served from dispensers, pitchers, taken from cooling units. All food and beverage items are placed on a tray on the conveyor belt or other movable device. Full plates of food may weigh up to 2 pounds and are placed on a conveyor belt 33–38 inches in height. Cover plates of hot food an appropriate dome.
5. Loader position loads completed trays, weighing up to 10 pounds, into transport carts. Shelf heights are 8 to 50 inches from the floor. This will vary depending on the number of room service trays to be served at one time (See chapter) May be part of a room service team which takes the food order, gather supplies, food and set tray up according to protocol. (This may be an individual or a small team.) Tray is delivered to the patient's bedside within the allotted time.
6. Cleaning tech position or tray line server transports food carts weighing up to 730 pounds to patient floors for distances up to 50 feet. Also returns carts with empty trays to the dish room. Porter duties include dish room duties and emptying 50-gallon trash cans in an outside dumpster. Trash can lift is 48 inches from ground. This is variable room service trays will need to be retrieved from patient units as needed or requested.
7. Performs floor stocking duties. Requires reaching overhead to a 73-inch height and a forward reach of 13 inches. Boxes lifted may weigh up to 25 pounds.
8. Checks assigned stations hourly for cleanliness and operates equipment as required. Check with diet office concerning any room service request.
9. Performs dish room duties as assigned, including unloading and loading dishes between carts and various workstations. Maximum weight lifted is 50 pounds occasionally to move loaded bins to different shelves on cart (11 to 34 inches). Duties require a forward reach up to 40 inches, and lifting ranges from 11 to 75 inches from the floor. Inspects dishes for cleanliness before taking to the serving line and before use.
10. Washes, drains, and dries empty food carts. Includes using spray hose and tilting 289-pound cart to drain water.
11. Cleans and sanitizes station before leaving area with approved cleaning solution.
12. Completes all line server shift assignments by end of shift. Responds to changes in the workload as assigned by the supervisor or manager. No eating or drinking in work area.
13. Uses disposable gloves and hair coverings. Facial hair and sculptured nails are not permitted in foodservice areas. Observes all sanitation, safety, and infection-control procedures.
14. Complies with policies and procedures in departmental manual and employee handbook.

Job-Related Equipment: Carts, trays, delifter, beverage dispensers, reach-in and walk-in refrigerated and freezer units, hot food storage units, steam tables, cart lift, microwave, dish machine, pulper, conveyor belt, serving utensils, blender, knives, disposable gloves, hair coverings, and safety belts.

EXHIBIT 6.2   (*Continued*)

Work Environment: Working in health care nutrition and foodservice increases the risk of exposure to sharp instruments and noise. Temperature varies in the area due to refrigerating and heating equipment. Cleaning duties include using various solutions to clean, disinfect, and polish surfaces. Tray line servers may be required to work different shifts including evenings and weekends. Standing and walking required for approximately seven hours out of an eight-hour day.

Safety Responsibility: All nutrition and foodservice employees must use good body mechanics and follow safe working procedures including infection control, OSHA guidelines for safety and proper ergonomics. The employee must report any unsafe and unsanitary conditions to a supervisor and demonstrate no on-the-job injuries due to a lack of good safety practices. On-the-job injuries must be reported immediately to the supervisor and an occurrence report completed. The environment must be protected; discard used products in appropriate containers—remember the 4Rs: Reduce, Reuse, Recycle, and Rethink.

Conditions of employment: Physical examination and drug test. Must provide proof of U.S. citizenship. No felony arrest. No visible signs of tattoos or body piercing.

Career Ladder: Through on-the-job training, advancement is possible to other positions including, but not limited to: hostess, cashier, vending, catering, cook, or clerk.

This job description reflects the general duties and principal functions of line server. It is not a detailed description of all the work requirements that may be inherent in the position. This example may not be applicable in your organization; however, it contains the major categories needed in a job description.

Every job description and job specification form must include the following elements:

- Job title and its classification or code (usually established with the help of the human resources department and used in defining salary levels and routes for promotion)
- Summary of major responsibilities of the position
- Clear statement of the minimum standards of performance for each essential function
- Description of the work environment—equipment used, possible health hazards involved, responsibility to safety, and other such essential information
- Outline of opportunities for promotion that are relevant to the position
- Minimum qualifications for eligibility to hold the job—education, training, experience, and any other special considerations such as skill set, task to be completed, autonomy, feedback

A job description and specification for every position in the foodservice department should be on file in the department director's office, as well as in the human resources department. In addition, employees should be given copies of their job descriptions and specifications on their first day of work and whenever the job requirements are changed. Using this document can lead to improved efficiency in the foodservice department by increasing the current employees' understanding of their responsibilities and by providing guidelines for training new employees.

As managers reevaluate current job descriptions and specifications or develop new ones, they must avoid establishing requirements that do not match the actual demands of the job. To cite an extreme example, managers cannot require that a patient nutrition aide have a college education or be a certified dietitian. Setting too high a standard for a position may violate certain regulations of the Equal Employment Opportunity Commission. Job descriptions should clearly identify physical requirements for the position as a reference in screening job applicants with disabilities. The Americans with Disabilities Act requires that Americans with disabilities be employed when they can perform essential functions and that reasonable accommodations be made to assist them in performing essential job functions. To ensure that job descriptions and specifications are in compliance with all federal and state laws, the foodservice director should work closely with the human resources department.

Work Division and Job Enrichment

The writing of job descriptions and specifications provides managers with the opportunity to consider how the work can be divided in such a way that employee productivity and satisfaction are maximized. At one time, the traditional method of assigning work in the foodservice department was to have employees perform specific jobs that they followed through on from start to finish. Therefore, a cook was responsible for preparing, portioning, and serving specific menu items as well as for cleanup of the equipment and workspace. In recent years, many institutions have replaced this method of assigning work a greater division of labor that makes more efficient use of skilled employees. In this system, skilled employees are assigned work according to the degree of skill needed to complete each task. This division-of-labor method allows highly skilled employees to perform fewer unskilled tasks, such as preliminary preparation of recipe ingredients and cleanup. Instead, skilled employees are responsible for tasks that use their skills to greater advantage.

Both the traditional approach and the division-of-labor approach have inherent advantages and disadvantages. In the traditional approach, employees who can do a task from start to finish have more personal commitment to their job and may be more highly motivated and accountable for the quality of the work. However, skilled employees must spend a lot of work time on portions of the job that do not require all of their expertise. From a manager's perspective, a greater division of labor is a more efficient use of the department's resources because preparation and cleanup tasks can be assigned to unskilled employees who are paid less than skilled employees.

The traditional approach is once again finding favor in foodservice departments. However, a combination of both approaches may be the most beneficial arrangement for managers and workers. In the foodservice department, for example, the measuring, weighing, and preparing of ingredients in a centralized ingredient area permits greater control of inventory and quality and modifies the division of labor so that all employees have more than one narrow set of tasks to perform. The repetitive tasks of measuring, weighing, and preparing the ingredients used in all recipes are transferred from skilled to less-skilled employees. Cleanup and maintenance responsibilities are also reassigned to those who are less skilled. To make the work of less-skilled employees more varied, their work assignments are typically enlarged to include greater responsibility, accomplishment, and achievement. This process is called *job enrichment* or *job enlargement*. For example, a tray line employee may be assigned to patient service for part of the workday, or he or she may work in the ingredient area for some portion of the workweek.

Research on work in different kinds of organizations has demonstrated the feasibility and benefit of job enrichment to provide greater employee satisfaction and to increase productivity. Both benefits can help an organization better meet the pressures of rising labor costs and diminishing availability of skilled employees. Most employees are happier when work incorporates a challenge to them and permits reasonable flexibility in determining how an assigned task is to be performed. Worker satisfaction tends to reduce turnover and the costs associated with recruiting and training new employees.

To implement job enrichment effectively, managers must be aware of the work to be accomplished, the most efficient methods for accomplishing that work, the skills each task requires, and the best means of motivating employees. The processes of job analysis and work division, which is also referred to as *job design*, means assigning specific work task to groups or individuals, must be an ongoing part of the manager's responsibility. They are also the bases for making decisions about staff size, schedules, and performance standards to be met. Chapter 11 discusses performance standards in the context of financial management and control for the foodservice department.

Determination of Staff Size

Once the type and number of foodservice tasks have been determined, job analyses have been performed, and job descriptions and specifications have been written, managers can begin to estimate the number of employees required by the operation to perform work that needs to be accomplished. This is called *staffing*. By answering the following, variables that specifically affect how much labor time the foodservice department requires can be identified.

- How much time is allocated for meal preparation and service? Is there a need for additional staff at peak periods?

- Is the service system centralized or decentralized? Traditional tray line service, room service, or a combination? (Decentralized systems usually require more personnel owing to the staffing needed in areas outside the foodservice department.)
- How efficient are the department's physical layout and equipment?
- What type of washing system is to be used for service ware and dishware? (When disposable service ware is used, the time required for washing is greatly reduced.)
- What quality of work is expected from the employees?

Careful consideration of these variables helps ensure that the foodservice department has sufficient staff. The manager must next calculate productivity, full-time equivalent (FTE), and overtime needs based on the number of staff projected.

Estimating Productivity Levels

Staffing requirements must be based on the department's output. *Output* is defined as the end result of a work process, or the transformation of inputs. Output in the nutrition and foodservice department includes a variety of meal types and nutritional units of service. Input includes food and other resources, including labor. Transformation refers to the processes that convert input to output. The ratio of input to output is defined as *productivity*.

The use of a preestablished productivity factor allows a foodservice manager to determine the staffing required to produce the number of meals provided. The first step in determining a productivity level is to establish guidelines for calculating a single unit of service or a meal. Output can be determined as actual meals/count, which is usually the case for patient meals, guest trays, late trays, between-meal nourishments, and infant formulas and feedings when the foodservice department purchases and delivers the product. However, for areas such as a cafeteria, a meal equivalent is used. Some health care facilities may determine cafeteria meals using the number by raw cost:

Raw food cost ÷ meal equivalent factor = Meal equivalents.

Meal equivalents are determined by first calculating a meal equivalent factor (MEF).

One accepted method of determining an MEF for a cafeteria is to use an average meal ticket. The average meal ticket is determined by dividing total sales by the number of customers over a predetermined length of time: average meal ticket = total sales ÷ number of customers. Special functions (catering, facility-served vending, and coffee shops and other non-cafeteria meals) would be figured as raw food cost ÷ MEF. This figure represents the average ticket for meal service and can be used to establish meal equivalents. For example, if total sales for the cafeteria equal $550 for lunch and 200 customers were served over a defined period of time, the meal equivalent would be $2.75 ($550 ÷ 200 = $2.75). The average meal ticket meal equivalent should be established after gathering at least one week of ticket averages for lunch. The meal equivalent should be verified on a quarterly basis. Another method of determining an MEF is to use the sum of the selling price for an entrée, starch, vegetable, salad, dessert, bread, butter, and beverage at the noon meal.

Once the MEF is determined, the number of meals produced can be calculated. Equivalent meals are calculated by dividing cafeteria sales for the period by the MEF (equivalent meals = sales ÷ MEF). Using the $2.75 MEF calculated above and a sales figure of $45,000 for the month, equivalent meals can be calculated as follows:

$$\text{Equivalent meals} = \$45,000 \div \$2.75 = 16,364 \text{ meals}$$

The number of equivalent meals is used to calculate productivity. Productivity in foodservice is usually expressed as meals produced per labor hour or labor hours per meal produced:

$$\frac{\text{Meals per labor hour}}{\text{Number of labor hours}} = \text{number of meals produced}$$

For the 16,364 equivalent meals produced in the cafeteria in the preceding example, a total of 2,975 hours were worked. Using the meals per labor hour calculation:

$$\text{Meals per labor hour} = 16,364 \text{ meals} \div 2,975 \text{ labor hours}$$
$$= 5.5 \text{ meals per labor hour}$$

Expressing this same productivity as labor hours per meal:

$$\frac{\text{Labor hours per meal}}{\text{Number of meals}} = \text{number of labor hours}$$

Using the same numbers as in the preceding example:

$$\text{Labor hours per meal} = 2,975 \text{ labor hours} \div 16,364 \text{ meals}$$
$$= 0.19 \text{ labor hours per meal}$$

$$\frac{\text{Payroll cost/meal served}}{\text{Meals served/day}} = \text{total daily payroll}$$

$$\text{Labor cost/day} = \text{total payroll cost/day} + \text{total of all other direct}$$
$$\text{labor cost (fringe benefits, etc./day)}$$

$$\frac{\text{Labor cost/meal served}}{\text{meals served per day/day}} = \text{total labor cost/day}$$

Guidelines for small hospitals use the standard of three to six meals per labor hour and for large hospitals, 12 meals per labor hour. Puckett suggested 14 minutes per meal. Others have suggested 11 to 12 employees for each 100 beds. For larger institutions, each employee can produce 7,200 meals per year.

The best and most accurate method of determining a meal equivalent is the adjusted occupied beds. *Adjusted occupied beds* is based on a mathematical formula used to correct the number of occupied beds to include care given to patients who are officially admitted as inpatients for at least 24 hours. At the end of each month, the accounting or admissions department provides the foodservice department with the number of adjusted beds for the month. To figure meals, 2.7 meals per adjusted day would equal number of patient meals for the month.

Because nonpatient services are similar to commercial food-service establishments, the best and most accurate method of calculating the profit margin is that used by the restaurant industry. The figures for patients and nonpatients should be reported separately.

Calculating FTE Needs

Full-time equivalency refers to an employee who works on a full-time basis for a specific period of time. The following hours and specific time periods are used in reference to FTEs:

- 8 hours per day
- 40 hours per week
- 173.33 hours per month
- 2,080 hours per year
- 1.55 employees are necessary for 7 days of one FTE position

Staffing needs are usually expressed as the number of FTEs needed for the department. FTE needs are calculated using the productivity factor in the preceding section.

1. First, the total number of labor hours must be calculated for the time period in question.
2. Second, the number of labor hours is converted to FTEs needed.

For example, if the cafeteria produced 16,364 meal equivalents in a month and the productivity standard being used is equal to 5.5 meals per labor hour, FTE needs are calculated as follows:

$$\text{Labor hours} = 16,364 \text{ meals per month}$$
$$= 2,975 \text{ labor hours per month}$$

$$5.5 \text{ meals per labor hour}$$

$$\text{Number of FTEs} = 2,975 \text{ labor hours per month} = 17.2 \text{ FTEs}$$

$$173.33 \text{ hours per FTE per month}$$

The number of FTEs is calculated for the day, week, month, or year by determining the number of labor hours needed in the period and dividing by the FTE factor identified earlier. For example, if department responsibilities require 40 hours of work per week, 40 hours ÷ 8 hours per FTE per day = 5 FTEs. For a department that needs 300 hours per week, 300 hours ÷ 40 hours per FTE per week = 7.5 FTEs. The monthly need of FTEs would be 2,113 hours per month ÷ 173.3 = 12.2 FTEs. Yearly the number of FTEs would be 25,536 hours ÷ 2,080 hours = 12.1 employees. FTEs required for the department do not necessarily reflect the number of staff members employed by the department. For example, if the department needs 10.5 FTEs on an annual basis to run the department, it may have a total of 13 employees. Nine of the employees may be full-time employees working a total of 40 hours a week, and three of the employees may be 0.5 FTEs, or those who work 20 hours per week.

$$9 \times 40 = 360 \text{ hours per week}$$

$$3 \times 20 = 60 \text{ hours per week}$$

$$420 \text{ hours per week}$$

$$420 \text{ hours per week} \div 40 \text{ hours per FTE per week} = 10.5 \text{ FTEs}$$

Anticipating Overtime Needs

In the preceding examples, the number of FTEs required as regular productive hours was calculated. This figure represents core staffing based on the number of meals served. To determine complete staffing, the manager must consider the number of overtime, benefit, and nonproductive hours to be paid. (Budgeting is covered in detail in Chapter 11.)

The amount of overtime used in the foodservice department depends on several factors, including fluctuations in demand, inefficient work processes or equipment, employee injuries, availability of workers, and department size. Some industry experts consider overtime above 2 percent of productive hours paid to be excessive and in need of attention. Most organizations establish an overtime percentage based on historical data and environmental information before completing the annual operating budget. In an effort to lower the amount of overtime, the number of part-time or occasional (on-call) employees can be increased. To determine the number of FTEs required to cover overtime, the following formula is used:

$$\text{Total FTEs} \times \text{overtime percentage} = \text{number of FTEs for overtime}$$

For example,

$$10.5 \text{ FTEs} \times 1 \text{ percent overtime} = 0.11 \text{ FTE}$$

Preparation for Outside Consultants

Effective control of labor costs requires a productivity measurement system to facilitate decision making. Many health care organizations are using outside consultants who attempt to generate productivity standards for the foodservice department. To prepare for outside consultants, it is incumbent on foodservice directors to identify and establish productivity measurements for their departments. Having departmental statistics available for outside consultants allows the foodservice manager to be in control of productivity demands. Exhibit 6.3 shows a productivity form that can be used to track internal productivity. This type of internal monitoring provides the foodservice manager with information for consultants or support documentation for staff or service changes.

SCHEDULING WORK IN A FOODSERVICE DEPARTMENT

Because health care institutions require round-the-clock staffing, the foodservice director must make sure that the jobs in his or her department are filled at the appropriate times in each 24-hour period. *Scheduling* is having an adequate number of staff on duty to perform work that needs to be completed. Therefore, scheduling the workweek and specific hours each employee must be on duty is a key step in achieving efficiency in the use of labor dollars while meeting the institution's service objectives.

When developing schedules they need to meet the needs of the department, not the employee; however, when possible the employee's preference should be considered. When schedule conflicts happen, honor requests in the order in which they were received. If the department employs PRN (personnel as needed) perhaps one of these individuals could be called in to cover the conflict.

The 40-hour workweek is common for full-time employees in most of the nation's businesses. Actually, this period includes only 35 working hours because each hourly employee has a 15-minute paid rest period every 4 hours and a 30-minute unpaid meal period each day. Although the workweek has commonly been divided into five equal workdays, some innovative foodservice directors have developed schedules in which employees work 10½ hours per day and 4 days per week. Such schedules have produced notable improvements in employee productivity, fewer called-in-sick days, less overtime, and job satisfaction. Four-day schedules may not work in all foodservice departments. At the present time more than one-third of U.S. employers now give the option to its employees. Another type of schedule calls for employees to work 4 days, take 3 days off, work 5 days, take 2 days off, and then begin the cycle again without working more than 8 days in any two-week pay period.

EXHIBIT 6.3   Sample Productivity Form

ABC Hospital

Foodservice Department Productivity Report for the Year:

Variables	Jan	Feb	Mar	Apr	May	Jun	Jul	Aug	Sep	Oct	Nov	Dec	Annual Average
Worked hours													
Paid hours													
Inpatient meals													
Outpatient meals													
Other meals													
Cafeteria meals													
Cafeteria sales													
Meal equivalent													
Total meals													
Payroll costs													
Food costs													
Supply costs													
Other costs													
Total direct costs													
Adjusted patient days													
Internal Trends													
Worked hours/meal													
Meals/labor hour													
Paid time (%) off													
Total salary/meal													
Food cost/meal													
Supply cost/meal													
Total cost/meal													
Other meals (%)													
(%) labor/total cost													
Labor cost/adjusted patient day													
Total cost/adjusted patient day													
Total meals/adjusted patient day													
Worked FTEs													
Paid FTEs													

Flexible Schedules

Retraining employees to perform a broader range of duties by overlapping schedules is a part of a job enlargement plan. For example, tray line workers could learn to perform production tasks and some sanitation duties, and sanitation workers could learn to perform some food production and tray line duties. This flexibility in scheduling significantly reduces the total number of employees needed to meet labor needs. It also may result in less absenteeism and turnover because of improved employee morale and job satisfaction. The new schedule provides each employee with the opportunity for a wider set of duties and is an important element in any job enrichment effort.

Professional employees in the department also may wish to take advantage of flexible scheduling. For example, a registered dietitian might choose to work during the institution's most active period, between 6:30 A.M. and 3 P.M. Two part-time professional employees might arrange their schedules so that together they meet the requirements of an FTE position; that is, one might work three 8-hour days, and the other two 8-hour days. *Flex time* or flexible working hours provide the employee some choice in their daily working hours such as when to begin and end work while still working a full eight hours. This type of schedule allows employees to attend to personal needs such as medical visits and personnel affairs. This arrangement is called *job sharing* or *job splitting*. A nutrition host might choose to work four 10-hour days instead of five 8-hour days so that he or she could cover all three meals served on the days worked. Others might choose to work 9 hours for four days and then take half a day off on the day of the week when there are fewer rounds and admissions. This type of flexible scheduling is referred to as *compressed workweek*.

Another expansion of flexible scheduling is *telecommuting*. This type of schedule is used when an employee spends some working time *outside* of the office. They are linked to the office, supervisor, and customers. They use a variety of IT tools. This type of work decreases interruptions and distractions and increases productivity. It provides freedom as to when work is completed and more time for the employee to plan and be creative.

Master Schedules

No matter which system of scheduling is best suited for a particular institution, the work schedule must be outlined by position (names), times for duty, and days off, and posted where employees have ready access. (This is a surveyor requirement.) The schedule should indicate the days on duty for each employee, daily scheduled hours (when they vary from one day to the next), days off, vacation days, and so forth. A *rotating master schedule* should be developed to reduce the amount of time the director spends in scheduling employees each week. Rotating master schedules ensure that employees have regularly scheduled days off without working more than 80 hours in a pay period or work hours per week. A rotating master schedule may complete the scheduling cycle every three, five, six, or seven weeks. Schedules must ensure that employees share responsibility for working weekends and holidays so that the same people are not scheduled to work every weekend or holiday.

Master schedules are designed to correspond to the length of the pay period so that each employee is assured of working an equal number of hours during each period. In addition, the number of overtime hours can be minimized when the schedule is designed to coincide with pay periods.

The foodservice director should examine the schedule of every employee. The daily hours to be worked and the scheduled days off should be assigned fairly, without favoritism. Also, situations in which an employee has the late shift on one day and an early shift the following day should be avoided, as should split shifts because most employees prefer a continuous workday. Rotating shifts (in which an employee is scheduled for varying work periods from one week or pay period to the next) are frequently used to provide more flexibility for management and employees. Once the master schedule has been set, frequent major revisions should be avoided. Although rigidity is not the goal here, a relatively consistent work schedule that repeats with every pay period helps establish smooth work patterns for individual employees. Furthermore, within certain work groups, employees must depend on being familiar with one another's pace of work to both ensure an adequate level of productivity and minimize the risk of accidents and injuries. Finally, consistent schedules permit employees to plan their personal time better, thus reducing the likelihood of absenteeism and employee turnover.

Other Schedule Types

In addition to scheduling employee workweeks, the foodservice director and his or her managers need to construct several types of schedules to ensure that all department work flows smoothly during a given day. The *daily schedule* pattern illustrated in Figure 6.10 indicates the different foodservice positions that need to be occupies within the department and the daily hours during which the functions of those positions usually must be accomplished.

Figure 6.11 shows an example of a *shift schedule* for eight cooks working in a department that serves three meals per day seven days per week. Cooks A, B, and C together cover the morning shift from 6 A.M. to 2:30 P.M. during which two cooks are on duty. On the one day per week when all three cooks are scheduled to work—Thursday on this schedule—they may perform extra cleaning duties or prepare special foods. The cooks on the afternoon shift, 10 A.M. to 7:30 P.M., are scheduled in the same way. Cooks D and E relieve each other so that four days per week, only one of the two cooks is on duty. Cooks D and E prepare foods for modified diets or special salads and desserts.

Written daily work schedules guide each employee's activities during the workday, listing the duties to be performed during specified time periods and the routine cleaning tasks that must be completed. An example of an individual employee work schedule is shown in Figure 6.12. Providing this type of breakdown for employees has several advantages:

- The employee has written instructions on hand for each task and does not need to rely on verbal orders, which are more easily misunderstood or forgotten.

FIGURE 6.10 Example of a Daily Schedule Pattern

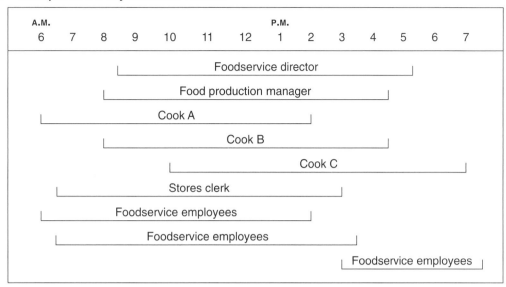

FIGURE 6.11 Example of a Shift Schedule

Week Ending: _____

Name/Classification	Sun.	Mon.	Tues.	Wed.	Thurs.	Fri.	Sat.
J. Lloyd–Cook A	6:00–2:30	6:00–2:30	Day off	Day off	6:00–2:30	6:00–2:30	6:00–2:30
T. Walker–Cook B	6:00–2:30	6:00–2:30	6:00–2:30	6:00–2:30	6:00–2:30	Day off	Day off
J. Foot–Cook C	Day off	Day off	6:00–2:30	6:00–2:30	6:00–2:30	6:30–2:00	6:30–2:00
I. Shenk–Cook D	9:30–6:00	9:30–6:00	9:30–6:00	Day off	Day off	9:30–6:00	9:30–6:00
M. Smith–Cook E	8:30–5:00	Day off	Day off	9:30–6:00	9:30–6:00	8:30–5:00	8:30–5:00
A. Frank–Cook F	10:00–7:30	10:00–7:30	10:00–7:30	Day off	Day off	10:00–7:30	10:00–7:30
B. Tyler–Cook G	10:00–7:30	Day off	Day off	10:00–7:30	10:00–7:30	10:00–7:30	10:00–7:30
B. James–Cook H	10:00–7:30	10:00–7:30	10:00–7:30	10:00–7:30	10:00–7:30	Day off	Day off

- Deadlines help an employee set objectives for each portion of the workday.
- Work can proceed more smoothly, with less time spent waiting for a new set of instructions or explanations.
- The manager can use the individual schedule to maintain workload balance among employees.

Some organizations set up separate cleaning schedules and rotate cleaning duties among employees. Rotating unpleasant jobs is usually desirable, but most of the daily and weekly cleaning tasks should be incorporated into individual schedules.

Computerized Scheduling

Scheduling for the foodservice department is a complex task requiring a large amount of information. Because of the complexity and time involved in scheduling, some departments have turned to computer software for this activity. Scheduling software can track the number of full- and part-time employees, the number of hours worked, vacation or other days off, specific times requested off by employees, and when an employee goes into overtime. *Computerized scheduling* also consistently provides management with timely reports of hours worked, which is necessary to track department productivity. In addition, workload and peak times can be predicted, allowing flexible staffing; management time is freed for other duties; and computer objectivity ensures scheduling equity among employees. Unlike manual schedules, computer scheduling can accommodate last-minute changes with little effort and time.

Scheduling software usually includes information about the job requirements for each position and information regarding employee capabilities. Based on this information, the manager can set features that allow the software to make the match of employees to days,

FIGURE 6.12 Example of a Work Schedule for an Individual Employee

Work Schedule for Cafeteria Counter Employee

Name: _____

Hours: 5:30 A.M. to 2:00 P.M.

30 minutes for breakfast

15 minutes for coffee break

Position: Cafeteria Counter Employee No. 1

Supervised by: _____

Day off: _____

Relieved by: _____

5:30 to 7:15 A.M.	1. Read breakfast menu
	2. Ready equipment for breakfast meal
	a. Turn on heat in cafeteria counter units for hot foods, grill, and dish warmers at 6 A.M.
	b. Prepare counter units for cold food at 6 A.M.
	c. Obtain required serving utensils and put in position for use
	d. Place dishes where needed, those required for hot food in dish warmer
	3. Make coffee (consult supervisor for instructions and amount to be made)
	4. Fill milk dispenser
	5. Obtain food items to be served cold: fruit, fruit juice, dry cereals, butter, cream, etc.; place in proper location on cafeteria counter
	6. Obtain hot food and put in hot section of counter
	7. Check with supervisor for correct portion sizes if this has not been decided previously
6:30 to 8:00 A.M.	1. Open cafeteria doors for breakfast service
	2. Replenish cold food items, dishes, and tableware
	3. Notify cook before hot items are depleted
	4. Make additional coffee as needed
	5. Keep counters clean; wipe up spilled food
8:00 to 8:30 A.M.	Eat breakfast
8:30 to 10:30 A.M.	1. Break down serving line and return leftover foods to refrigerators and cook's area as directed by supervisor
	2. Clean equipment, serving counters, and tables in dining area
	3. Prepare serving counters for coffee break
	a. Get a supply of cups, saucers, and tableware
	b. Make coffee
	c. Fill cream dispensers
	d. Keep counter supplied during coffee break period (9:30–10:30)
	4. Fill salad dressing, relish, and condiment containers for noon meal
10:00 to 11:30 A.M.	1. Confer with supervisor regarding menu items and portion sizes for noon meal
	2. Clean equipment, counters, and tables in dining area
	3. Prepare counters for lunch
	a. Turn on heat in hot counter and dish warmers at 11 A.M.
	b. Set up beverage area
	c. Place service utensils and dishes in position for use
	4. Make coffee
	5. Set portioned cold foods on cold counter
11:00 to 11:15 A.M.	Coffee break
11:30 A.M. to 1:30 P.M.	1. Open cafeteria doors for noon meal service
	2. Replenish cold food items, dishes, and tableware as needed
	3. Keep counters clean; wipe up spilled food
	4. Make additional coffee as needed
1:30 to 2:00 P.M.	1. Turn off heating and cooling elements in serving counters
	2. Help break down serving line
	3. Return leftover foods to proper places
	4. Clean equipment and serving counter as directed by supervisor
2:00 P.M.	Off duty

FIGURE 6.13 Example of a Manager's Daily Planner

Time of Day	Already Planned	Must Do	Comments/Carryovers
8:00	Staff meeting	1. Budget review	
:15		2. Write QA report	
:30		3. Procedure for use of new dishwasher	
:45			
9:00			
:15	Start budget review		
:30			
:45			
10:00			
:15			
:30			
:45			
11:00			
:15	Break		
:30			
:45			
12:00–1:00	Lunch		
1:15	Write QA report	Complete tomorrow	
:30			Complete QA report tomorrow
:45			See DB about figures
2:00	Complete budget review		Call engineer–dish machine
:15			Infection Control Committee
:30			on Wednesday
:45			
3:00			
:15			
:30			
:45			
4:00			
:15			
:30			
:45			
5:00			

times, and tasks to be performed. Scheduling software can offer many benefits to a department, as long as program users are adequately trained.

Managing Time Effectively

Although managers assume responsibility for developing work schedules for their employees, they often fail to schedule their own time to best advantage. One step toward effective time management is for managers to analyze the way they currently use their time. A detailed *log of daily activities* helps managers keep track of what they do, the amount of time spent on each activity, others involved in the activities, and how important each act is to the day's objectives. Analysis of these logs helps managers determine how effectively they spent their time and some of the reasons they do not reach their objectives during a particular week. For example, unnecessary

phone calls, avoidable interruptions, or lack of a good work plan all contribute to an inefficient use of time. Using this analysis allows the manager to do first things first. Maintaining a daily planner allows a manager to keep track of necessary activities and aids in the appropriate use of time (Figure 6.13).

Much of the manager's time is spent in meetings, working on departmental business, counseling employees, and walking around interacting with employees.

Prioritizing Work

Once managers have monitored their daily activities, they are in a better position to list the essential tasks of the coming week and assign each a priority: **A** for tasks that are critical, **B** for tasks that are important but not critical, and **C** for tasks that might be delegated (Figure 6.14). Look for duplication of efforts and eliminate

FIGURE 6.14 Example of a Foodservice Director's Weekly Planner

Goals (Priorities)	Estimated Time	Day Completed	Comments
1. Complete budget (A)	6½ hours	Wednesday	Give budget to secretary to type by Wed, noon; review Thurs.; turn in by Fri., 3 P.M.
2. Discuss disciplinary action (A)	2½ hours	Thursday	Meet with Human Resources Department
3. Attend meetings (B)	3½ hours	Monday, Thursday	Be sure to go to staff meeting
4. Handle mail, meet with employees (B)			
5. Review magazines (C)	1 hour	Thursday	

	Monday	Tuesday	Wednesday	Thursday	Friday
9:00	Attend				Attend
9:30	nutrition	Complete	Complete		staff
10:00	support	budget	budget	Review	meeting
10:30	meeting			budget	
11:00					
11:30					
12:00					
12:30					
1:00		Complete	Discuss		
1:30		budget	disciplinary		
2:00			action		
2:30					
3:00					Turn in budget!
3:30				Review	
4:00				magazines	
4:30					
5:00					

them. Priorities should be set for the tasks to be accomplished daily and for longer-term projects, such as recruiting a new staff member, developing a budget, or gathering information to plan a new program. Large projects need to be prioritized and broken down into their component parts and tackled one step at a time. Adjust estimated time to do a job. Build in time for emergencies.

Another method of prioritizing work has been suggested by Stephen Covey in his book *7 Habits of Highly Effective People*. The focus of Covey's priority system is to manage "self" rather than time, using four quadrants for time management:

1. *Urgent and important.* This quadrant encompasses crisis situations or problems. Being problem-oriented and driven by deadlines prevents managers from focusing on more important tasks.
2. *Not urgent and important.* This quadrant has to do with effective personal management as represented by planning functions. Functioning in Quadrant 2 requires the manager to seek balance in work and personal activities and to undertake important activities that are not urgent.

3. *Urgent and not important.* Like Quadrant 1, the driving force for Quadrant 3 is urgency. Unlike Quadrant 1, however, task urgency here is determined by others. That is, these tasks may be urgent to someone else but not for the manager's goals and focus.

4. *Not urgent and not important.* The activities in this quadrant are referred to as "comfort" activities, those tasks that require no great amount of thought and may be relaxing. The biggest problem with focusing on tasks in this area is that comfort tasks prevent managers from focusing on the tasks in Quadrants 1 and 2.

With the self-management theory, time management is the responsibility of the manager and not determined by the tasks. Managers must choose the activities they will spend time on. To meet the challenges of a rapidly changing health care environment, managers should focus energy on the tasks of planning outlined in Quadrant 2.

Setting Limits

Managers should avoid the four biggest time wasters: (1) excessive telephone calls, (2) unnecessarily long meetings, (3) unexpected visitors, and (4) paperwork. To reduce the time spent on each, managers should set their own limits:

- Develop a system to screen and answer telephone calls and e-mail. Delete items that do not apply to the job.
- If possible, schedule no more than one hour each day for returning telephone calls. Each conversation should be related to the work at hand.
- Control your calendar—set time limits for necessary activities; do not let someone else control your request for meetings.
- Although meetings can be useful, make sure that the meeting time is used productively by planning an agenda or proposing an outcome and by ending the meeting at a predetermined time.
- To better minimize unexpected visitors, avoid making them feel too welcome or too comfortable. When possible, a closed door and being screened by a secretary should do much to discourage unscheduled visitors. If that does not suit a manager's style or the institution's working climate, a manager might stand when an unscheduled visitor enters the room and remain standing until he or she leaves. Other options are to suggest a better time for a meeting, make an appointment to see the person in his or her own work area, and end the meeting as soon as the business is completed.

- Managers can reduce their share of paperwork by using several tactics. Have someone screen the paperwork and sort it according to its relative importance. Do not handle any piece of paper more than once. Write responses directly on memos and return them to the sender. Whenever possible and appropriate, delegate responsibility for handling paperwork.
- Minimize details by trying to find a way to handle them accurately and with a minimum effort. Delegate some of the details to staff.
- Say no to a request that deters you from what you need or should be doing.
- Do not search the web for information that does not apply to your job. Avoid playing games on the computer or performing personal individual tasks such as paying bills online.

Time management, like any other management skill, can be learned with practice. Managers need to begin applying time-management techniques to their own schedules to achieve the full range of their professional and personal objectives.

SUMMARY

The organizing function of management involves designing appropriate organizational structures, grouping work according to some common criteria such as function or product, and establishing relationships between the organization's activities and its job positions. In addition to divisions of authority and responsibility according to departments or units, managers often find that work groups such as committees, task forces, and project teams are useful in completing certain types of activities that require the expertise and cooperation of several departments. Foodservice departments benefit in many ways from participation in such work groups.

When coordinating work, managers also must organize the way authority is distributed throughout an organization. The sharing of authority by managers with their employees is called *delegation* and is instrumental in obtaining for managers the support, advice, and special knowledge of staff outside the direct chain of command.

The building of a competent staff to carry out the work of an organization involves assessment of the tasks to be performed and the employees needed for performing those tasks. Managers determine staffing needs by assessing workload, undertaking job analyses, and preparing job descriptions and specifications. The smooth flow of work throughout an organization is ensured through the careful scheduling of employees' time and by the managers' vigilance over the expenditures of their own time.

Ad hoc committee
Accountability
Chain of command
Closed system
Compressed schedule
Computer-assisted schedule
Cross-functional team
Departmentalization
Flat organization
Flexible schedule
High-performance team
Job analysis
Job description
Job enrichment
Job specification
Line and staff
Line of communications
Matrix model

Open system
Organizational culture
Organizational structure
Productivity
Project team
Reintegration
Self-managed team
Span of control
Standing committee
Systems approach
Tall organization
Task force
Telecommunicating schedule
Time management
Unity of command
Virtual team
Work schedule

DISCUSSION QUESTIONS

1. What is the best method to use to draw an organizational chart that would show line and staff and the span of control?
2. Compare the different work teams as to needs, advantages, and disadvantages of each.
3. Describe the high-performance teams and the manager's responsibility to this type of team.
4. What is the difference of self-managed teams as compared to other types of teams? Why is it important to develop self-managed teams?
5. Explain the importance of a system approach for foodservice.
6. What is the importance of developing an organizational culture and the advantages of such a culture?
7. Define authority, delegation, and responsibility and describe how each is used in distributing authority.
8. What is the best method for calculating productivity levels and comparison of benchmarking with peers?
9. Develop a self-time-management program.

CHAPTER 7

COMMUNICATION

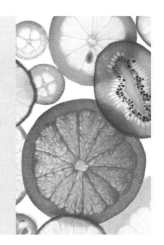

LEARNING OBJECTIVES

- Describe the communication process and barriers to it.
- Select both verbal and nonverbal communications.
- Choose correct spelling, punctuation, and grammar when writing memos, business letters, justifications, and reports.
- Analyze barriers to communication and find methods to overcome them.
- Prepare and conduct effective meetings, communicate daily with staff.
- Learn the process of making effective presentations.
- Actively learn to listen to what others are saying.

COMMUNICATION CAN BE defined as the process of conveying verbal or written information from one party to another; it involves a sender transmitting a message and a receiver understanding it. Effective communication plays a vital role in how well employees will work together to complete a task and to accomplish outcome goals. Communicating effectively is both a language process and a people process that requires interpersonal skills. Communication skills are vital to performing the basic functions of management: planning, organizing, controlling, and especially leading. In fact, managers spend most of their time in activities that involve some form of communication. The strength of your communications will directly reflect on the effectiveness of your performance efforts.

To run smoothly, organizations must have efficient information distribution systems that ensure that messages are received in the manner intended. The kinds of information disseminated throughout an organization include goals and objectives, change strategies,

policies and procedures, behaviors and concerns, and problems and solutions. Communication is essential for obtaining information from customers because it allows managers to enhance service delivery. Furthermore, harmony, cooperation, and efficiency within a work team depend on effective communication as a means of ensuring that all members understand the team's objectives and the tasks to be performed.

Communicating in health care organizations requires the manager to fulfill the following roles:

- Receptive listener in interactions with customers, superiors, peers, and employees
- Distributor of information in both sending work plans and instructions to employees and reporting activities and results to peers and superiors
- Spokesperson for top-level managers in communicating with employees and spokesperson for employees in communicating with top-level managers

This chapter examines the elements and process of communication, that is, factors that affect how messages are sent and how they are received and interpreted. Three barriers to effective communication—environmental, experiential, and behavioral—are looked at. The two means of communication, the spoken word and the written word, are discussed, as well as a third medium of nonverbal communication through body language. In discussing methods of communication, pointers are provided on how to plan and conduct meetings, make oral presentations, and design effective written communications. The chapter closes with a brief description of the manager's role in mediating and resolving conflict.

FIGURE 7.1 Communication Process

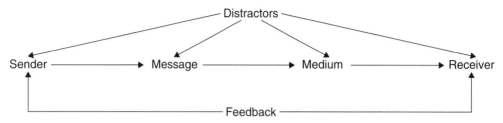

COMMUNICATION PROCESS

The communication process is complex, consisting of the formation, transmission, and translation of information. Five basic elements are involved in the communication process:

1. The message sender—the person who creates and transmits a message to another person or people
2. The message (information)
3. The medium used to transmit the message, such as print, telephone, fax, or e-mail
4. The message receiver who receives message from sender
5. The feedback exchanged between receiver and sender (Figure 7.1)

The *message* is the actual physical product that may be typically words and nonverbal cues. The *medium* or channel is how the message travels. The *sender* not only determines the message to be sent but is also responsible to deliver the message in a way that minimizes the chance that the message will be distorted.

The *receiver* is the person who receives the message and decodes (deciphers) the message that was received. The receiver must also interpret the message based on personal experience. *Feedback* is exchanged between the sender and the receiver to determine whether the message received was the message intended (see Figure 7.1). It is also the reaction to the message.

Feedback is necessary to let the sender know that the message has been received and is understood. It can have a negative or positive effect on business and personal relationships. Positive feedback confirms and reinforces desirable behavior. Positive feedback should be specific, for example feedback to a cook—the beef stew was excellent, the garnish added to the appearance and taste. Negative feedback has the opportunity to allow employees to evaluate themselves and make changes in their behavior. Negative feedback will need to be handled with respect and care. Negative feedback could relate to an employee's job skills. With care, the manager could advise the employee on a program that includes additional education and skill development. If followed, the feedback may have an impact on the employee's future. Sometimes feedback is hard to decipher; managers will need to observe behavior, listen to what is said, and check for nonverbal cues.

All feedback needs to be given with a positive attitude, be specific. Before giving feedback, be sure it is accurate.

When messages are sent there are *interferences*. This interference is in the flow of communications between the sender and the receiver. There are many forms of interference and include:

- *Apathy*, when either the receivers or senders think no one cares about their performance, whether they are performing well or not.
- Difference in *perception*—the sender must send a clear message that is understood by the receiver.
- *Semantics*, the meaning of words. Words have different meanings to different people.
- *Lack of knowledge*, when the senders or receivers do not have the knowledge to understand each other due to language or word use.
- *Defensiveness*, when the senders or the receivers are given information that may clash with their self-concept—a way to try not to lower their self-esteem.
- *Emotions*, such as anger or anxiety, may cause either the sender or the receiver to not concentrate on the message.
- *Lack of interest*, when neither the sender or the receiver has any interest in the message.
- *Perception*, when senders and receivers perceive the message in a different way, a reflection on what they believe.
- *Personality*, clashes may occur between the senders and the receivers, especially if they do not like each other. If they are friends and like each other, communication is likely to go well.
- *Appearance*, especially when using oral communications, may interfere with the communication cycle. Bias against obesity, for instance, will more than likely show.
- Each element affects the creation, transmission, and translation of information in the communication process. Influences outside the communication process, called distracters or *barriers*, can affect each element of the process.

Senders and receivers are influenced by their respective personal characteristics, shaped over a lifetime by language, education, religion, life experiences, culture, environment, work, and physical traits. Because lifetime experiences affect the perception of both sender and receiver, understanding the message sent means understanding the sender. Likewise, ensuring that the message is interpreted as intended implies understanding the receiver.

The *medium* selected often depends on the message to be conveyed. Sometimes—for example, when immediate feedback is desired—it is appropriate to convey a message verbally in person rather than by a written memorandum. Feedback is exchanged between sender and receiver to confirm whether the message received was the one the messenger intended. Feedback may be negative or positive. It should be provided as soon as possible and should be problem-oriented, not people-oriented. The feedback process is affected by the medium used and by the personal characteristics of sender and receiver. In other words, the five elements of the communication process are interrelated.

Communication may be one-way or two-way. In one-way communication the sender does not expect feedback from the receiver. For example, the receiver is sent a notice stating there will be a meeting at a specific time. Two-way communication is where feedback from the sender to the receiver is required. This can be accomplished face-to-face or by a written response.

Communication Barriers

At any point the communication process can be interrupted or interfered with by distracters. *Distracters* are circumstances that interfere with the sender's or receiver's attention and draw it away from the message sent or that alter or otherwise compromise the message. Distracters can include absence of feedback, physical distracters, status, cultural differences, and language problems. Barriers can cause miscommunication of even the simplest facts in the communication process, and as messages increase in complexity, the potential for miscommunication increases. Communication barriers can be divided into four broad categories: environmental, experiential, behavioral, and cultural.

Barriers Due to the Environment

An obvious distracter in the communication process is an *environmental interference*, which distorts or breaks the information flow between sender and receiver. Two types of environmental barriers exist: physical (or mechanical) and operational.

Examples of *physical* or mechanical environmental barriers are broken connectors or static on telephone lines, conversations interrupted by ringing phones or knocks on office doors, or loud laughter that disrupts a meeting. *Operational* barriers have to do with system breakdowns. Examples are letters that are lost in the mail, misplacement of a critical memo due to an inadequate filing system, or loss of data due to a programming error.

A foodservice manager whose office is near a cafeteria entrance can anticipate certain physical environmental barriers (such as noise). Therefore, the manager should schedule a one-on-one, manager–employee conference in a private conference room. Otherwise, it could be difficult for the sender (the manager) to communicate the message (the consequences of a specific inappropriate behavior and what must be done to change it) to the receiver (the employee) because the medium (the sender's voice) might be drowned out by the cafeteria's noise. Unless the message is conveyed and received accurately and without distraction, feedback can be virtually impossible.

Managers cannot anticipate *all* environmental distracters. In a situation where a patient with diabetes was given the wrong meal tray, the manager's responsibility is to recognize the probability of an operational environmental barrier. The manager should then investigate the foodservice department's information systems to discover the reason for the miscommunication of patient tray information.

Barriers Due to Experience or Personal Perception

In Chapter 1, the increasing cultural diversity of the workforce and the effect this has on daily management functions and service operations were noted. In the communication process, both sender and receiver are products not only of life experiences but also of accumulative cultural experiences. Collectively, these experiences define their personal perception in terms of who they are, how they feel about themselves, and how accepting they are of similarities and differences in customers, peers, coworkers, superiors, and subordinates. Words, actions, and situations are perceived by different people and groups and who may react differently to the same message.

Personal bias can create barriers to communication. For example, a cook asked to clean up a spill on the floor during lunch meal preparation to prevent someone from falling might interpret the request as a waste of time, even a form of punishment if the cook perceives the job of a cleaning technician to be less important than his or her own.

In the situation described earlier, the same message also might be received negatively if the cook is already busy preparing meat loaf. In addition to being influenced by personal outlook, messages and their interpretation can be affected by the circumstances of the moment. Pressures and stressors—those imposed by the work environment and those that are the result of personal perception—can affect all five elements of the communication process. Therefore, managers must be in touch not only with their own stress levels but also with those of others with whom they come in contact.

Savvy managers make every effort to suspend judgments that are based on differences in appearance or use of language, for example. Otherwise, they risk a loss of opportunity that may be conveyed in information exchanges. A menu planner's suggestion to incorporate more ethnic entrées into patients' menus can be seen as a business opportunity because these managers are able to interpret the message with objectivity. Such managers demonstrate the valuable skill of separating the message from the messenger.

Barriers Due to Behavior

Personal perspectives and life experiences may precipitate certain behaviors that can block or distort the flow of information. Sometimes the *behavior* (the action) is the product of an emotion (a feeling). Emotions can affect the transmission and interpretation of messages. Emotions can be conscious or unconscious. A tray assembler angry at being refused a promotion might deliberately miscommunicate patient menu orders. A cook denied approval to purchase precooked roast beef rather than preparing it might fail to take the meat out of the oven before it burns. In both cases, the flow of information is impeded because of what can be described as an *emotional behavior barrier to communication*. The emotions in the earlier examples are anger and disappointment, respectively.

An effective tool for removing the negative influence of emotional behavior is acknowledgment. Acknowledgment does not mean making judgments about the legitimacy of the feeling. If the tray assembler and the manager are "found out" and held accountable, their respective superiors should not judge the unacceptable behavior but simply state that the listener understands: "I understand that you are upset about _____ ; however, it is important to discuss how the situation can be handled."

Another method of handling emotional behavior is to continue the conversation while allowing—but not acknowledging—the behavior. For example, if an employee cries while the manager attempts to discuss a performance problem, the manager can simply continue the conversation. This is effective only if both manager and employee can continue to focus on the issue without allowing it to influence the outcome. If not, the conversation should be rescheduled. In emotional situations, it is important that the manager understand the other person's position before he or she can be expected to hear and understand the manager's message.

Barriers Due to Culture

Cultural factors can ease or hinder communication. A similarity in culture between senders and receivers facilitates successful communication, and the intended meaning has a higher probability of getting transferred. A difference in culture hinders the communication process, and the greater the cultural difference between sender and receiver, the greater the expected difficulty in communicating. This is especially the case in states such as California, Florida, New York, Texas, and Michigan where language (words) may not translate directly. Other cultural differences that managers need to be aware of when dealing with a culturally mixed work group include the following:

- The other's communication approach is interpreted negatively.
- The rank, status, education, and socioeconomic of the receiver may affect the message and the process.
- Nonverbal cues such as spatial separation, body language, touching, behavior, and customs may be distracters.
- The message and method used to send it may be misinterpreted if the receiver is not fluent in English.
- Interpreting words differently. The English language is difficult and words may have different meanings to different people.
- *Ethnocentrism*, the belief in the superiority of one's group and the related tendency to view others in terms of the values of one's own group, is probably the largest single barrier.
- *Stereotyping*, the tendency to oversimplify and generalize about a group of people, is another major barrier to effective communication. Stereotyping occurs between and within cultures. For example, some people think all people who work in foodservice are lazy and uneducated and could get a better job if they wanted to.
- Differences between "the haves" and the "have-nots" create barriers predicated on language, economics, social standing, location, job status, and general cultural and custom differences.

Use "politically correct" (that is, culturally sensitive) terms when communicating with coworkers. A manager should use terms that are nonoffensive or neutral to replace words or phrases in common usage that are disparaging, offensive, or insensitive.

When working with diverse cultural groups, a manager should know and learn that cultural differences will likely exist. When a misunderstanding occurs, and the other categories of barriers to communication have been eliminated, the manager should be aware that the cause may be cultural. For example, people from Japan rarely speak first in meetings because they think it is unwise. Avoid ethnocentrism and stereotyping. Be objective and appreciate the differences in the members of the work group. Be conscientious of how individuals or groups are designated. Many politically correct words have replaced many terms that were offensive. However, racial, sexual, and other slurs that hurt and offend individuals and groups are still commonly used. Managers should learn the preferred ethnic terms of their workers. Some people of African heritage may prefer being called "black," whereas others may want to be called "African American." Depending on ancestry, Spanish-speaking persons may be called "Latino," "Chicano," "Hispanic," or other terms related to their country of origin (such as Puerto Rican). People from the Pacific Rim may wish to be referred to as "Asian American" or a term reflecting their country of origin (such as "Korean," "Japanese," "Filipino").

Barriers Due to Other Factors

Often behavior called *nonverbal communication* can communicate just as effectively as emotional displays. This behavior is conveyed through body language rather than spoken or written words. Facial expressions, gestures, and posture send "wordless transmissions" about attitudes, perceptions, and emotions. Smiling, shrugging, or sitting slumped in a chair are common expressions in the nonverbal vocabulary. Sometimes nonverbal communication can serve to support verbal communication, such as when a manager's words of encouragement to an employee are accompanied by smiles and nods.

When either the sender or the receiver does not have adequate knowledge to understand the other, the process is not effective. Other barriers include:

- *Lack of interest.* Either the receiver or the sender does not have an interest in the message being conveyed.
- *Use of jargon.* Physicians or administrators may use technical language, terms, and phrases that are unique to foodservice or health care operations that can be mystifying to foodservice employees not familiar with terms.
- *Source of the message.* Evaluating the source of the message can cause the receiver to "filter" or manipulate the information as to its importance.
- *Personality conflict.* When there is a conflict between the sender and the receiver, problems can arise. If the receiver does not like the sender, the message is less likely to be received.
- *Selective communications.* Receiving communications on the basis of what one selectively hears and sees, depending on his or her needs, motivation, experiences, background, and other personal characteristics.

- *Information overload.* This occurs when the amount of information is so great and detailed that it exceeds a person's processing capacity.
- *Regional language.* Despite the pervasiveness of the popular media, regional phrases are still common throughout the United States. For example, in some regions, "hurry up and fix it" may mean "repair it quickly." Each region has its own particular variations that should be carefully avoided when messages are widely distributed out of the region.
- *Disorganization.* When the sender and receiver disagree about what message to send, a problem arises. The receiver may be disorganized due to not being aware of the procedure or may have a problem reading and understanding.

Nonverbal behavior also can contribute to another behavioral barrier known as the *mixed message*, which results when a verbal message and a nonverbal message do not coincide. For example, while leaning back in a chair and shuffling papers without looking up, a manager might say to an employee, "I'm very interested in your suggestion." The employee leaves the office confused, having received two seemingly contradictory messages: Although the manager's words convey interest, the manager's body language (absence of eye contact and preoccupation with desk papers) conveys apathy.

Workers throughout an organization rely daily on one another's nonverbal cues in gauging intent, acceptance, and comprehension of messages. All groups must remain alert to the information—verbal and nonverbal—that they send.

METHODS OF COMMUNICATION

Direct communication can take two forms as determined by the medium used in the process. *Verbal communication* uses the medium of the spoken word: in face-to-face conversations, telephone conversations, and meetings. *Written communication* includes letters, reports, proposals, e-mail messages, justifications, and memos.

Verbal Communication

Verbal communication involves face-to-face contact between people in conversations or group discussions, sharing information through words, either written or spoken. Telephone calls are also common forms of verbal communication. The central avenue of communication for most managers, verbal communication is immediate in that it permits prompt feedback about the message, and it does not require the technical skills of typing or word processing. However, verbal communication is not always the best way to communicate messages in management situations. Aside from the environmental distractions of noise and static mentioned earlier, verbal exchanges provide no written record of conversations. Therefore, decisions and compromises reached verbally could be subject to debate later on. Verbal communication also may not give communicators time to reflect on their responses to questions raised and decisions discussed.

In organizations, verbal communication is used extensively when managers direct employee work activities, give instructions to employees, conduct meetings, lead work or process improvement teams, and make formal presentations. These formats are discussed in the following subsections.

Use of Persuasion

Persuasion is an effective mode of communication when you need the help of employees, nurses, administration, and the medical staff. Persuasion means an effort to influence another person or group to change their beliefs, attitudes, religion, or feelings. Persuasion can be subtle or via the use of force.

When using persuasion the manager will need to:

- Be honest in their "request."
- Be credible.
- Explain the values, vision you share with the person or group.
- Use examples, stories, experiences that will help the person or group relate to what you need.
- Use animation and enthusiasm when presenting your request.
- Stand up, speak up, and shut up—but be positive.
- Remind the person or group that the final decision will be for the person or group benefits.
- If you feel that your persuasion techniques may not be working or understood, repeat stories, suggestions, and reemphasize that the benefits are for the person or group.

When using persuasion techniques *do not* come across as phony or your desire will not be accepted.

Directing or Instructing Employees

Managers' verbal directions and instructions to employees should be thoughtfully prepared and carefully delivered to keep misunderstandings to a minimum. Every verbal direction given to an employee should be framed so that its meaning is clear, complete, and reasonable. The manager should always keep the employee's viewpoint in mind. New terms should be explained and simple words and sentences used. The manager should ask employees regularly whether they have any questions about the directions given.

When it is clear that the employees understand the directions, the manager should indicate when the task is to be completed and how the employees are to report back after it is completed. Complicated directions may require the manager to follow up and, if necessary, clarify the instructions to ensure that tasks are completed as directed. However, it is important that the manager show confidence in employees and allow them reasonable independence in performing their regular duties.

New or particularly complex tasks should be described in written detail in addition to being explained verbally. The manager should be careful to ensure that the written information matches the information given verbally. Conflicting sets of instructions for the same task can only cause misunderstanding and confusion.

Planning and Conducting Meetings

Managers spend a great deal of time attending meetings with superiors, peers, and employees in the organization. Many complain that most meetings are a waste of their time. However, meetings are the means by which organizations conduct a large part of their business. Planning is the key to conducting productive, informative, and cost-efficient meetings. There are several types of meetings that include informal, formal, committee, problem solving, and information passing. For the purpose of this text, meetings will be categorized as business meetings and team meetings.

Business Meetings   The purpose of *business meetings* is to provide or share information and to delineate planning or development functions. These meetings are usually formal. For the most part, the department-level planning and development meetings that foodservice directors attend deal with menu planning, production planning, and nutrition care planning. The director or manager also attends informational meetings of the management staff and, depending on the size of the department, employee meetings. Meetings held for the sole purpose of providing information should be carefully evaluated. If the information could easily be shared in a memo, or via e-mail, fax, conference call, or chat room (a real-time online discussion group), a meeting may not be necessary. However, many foodservice department employees appreciate and enjoy hearing information from the department manager. Also, this type of meeting allows for questions and discussion of the information presented, ensuring understanding.

Each meeting requires a coordinated plan for conducting business and for decision making. The director or manager responsible for conducting such meetings should plan the meetings by routinely following a simple eight-step process:

1. *Decide who should attend the meeting.* Factors to consider are the authority levels of the participants and the most cost-effective and efficient size for the group. Participants must have authority to make and act on decisions that come out of the meeting. The number of attendants should be kept to a minimum to control the cost in time expenditures. It should also be kept in mind that the larger the group, the less likely it is that the meeting's goals will be fulfilled.

2. *Set a time* and day for meeting that is the most convenient for everyone. Two meetings may be necessary to cover all employees on all shifts.

3. *Clearly define the goal(s) of the meeting.* Be careful to avoid covering too much in any one session. It is better to discuss thoroughly and solve one problem than to discuss many subjects but reach no clear-cut conclusions.

4. *Determine how much time should be allotted for accomplishing the meeting's goals.* Most meetings should last no longer than 60 or, at most, 90 minutes. When longer meetings are planned, a break should be provided after the first hour.

5. *Determine the format that will best suit the goal of the meeting.* If the goal is to solve a problem, the meeting should be a free exchange of ideas and suggestions. If the goal is to distribute information, the meeting should be a preplanned discussion and explanation of data or other information. If the goal is to win the group's acceptance of a new proposal, the meeting should be a carefully constructed presentation of background materials and projections.

6. *Plan a strategy for accomplishing the goal of the meeting.* Anticipate potential resistance to change, conflict within the group, and other problems. Formulate methods for handling such problems and securing the support of other group members before the meeting.

7. *Write an agenda for the meeting.* An agenda is a written statement of the order of events in a meeting and is called an operational agenda (Figure 7.2). If anyone other than the meeting planner is to be responsible for presenting topics, that person should be notified ahead of time. The final agenda should be distributed in advance to everyone who is to attend the meeting. To save time, combine routine items into one item for the group's approval. This is called a *consent agenda.* Items in the consent agenda should be things that are generally agreed upon and that do not need to be discussed before a vote. Items to be included in a consent agenda include:

    Approval of agenda
    Committee and previous meeting minutes
    Minor changes in procedure
    Routine revision of a policy
    Updating of documents
    Treasurer's report (as appropriate)
    The items should be standard, noncontroversial, and self-explanatory.

The *consent agenda* and any supporting materials should be distributed before the meeting. When using a consent agenda, make sure everyone knows the rules. Any member can ask for any item to be removed from the consent agenda and open for discussion. If no one asks for the removal of an item, the entire group is voted on without discussion (see Figure 7.3).

8. *Record the meeting minutes.* If a written record of the meeting is required, appoint a group member before the meeting to be the secretary. Clearly state any action taken, what follow-up is needed and who is responsible for the follow-up. If another meeting is to be scheduled, state the date, time, and place of the next meeting.

The person designated to conduct the meeting (referred to as the *chairperson or chair*) is responsible for moving the meeting toward accomplishment of its goals. The chairperson should schedule the meeting room and the meeting room setup well ahead of time, making sure that it is large enough to accommodate the group

FIGURE 7.2   An Operational Agenda

Type:	Clinical Management Meeting	Place: Conference Room H20
Date:	January 20	Time: 1:30 P.M. – 3:00 P.M.

A.   General Business   (30 minutes)

    a.   Call to order, attendance

    *b.   Approval of agenda

    *c.   Approval of minutes

    *d.   Report of director's retreat

    *e.   Approval and discussion of policy Q16

    *f.   Approval of update call list

B.   Programs   (45 minutes)

    a.   Diet manual revision

    b.   Update formulary

    c.   Quality Indicators for Food and Drug Interaction

C.   Announcements   (15 minutes)

    a.   National Nutrition Month

    b.   New RN on 4th West

    c.   Special event in cafeteria

    d.   Next meeting

D.   Adjournment

Note: An asterisk indicates that the item needs individual motions or approval rather than one motion as in a consent agenda.

FIGURE 7.3   A Consent Agenda

Type:	Clinical Staff Meeting	Place: Conference Room H20
Date:	January 20	Time: 1:00 P.M. – 2:00 P.M.

A.   Call to order

B.   Consent agenda* (materials sent Jan. 10)

    a.   Approval of minutes from previous meeting

    b.   Approval of agenda

    c.   Report of director's retreat

    d.   Approval of policy #Q106

    e.   Approval of updated call list

C.   Diet manual revision—Jones

D.   Update on enteral formulary—Smith

E.   Quality Program Indicators for Food and Drug Inactions—Brown

F.   Announcements

G.   Adjournment

Note: An asterisk indicates that it needs a motion and approval.

and that the physical environment is comfortable (Table 7.1). Any audiovisual equipment, displays, and handouts should be arranged for ahead of time. Equipment should be checked in advance to ensure that it is in good working order.

During the meeting, the leader should follow a few simple rules of courtesy:

- Arrive early so that he or she can greet people as they arrive. Turn off cell phones, pagers.
- Start the meeting on time unless several people are late, in which case the leader should send out reminders, such as a telephone call, and then proceed with the meeting.

- Direct discussions with open-ended questions that give everyone a chance to contribute.
- Stick to the agenda and make sure that other group members do so as well. If items or issues are raised that are not on the agenda, a "parking lot" can be created by writing on a board or flip chart a list of items that may need further discussion outside the meeting or to be added to the agenda in the future. The meeting can then move forward while providing a record of issues that require future attention.
- Use consent agendas.
- Limit the discussion to one point at a time to avoid conflict.

TABLE 7.1 Meeting Room Setup

Schoolroom or classroom	Rows of tables with chairs: Allows participants to take notes and spread out materials but limits interaction with other attendees
Banquet round	Usually used for food functions but works well for small groups
U-shape setup	A hollow square or rectangle with one side removed works well for visual aids
Theater or auditorium	Features a platform with a podium as a focal point and maximizes the number of people that can be accommodated
Conference boardroom	For small groups that require a lot of interaction
Crescent round	Round banquet tables with chairs around half- to three-quarters of the table, all facing the front; use when networking and note taking are important
Hollow square	Works for a schoolroom-type presentation; no one sits inside the hollow

- Avoid unnecessary interruptions (such as telephone calls) and discourage distractions (such as shuffling of papers and whispering among attendees).
- The chair should remain neutral. If he or she has a strong opinion on a topic, the chair should relinquish authority to provide input into the discussion.
- Ask for input from attendees regarding how the meeting went, its structure, and whether they feel goals were met, topics were given appropriate time, and their participation was valued. Express sincere thanks to the group's members for their attendance and participation. Taking time to ask members to evaluate effectiveness can enhance future meetings of the group.
- End the meeting at the appointed time by reviewing key points, assigning follow-up tasks, and setting the date, time, and place for the next meeting.

When conducting surveys, most surveying agencies' standards require that meetings should be conducted for *all* employees on *all* shifts. Sign-in sheets with the date and other pertinent information concerning the meeting must be filed. Supervisors of employees who were off duty when the meeting was held have a joint responsibility, with the employees to be informed by minutes of the meeting or by an oral report from the supervisor. These employees will need to sign that they have received the information. The form should be dated and signed by supervisor and employee.

After formal meetings, the minutes need to be reviewed and then distributed to the participants to ensure accuracy. Use the minute recording format used by the organization. The names of those attending need to be recorded as part of the minutes. Minutes should be sent to all members for approval. When members suggest a correction, these corrections need to be sent to the secretary who

will make the corrections and resubmit them. Approval of the minutes will go on the next meeting agenda. The approved minutes should be signed by the chairperson and secretary and kept on file for future reference and follow up. Minutes may become legal documents in cases of ligation.

At least once a year, the foodservice director should evaluate all formal meetings held in the department. Committees, task forces, and other formal groups will be dissolved if their goals have been met. The director should also review the cost of the department's meetings in terms of the supplies used, the salaries of the staff members who attended, the refreshments provided, and so forth. The director should ask basic questions about the meetings to determine their effectiveness: Did too many people attend? Were the costs of the meeting justified by its results? Did the meeting meet the mission of the department? Did the meeting define outcomes and were they met? If not, how can future meetings be planned to meet outcome goals?

Team Meetings *Team meetings* are conducted with employees in the department or as cross-functional teams with employees across the organization. Team meetings, which may or may not have a manager as the team leader, can be designed to discuss work methods, customer satisfaction, or process improvement. Their goal is to improve quality, that is, quality of work life, quality of customer satisfaction, or quality of work accomplishment. Before a quality improvement team can be initiated, several questions must be answered.

- What is the purpose or mission of the team? This question helps identify the process or issue under discussion, the background information surrounding the process or issue, and what information or data are available regarding the process or issue.
- What is the scope of the project? It is important to understand what is not being included in the activities. Once boundaries are identified, budget constraints must be explored. The decision-making authority of the team members and leader also must be clarified.
- Who should be on the improvement team? This question involves identifying who has ownership of the process, who knows what the issues and concerns are for the customer, and who is needed to offer a different perspective. This is the time to decide whether a facilitator is necessary.
- What are the expectations for improvement? Questioning the expectations identifies the outcome or goals, timelines for recommendations, the magnitude of improvement expected, and who is responsible for approval and implementation of the recommendations.
- What resources are available to the team? Resources may include consultants or internal experts, facilitators, coworkers who perform extra work so that team members can attend meetings, and support staff who can create presentation materials. Data collection and analysis also are needed. They may include computers and software.

Answering these questions provides team members with a clear picture of their charter or mission. When the team meets for the first time, the information compiled from these questions is presented for review and discussion by the team leader. It also may be necessary to provide the answers in the form of a proposal to the administrator and other department administrative personnel for its approval before the meeting, especially if the process requires a cross-functional team (see Chapter 4). Once approved and the team members are clear about the team's mission and purpose, ground rules for the meetings should be discussed. Ground rules may be a part of the training program provided for all employees involved in quality improvement but should be covered as a reminder in the first team meeting. Ground rules include the following:

- *Attendance*: Time and place for meeting, how to notify team of absence, acceptable number of absences, designation of a replacement, and so on
- *Time management*: Punctuality with regard to meeting start and end, timekeeper responsibilities, appointment of timekeeper, what must be accomplished during meeting, agenda for meetings
- *Participation*: Being prepared for meetings, completing assignments, sharing responsibilities, and so on
- *Communication*: Confidentiality, candor, orderly and focused discussion, one speaker at a time, active listening, respect for others' opinions
- *Decision making*: How decisions are made (majority vote), open discussion permitted before voting, conflict acceptable and handled in the open, number of members who must be present for decision making
- *Documentation*: Format for agenda, format used for minutes, distribution of agenda and minutes, storage of and access to documentation
- *Miscellaneous*: Breaks, refreshments, room setup and cleanup, need for support services, how they will be coordinated

The same guidelines need to be followed for conducting team meetings as for business meetings. The leader (not necessarily the manager) is responsible for conducting the meeting, setting up the next meeting, and providing follow-up information or information needed before the next meeting. When conducting team meetings, the leader must keep individuals on target to reach established goals.

Making Presentations

Sometimes the foodservice manager may be asked to provide information in a formal presentation. Presentations may include training sessions for employees or students or delivery of information regarding the department business plan, budget, or special project to decision makers. Managers can give successful presentations by being prepared and by understanding how to deal positively with the anxiety or stress related to this activity.

A substantial body of literature is available to assist managers with gaining skills in business or technical presentations. The limited scope of this text prevents a detailed review of technique, but the following basic guidelines can serve to help managers prepare to present information to a group.

- *Plan the presentation by identifying the objectives to be achieved.* Next, assess the needs and level of knowledge of the audience. For example, in speaking to students regarding the cook-chill process, a manager might relate the history or evolution of this food production method. On the other hand, in presenting a request to decision makers for conversion of the food production system to cook-chill, the focus might be on costs associated with the current system versus savings to be realized on conversion. Know the audience before you begin your presentation
- *Organize the information to be presented.* Using the objectives for the presentation will help determine the order of presentation. Organizing should include the development of an outline, and main ideas with their subpoints. The presentation should have an introduction and a conclusion. The introduction provides the setting for the rest of the presentation. It should relate to the topic of the presentation, establish a common ground between the speaker and the audience, and be a preview of the remainder of the presentation. The conclusion should summarize what the speaker hopes the audience will do; and is an effective way to terminate the presentation. In other words, to use a well-known phrase: "Tell them what you're going to tell them; tell them; then tell them what you told them." Deliver the most important point(s) first. Concentrate on the listener. **Practice** ahead of time to become familiar with material.
- *Conquer your fears.* This can be reduced if you know your topic, you are confident in the quality and appropriateness of the topic, and the topic is what the audience is expecting to hear. Be prepared for "What if . . . ?"
- *Use handouts and visual aids to enhance the presentation.* Visual aids focus the audience's attention, reinforce the verbal message, stimulate interest in the topic, or illustrate hard-to-visualize factors. They should not be used if they do not improve the presentation's effectiveness. Nor should they be used to avoid interacting with the audience. If handouts are used, the manager must decide at what point to distribute them: If they are handed out in the beginning, the audience may spend time reviewing rather than listening; if they are handed out during the presentation, they should be distributed quickly to prevent distracting from the presentation. It also may be appropriate to distribute handouts at the end to provide written support of the verbal presentation.
- *Add variety* to a presentation. Use demonstrations, such as how to clean a new piece of equipment. Role-play a situation, or use case studies or panel discussions. Make eye contact with the group and walk around the room, but do not pace. Use persuasion to change beliefs, feelings, or attitudes of the audience.
- *In advance*, gather all handouts, visual aids, supplies and equipment needed. Visit the meeting room ahead of time to be familiar with the room layout. Make sure the room is comfortable and free of distractions. If this is not possible, arrive early and organize notes, handouts, and visual aids. Practice the entire presentation beforehand to uncover possible difficulties with terminology or ambiguous points. Practice also gives a clue as to whether the predetermined time frame is realistic.

- *Be aware of your personal appearance.* Use moderation in dress—for business wear business attire (dress, suit, or business pantsuit). Go easy on the makeup and perfume. Make sure shoes are clean/polished, appropriate foot covering (socks or hosiery). Be sure body, hair, nails, and teeth are clean.

Knowing the audience will dictate the dress code.

- *Relate to the audience.* Most audiences will determine who you are before you speak. When being introduced, remember that your introduction is part of the presentation. Work with the person who will introduce you and decide on what the introduction will be. Do not make the introduction too long, too short, or too boring. Draw attention away from yourself and give the audience the opportunity to become personally involved in the presentation. Always let the audience win. When necessary make adjustments to the presentation to keep the audience focused. Remove yourself, involve your audience.

- *Be natural and show enthusiasm for the topic.* Avoid standing stiffly or speaking in a monotone. Maintain eye contact with the audience and move naturally using hand movements and a conversational style of speech. Show confidence, objectivity, tact, and as appropriate, humor. Be careful in using jokes to avoid offending someone, be knowledgeable on the topic, use simple and understandable language, be prepared to answer questions to back up the topic, use a pleasant voice, control emotions, and use charisma. Be well groomed. Know and understand the needs of the audience. Stay on timetable. Finish early so there is plenty of time for questions and discussion. When a question is asked, repeat each question for the audience before answering. When using copyright material give the author and the material credit. This can be accomplished by saying, "And I quote xxx from xxx . . . " and saying "End of quote" when the quotation is complete.

It is natural to have some anxiety about presenting to a group. However, effective speakers have learned to use this anxiety to their advantage. Following the steps listed earlier helps to decrease anxiety by being prepared for the presentation. In addition, use positive visualization and imagery, which have been shown by researchers to ensure success in accomplishing a task. Other techniques for decreasing anxiety include deep breathing and tightening and relaxing muscles.

Nonverbal Communication

Some of the most meaningful communication is neither verbal nor written. These are nonverbal communications. Managers and subordinates use a number of nonverbal communications on a daily basis, such as "props" that are used to send a message. This could include frequent looking at a wall-mounted clock during an interview or meeting ("let's get this over with") rather than looking at a small clock on the desk. The amount of personal space between the sender and receiver is another example. Small space is more personal, and conversation can be more intimate. Invading one's personal space can cause discomfort and even resentful feelings, depending on the culture of the people involved.

Perhaps the best-known and most frequently used nonverbal language is body language. *Body language* may be unconscious behavior, but some of it may be due to nervous behavior or cultural or ethnic customs. Some typical body action includes smiling, blushing, frowning, shrugging, shaking the head, putting hands on hips, kicking the foot, pointing a finger, sighing, stomping the foot, making steeple fingers, winking, slamming doors, tightly crossing the arms against the chest, or nodding and patting another on the shoulder. Even though scientists have studied nonverbal actions of people and have correlated certain actions with specific nonverbal language, managers must be careful not to misinterpret meanings. Some actions are subtle, and it is difficult to determine their meaning. Interpreting the meaning wrongly can cause problems for both the sender and receiver.

Touching is also a form of nonverbal communication. Touching involves handshaking, pats on the back, hugs, or hand-holding. Touching is usually unplanned and can convey warmth, acceptance, strength, or authority. Touching an employee who has had a bad day can convey understanding or authority, sexual harassment, or invading personal space.

Written Communication

Written communication has benefits for writer and reader alike. The writer has the satisfaction of immediacy, of communicating his or her message right away without waiting to see the receiver in person. The receiver benefits from having a written record, especially of complex information. Although written communication is unavoidable much of the time, it has some disadvantages. One key disadvantage is that written communication takes longer to reach its destination than verbal communication. A second and related disadvantage is that feedback for written communication can be delayed. However, when important details must be communicated, written messages provide a record of facts that can be referred to again and again, and they give the receiver time to study and absorb those facts before responding to the communication.

At its best, good written communication is clear and concisely worded, with short sentences and simple words. There should be no obvious mistakes in grammar or spelling, Sentences and paragraphs should not be overloaded with too many ideas; it is best to present one idea per paragraph. Be positive, not negative. Jargon should be avoided except, of course, for the use of appropriate technical language. The ultimate measure of a good exchange is that both sender and receiver understand the message.

Effective written communication anticipates and answers any questions the reader might have, not only to better communicate the whole message but also to avoid delays in the receiver and response. The tone of the written message is also important, in the same way that it is important for a sender to consider the receiver's point of view. Writers should be tactful and focus on the reader's concern rather than on their own. In the age of word processors and personal computers, managers should use all the technical support that such equipment provides to make sure that their written messages are not distorted by poor spelling and grammatical errors that might reflect poorly on their abilities to communicate with and influence others. There are computer programs available that will assist the writer to improve sentences, spell words correctly, and provide other assistance to improve written communications.

Types of Written Communication

The kinds of written communication used most often in the food-service department, and in most business operations for that matter, include letters, internal memorandums, proposals, justifications, reports, policies and procedures, and materials for distribution to customers. Figure 7.4 shows a sample format for formal business correspondence. Figure 7.5 shows a sample format for an interoffice memorandum.

In *writing a business letter*, the sender should clearly state the purpose of the letter in the first paragraph or sentence. The rest of the letter needs to be organized logically, and each paragraph should contain one main idea. Short paragraphs are usually better than long paragraphs. A letter should be no longer than it needs to be to make its point. Extra information or materials should be attached as addenda to the main letter.

Internal memorandums are an efficient way to communicate with department employees, with higher levels of management, and with peers in other departments. Note that everyday communications with employees for the purpose of giving directions and feedback should be more informal and verbal communications are best on the supervisory level. A few basic guidelines for writing memorandums follow:

- Each memorandum should have just one subject.
- The memorandum should be direct, concise, and to the point.
- It should be typewritten or prepared on a word processor.
- It should be kept to one page in length, if possible.
- It should ask for a response and feedback, if required.
- It should close with a thank-you.
- A copy of the memorandum should be kept on file in the manager's office for future reference.

Written communication is often used to make a position known or to persuade someone of something—for example, written proposals and justifications. Skills for writing persuasive communications are increasingly important to foodservice directors, whose purpose might be to inform and provide rationale for a decision that may require input from upper management. For example, a manager may wish to develop an outpatient nutrition education program in conjunction with the rehabilitation department or outside fitness center. To move forward with this decision, a proposal must be submitted to top managers to outline the need for such a program, the benefits of the program for the organization and community, the costs of the program, and the resources needed to implement the program.

A *justification* may be necessary to receive approval for capital equipment investments or for the addition of staff. With each of these types of justifications, the manager must present the facts used in making the decision for the request and answer questions that may be asked by administration. Anticipating questions will prompt the director to include information that can speed up the approval process. Justifications and *proposals* are designed to influence the decision maker based on the needs of the department. A sample justification for an additional cook's position is provided in Figure 7.6. When writing justifications or proposals, the sender should clearly state the action expected from the receiver. For example, if it is necessary to have a signature on a requisition for an additional position, clearly state that the requisition is attached for signature. A statement inviting questions or requests for further information can be helpful, as would an offer to pick up the requisition on being notified that it has been signed. This type of clarification allows the manager to know when the next step has been taken and when the issue has been closed.

Reports are another form of written communication frequently prepared by managers. Financial and departmental activity reports are generally completed on a monthly basis. (Financial reports are discussed in Chapter 11.) Employee handbooks are written documents produced by the organization or department to provide

FIGURE 7.4 Sample Business Letter

ABC Hospital
300 Main Street
Any City, State 55555

August 20,XXXX

Jane Smith, Sales Representative
XYZ Foodservice Company
xxx Street
Any City, State 55555

Dear Ms. Smith:

I am writing to follow up on our telephone conversation on August 5, regarding . . .

During our conversation, you indicated that your company would be willing to supply the following items . . .

Please contact me if any other information is needed regarding . . .

Sincerely,

Hollie Walker, RD
Director, Nutrition and Foodservices

FIGURE 7.5 Sample Memorandum

MEMORANDUM

To: All Department Managers
From: Vera Brown, RD, Director Nutrition and Foodservices
Re: Ordering Food Supplies via the Fax Machine or E-mail
Date: August 20, XXXX

Attached are the new forms for obtaining food supplies for your department or unit. Use of the forms will be effective September 1, XXXX. Additional forms can be obtained by calling extension 0000. The completed form can be faxed to the department storeroom by _____AM. Your order will be filled by next day_____AM.

If you should choose to use e-mail the forms may be found under Food and Nutrition; using the red tab marked Ordering Supplies, cut and paste and send your order at least 3 days before the items are needed.

Thank you in advance for supporting this new order system designed to benefit the department in better meeting the needs of our customers. customers. Please contact _____ at _____ if you have any questions or problems with the new process.

FIGURE 7.6   Sample Justification Statement

Justification for an Additional Position
August 20, XXXX

Need for an Additional Cook's Position

Based on departmental productivity and meal equivalents, I would like to add 1 FTE as a cook's position. Maintaining coverage for the production area for meal preparation and sanitation has become increasingly more difficult as the number of meals prepared and served continue to increase.

Productivity for the department has met or exceeded the 1,000% goal set with labor hours per meal at 0.21. The labor hour per meal goal set for this year is 0.23. The total complement for paid FTEs is currently 70, which is well below the 73 to 77 shown, as required on the productivity reports.

Validity of Production Figures

I have reviewed the validity of the paid FTE number with the changes made in the cafeteria renovations. It stands to reason that enough efficiencies have been gained with the renovation and number of meals served to make adjustments in the factor used to measure departmental productivity. The following steps have been taken or are in the process of being taken to ensure accuracy of our productivity numbers.

1. A two-week review of sales and counts in the cafeteria was conducted using figures from _____ through _____. The attached chart shows the current average meal or meal equivalent to be $_____, slightly below the $_____ now used to determine cafeteria meals. These numbers also indicate that roughly 2,000 more individual customers enter the cafeteria than is verified by the average ticket or meal.

2. The number of meals prepared for patient and all nonpatient areas have been charted and compared with the counts from a year ago. The attached table shows an increase in meals for all areas except vending. The total increase is 4.11% over last year. Patient meals show a 2.4% increase; these meals are the most labor intensive.

3. In addition to the above two steps, observations will be made to determine the overall effect of changes made with the layout of the new cafeteria service area. If it is determined that these meals are now being served more efficiently, I will evaluate and modify the other meal factor used to determine departmental productivity.

Benefits and Rationales for Adding a Cook

The cook's position is being requested at this time based on the following:

1. Meal preparation for the physicians' dining area is consistently being done by the production supervisor.

2. Either the production supervisor or the purchasing supervisor must fill a line slot when time off is granted to a cook, baker, or salad maker. This means these employees are working out of jobs specifications.

3. Cooks are voicing concern that they are unable to complete their meal preparation in a timely manner. They also state they are under excessive stress and feel overworked.

4. Although we have been able to decrease our injuries, last year's experience revealed that a high level of productivity directly affects the number of injuries.

5. Efforts to increase sales and therefore the number of customers in the cafeteria will continue. These efforts have been shown over the past three months to increase counts.

6. Meal counts are higher in all areas other than vending. Patient meals are more labor intensive and are higher than budgeted due to an increased census.

Effects on Department Budget

The budget for this fiscal year will not be negatively affected by the addition of a cook for the next six months. We are currently $50,000 under budget for the year. Adding a cook for the remainder of the year will cost $20,800 (this does not include fringe benefits).

Average cook salary = $20/hour x 1,040 hours = $20,800

Thank you for your consideration in filling this position Please let me know if this position is approved or if additional justification is needed.

Laurie Brown, RD, Director
Nutrition and Foodservices

---

information that relates to the mission, values, policies, rules, benefits, and other pertinent information. Written departmental policy and procedures manuals need to be developed to guide the department.

Written materials are often prepared and distributed to patients and other customers of the department. These materials include dietary instructions, menus, brochures of services offered, and in some cases, department newsletters. Because these materials represent the department, it is important that the materials be professional in appearance. Although many large organizations have in-house print shops, most small organizations use outside sources.

Regardless of where printing occurs, development should be the responsibility of individuals professionally trained to create high-quality materials. Large organizations generally have a marketing department to assist managers. Small organizations can take advantage of preprinted materials or support from food vendors willing to supply materials, or they can work with outside printing companies.

Although most written communication is in paper form, it also can be in the form of output from personal computer networks. Electronic mail (e-mail) can communicate information to a single department or distribute information to every department. E-mail is fast, convenient, and cheap, and the same message can be sent to several persons at the same time. It is the fastest-growing and most widely used way for organizations to communicate. E-mail is public information and should never be used for sending sensitive information. When using e-mail, the following etiquette should be followed:

- Use subject heading.
- Proofread all messages before sending.
- Check spelling for accuracy.
- Use name, position, or signature to identify yourself to recipients.
- Send e-mail only to those who need the information.
- Keep messages and attachments short.
- Learn how to send and receive attachments.
- Do not react if message does not apply to you, your organization, or department; simply delete it.
- In replying to e-mail, use the appropriate reply key to verify that the message is going to the intended person(s). When replying to a group message, use the key for replying to all.
- Maintain copies of outgoing mail even if you have to send it to yourself.
- Set up a filing system to sort and organize e-mail.
- Use the address book and update periodically.
- Run virus checks frequently.
- If desired, subscribe to listservs.
- Delete any unnecessary or dated messages.
- Be courteous and use business etiquette when sending and receiving messages.
- It is not necessary to reply to every e-mail.
- Do not forward messages to other groups unless necessary and with the approval of the sender.
- Do not send copyrighted materials unless so noted or used by permission; do not put your name first on a project or written reports, articles, books where you were **not** the lead or first author.
- Never send confidential information.

With the use of handheld computers that are capable of sending pictures as well as messages, the sender needs to be aware of invading the privacy of others. In a recent court case that involved an employee sending personal and confidential information concerning a fellow employee resulted in a major fine, jail time, and loss of position. A *listserv*, an electronic mailing list that is used as a means of communication among colleagues wishing to interact with one another in areas of mutual interest, is another form of written communication. Facsimile (fax) machines also have enhanced the capability to send information within and outside organizations. A memorandum may be typed but the information is distributed not through the mail system but through a facsimile machine. Hard-copy fax machines have enhanced this form of written communication, making permanent copies available

Most companies as well as health care facilities have established harsh rules concerning the use of electronic communication while on duty. When using this type of communication the sender **must**

be aware of privacy issues and avoid breaking the policy. Sending false information can be dangerous. Sexual communication should never be sent on company IT network. Before using e-mail or websites it is extremely wise to know the organization's rules and follow them. **Never** assume that your e-mail or website is private. In a recent American Management Survey of 304 companies it was discovered that management monitored how employees were using the telephone (checked telephone records), web, and e-mail while on duty. About 25 percent of those monitored were fired for misuse of telephone, e-mail, and web. *Know the policies* before you hit the send button.

RULES FOR EFFECTIVE COMMUNICATION

It is important to remember that communication depends on two dynamics. One has to do with how a message is sent, and the other has to do with how the message is received. As senders of messages, managers should consider the following guidelines:

- Plan the message by identifying the outcomes to be achieved through the communication. For example, if the objective is to seek information, formulate specific questions about the subject on which information is needed. When the objective is to change employee behavior or persuade decision makers, plan well-reasoned arguments in support of the change or decision.
- Determine the type of language appropriate to the communication. For example, if a manager is seeking to persuade hospital administrators to approve implementation of a cook-chill system, the language should be in lay terms. But in a conversation between two technicians, technical language is entirely appropriate.
- Seek to maintain credibility by being honest and accurate, by gathering facts to support opinions, and by not pretending to be an expert on subjects on which the sender has limited knowledge. Managers who fail to follow this simple rule are likely to find their messages met with suspicion from employees, peers, and superiors.
- Be aware of the message behind the message—that is, the one conveyed by tone of voice and body language. Ensure that body language is congruent with the spoken message. Anticipate different ways the message could be interpreted and ask questions to ensure that it is received as intended. Avoid letting minor points of disagreement distract from the message.
- Be sensitive to the receiver's perspective, especially when the message deals with a sensitive issue, such as an employee denied a promotion. Avoid raising emotionally loaded issues when the receiver appears preoccupied or when time does not permit dealing with the issue adequately.
- Ensure that the setting is appropriate to the conversation. If it is too public and surrounded by distractions, relocate. For example, it would be inappropriate to discuss performance with a cafeteria tray line worker during a heavy-traffic period.

- Encourage feedback in communications. Invite receivers to ask questions, request clarification, or express opinions.

As receivers of messages, managers should fine-tune listening skills, try to remain open and receptive, and accommodate the sender.

Listening

Listening and hearing are two different things. *Hearing* is a physical sense that takes place automatically. People hear noises around them, such as music, car horns, and dish machines, without paying much attention to them. *Listening* is an active process that requires effort or attention from the listener. Listening completes the communication cycle. Listening demands concentration on the implied meaning as well as the stated meaning. The undertones or unspoken words are gleaned by developing listening power. With today's non-personal automated telephone messages, a person has to listen actively to push the correct button before proceeding to the next instruction. The listener must be attentive to the prompting or risk having to start the procedure again.

To become effective listeners, managers need to:

- *Be attentive.* Concentrate on what the person is saying. A manager should not turn off the speaker as uninteresting or because it is a subject that he or she is not interested in or already knows. A manager should listen without making premature judgments about the speaker's message.
- *Be open-minded.* Stereotyping, ethnocentricity, and rigid frames of reference are barriers that interfere with receiving an intended message.
- *Develop empathy.* Empathy means understanding others' feelings, situations, and motives. Why are they motivated to speak on this issue? How do they really feel about the issue? Respond to feelings by letting the employee know that feelings are recognized.
- *Wait before responding.* A manager should not rush an employee when only a portion of what has been said but wait until everything has been said. While forming the response, the manager may miss a salient point.
- *Observe nonverbal cue.* Observe gestures, tone of voice, body position, eye movement, breathing patterns, and verbal cues without underreacting or overreacting and relating them to the ethnicity or culture of the speaker.
- *Listen to the whole message.* Managers should listen not only for facts but to the whole message before making a judgment or formulating a response.
- *Keep distracters to a minimum.* The manager should try to find a quiet, private place. Face the person who is talking. If the listener is near his or her desk or work area, the listener should turn his or her back to it. Listen actively, and do not fiddle with papers or take phone calls.
- *Be aware of impatience.* Do not rush the speaker in order to reply.
- *Do not pretend to listen.* This type of listening frequently leads to "Pardon me, what did you say?" The manager

should be sincere, and listen attentively. Lending undivided attention may solve problems.
- *Be prepared to compromise.* Compromise may be necessary to achieve agreement or understanding.
- *Do not show favoritism.* Managers must listen to all employees.

Four good rules to follow will improve listening skills and help to uncover a whole new world of useful information:

1. *Repeat what you have been told.* Repeat what was heard using neutral tones. This is not a sales job but a way to determine if what was heard is to be believed.
2. *Consider the source.* Is the speaker biased? Is the speaker exaggerating? Is the speaker looking for attention? Does the speaker really want an answer?
3. *Use self-discipline.* Lack of empathy or sympathy and an angry manner cause loss of objectivity and cloud the message.
4. *Summarize.* Ask exploratory, open-ended questions to confirm the meaning of the message. "Is this what I heard?" or "What I hear you saying is. . . ." This technique, called mirroring, validates the speaker's effort to communicate by allowing him or her to confirm, correct, or clarify intent.

Senders and receivers should remember to:

- Follow up on a message to make sure it was sent as intended and received as intended. In face-to-face communication, this is simply a matter of asking a question. In written communication, follow-up can be accomplished with a telephone call, a brief office (or hallway) conference, or written confirmation.
- A manager should avoid the temptation to provide too much information in sending a communication or in giving feedback on it.

This last guideline suggests a common problem, especially in large organizations: the burden of handling too much paperwork and trying to process too much information. Simple written messages probably do not require written responses, and it wastes everyone's time to ask for them. Not all telephone conversations require confirming letters. In addition, a manager should not expect to read from cover to cover every journal that crosses his or her desk. Some sensible decisions must be made about what kind of information exchange is essential, what kind must be committed to paper, what types of information employees need, and what might be left to casual conversation.

As noted earlier, managers should choose the medium that is best suited to a particular message. For example, a sudden and drastic change in an employee's work schedule might best be discussed in a face-to-face conversation rather than in an impersonal memorandum. However, a request for funds to hire a consultant for a special project needs to be formally presented in writing, with solid supporting evidence for the request, rather than in a drop-in conversation. The choice of the appropriate medium should always be made with the receiver's perspective in mind.

CHANNELS OF COMMUNICATION WITHIN ORGANIZATIONS

Because information exchange is essential to the operation of an organization, formal and informal channels of communication ensure that information moves from one point to another efficiently. Formal channels include a vertical track and a horizontal track of communication. The vertical track runs in two directions, *upward* and *downward* between the top of the organizational structure and the bottom. The horizontal track carries communications laterally across the organizational structure between departments and individuals on about the same levels. The most common informal channel of communication in organizations is the *grapevine*.

Another channel of communications that helps to build trust and improve communications is called *walk the talk* or *management by walking around* (MWA). Walk-the talk means leaving your office by walking around and talking face-to-face to employees. This method provides the employer the opportunity to encourage employees to discuss problems or provide solutions to problems about their work, equipment, or other needs. It also gives the employer an opportunity to let employees know the status of events that related to the organization/department. This method also allows the breakdown of status barriers. Posting office hours, which allows employees an opportunity to meet with the director at a specific time and specific day(s), is another effective method. These meetings are to be set up for discussion of events, problems, suggestions, and information. These types of communication can use up a lot of the employer's time and needs to be carefully monitored. Employers and employees may also communicate via e-mail. When this method is used procedures must be developed and followed.

Upward Communication

Upward communication includes verbal and written messages (problems, perceptions, or suggestions) that subordinates send to superiors. Sometimes messages may seek clarification of instructions or advice. Top-level management depends on this vertical flow as a way to monitor each department's or unit's performance to make the best decisions possible in planning future activities of the organization.

Activity and *performance reports* are the most frequent form of upward communication. These provide information necessary for making decisions regarding capital purchases, FTE additions, or other such operational changes. Directors are responsible for adequately communicating to upper management the goals and objectives of the department and how these interface with other departments and with the broader vision of the organization.

Research has shown that the greater the difference in level between an employee and the superior to whom the message is being sent, the more likely it is that the message will be distorted or incomplete. Although department directors should communicate a sincere desire to listen to employees' suggestions and ideas, they must be conscious of employees' tendencies to provide incomplete or inaccurate information. The director should also avoid depending on lower-level employees for essential information.

Downward Communication

Downward communication occurs when information flows from superiors in the organizational hierarchy to employees. Top-level managers communicate the organization's goals and objectives and specify policies and procedures. They also explain the rationale for various operational decisions, give instructions about specific tasks, provide feedback to employees about their performance, and respond to messages from employees. Research suggests that most managers believe that they communicate information to their employees better than they actually do. Because information is often the lifeline of an operation and because accurate information is especially crucial in health care institutions, foodservice directors should examine their own patterns of downward communication for any possible shortcomings. For example, they should never assume that information supplied to higher-level managers will automatically be communicated to lower-level employees. Information that affects employees should be communicated to them deliberately and directly.

Horizontal Communication

Communication that follows the horizontal channel consists of verbal and written information flow between organizational units that are at about the same level. This flow is particularly important in health care institutions because service to patients depends on efficient communication among several different departments. For example, the foodservice department cannot provide appropriate nutrition care services without information about patients from nursing staff. Such interdependence is apparent in daily activities such as meal service, but it also influences the department's long-term ability to plan major projects.

In addition, horizontal communication between units is more direct, thereby relieving some of the strain imposed on the vertical track. Interdepartmental communication minimizes the distortion and slowness of message relay that can hamper upward and downward communication. For example, the foodservice director and the nursing service director can communicate with one another directly and more immediately about a common project without necessarily exchanging information through their respective superiors.

Grapevine

The grapevine is an important route for informal information flow in organizations. *Grapevine communications* are also called rumors, gossip, or scuttlebutt. It is present in all organizations and is usually the result of lack of communications from the "boss," curiosity, and insecurity. It is a natural result of the universal human need for social contact and what the employees feel and think. Unlike formal communication channels, the grapevine operates without planning or documentation. Despite its haphazard nature, the grapevine is sometimes more informative than the messages sent through formal channels. In this sense, the grapevine can work either for or against the interests of management and the well-being of the organization. Some of the information on the grapevine can become dangerous when false information is circulated about an organization, personnel, and policies. Electronic grapevine communications is used to transmit information (true or untrue) around an informal network both inside and external to the organization.

Managers can use the grapevine to get a sense of the attitudes and perceptions among their subordinates and respond to them more quickly than if they waited for problems to surface through formal methods. To minimize the potentially negative effects of grapevine information, managers should share as much information as possible with subordinates about organizational activities. If everyone in the organization has appropriate access to up-to-date and accurate information, the speculation that leads to rumor can be dispelled.

Business Etiquette

Business etiquette contains a number of rules. *Etiquette* means manners that are followed, accepted, or required in society, business, and professions. *Manners* means a way in which something is done or happens; a usual way of acting. Business manners include:

- When on duty wear your name tag in a manner that the photo and name are visible.
- Use proper methods of introduction. A younger person is introduced to an older adult. A person of a high rank is named first and receives the introduction. When introducing others to family members the other person's name is generally first. Men are introduced to women.
- Introduce yourself before addressing someone you do not know, as appropriate exchange business cards.
- Communication etiquette protocol is important in business, such as returning phone calls, answering e-mail, and avoiding gossiping, telling ethnic jokes, flirting with subordinates or your supervisor. Discretion is always the best way to proceed.
- When communicating, look the other person in the eye; when necessary, repeat the person's name often as this helps to remember the name.
- Moderate the tone of your voice, speak calmly, allow the other person to speak without interrupting.
- Listen passionately.
- Always follow the chain of command.

Conflict Resolution

Occasionally a manager must act as a mediator and resolve conflicts between employees or between an employee and a supervisor. A *conflict* is a perceived incompatible difference resulting in interference or opposition. (*Mediation* is the process of working with conflicting parties to suggest settlements and compromises.) Although full treatment of conflict resolution is beyond the scope of this book, this is one of the most important management skills a manager needs to possess. Mediation should be conducted, if

possible, when both parties can be winners. There are times when a manager will be required to end a conflict by making a decision that will be unpopular with one of the parties involved.

Generally, when conflict arises, most people make a "fight-or-flight" decision. If they choose fight, they expect to win. If they choose flight, they will ignore the person with whom they are in the conflict and refuse to talk about the issues. For effective teamwork and management, the manager must have an empowered response to conflict resolution and should understand that neither fight nor flight is appropriate for creating winning solutions to conflict.

There are other methods that can be used by management to assist the individuals or the group to reach a mutually agreeable *consensus*. Although not everyone will agree with the resolution, the individuals or group should have made the most acceptable resolution for everyone.

Other methods that may be used to reach a resolution include:

- *Aggressive* resolution is not the best choice because there will always be a winner and a loser.
- *Submissive* individuals will not participate in a solution due to the dominance of the aggressive individual; usually one or both parties are uncomfortable with the outcome.
- *Avoidance/ignorance* is refusing to discuss the conflict or being ignorant of the real issues.
- *Accommodation* is giving in to stop the conflict.
- *Compromise* is both parties settling the conflict through mutual concessions.
- *Collaboration* is where both sides work together to achieve a resolution.
- *Forcing* is where a decision is forced on the group by management or by a negotiator who was hired to settle the conflict.

Methods for Resolution

The following suggestions are helpful in coming to a resolution:

- Use the decision-making tools as outlined in Chapter 5.
- Be respectful during the process.
- Avoid judgmental comments or criticism.
- Deal with behavior, not the people, and maintain relationships.
- Observe nonverbal behavior.
- Listen to the discussion; give both sides time to speak and give their perspective.
- Be fair; do not go to the meeting with a perceived solution.
- Seek participation from all the members of the group or each individual; do not allow one person to dominate the discussion.
- Establish outcomes for the resolution that everyone will commit to follow.
- Try to reach a balance.
- Ask members of the group for commitment to the resolution.

Communication is the key to resolving conflicts. In meeting privately with opposing parties to mediate issues, the manager should make it clear at the beginning that both parties will have an opportunity to state their point of view. He or she also must emphasize that it is unacceptable for one party to interrupt the other. The meeting should be held in an appropriate location, such as the manager's office or a conference room. Adequate time must be set aside to work out the conflict.

When the mediation session begins, the manager should express concern about the effects the conflict has on both individuals. The manager also should express optimism that a solution can be reached that is in the best interest of both parties. The outcome should be a solution that both can agree to. Once a solution has been reached the manager should clearly and concisely explain to both parties the expectation, standards, and policies for future action. The manager needs to define acceptable and satisfactory behavior and poor performance or interpersonal conflict. The director or manager needs to express confidence that the situation will be resolved and what assistance may be given. It may become necessary to take further action such as probation or corrective action, including termination. It may become necessary to involve human resource management if you think there may be a continuing problem.

In a conflict situation, reactions can be displayed in an eruption of emotions and hurt feelings. Again, these feelings probably are tied to past experiences. The issue at conflict may remind the parties involved of previous situations or topics that, although unrelated, are present in their subconscious. In dealing with conflict, it is important to get individuals to understand why they are angry and what they would consider a suitable outcome.

SUMMARY

Communication is the process of sending and receiving verbal and written information from one person to another. Effective communication is achieved when the message received is in harmony with the message sent. The basic management functions all depend on the communication of information, especially the function of leading and directing employee activities. Active listening is a vital component of communication.

Communication among people on all levels in an organization is vital to accomplishing the organization's work and achieving its goals. In their working relationships, successful managers tend to find and use the most appropriate and effective channels for communication within their organizations. They also develop and use effective interpersonal communication skills while remaining objective and nonjudgmental, always separating the message from the messenger. Employees must also know the policies and procedures for the use of electronic communications.

KEY TERMS

Business letter
Channel of communication
Communication barrier
Conducting meetings
Conflict
Consent agenda
Downward communication
Electronic communication
Horizontal communication

Justification
Listening
Memorandum
Planning meetings
Presentation
Upward communication
Verbal communication
Written communication

DISCUSSION QUESTIONS

1. Determine the best method to use when holding a business meeting, a production meeting, and an all-employee information-passing meeting.
2. Practice communicating with a group of friends and try to determine how many barriers you observed during the conversation.
3. Discuss how a presentation on *Food Code 2009* can be made to ensure safe handling of food.
4. Write a business letter, memorandum, and a justification for hiring a part-time room-service employee.
5. Closely listen (follow the guide in the text) to a group of friends. What did you learn?
6. Explain an ongoing conflict between two employees and give steps to reach an agreement with the two employees.

CHAPTER 8

HUMAN RESOURCE MANAGEMENT
Laws for Employment and the Employment Process

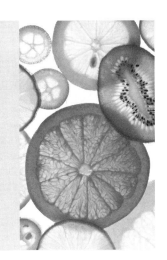

LEARNING OBJECTIVES

- Gain knowledge concerning the legal ramifications of improper actions that may lead to ligation when laws are not followed.
- Develop an interview checklist that complies with all federal laws, rules, and regulations.
- Follow established standards in hiring, orienting, and training.
- Implement training programs for all employees.
- Maintain individual personnel records of the hiring procedure, orientation, and in-service.
- Work closely with human resources to maintain compliance with law and the facility personnel policies and procedures.

A N ORGANIZATION'S MOST valuable resources are the people who perform the work—its *human resources*—without whom no organization could function. Employers who recognize this fact understand the importance of involving employees in meaningful work to ensure their long-term retention. Consequently, human resource departments have become a mainstay in organizations of all kinds. The department advocates employee rights and serve as a source of counsel for managers on all levels.

The structure of a health care organization's human resource department varies with the size of the institution. Specific departmental activities also vary with type and size of the facility. In any case, a foodservice director must work closely with human resource specialists to make sure that the department's service delivery complies with labor laws and with the organization's personnel policies and procedures.

This chapter discusses the following specific areas of concern in human resource management:

- Laws that affect the employer-employee relationship
- The role of the human resource department
- The employment process (recruiting, screening, interviewing, hiring, orienting)
- Employee training and coaching

Although foodservice directors may not be directly responsible for performing all of these activities, they are involved in or affected by each one in some way. In small health care organizations, the foodservice department may be directly responsible for performing some of the activities usually performed by human resource departments in large organizations—for example, conducting its own training and orientation programs. In addition, foodservice supervisors may be charged with interviewing and hiring new employees they will supervise directly.

LAWS THAT AFFECT THE EMPLOYER-EMPLOYEE RELATIONSHIP

Federal, state, and local laws and regulations affect the way employers hire, pay, and manage their employees. In most health care organizations, the human resource department is primarily responsible for making sure the organization's personnel policies are fair and legal. However, anyone whose job is to supervise or manage other people must also be aware of workers' legal rights.

Most of the laws that affect human resource management fall into one of the following five areas:

1. Equal employment opportunity
2. Compensation and benefits

3. Labor relations
4. Health and safety
5. Immigration reform

The remainder of this section briefly describes the major federal laws that affect human resource management.

Equal Employment Opportunity Legislation

Equal employment legislation forbids employers to discriminate against employees on the basis of race, color, religion, sex, disability, or national origin. The Equal Employment Opportunity Commission (EEOC) is the federal agency charged with making sure that workers are not discriminated against. All areas of employment are regulated, including:

- Hiring
- Dismissals, work reductions, and layoffs
- Disciplinary actions
- Compensation policies
- Access to training and advancement

The EEOC's regulations are based primarily on Title VII of the Civil Rights Act of 1964. Several other laws have made other kinds of discrimination illegal as well.

Civil Rights Act of 1964 (Amended 1972)

Title VII of the Civil Rights Act of 1964, and later laws that amended (or legally changed) the act, regulates the employment practices of most U.S. employers having 15 or more employees. (The Equal Employment Opportunity Act is one of the laws that amended Title VII.) Under Title VII, it is illegal for employers to discriminate based on race, color, religion, sex, or national origin in hiring, firing, promoting, compensating, or in terms, conditions, or privileges of employment.

Age Discrimination in Employment Act of 1967 (Amended 1978 and 1986)

The Age Discrimination in Employment Act protects persons aged 40 years or older from age discrimination in selection, discharge, and job assignments. The law prohibits employers from replacing employees with younger workers, regardless of whether the purpose is to save money in wages or to give a company a more youthful image.

Vocational Rehabilitation Act of 1973

Section 503 of the Rehabilitation Act of 1973, as amended by the Rehabilitation Act Amendments of 1986, affects all companies that hold federal contracts for $2,500 or more. According to the amendments, such employers must take affirmative action to avoid breaking the law. That is, they must seek out, hire, and advance reasonably well-qualified individuals who belong to racial, sexual, or ethnic groups that because of discrimination have been under-represented in the past. Also protected by the affirmative action mandate are individuals with physical and mental challenges.

Vietnam Era Veterans Readjustment Assistance Act of 1974

Section 402 of the Vietnam Era Veterans Readjustment Assistance Act prohibits discrimination against disabled veterans in general. It applies specifically to veterans of the Vietnam War.

Pregnancy Discrimination Act of 1978

The Pregnancy Discrimination Act represents an amendment to Title VII of the 1964 Civil Rights Act. This law prohibits discrimination against workers on the basis of pregnancy, recent childbirth, or related medical conditions. It applies to employment practices and to qualification for employee benefits.

Interpretive Guidelines on Discrimination Because of Sex, National Origin, and Religion

Under Title VII of the Civil Rights Act amended in 1972, the EEOC generally prohibits discrimination in employment on the basis of gender. The EEOC has issued interpretive guidelines that state that employers have an affirmative duty to maintain a workplace free from sexual harassment and intimidation. Under these guidelines, employers are totally liable for the acts of their supervisors, regardless of whether the employer is aware of the sexual harassment. The guidelines state that harassment on the basis of sex is a violation of Title VII when such conduct has the purpose or effect of substantially interfering with a person's work performance or creating an intimidating, hostile, or offensive work environment. *Sexual harassment* in the workplace is defined as subjecting a person to unwelcome sexual advances, requests for sexual favors, and other verbal or physical conduct of a sexual nature. Sexual harassment is illegal under any one of the following conditions:

- When an employee is required to submit to such conduct as a condition of his or her continued employment
- When an employee's submission to such conduct is made the basis of a hiring decision
- When an employee's subjection to such conduct has the purpose or effect of unreasonably interfering with his or her work performance
- When such conduct creates an intimidating, hostile, or offensive working environment for employees

In 1993 EEOC issued a definition of harassment:

It is unlawful harassment if there is verbal or physical conduct that denigrates or shows hostility or aversion towards an individual because of race, color, religion, gender, national origin, age or disability, or that of their relatives, friends, or associations and that:

- Has the purpose or effect of creating an intimidating, hostile, or offensive working environment;
- Has the purpose or effect of unreasonably interfering with an individual's work performance
- Otherwise adversely affects an individual's employment opportunities.

Ethnic slurs and other verbal or physical conduct relating to an individual's national origin constitute harassment. Racial jokes are an example of what might constitute ethnic harassment.

Employers have an obligation to accommodate religious practices unless they can demonstrate a resulting hardship. The guidelines identify methods that would accommodate religious practices that include voluntary substitutes, flexible scheduling, lateral transfer, and change of job assignment.

EEOC policy guidelines on sexual harassment require employers to install a distinct policy against sexual harassment. To meet this requirement, the policy should demonstrate examples of exactly what is considered sexual harassment, an explanation of whom to talk to (other than a direct supervisor), the importance of confidentiality, and the fact that reprisal actions against a person claiming sexual harassment are not tolerated by the organization. The policy also should state that disciplinary action could include termination and that management is responsible for monitoring and preventing sexual harassment in the workplace.

Civil Rights Act of 1991

In 1991 Congress passed a comprehensive set of amendments to Title VII. Among the most important aspects of the law is this passage: "*Quotas*—are prohibited under this law. Quotas have been used by employers to adjust the hiring decision to ensure that a certain number of people from certain protected classes are hired. . . . Collection for damages either punitive or compensatory are allowed. *Punitive damages* are fines awarded to a plaintiff to punish the defendant; *compensatory damages* are fines awarded to a plaintiff to compensate for financial or psychological harm the plaintiff has suffered as a result of discrimination act."

The term *glass ceiling* is included in the 1991 Civil Rights Act. The glass ceiling is the invisible barrier of an organization that prevents many women and minorities from achieving top-level management positions. An aspect of the act was the establishment of a Glass Ceiling Commission to study how management fills higher-level positions, the qualifications needed for advancement, and the compensation plan and reward structures that are in place.

Executive Order 11246, Amended by Executive Order 11375

In 1965 Executive Order 11246 was established by then-president Lyndon Johnson. It prohibits discrimination in employment due to race, creed, color, or national origin. The major provision of Executive Order 11246 was the affirmative action that requires covered employers to take positive steps to ensure employment of applicants and treatment of employees during employment without regard to race, creed, color, or national origin. In 1968 Executive Order 11246

was amended to Executive Order 11375, which changed the word "creed" to "religion" and added "sex discrimination" to the other prohibited terms.

Privacy Act of 1974

Employees of the U.S. federal government have the privacy of their personnel files protected as well as lockers and personal inspections, background investigations, and other matters. The act requires federal agencies to permit employees to examine, copy, correct, or amend employee information in their personnel files. The act includes a provision for an appeal over disputed material in the file.

Americans with Disabilities Act of 1990 (Title I)

Title I of the Americans with Disabilities Act became effective July 26, 1992, for employers with 25 or more employees and July 26, 1994, for employers with 15 to 24 employees. Title I of the act prohibits employment discrimination against disabled workers who are qualified to perform the essential functions of a job. The law in this regard covers all aspects of employment, including the application process and hiring, on-the-job training, advancement and wages, benefits, and employer-sponsored social activities. An employer must provide reasonable accommodations unless it can be proved that such accommodations would impose undue hardship on the employer.

Disability under the Americans with Disabilities Act is defined as:

- Any physical or mental impairment that substantially limits one or more major life activities
- A record of such impairment
- An individual regarded as having such an impairment

In this definition, major life activities include—but are not limited to—seeing, hearing, speaking, walking, breathing, learning, working, performing manual tasks, and caring for oneself.

Employers are required to make reasonable accommodations or modifications that help impaired individuals in completing essential functions of a job. *Reasonable accommodations or modifications* are identified as adjustments to a job or the work environment that will allow a qualified disabled person to perform essential job functions if these accommodations do not create undue hardship. With respect to the provision of an accommodation, undue hardship is defined as significant difficulty or expense incurred by a covered entity.

As related to nutrition and foodservice, department directors are required to consider carefully what are outlined in job descriptions as essential job functions and what could be reassigned to provide reasonable accommodations. During an interview, neither employers nor their representatives can ask whether an applicant has a disability, but they may ask whether the applicant can perform the job with or without accommodation.

Bona fide occupational qualifications (BFOQ) are based on criteria for employment that can be clearly justified as being related to a person's capacity to perform a job. It is the right to employment and advancement without regard to race, religion, sex, age, color, or national origin. However, an employer has the right to establish BFOQ. The criteria must be justified as relating to a person's capacity to perform the job.

Compensation and Benefits Legislation

Several important federal laws regulate how employers pay their employees and provide employee benefits. The following subsections briefly describe this body of legislation.

Social Security Act of 1935

The Social Security Act of 1935 created a system of retirement benefits. The act established a federal payroll tax to fund unemployment and retirement benefits. Employers are required to share equally with employees the cost of old age, survivors, and disability insurance. Employers are required to pay the full cost of unemployment insurance.

Social Security provides retirement income to people who retired at age 62 in 2000; the retirement age will gradually increment until 2007, when it reaches age 66. After stabilizing at this age for a period of time, it will increase again.

For people who become disabled and cannot work for at least 12 months, Social Security provides a monthly income comparable to retirement benefits.

Medicare is a part of the Social Security program that provides health insurance coverage for people aged 65 and older. Medicare has two parts: Part A covers hospital costs, and Part B covers medical expenses. People pay an annual deduction for Parts A and B. Survivors' benefits are paid to the deceased employee's family members if they qualify.

Fair Labor Standards Act of 1938

The Fair Labor Standards Act (FLSA), also called the Wage and Hour Law, requires all organizations covered by the act to pay non-salaried employees at least the *minimum wage*, an hourly wage that is fixed by the federal government and is considered to be the lowest wage on which an individual can live under current economic conditions. The federal minimum wage was $4.25 per hour in 1993. However, in August 1993, a bill introduced in Congress raised the federal minimum wage to $4.50 and further increases would be tied to the rate of inflation. In 2009 the minimum wage was $7.25 for nonexempt employees. Congress sets the minimum wage for non-exempt employees. States may have a legal rate that is higher than the federal rate; where such laws exist, the higher rate prevails.

The FLSA defines two categories of employees: *exempt* and *nonexempt*. Exempt employees include professional, executive, administrative, and outside sales jobs. The Department of Labor provides guidelines to determine if a job is exempt or nonexempt. Exempt employees are not covered by the provision of the FLSA. Nonexempt employees are covered by the FLSA. Nonexempt employees who are paid an hourly salary must be paid overtime at the rate for the number of hours worked beyond 40 hours in one week. The usual overtime rate is time and a half. Congress is in the process of redefining overtime, the rate of pay, and employees who are eligible to receive overtime pay.

Equal Pay Act of 1963

The Equal Pay Act, an amendment to the FLSA, requires employers to pay equal wages to men and women for doing the same jobs. The jobs must require equal skill, effort, and responsibility, and they must be performed under similar working conditions.

There are four exceptions that allow employees to pay one sex more than the other—more seniority, better job performance, greater quantity or quality of production, and certain other factors such as paying extra compensation to employees working a night shift. Although sexual equality is law, the federal government in 2009 stated that of the 122 million women age 16 and over in the United States, 72 million or 59.2 percent were working; of the 66 million women employed, 74 percent worked full time and 26 percent worked part time. The median weekly earning of women who were full time wage and salary workers was $657—or 80 percent of men's $819. When comparing the median weekly earnings of persons age 16 to 24, young women earned 93 percent of what young men earned ($424 and $458, respectively).

In all instances women earned less than men. Women are moving forward in the workplace with an increase in executive/managerial positions, and women hold the majority of the jobs in the field of technical and related support service. In some occupations, women's salaries surpass men's.

Lily Ledbetter Fair Pay Restoration Act

In 2009 President Obama signed the Lily Ledbetter Fair Pay Restoration Act, which allows victims of pay discrimination to file a complaint with the government against an employer within 180 days of their last paycheck. The president has vowed to reduce the wage gap between genders. At present women make $.78 to every man's $1.00.

Unemployment Insurance

The Social Security Act of 1935 established unemployment insurance to provide temporary income for people during periods of involuntary unemployment, such as a layoff. Compensation is usually for 26 weeks but the government can extend the time. Unemployment insurance is funded by a tax paid by employers on all employees' earnings. Unemployment benefits are administered by the state. The proceeds of the tax are split between the state and federal governments, which provide different services for the unemployed.

To be eligible for unemployment insurance, employees must meet these qualifications:

- Must be available for and actively seeking employment.
- Must have worked a minimum of four quarter-year periods out of the past five quarter-year periods and earned at least $1,000 during the four quarter periods.

- Must have left the job involuntarily or became unemployed through no fault of their own.

The following conditions render employees ineligible for unemployment insurance:

- Quit their job voluntarily.
- Discharged for gross misconduct.
- Participated in a strike.

Workers' Compensation Insurance

Both state and federal workers' compensation insurance compensates employees or their families for the cost of work-related accidents and illnesses. In most states, workers' compensation insurance is compulsory. Workers' compensation laws typically stipulate that insured employees will be paid a disability benefit that is usually based on a percentage of their wages. Benefits vary from state to state, but there are usually four types of disabilities: permanent partial disability, permanent total disability, temporary partial disability, and temporary total disability.

Disabilities may result from injuries or accidents, occupational diseases, radiation illness, and asbestosis.

Employee Retirement Income Security Act of 1974

The Employee Retirement Income Security Act (ERISA) sets standards for companies that protect private pension plans for employees from mismanagement. However, ERISA does not require companies to offer employee pension plans. As mandated by the act, employers must have a system for providing federal retirement insurance for cases in which employers' pension plans go bankrupt. The goal of ERISA is to ensure that employees who are covered by pension plans receive all of the benefits to which they are entitled; this is called *vesting*.

Family and Medical Leave Act of 1993

The Family and Medical Leave Act requires employers with at least 50 employees to provide up to 12 weeks of unpaid, job-protected leave to eligible employees for certain family and medical reasons. Employees are eligible if they have worked for a covered employer for at least one year and for 1,250 hours during the previous 12 months. Reasons for taking the leave include the employee's need to care for his or her newborn child or a child placed with the employee for adoption or foster care; to care for a spouse, son, daughter, or parent who has a serious health condition; or to attend to the employee's own serious health condition that makes the employee unable to perform his or her job.

Labor Relations Legislation

The federal government regulates how unions conduct their activities and how companies deal with unions. Managers should understand the requirements of the three main labor relations laws, as described below.

National Labor Relations Act of 1935 (Wagner Act)

The federal National Labor Relation Act of 1935 (NLRA) "protects the rights of workers to organize and bargain collectively and prohibits management from engaging in unfair labor practices that would interfere with these rights." These rights include "employees' rights to join a union, to engage in such activities as strikes, picketing, and collective bargaining." Unfair management practices include "firing employees who support unionization, threatening or bribing employees, and sending spies to union meetings."

Labor unions are organizations that employees join that act as spokespeople on behalf of the employees. Labor unions are a collective voice of employees that can be heard when a single voice may not. Labor unions develop *labor contracts* that detail the rights and obligations of employees and management that deal with wages, work hours, work rules, seniority, hiring practices, grievances, and other work-related rules.

Labor unions also use *collective bargaining* to bring management and union representatives together in negotiating, administering, and interpreting the labor contract. Among the worker's rights legalize by the NLRA was the right to enter into a *closed shop* agreement. A closed shop differs from a *union shop*, in which all workers, once employed, must become union members within a specified period of time as conditions of their employment. *Closed shop* agreements ensure that only union members who are bound by internal union rules, including rules enforcing worker solidarity during strikes, are hired.

The National Labor Relations Board has the power to enforce the act. The National Labor Relations Board can look into any labor dispute that affects interstate commerce (business dealings between companies in different states).

The Obama Administration and the NLRB made major changes in rules concerning the role of management and unions. These changes:

- Require employers to hang posters which inform employees that they have the legal right to form unions
- Strengthen a union's ability to retain representation after a business is sold
- Prevent rival union or group of antiunion employees from trying to toss out a new union

The posters state that the employee can "join or assist a union" and that employers are **not** allowed to "fire, demote, or transfer you . . . because you join a union." They also state that unions cannot "threaten or coerce you in order to gain support for the union" and that unions may **not** "refuse to process a grievance because you have criticized union officials." These changes have an effect on all foodservice departments whether they are or are not unionized. (See http://unionreview.com/NLRB_Get_Heard_Now; posters may be downloaded from the NLRB's website.)

Labor-Management Relations Act of 1947 (Taft-Hartley Act)

In 1947 Congress amended the National Labor Relations Act and the amended version became known as the Taft–Hartley Act. This new law placed many restrictions on union activities. It limited picketing rights, banned supervisory employees from participating in unions, and restricted the right to strike in situations where the President and Congress determined that a strike would endanger national health or safety. The law allowed states to ban union shops by passing the *Right-to-Work law* that prohibits employees from being required to join a union as a condition of receiving or retaining a job. Another condition of the law was the outlaw of the *closed shops*, but did allow collectively bargained agreements for union shops, provided certain safeguards were met. It also establishes procedures for *secret ballot election*. In secret ballot elections, employees decide whether a union will represent them in collective-bargaining negotiations with management.

Labor-Management Reporting and Disclosure Act of 1959 (Landrum-Griffin Act)

The Labor-Management Reporting and Disclosure Act was passed to strengthen democracy within unions. The act protects the individual rights of union members and limits the economic and political power of unions. It also requires that unions report their financial status to the government. Regulations based on the law affect secondary boycotts, informational picketing, and recognition and jurisdictional strikes.

Health and Safety Legislation

Many federal and state laws protect the health and safety of employees in the workplace. Regulations that affect foodservice departments in health care organizations are discussed in other chapters. However, the most far-reaching federal law that affects the health and safety of U.S. workers is briefly described below.

Occupational Safety and Health Act of 1970

Under the Occupational Safety and Health Act (OSHA), employers are required to provide employees with "employment and a place of employment which are free from recognized hazards that are causing or are likely to cause death or serious physical harm." Employers also are required to obey all safety and health standards established by the Occupational Safety and Health Administration (OSHA). One such standard deals with blood-borne pathogens. The OSHA standards are enforced through on-site inspections, and employers found to be in violation are subject to fines and other penalties. (The OSHA standards related specifically to the foodservice department also will be discussed in Chapter 15.)

Fringe Benefits or Discretionary Benefits

Most organizations offer their employees *fringe benefits* that provide security for employees and their families. The cost to employers for each employee per year varies from approximately $10,000 upward to $250,000 as is seen in some financial institutions. These benefits account for 30 percent or more of a typical worker's earning. Legally the U.S. law requires the employer to provide for only four benefits to all employees, with a few exceptions: (1) Social Security, (2) worker's compensation, (3) unemployment insurance, and (4) family and medical leave. Other benefits are provided voluntarily by the employer. All of the following voluntary benefits may not apply to all organizations/employers. These benefits include:

- Health insurance (This is subject to change under President Obama's health care plan. You will need to keep up with these changes.)
- Retirement pay after employee retires
- Various types of insurance (life, disability, death, long-term care)
- Employee stock options
- Paid time off (vacations; sick leave; a certain number of days per year that employees can use as they wish; obligations like civic duties, jury duty, and National Guard or military reserve; voting time; bereavement time; coffee breaks; lunch periods)

Another benefit plan is a required amount of money from the employer to be added to a retirement or saving account that has been established for the employee. There is a shift away from benefits and contributions plans to a *Roth plan* and/or *401(k) plan*. The 401(k) plan is where employees defer income up to a maximum amount allowed. In some organizations the employer matches the employee's contribution for 50 cents for each dollar deferred. Under this system employees set up their own retirement plans.

Immigration Reform Legislation

Federal legislation affects all U.S. employers. It has specific effects on those employers who employ or seek to employ citizens of countries other than the United States. The body of law that covers employment of immigrant (or alien) workers in the United States is described in the following subsection.

Immigration Reform and Control Act of 1986

The Immigration Reform and Control Act of 1986 was passed to stop the unlawful employment of unauthorized immigrants in the United States. The act requires employers to verify the citizenship status and employment eligibility of all employees hired after June 1, 1987, as well as all current employees hired after November 6, 1986. To comply with this law, employers must request that all new employees supply proof of their identity and employment eligibility. Proof may be in the form of a valid driver's license, a Social Security card, or an unexpired reentry permit, among others. They also must complete a Form I-9 certifying that they are eligible for employment.

The Immigration Reform and Control Act imposes substantial civil and criminal penalties on employers who knowingly violate this law. In addition, the law makes it illegal to discriminate against any individual other than unauthorized immigrants on the basis of national origin or status as a citizen or an "intending citizen." All areas of human resource management are covered, including hiring, recruitment, referral, and discharge. A separate enforcement procedure has been established to handle discrimination violations. However, any alleged discrimination that is covered under Title VII of the Civil Rights Act of 1964 would still be addressed under the provisions of that act.

Illegal Immigration Reform and Immigrant Responsibility Act

In 1990 the Immigration Act revised U.S. policy on legal immigration, increasing levels of immigration of highly skilled professionals and executives. In 1996 the Illegal Immigration Reform and Immigrant Responsibility Act became law. This law placed limitations on persons who have come to the United States and remained in the country longer than permitted by their visas or persons and who have violated their nonimmigrant status. (It is your **responsibility** to keep informed on the status of this act as many states are establishing various laws that limit illegal persons to hold jobs, rent homes, and so on. With the high unemployment rate and the anger and concern of U.S. citizens regarding the benefits offered to illegal immigrants, many states are drafting laws that hinder the status of illegal immigrants. As of April 2012, the Supreme Court is hearing cases, especially Arizona law.)

ROLE OF THE HUMAN RESOURCE DEPARTMENT

Most organizations today have some form of human resource department. In large organizations especially (those with more than 200 employees), this department is a separate, discrete entity whose role is to perform unique functions. In some organizations, the human resource department may be called the personnel department or employee relations department.

Health care human resource departments are charged with five major areas of responsibility:

1. Recruitment and employee activities
2. Performance evaluation policies and procedures
3. Compensation and benefits administration
4. Labor relations
5. Analyzing staffing needs—benchmarking for staff required

Specific responsibilities of the department vary from one organization to another, depending in part on the organization's structure and number of people it employs. For example, in a large teaching hospital, the human resource department might be responsible for the initial screening and interviewing of potential employees. In addition, it might be active in developing standards for evaluating employee performance, maintaining employee records, and operating employee training and orientation programs. In most health care organizations, the human resource department is directly responsible for administering the compensation and benefits program, managing the overall employment process, and overseeing labor relations.

Functions of the human resource department revolve around recruitment and retention of competent employees to staff the organization. Responsibility for successfully performing these functions generally is shared with department and unit managers. Human resource specialists advise, counsel, and assist health care managers from all departments in a variety of activities related to employee management. For example, human resource specialists may perform the following functions:

- Recruit new employees and offer advice on hiring decisions.
- Conduct organization-wide orientation.
- Help determine what new employees should be paid.
- Set up standards for evaluating the performance of current employees.
- Help initiate corrective action procedures.
- Handle employee grievances.
- Resolve benefit issues.
- Interpret personnel policies and procedures.
- Coordinate the negotiation and implementation of labor contracts.

In health care, as in other businesses, the human resource department acts as a communications link between employees and their managers. As a trusted employee advocate, a human resource representative is available to help resolve employee issues and problems. For example, an employee may wish to discuss a work-related issue, such as perceived discrimination, or a personal problem that affects work performance, such as stress or chemical dependency. In this capacity, the representative works to resolve the issue or problem by taking appropriate action.

Another key function of a human resource department is to ensure fair treatment to all employees. Accomplishment of this priority depends on having the support and cooperation of management, administration, and the board of directors. The department also is responsible for ensuring compliance with federal, state, and local laws regulating employment, prohibiting discrimination, and promoting equal employment opportunities for protected classes, such as women, minorities, and persons with disabilities. If the organization is required by law to have an affirmative action plan, the human resource department is responsible for its development and implementation.

The foodservice director must work closely with human resource specialists to keep the nutrition and foodservice department in compliance with the law and with the institution's personnel policies and procedures. In addition, the director should make sure that his or her department's employee performance records contain all information required by law. In managing conflict resolution, the director must carefully follow human resource policies on disciplinary, probation, and grievance procedures. Finally, the director should discuss special problems—for example, claims of sexual harassment within the department—with representatives of the human resource department. In addition, the organization's legal affairs staff may need to be consulted at times to ensure nondiscrimination.

FIGURE 8.1 The Employment Process

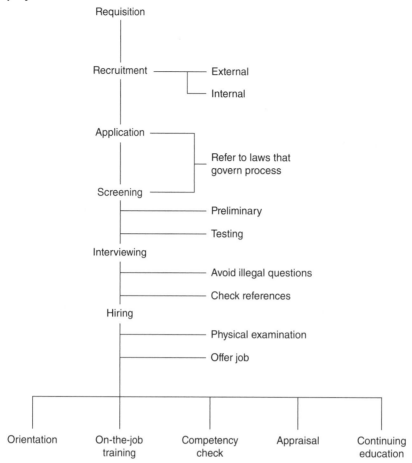

Source: Ruby P. Puckett. Developed by Ruby P. Puckett©.

Employment Process

The foodservice director may share responsibility for recruiting and hiring new employees with the human resources department. No matter where this responsibility falls, nine basic steps are almost always followed in the process of recruiting and hiring employees (sometimes referred to here as the employment process) (see Figure 8.1). These include the following:

1. Prepare the personnel requisition (request for a specific job and job description number).
2. Recruit qualified applicants.
3. Take applications.
4. Screen applicants.
5. Interview applicants (may require more than one interview and various interviewing methods).
6. Check references—reference checks are usually performed by human resources to avoid invading the privacy of an individual.
7. Make the final hiring decision in most cases the foodservice director or designee makes the final decision.
8. Arrange for a physical examination and drug screen, if applicable. This is a human resources responsibility.
9. Conduct a new employee orientation program (to the facility, human resources; to the department, foodservice director or designee).

The operation of a foodservice department is like the operation of any business organization in that its success depends on the skills and commitment of its human resources—the people who do the work. For this reason, it is extremely important that the recruitment and hiring process be conducted with careful adherence to the letter and spirit of the law. When recruiting for foodservice personnel, the human resource department needs to be knowledgeable concerning the types of personnel required and the hours worked. The foodservice department is composed of a variety of *professional* and *nonprofessional* employees. Professional employees have extensive academic training, experience, and skills to make independent judgments and work with minimum supervision. This group is made up of directors, dietitians, dietetics technicians, and dietary managers. Some foodservice jobs may be entry level, that is, suitable for persons just entering the profession who have the education and basic skills required to do the job, but who may need additional supervision in the beginning. Some of the professionals may have advanced education, training, or skills and be specialized, such as a certified diabetes educator. Supervisory personnel have the authority and responsibility for a group of subordinate workers and are accountable for their own work. The supervisor is responsible to ensure that standards are maintained and for the output of the group. The department also employs skilled and unskilled workers. *Skilled workers* have received special training or have the ability to perform the job functions. A skilled worker is a cook or baker. *Unskilled workers* usually have no marketable skills and are trained on the job. The department also employs full-time employees. A *full-time employee (FTE)* is one who usually works 40 hours a week. Some organizations consider 32 hours per week as full-time. *Part-time employees* are those who work a set number of hours per week, usually 16 to 20 hours. Some employees *job share*: two or more people work together in the same job to equal the hours of a full-time employee. Some dietitians like this type of position, with the hours and days being decided by the dietitians and directors.

Temporary employees may be used during times of high census, to complete a project, to fill in for illness, or for other leave reasons. Temporary employees may be professional or nonprofessional.

Contract employees are hired for a specific task or project such as a dietitian or engineer to install a new tray line system. These people are usually consultants who are paid a set fee. Consultants pay their own benefits and taxes.

Foodservice personnel may be paid by the hour. An **hourly employee** receives a set fee for the hours worked. This may be minimum wage or a higher scale determined by the competition, the organization's compensation plan, or both. Other foodservice employees may be paid a salary and are considered **salaried employees**; they are paid for the job.

A foodservice department also employs a diverse work group. Workers may have different ethnic backgrounds, racial diversity, age, gender, religion, and other differences. All of these factors must be considered by the human resource department and the foodservice professionals during the employment process.

Hiring employees who lack the skill, experience, and incentive to perform their jobs contributes to an organization's turnover rate. Turnover is expensive because the process involved in recruiting, hiring, and training new employees draws on many resources, including time, energy, staff, money, and materials. During this process, the department's productivity can fall and so can employee morale. Therefore, excessive repetition of this cycle should be guarded against.

Earlier chapters described the legislation regarding treating employees fairly in the employment process. To avoid illegal discrimination against applicants on the basis of sex, age, race, color, religion, or national origin and to refrain from asking illegal questions on application forms and during interviews, managers who take part in this process must remember one critical fact: their organization can be sued by unsuccessful applicants who claim unfair treatment or discrimination.

Preparing a Personnel Requisition (Request for Employee)

A foodservice department's operating budget specifies how many full-time-equivalent employees it may employ. A position becomes vacant when an employee resigns or is dismissed or when a new position is added because of increased workload. At this point, the foodservice director should start the recruitment and hiring process to avoid problems associated with understaffing.

The first step is to fill out a *personnel requisition*. The official title of the vacant position, the pay grade, job description and number, qualifications and experience required, and any other information needed by the human resource department should be completed on this form. The director then signs the request and, if applicable, submits it to his or her immediate supervisor for approval.

Once approved, the personnel requisition is sent to the human resource department, where it is checked for accuracy and completeness. In large organizations, the requisition is handled by an employment manager; in small facilities, it may be handled by the director of the human resource department or by one of the department's clerical assistants. The next step is recruitment.

Recruiting Qualified Applicants

Recruitment is the process of identifying and attracting qualified potential employees on a timely basis and in sufficient number. Usually the human resource department is directly responsible for recruiting applicants from inside and outside the organization. However, qualified candidates may be recommended or referred by members of the foodservice staff or by outside referral sources (for example, another health care facility).

In filling job openings, many organizations have a policy of hiring from within the organization. This policy encourages employees' commitment and allows them to advance within the organization. Also, such a policy may be part of the organization's contractual agreement with an organized labor union. With a policy of *internal recruiting*, the vacancy must be publicized in-house before outside applicants are sought. For a certain length of time as specified by policy, job openings are routinely posted on bulletin boards in the human resource department, the human resource in-house website, in staff lounges, or in other designated posting places in the facility. *Job posting* is publicizing the open job; it lists qualifications, supervisor, working schedule, and pay grade (rate).

Job bidding is a technique that permits employees, within the organization, who believe that they possess the required qualifications to apply for the posted job.

Once internal candidates have been provided the chance to apply, the department begins the *external recruiting process*. One possible source for external applicants is current staff members who may recommend people they know. Government and private employment agencies are another source. Public and private employment agencies help organizations recruit employees. *Private* agencies usually recruit employees for white-collar jobs. Private employment agencies charge a fee that may or may not be paid by the recruiting organization. *Public* employment agencies' main recruitment is for operative jobs, but they also recruit for technical and management positions. Public employment agencies provide their services without charge to either the employer or the prospective employee. High schools, vocational schools, and community colleges are a good source for recruiting full-time and part-time employees.

Executive search firms are organizations that seek the most qualified executive available for a specific position and are generally retained by an organization or company needing specific types of individuals. These firms usually search nationwide. A search firm's fee is usually a percentage of the individual's compensation for the first year. The client pays expenses as well as the fee.

Professional associations such as the Academy of Nutrition and Dietetics (AND), Association of Nutrition and Foodservice Professionals (ANFP), and others provide recruitment services for their members by including job advertisements in journals and job markets at national meetings.

Some health care organizations hold *open houses* as a means of recruiting. Due to the short supply of health care personnel, this method is held on college campuses, health fairs, and in health care facilities.

Colleges with foodservice programs and dietitian training programs have *placement offices* that are eager to help students and graduates find jobs. Advertisements can be run in local and out-of-town newspapers and in foodservice industry publications. Job fairs are usually held on college campuses. People seeking employment meet recruiters face-to-face to discuss job availability and to match individuals to specific jobs. The *Internet* is used by organizations to post jobs, and individuals use it to post their résumé. This is among the newest methods of recruiting.

Advertisements in local newspapers, magazines, television, radio, and professional journals should briefly describe the duties and responsibilities of the position and the qualifications required. Such information is taken from a current job specification that corresponds to the official job description for the position. For a new position, a job description and job specifications must be developed by the appropriate team. (Job descriptions and specifications are discussed in Chapter 6.) All recruitment activities must comply with equal employment opportunity law as outlined earlier in this chapter.

Taking Applications

The *application blank* provides an opportunity to gather basic nondiscriminatory information on all persons who apply for a job position. Each external applicant should personally fill out a written employment application. Internal candidates should fill out whatever forms are required by the institution's personnel policies and procedures. Application forms should ask only for job-related information needed to determine an applicant's qualifications for the position. Forms should be supplied or approved by the human resource department to ensure compliance with EEOC guidelines, immigration regulations, and affirmative action program requirements.

The application blank is a useful tool in the employment process. The form contains name, address, telephone number, Social Security number, and who to contact in case of an emergency. The information on education, military service, experience, work record, and references is used to determine if the applicant meets the job requirements and needs to be given further consideration for the

position. The main purpose of the application blank is to aid in the selection process.

No application may ask questions that violate the legal rights of an applicant. For example, employers may not ask—on written application forms or during personal interviews—whether an applicant has an arrest record or has organizational affiliations that do not relate directly to the position applied for. Civil rights laws forbid employers from asking questions related to age, race, religion, or national origin. However, the *application form* may include questions similar to "Have you ever been convicted of a felony or a misdemeanor involving any violent act, use or possession of a weapon, or act of dishonesty for which the record has been sealed or expunged?" It is recommended that the application contain certain language that the conviction of a crime will **not** automatically result in a denial of employment. Automatic disqualification could be a violation of state and federal laws. However, the employer may deny employment **if** the employer can establish a business-related reason for the refusal to hire. Questions related to disabilities or medical conditions also may not be asked as part of the hiring process. Applicants may not be asked about their familial status or whether they plan to have children. However, questions about age, medical condition, marital status, and number of dependents may be asked **after** an applicant has been officially hired. This is because such information is needed on applications for health insurance and life insurance coverage offered to new employees as part of their employee benefits.

Screening Applicants

The sequence of activities in the screening stage may vary. Many times, unqualified applicants are screened out, or eliminated, when they ask about the position by telephone or mail before filling out an application. Furthermore, the human resource representative may either screen out unqualified applicants soon after they apply or wait until all potential candidates have filled out applications and then eliminate those whose skills, training, or experience do not match requirements for the position.

If the position requires special skills, such as typing, computer literacy, or experience using technical office equipment, the human resource department may test the applicants to determine whether their skills meet the criteria specified for the job. Some organizations may employ qualified persons to administer intelligence, personality, and aptitude tests as well. However, test results cannot be used for purposes of discrimination. In addition, these tests must be standardized and proved to be ethnically and sexually unbiased by independent testing authorities. The use of all such tests must be coordinated and monitored by professionals trained in their administration and fair interpretation.

The foodservice director may further screen qualified applicants to determine which individuals will be interviewed. Interviewing is time-consuming and costly and should be reserved for the best-qualified applicants. There is no magic formula for the number of candidates who should be interviewed, but enough people should be seen to ensure that the best candidate available is offered the job.

Interviewing Applicants

After unqualified applicants have been screened out, interviews with potential employees are scheduled by the human resource department. In some organizations, the employment manager interviews the candidates before the foodservice manager does. In others, the foodservice director or a designee may be the only person who actually interviews the candidates. An organization's personnel procedures dictate who has this responsibility.

Several methods may be used to interview a job professional candidate who may be from out of state. Preliminary interviews may include a *telephone interview*. Telephone interviews are made to keep costs down, to exchange information with applicants in distant places, and to screen a large number of applicants.

Videotaping can also reduce cost. The applicant is provided questions that are answered while the applicant is being videotaped. This can be expensive if outside consultants are used.

Other methods include *panel* or *group interviews* when the applicant is screened by a panel of administrators, employees, or both that will be working with the selected applicant. The method reduces single-bias. The most common method is the personal interview. Another type of interview is *behavioral interviewing* (discussed later in the chapter).

Interviewing is not an exact science. Interviewers have responsibility for treating candidates fairly, cordially, and professionally. They must make every effort to suspend negative judgment of candidates based on appearance or language and conduct the interview with an open mind. Interviewers should remember, too, that the candidates are judging them as well. The interviewer must dress professionally and give the candidate a positive impression of the job and the organization.

The interview should be a positive experience for both managers and prospective employees. A well-conducted interview is the first step in establishing a constructive and professional relationship with new employees and in creating goodwill with those who are not hired. Unsuccessful applicants may be qualified for future openings or may recommend the organization to others who may be interested in applying for future openings.

Well before the scheduled time for the interview, certain preparatory steps should be taken:

- The human resource department should give the interviewer copies of all information available on individual candidates. The information must include application forms, screening notes, letters of reference, résumés, and test results, as applicable.
- The interviewer should review the job description for the vacant position, making notes on the specific qualifications required and ranking them in importance.
- The interviewer should write an interview plan that includes direct questions intended to elicit information on each candidate's qualifications as compared with the qualifications shown on the job description.
- Next, the interviewer should thoroughly review all candidate information supplied by the human resource department, looking for points of compatibility between the candidate and the position requirements.
- The interviewer should compile a list of open-ended questions designed to reveal or clarify information about the candidate's education and training, work history, and career goals. Questions about the candidate's lowest to highest salary expectations need to be planned.
- The interviewer should develop an *employee application interview questionnaire*. The use of this questionnaire will ensure that the *same* questions are asked of each applicant. Answers from each applicant, as well as other notes the interviewer makes during and after the interview, can serve as a record of the interview and help make the decision about which applicant to delete and others you may want to reinterview. The questionnaire needs to have open-ended questions as this provides an applicant the chance to demonstrate his or her knowledge, experience, and ability to communicate that yes-or-no questions do not.
- The interviewer should reserve a private setting in which to conduct the interview. Interruptions from phone calls and would-be visitors interfere with privacy, making it difficult for both candidate and interviewer to give their full attention to the interview.
- The interviewer should set aside enough time to make sure that all questions planned are asked of the candidate and that the candidate has enough time to ask questions he or she has about the job and the organization.

Following are some questions that could be asked of candidates for foodservice jobs:

- Why did you choose health care foodservice as a field of work?
- What type of position are you most interested in? Why?
- What qualifications do you have that would make you a success in this job?
- What are your strengths and weaknesses as a foodservice worker?
- What hours of work do you prefer? Why? Could you work overtime in case of an emergency?
- What did you like and dislike about your previous job? Why?
- What did you do in your last job?
- Why did you leave your last job?
- What job do you enjoy doing most in foodservice?
- Do you work better in a group or alone? Please explain.
- What do you know about foodservice in a health care operation?
- What do you think is good customer service?
- What are your goals in this position?
- Where do you see yourself five years from now?
- Describe your ideal supervisor.
- Why do you want to work here?
- If you could find a perfect job what would it be? Describe.

During the interview, certain steps establish an atmosphere conducive to conducting an effective session. Interviewers can follow the eight steps outlined below.

1. Greet the candidate cordially while shaking the candidate's hand, identifying yourself, and telling the candidate what position you hold. Ask the candidate what name he or she prefers to use. Ask if the applicant would like a beverage.

2. Describe how the interview will proceed so that the candidate knows what to expect. Ask whether the candidate minds if the interviewer takes notes during the interview. Notes are extremely valuable for making evaluations and comparisons of candidates after the interview process. However, note taking can make some candidates apprehensive. In addition, interview notes may be examined as part of legal proceedings if an unsuccessful candidate later sues the organization for discrimination. Therefore, interview notes must contain only objective and relevant comments. **All** applicants must be asked the same questions.

3. First, ask general questions about training and work history, but questions already answered on the application form should not be repeated unless clarification or additional information is needed. For example, the interviewer might ask, "I notice that you left your previous job for personal reasons after just six months there. Can you tell me why you stayed at that job for such a short time?" Because most interviewers make the mistake of talking too much, the interviewer should be careful to allow the candidate to answer all questions completely and be given enough time to ask questions in turn.

4. After the candidate's educational background and work history have been explored fully, describe the position and give the candidate a copy of the job description.

5. Ask a series of open-ended questions to see whether the candidate understands what the position involves and whether he or she has the skills and knowledge needed to perform the job. Avoid questions that can be answered with a simple yes or no.

6. Encourage the candidate to ask questions about the job itself, the organization, wage levels and work schedules, the employment benefits available, and opportunities for advancement or promotion.

7. Once the candidate has been given every opportunity to ask questions and seems satisfied with the information provided, move the interview toward conclusion. Tell the candidate what will happen next and when he or she may expect to hear a decision. Be friendly and positive, but be careful not to give the impression that the candidate definitely will be offered the job. It is especially important not to create false hopes for candidates who did not perform well in the interview or who obviously are much less qualified for the position than other candidates being considered. Disappointed candidates may feel that they have been treated unfairly when they are not offered employment.

8. Express sincere appreciation for the interest the candidate has shown in working for the organization.

The following are things an interviewer should *not* do:

- Interrupt the applicant, talk too much about self, job, organization, or the like.
- Rush the interview or appear disinterested.
- Ask leading or embarrassing questions.
- Ask personal questions about applicant's life, religion, medical condition, marital status, number of children and plans to have more, age, sexual orientation, arrest record, credit score, or credit record.
- "Talk down," preach, or argue.
- Agree or disagree with the answers the applicant gives.
- Lose self-control or become angry with the applicant.

After the interview, the interviewer should take the following four additional steps:

1. Review the notes taken during the interview immediately, adding missing information and noting final impressions of the candidate. Make a preliminary notation on the candidate's qualifications and a preliminary ranking compared with other candidates. For example: "Mary Johnson appears to be well qualified for the job. She has four years' experience and a steady work record. One of the top three candidates so far." In making such appraisals, consciously try to overcome biases based on the candidate's personal qualities and physical characteristics.

2. After all candidates have been interviewed, review all notes and preliminary rankings again. Then rank the candidates a final time according to their skills, knowledge, and experience. The rankings also should take into account the candidates' degree of interest, usually expressed during the interview by the number of questions candidates ask and by their general attitudes toward the interview process and the position being offered. An enthusiastic candidate with two years' experience may make a better employee than a disinterested candidate with five years' experience. Such decisions are always based on the experience and judgment of the interviewer.

3. Decide which candidate seems to be best suited for the job. At this point, it may be appropriate to seek the advice of the human resource department, especially if one of its representatives also interviewed candidates. For professional positions, it is customary to conduct more than one interview with one or more candidates before a decision is finalized. It is also important to have others in the organization and department to interview the candidate. This may be by individuals or by a group such as a group of dietitians interviewing a dietitian for a position.

4. Inform the human resource department of the decision to offer a particular candidate the position.

Background Check

After the decision is made to offer the job, a human resource representative is informed so that the human resource department can check the chosen candidate's background record. The background check involves contacting at least the candidate's most recent employer by telephone or letter. The present employer should not be contacted before the applicant resigns, unless there is written permission to do so, because if dismissal results, the applicant may take legal action. Often other former employers are contacted as well. Verification of credentials of professional employees is made at this time.

Because employers are sensitive to the legal liability associated with supplying potentially damaging information about former employees to prospective new employers, many organizations have a personnel policy that forbids disclosure of employee information beyond dates of employment, job titles, and final salaries or wages. If there is any doubt about the candidate's work record or personal integrity, the human resource representative may contact all previous employers, confirm the candidate's personal references, or check the candidate's record with legal authorities.

In checking backgrounds, there are questions prohibited by law that employers (human resource representative) must avoid. Questions that relate to the federal Privacy Act and the Fair Credit Reporting Act must not be asked. The background check may seek information on:

- Criminal records (The background checker must be careful in checking criminal records. People with criminal records should only be excluded when there is a *legitimate disqualification*.)
- Credit records, including bankruptcy
- Driving record
- Education record

For a potential employer to get an applicant's personal records, such as credit history or educational records the prospective employee **must** give the employer **permission** to do so. If the employer's decision not to hire is based on information in the applicant's credit report the employer **must** comply with all the notice and disclosure requirements of the Fair Credit Reporting Act. If a job applicant believes information on the credit report is wrong, he can notify the firm that ran the background check. The firm is then required to remove or correct inaccurate or unverified information within 30 days.

It is for this reason that most organizations have a personnel policy that requires the human resource department, instead of the interviewing department manager, to check the references of potential employees. Human resource specialists usually are fully aware of what questions may and may not be asked in the employment process.

Behavioral Interviewing

Behavioral interviewing and behavioral simulations combine the in-depth personal interview and behavioral simulation. Behavioral simulation is asking clients to demonstrate how they can perform key responsibilities that are on the job description. Behavioral simulations are how applicants would behave in the position in which they are applying. It is not a test to determine intelligence or personality but an objective measure of job skills; nor is it discriminatory or used to rule out race, gender, age, or religion.

Behavioral simulation works this way: the applicant is given a situation and asked how he or she would handle it. The simulations could be through role playing, case studies' problem solving, or by a specific task from the job description.

Behavioral interview includes questions that require the applicant to answer. These questions give specific examples of previous job skill performance. Questions usually are worded "Tell me about . . . , Give me an example . . . , Describe a situation . . . ." This type of questioning gives applicants the opportunity to exhibit their job skills as well as potential. Any question must be based on the skills and abilities needed for the position. If you use this type of behavioral questioning, be sure to give the applicant adequate time to answer. Some applicants who have experience will have less trouble answering questions than applicants who have less experience.

Making the Final Hiring Decision

The final decision to hire a new employee is one of the most *important* any manager will make. Hiring unqualified or uncooperative employees can waste training dollars and damage department morale. The wrong decision also may cost the organization hundreds or thousands of dollars. The employment process is expensive because it requires a great deal of the manager's and the human resource department's time, plus advertisements in publications and fees charged by private employment agencies and recruitment firms are increasingly expensive.

Therefore, the hiring decision must be based on careful screening of all candidates available, a fair and well-thought-out interview, and thorough reference checking. The hiring decision should never be rushed, and it should never be based on superficial first impressions or personal biases.

Once the final hiring decision has been made and the best-qualified candidate has been chosen, the human resource representative and the foodservice director jointly decide the starting salary or wage the candidate should be offered. The starting salary is based on the wage or salary range for the position and on the candidate's work experience and educational training. The 2009 Joint Commission Standards state, "[T]he hospital verifies staff qualifications and must verify credentials with the primary source upon hire and renewal. This may be accomplished electronically or via phone with documentation." The human resources representative then contacts the candidate (by letter or telephone) to offer the position at the salary assigned. In some organizations, the employing manager may make the actual job offer. However, because human resource specialists are trained to address sensitive legal issues that surround the employment process, the trend is toward having them make job offer contacts with candidates. One important area of concern is that the offer of employment be made in such a way that the candidate is not led to misconstrue the offer to be an employment contract.

Making the job offer includes giving the candidate specific information about the starting salary or wage, anticipated date of employment, official job title, and other information about employment with the organization. Other information might include details about qualifying for health benefits and vacation time. Often the candidate may ask for some time to think about the offer. Setting a definite time for a follow-up contact for a final decision prevents delays in filling the position.

If the candidate accepts the offer, the human resource representative arranges for the new employee to undergo a physical examination and other tests as designed by the organization. If the candidate decides not to accept the position, the representative notifies the foodservice director so that a second candidate can be chosen and the cycle repeated.

The application forms, test scores, interview notes, reference-check notes, and any other information on unsuccessful candidates should be filed in the human resource department. Such materials will be extremely valuable in the event that unsuccessful candidates take legal action against the organization. (However, this material can become a double-edged sword if records reveal that the organization failed to follow its own policies and procedures—for example, to check references.) In addition, the files may be a source of information on potential candidates in recruitment efforts to fill future openings for similar positions. The files should include clear statements indicating the reasons the candidates were not hired. The application forms and other information gathered on successful candidates must be kept as part of the permanent personnel records, discussed later in this chapter.

Arranging for a Physical Examination and Other Tests

Before the implementation of the Americans with Disabilities Act of 1992, employees were usually given a preemployment physical before a job offer was made. Because organizations must be careful not to discriminate against disabled individuals, especially disabled veterans, most now make a preliminary job offer pending completion of a medical examination, agility evaluation, or other testing. On the applicant's acceptance of the initial job offer, the human resource department schedules the candidate for a physical examination to be performed by a physician, nurse, or nurse practitioner, who should be given a copy of the candidate's job description.

The examination is to determine whether the new employee can meet the physical demands of the job or needs reasonable accommodations, to detect health conditions that might pose a risk to the employee if he or she were placed in a specific job or area, and to protect the organization's customers and staff from exposure to potentially infectious illnesses. This step is especially important for foodservice workers because of the danger of spreading communicable diseases through food handling and because much of the work involved is physically taxing. During the pre-placement examination, the employee generally is asked to provide a cardiopulmonary history and to take a tuberculin skin test. For some positions a series of hepatitis shots may be required.

Screening for illegal or controlled drug usage has been implemented by many health care organizations. Drug screens are meant to combat absenteeism, accidents, work-related injuries, equipment damage, and inefficient performance due to substance abuse among employees. Screening for substance abuse also can help employers control the cost of health care and workers' compensation. Employers may deny employment to individuals who are using illegal or controlled substances at the time of a preemployment screen, but applicants with prior addictions are covered under the Americans with Disabilities Act.

Organizations that decide to use drug screening must use a nationally approved laboratory and follow strict protocols for chain of custody to ensure the validity of the test results. Confidentiality is of critical importance and is generally ensured through minimal handling of the specimen as outlined in the organization's human resources policy and procedures. The manager of the foodservice department should become familiar with the policy and procedures of the organization to ensure compliance.

Other tests may be required by the organization and must be given to all applicants to avoid discrimination. Some organizations may require a *polygraph test* (sometimes called a lie detector test). The Federal Employee Polygraph Act of 1988 prohibits most private employers from using a polygraph as a selection device; however, in those situations involving cash or the manufacture of controlled substances, the use is sometimes permitted.

Graphology is a handwriting analysis in which a graphologist evaluates the applicant's handwriting using certain methods to make inferences about the applicant's personality.

Some organizations may require a *personality* and *interest test*, an indicator test such as the Myers-Briggs Type Indicator (a personality inventory that helps employees and employers understand how employees like to take in information or look at things, make decisions, use time, and in general organize themselves), or an achievement test. Some organizations may require an intelligence test (IQ).

Motor and physical abilities tests may be used if all applicants are given the test and the results are not used as a discrimination tool. Any skill test, such as computer use or simple arithmetic for recipes, should be administered by a qualified person using standardized testing methods.

Personnel Records

After the employee is hired, the human resource department will set up the organization's personnel file on the employee. The foodservice department should also set up a file that contains:

- Who to inform in case of an emergency
- Current address, telephone number
- Date of hire
- Job classification, rate of pay
- Orientation
- Insurance record
- Leave slips, and any other information the department may deem necessary

This file may be on cards, loose-leaf notebook, or computerized.

Conducting a New Employee Orientation Program

The first few days on the job are crucial for new employees as they must learn how things are done as well as the organization culture. Not only must they be introduced to the job, other employees, and the organization, but their future performance may depend on the attitudes and impressions they form during these first days. Therefore, well-organized orientation procedures are needed to help new employees quickly become productive members of the staff. A well-planned and implemented orientation helps to prevent or reduce turnover. Employees who are provided an orientation at the beginning of their employment are more likely to be loyal, content, and successful in their job.

Orientation to the Organization

In many medium-size and large health care organizations, the human resource department is responsible for explaining the organization's personnel policies, regulations, and employee benefit programs. During general orientation sessions, new employees fill out tax-withholding statements for the Internal Revenue Service and application forms for health insurance, life insurance, and other group benefits. This is usually done the first day.

Also during this time:

- New employees may be given a guided tour of the facility. This inspires pride in the organization, allows the new employee to get a feel for the organizational culture, and helps the employee understand his or her role.
- A brief history of the organization and an introduction to the organization's mission and goals also are common elements of employee orientation programs.
- The new employee may be given a copy of the organization's employee handbook at this time. (The employee handbook is discussed later in this chapter.)

In smaller health care facilities, the foodservice director may be responsible for conducting general orientation for new employees as well as their orientation to the foodservice department. When this is the case, the director should make every effort to make the general orientation an interesting and thorough introduction to the operation of the organization as a whole. Specific training for work tasks should be conducted only after the general orientation session.

Orientation to the Foodservice Department

A new employee's introduction to the foodservice department should be warm and friendly. Orientation is a form of courtesy. It helps a new employee feel welcome. The director and any other department managers who will work with the new employee should set aside time to welcome and to introduce the employee to others in the department. People should be introduced by name and a brief description of their duties given. Such introductions will make it easier for the new member to understand who does what in the department.

After all introductions have been made, the person who will supervise the employee directly should begin the gradual process of easing the new person into department operations and his or her specific job requirements. By conveying a sincere interest in making the orientation and training period a pleasant experience, the supervisor supports a new employee's eagerness to do the job well, be accepted by coworkers and supervisors, and overcome being nervous in a new situation.

The supervisor should not cover too much information at once, reassuring the new worker that additional information will be provided gradually throughout the orientation period. Information overload may cause a new employee to become confused and even more apprehensive. The new employee should be given a copy of the department's procedures handbook and be allowed enough time to read it thoroughly before beginning work.

In the next section of this chapter, we discuss in detail some methods for training new employees to perform their jobs. However, it first may be helpful to offer guidelines for a typical orientation and training program for a production worker. Managers should keep in mind that these guidelines would not be suitable for orienting professional or managerial employees. For example, an orientation and training program for registered dietitians and other nutrition professionals should be arranged on an individual basis so as to be suited to the various levels of experience and knowledge such professionals would have.

The following guidelines cover the first five days (one workweek) of a new employee's orientation as a foodservice production worker in a hospital:

- *Day 1.* The supervisor explains the general departmental routine and where the new employee's job fits in; shows the employee the general work area, the employees' lounge, and the employees' locker room; assigns the new employee to an experienced employee whose duties are identical or similar to those the new employee will perform; and gives the new hire a copy of the department procedures handbook. The new employee spends the rest of Day 1 observing and working with the experienced employee.
- *Day 2.* The supervisor checks with the new employee to see whether he or she has questions about yesterday's activities, clarifies any task or departmental routine, and reaffirms a friendly and supportive atmosphere by offering encouragement and helpful suggestions rather than criticism. The new employee spends the rest of Day 2 working with and observing the mentor employee perform tasks the new employee eventually will perform.
- *Day 3.* The new employee spends more time working independently. The supervisor observes his or her job behavior and corrects or clarifies work performance as necessary.
- *Day 4.* The new employee continues to work independently, but the supervisor and coworkers remain available to answer questions and offer advice. The supervisor begins to review the job description as well as key points of departmental policies—especially those on infection control, disaster planning, fire safety, and hazardous substance handling—offering the new member opportunity to raise questions and clarify points as necessary (for example, fine points of the department's or organization's personnel policies such as employee benefits, grievance procedures, and performance evaluation).
- *Day 5.* The new employee assumes job tasks independently. The supervisor may apprise the employee of training opportunities in specific production procedures and techniques once the employee has adjusted to his or her new work setting. All orientation checklists are filed in the department's employee personnel file.

TRAINING

Employee training and development is one of a foodservice director's most important responsibilities. *Training* is the process of providing skills or helping to correct deficiencies. *Developing* is providing employees with knowledge, skills, and abilities the employee/organization will need in the future. A continuous, well-organized training program for all levels of employees increases productivity, quality level, safety consciousness, and department morale. New employees may require a complete training regimen. Experienced employees may need training in new or updated production methods, equipment, and approaches to handling set job tasks. Most new employee training is conducted one-on-one, whereas experienced foodservice employees usually are taught new or updated skills and concepts during in-service group training sessions.

The department director responsible for the performance and training of unit managers and nonmanagerial employees in a health care setting has access to more resources than ever. Many health care human resource departments now employ training specialists (sometimes called *education coordinators*) who serve as instructors or advisers in helping facilities plan their training programs. These specialists coordinate department-level in-service programs or design individual training plans for all levels of department employees.

Nonprofessional employees in the foodservice department have varied educational and social backgrounds. Some may lack skill in foodservice work on being hired. Despite the differences in abilities, social backgrounds, and basic skill levels (for example, in math and reading), it is essential that all foodservice employees receive adequate training. It may become necessary to provide basic literacy skills such as teaching English, reading, and math skills. Technical skills may be taught for new technology, to improve existing skills, or due to a reduction in the work force, and cross-training. Other skills that need to be taught include interpersonal skills, how to communicate more clearly and how to be an effective team member.

Other training areas that may be taught to all employees include diversity training, the importance of ethics and values of the organization, workplace violence, and customer service. Part of any training is gaining an understanding of the responsibility of the foodservice department to provide safe, nutritious, and high-quality food to customers.

Training for physically or mentally challenged employees must be conducted on the basis of any accommodations needed by these individuals. For example, if an employee is learning disabled, training requires verbal instructions and demonstrations. If modifications are made to equipment to enable a physically challenged worker to complete a task, it might be necessary to train other staff to use the modified equipment.

In the United States, billions of dollars are spent annually on job training. This level of investment makes it incumbent on managers to ensure the highest return possible. Training can pay for itself many times over when an employee is consistently and adequately trained from day one. Training programs should be planned and designed with specific objective outcomes for knowledge or skills enhancement in mind. The purpose of training should include:

- Meeting the basic needs of employees and improving morale
- Improving productivity
- Improving customers' satisfaction
- Improving compliance with regulatory agents
- Meeting or exceeding established standards
- Reducing turnover
- Reducing accidents, injuries, and mistakes
- Maintaining cost

Planning and determining objectives are discussed later in this section.

Understanding the Instructor's Role

The instructor, a key to successful training, must maintain a positive attitude toward the work to be taught and toward the employees who must be trained to perform it. The instructor must know the subject to as well as the audience to be taught. To facilitate the learning process, the instructor must first earn employees' respect and confidence by demonstrating his or her skills, explaining convincingly why tasks are performed in particular ways, and showing fairness and patience. The instructor also should be careful to gauge the employees' knowledge beforehand to avoid unnecessary training as well as training for which they may be inadequately prepared. For example, training in the use of new cook-chill or cook-freeze procedures is futile unless employees understand the importance of maintaining the structural and textural integrity of the food prepared with these systems. Assessing employee knowledge may be accomplished through observation, demonstration, or written pretesting. For example, if training involved the proper method of steaming vegetables, the employee should be asked to demonstrate the technique. A written pretest asks questions regarding the key concepts the trainer wishes the employee to learn. For example, a pretest on proper food handling should ask specific questions regarding holding temperatures and proper labeling of the product.

The instructor also must understand basic principles of training adults. Some of these include the following:

- Know how to present material (use a variety of methods for the audience that is to be taught).
- Do not mumble, speak too fast, mispronounce words, use unfamiliar words, when a familiar word would be best, nor speak in a monotone.
- Avoid "er," "uh," "uh-huh," "you know," "okey-dokey," "right," "you understand."
- The desire to learn must come from the learner.
- People learn at different rates.
- All training does not progress smoothly but in up-and-down cycles.
- If treated with disrespect, adults resist taking part in activities.
- Learners become discouraged when they reach a plateau in their skill levels.
- Adults come to the learning situation with a great deal of life experience and want to contribute actively.

- A certain amount of apprehensiveness is a natural part of learning.
- Adults require practical outcomes from their learning experience.
- The whole task should be demonstrated before it is broken down into its component parts for learning purposes.
- Poor training methods hinder learning.
- Adults learn more efficiently in well-timed training periods that last no longer than an hour without a break.
- The reasoning behind every element of the skill being taught must be explained to help employees understand the whole process.
- Learners need to be told how well they are doing as the learning progresses.
- Observe body language as 65 percent of the message can be observed by the type of body language exhibited by the learner—watch for gestures, facial expression, body movements, whispering with fellow employees. Do not distrust the body language of the learners.
- Listen to what the employees are saying.

Although, as stated earlier, a positive attitude is important, instructors should not expect maximum skills to be attained by the end of the training session. Full learning of tasks requires on-the-job practice.

Conducting Individual Training Programs

In many foodservice departments, individualized training of new nonprofessional employees is delegated to experienced employees who perform identical or similar jobs. The employee selected for this task should know how to teach, so the manager must work with this person to plan step-by-step how the new employee is to be trained. This way, common errors made by inexperienced trainers can be circumvented. Some of these errors include:

- Trying to teach too much at one time
- Describing how to perform a task without first demonstrating it
- Lacking patience
- Failing to give and receive feedback as the learning progresses
- Failing to prepare adequately
- Forgetting, overlooking, or inadequately explaining key points

The director or manager who delegates training responsibility must check periodically to ensure that training is proceeding appropriately. Any shortcomings in the process need to be addressed at the time they occur, as this helps both employee trainer and manager to learn from mistakes.

The step-by-step plan will need to be developed and designed between manager and designated trainer to ensure maximum benefit to the new employee. Following are some basic guidelines for training new nonprofessional foodservice employees:

- Use the new employee's job description to plan the tasks and skills to be taught.
- Outline a step-by-step procedure for teaching each task or skill as the goal of each training session is stated and communicated to the trainee.
- Set aside a specific time for each training session so that interruptions are kept to a minimum.
- Gather and arrange all supplies, utensils, equipment, and teaching aids before the session begins. The workplace should be set up just as the employee will be expected to keep it.
- Prepare for each session by first learning what the new employee already knows about the task.
- Demonstrate each task before teaching it. Explain each step completely and clearly, stressing and repeating key points and demonstrating acceptable shortcuts that make the task easier, faster, or more effective.
- Ask and invite questions at each juncture of the demonstration to ensure the trainee's comprehension.
- Give the trainee ample opportunity to perform the task and explain its steps along the way while observing and correcting errors patiently. Have the trainee repeat the task until it is clear that he or she understands it fully.
- Allow the trainee to practice the task independently after all safety procedures have been fully learned. However, remain close at hand to answer questions and provide feedback or help if needed.
- Withdraw direct supervision gradually as the trainee becomes proficient at the task.
- Acknowledge the trainee's progress and congratulate him or her on successful completion of the assigned task.
- Discuss the schedule for additional training and set reasonable goals for learning related tasks.

Conducting Group In-Service Training Programs

An in-service training program is essential for maintaining an efficient and cost-effective foodservice department. Continuing education enables employees to grow in their jobs by learning new techniques or gaining new knowledge that will help them become more productive and increase job satisfaction and ownership. Well-organized group training sessions are the primary method of conducting in-service training. They are an efficient means of communicating vital information in a structured training environment. Most states require official in-service training programs for health care providers.

Program Planning and Scheduling

Programs or in-service sessions should not be planned or conducted until a needs assessment is made. *Needs assessment* is a tool, a fact-finding process. Needs assessment helps the supervisor determine where training efforts need be focused. It helps to determine whether a problem is caused by the job or the working conditions. Needs assessment allows the trainer to provide positive reinforcement for correct action. It also removes obstacles and provides the supervisor with an idea of what is needed for the employee, department, or both to perform correctly when determining needs. The main priority should be not only to provide quality service to the client but also to constantly improve the quality of that service as well. When developing training needs, consider the following:

- *Knowledge:* What is needed to perform the job. Information may include policies, procedures, budget limitations, and the like.
- *Skills:* How the job is to be done.
- *Assessment:* More training to increase skills and knowledge.

Once staff needs have been assessed, the topics for in-service training can be rated by importance, and the employees who require training can be identified. A successful program is based on employee needs: What problems, issues, or changes need to be explained? What attitudes, knowledge, and skills will help employees do their jobs effectively, now and in the future? Some topics may be relevant to the work of the whole department (for example, safety procedures). Other topics apply to only a few employees (for example, salad preparation techniques). A firm schedule for training sessions must be established several months in advance. The date, time, and subject of each session should be stated on the schedule and made available to all employees.

The foodservice director or education coordinator (or both) should plan the entire year's in-service program in conjunction with the organization's annual business plan. The program should take into consideration overall organizational requirements and legislative and regulatory agency requirements. For example, programs may cover disaster or emergency preparedness, fire and safety procedures, infection control, OSHA regulations, or quality assurance and quality control procedures.

Because most foodservice employees work in shifts, two or more sessions on each topic need to be planned. Work schedules and workloads should always be considered when designing training schedules. Whenever the work volume does not allow enough time to schedule group meetings during the workday, sessions should be scheduled at the end of the workday or between two overlapping shifts. Personnel policies should be followed to determine whether hourly employees are paid overtime for attending sessions outside their regular working hours.

The topic to be presented for each in-service meeting should be defined narrowly so that the subject can be covered adequately. Most sessions conducted during a regular workday should be short (20 to 40 minutes) because employees may be too fatigued to learn effectively.

Behavioral objectives are developed with a method to evaluate the results of training. Objectives and results can be identified by asking two basic questions: What do the employees need to know? How are the outcomes of training evaluated?

A *behavioral objective* states in specific terms what the outcome of the training should be and how it is to be measured. Behavioral objectives should be based on the kind of material to be learned. Should it be a skills objective, an attitude objective, or a knowledge objective?

A *skills objective* involves teaching some kind of manipulative skill; in psychology this is called a *psychomotor* skill. The level of psychomotor skill can be easily measured. An example of a skills objective could be the following: At the end of training, the employee will be able to disassemble the dish machine, clean it, and reassemble it correctly 100 percent of the time.

Attitude objectives involve developing in participants new or modified feelings (attitudes) toward the topic covered in the training session. (Such emotional components are called *affects* in psychology.) Attitude objectives also involve individual interests, values, and feelings of appreciation. The level of accomplishment in fulfilling attitude objectives is difficult to measure because personal emotions and beliefs are intangible and elude assessment. An example of an attitude objective could be the following: At the end of training, the employee will have an increased appreciation of the need to practice good guest relations when serving patients and other customers.

A *knowledge objective* involves teaching intellectual skills (called *cognitive skills* in psychology). The level of knowledge or understanding gained through in-service training is relatively easy to test and observe. An example of a knowledge objective could be the following: At the end of training, the employee will be able to correctly calculate the composition of a 1,200-calorie, low-fat diet 100 percent of the time.

No matter what skills or attitudes are being taught, all behavioral objectives should accomplish six things:

1. State the action to be accomplished.
2. State what the action is directed toward.
3. Describe how the action is to be accomplished.
4. State how accomplishment of the action is to be measured.
5. Include clarifications of the preceding components as necessary.
6. Include training method and materials.

After the type of objective is determined, the behavioral change or changes being sought as the goal of the training should be determined. This can be done by asking one of the following questions: What can the employees now do that they could not do before? What do they now understand that they did not understand before? What do they now know that they did not know before? What will they now do that they would not do before?

Training Methods The person who attends a training session must have the desire to learn. No one can be forced to learn. Training must meet the wants, needs, and goals of the trainee. Employees (adults) want an active part in training activities; they learn best by doing, not listening and reading.

The following are examples of training methods:

- *Lectures and videotapes* involve a one-way flow of communication. This type of training is the least effective unless follow-up activities are planned that help the learner to participate in a hands-on practice.
- *Computer-based or interactive computers* training can enhance motivation and feedback when the programs are

interactive and allows the trainees to progress through the materials at their own pace.

- *Teleconferencing* is an excellent way to bring together employees from various units of an organization for the purpose of training or a business meeting. It allows people at diverse locations to see, hear, and interact with each other by electronic technology. This method may also be referred to as Webinars.
- *Internet/web education–based courses* are formal, stated outcomes, assignments, textbooks, and other information concerning the course. These courses may lead to a degree and in some cases an advanced degree. They are individual study programs where an instructor and students may interact through chat rooms and e-mail. Specific course work is required. All course work and the final examination is completed online, is electronically transmitted to the institution offering the course.
- Informal education courses that do not lead to degrees include language, math, English, and so forth.
- *Conferences* are effective when used by in-house educators to meet a specific purpose such as explaining a new organization-wide safety program. They are also used by professional organizations where members meet to listen to expert speakers and share information.
- *Case studies* are used to present a case or problem, and the trainees analyze and discuss the problem and come up with a solution. Nursing and grand rounds are a good example of this method.
- *Incident reports* are training sessions using a recent incident, evaluating why it happened, and devising methods to avoid its happening again. An example would be a recent injury to an employee due to a wet floor.
- *Demonstrations* break a job down into its various parts. Once the job has been demonstrated, employees practice the procedure while receiving feedback from the trainer. This method of training is an excellent tool to use when new baking items are added to a menu.
- *On-the-job-training* (OJT) is used to teach a trainee how to do a job while on location. The trainee actually performs the job.
- *Coaching* is used to assist a trainee while practicing the job. The coach observes the task and makes friendly suggestions about the job. The coach should compliment the trainee when he or she meets the quality and quantity standards.

In all of these methods, the trainer will need to follow up to ensure that the trainee can do the job as taught without constant supervision. Feedback is important.

Evaluating In-Service Training Sessions To determine whether the desired outcome has been achieved at an in-service meeting, a method must be devised to evaluate its end results. Tests, reports, demonstrations, questionnaires, case studies, observations, and so forth can measure the level of employee competency. In some cases, post-training follow-up may indicate that some employees need individual training to achieve the level of competency required.

Once the outcome of training and an evaluation method are determined, a task analysis is completed. A *task analysis* is a written description outlining the main steps of a specific work activity in order of occurrence. Figure 8.2 is an example of a task analysis. The task analysis may be supported by notes on the main points to be emphasized in the training. These materials also are used as the basis for the instructor's plans for the training session.

If the session's instructor is from outside the department or the organization, a department representative must contact him or her well in advance to explain what skills or concepts are to be taught. The representative also should offer help in setting up demonstrations or obtaining audiovisual equipment.

Identifying In-Service Training Topics and Resources As a result of the employee needs analysis for in-service training, a number of issues or themes may surface. Some possible topics for a continuing education program for the foodservice staff include:

- Standards for personal hygiene, infection control, and other illnesses identified in *Food Code 2009*
- Advances in food-handling procedures, hazard analysis critical control points
- Changes in cleaning techniques and procedures
- Operation and maintenance of new equipment
- Current fire safety, disaster, and emergency preparedness procedures
- Injury or accident prevention
- Risk management
- Future operational changes in the department and in the organization
- Basic concepts of nutrition
- Procedures for preparing and serving foods for modified diets
- Changes in personnel policies, sexual harassment policies
- Meeting the needs of special patient populations (for example, the elderly and the physically or mentally challenged)
- Safety precautions related to equipment, hazardous chemicals, cuts, burns, falls, and right to know
- Customer satisfaction
- Diversity in the workplace
- Generational difference—what it means
- Workplace violence (new TJC requirement)
- Quality customer service, benchmarking, and productivity

It may be useful to maintain a list of people who demonstrate interest in teaching in-service training sessions in their areas of expertise. Speakers and instructors from the community and employees of state and local public health agencies, universities, and technical colleges may be helpful in training employees in specific skills and knowledge. Possible speakers also may be identified at meetings of professional organizations serving the foodservice and health care fields or through national speakers' bureaus. Staff members from other departments in the organization and from nearby health care organizations are additional resources.

FIGURE 8.2 Example of a Task Analysis for a Foodservice Department Training Session

Task Analysis

Positions: Dining room cashier
Task: Cash transactions
Frequency: For each cash customer
Equipment: 190 Cash register cash drawer
Contact: Café manager or head cashier

Important Steps in Job	Key Points
1. Tally each food item on the tray.	Tally each item under the proper food category.
2. Push subtotal button.	—
3. Push the tax button.	—
4. Push total button.	Be sure the tax has been added.
5. Check the amount on the indicator.	Be sure it agrees with the amount of sale.
6. Tell the customer the amount.	Speak clearly.
7. Take the money from the customer.	Hold the palm of your hand upward.
8. Punch value received.	Be sure to punch value in correctly.
9. Place the money in drawer.	Be sure to place in appropriate value category.
10. Punch the change indicator button.	Check the indicator for the amount of change to be returned to the customer.
11. Count bills back to customer.	Start with ones, fives, tens, and so on. Tell the customer to pick up change from counter.
12. Close cash drawer.	Do not lock cash drawer.
13. Give receipt to customer.	Do not drop it.
14. Say thank you.	Smile.

Training materials are available from a number of sources and in varying formats, including videotapes, filmstrips, slides, and printed materials. Employees from colleges, universities, vocational schools, and extension programs may be asked to present an in-service training session on a specific topic. Other groups such as sales representatives, equipment manufacturers, special counseling services, community service organizations, outside consultants, and government agencies have trainers or speakers who will present special training programs. Trainers should prescreen all materials before renting or purchasing them to ensure their appropriateness for the training planned. Screening further ensures that the department's training dollars are being put to good use.

Program Implementation

The instructor for a particular in-service training session should prepare a detailed instruction plan based on the objectives previously identified. A lesson plan, a written blueprint of how a lesson is to be conducted, describes key points to be covered and how they are to be taught (for example, by demonstration or discussion) and lists all materials needed to conduct the lesson. Lesson materials may include printed handouts, wall charts, audiovisual materials, equipment, and supplies, among others. The lesson plan also should include written questions to be discussed with the group. The instructor should be sure that the elements in the lesson plan can be covered adequately in the amount of time scheduled.

Well before the session is scheduled to begin, the instructor should check whether all audiovisual equipment needed is available and in good working order. Similarly, he or she should have any posters, charts, handouts, and other printed materials prepared in advance. Such materials should be well organized and neatly prepared. Posters and charts should be large enough to be seen from all areas of the training room.

The session should start on schedule. At the beginning of the session, the instructor should introduce himself or herself to the group, if necessary. Next, other members of the group should introduce themselves in the event they are not known by name to all present.

The session should begin with an overview of the topics to be discussed or demonstrated. Any supplementary teaching aids should be set up or passed out when appropriate. The instructor should involve members of the group in as many demonstrations and role-playing activities as possible, asking questions all along to encourage further discussion and involvement.

At the end of the session, the subject should be summarized, with time allowed for any additional questions to further ensure that all key points have been covered adequately and are understood by all participants. Finally, the group should be asked to give specific examples of how the skills and concepts learned in the session can be applied to the everyday work of the foodservice department.

Program Evaluation

Measuring the outcome of in-service training and evaluating the overall program are important to the training process. Employee performance should be assessed on an ongoing basis to determine the need for further training or retraining. Employees' skills can be tested and measured immediately before and shortly after a program to determine its effectiveness. On-the-job performance tests and observations, interviews, questionnaires, and department records also serve as indicators. Department accident and event reports, as well as quality control assessments, are reliable gauges of job-related skills and attitudes and, therefore, of the merits of the department's training program.

An instructor's training skills also may be evaluated by asking questions about how well the instructor knew the material and how well the material was presented. Were the teaching aids helpful and interesting? Was the class discussion informative? Did the instructor answer all questions thoroughly and respectfully?

Participants can be asked to complete written evaluation forms at the end of each training session. Survey questions might include:

- Will information from this session help me to improve my job skills?

- What did I learn that will help me in my job?
- Was this subject interesting to me?
- Was this session worthwhile?
- Did the session contain enough practical information, or was it too theoretical?
- Was the session long enough? Too long?
- How could the session have been better?
- What subjects would you like to learn more about in future sessions?
- Was the learning environment comfortable physically and socially (too crowded or too warm)?

Maintaining Records of Individual and Group In-Service Training Programs

Records of individual and group training efforts must be maintained by the foodservice department (Exhibit 8.1). Employees should sign attendance sheets for each training session they attend. A monthly report showing the number of sessions conducted and the level of staff attendance can be a valuable part of the department's continuous quality improvement program. Such records may be examined by surveyors from TJC and by state regulatory agents. The human resource department should also keep records of in-service training for the organization (Exhibit 8.2).

EXHIBIT 8.1   Sample of an Employee's In-Service Record

In-Service Record

Food and Nutrition Service
In-Service Record [year]

Name _____   Social Security [Employee] No. _____

Title   _____

Shift   _____

In-Services Title (required)	Date attended
Risk Management	_____
Patients' Rights	_____
Disaster Planning	_____
Fire Safety	_____
Infection Control and Sanitation	_____
Hazard Analysis, "Right to Know"	_____
Safety and Equipment Handling	_____
Improving Organization Performance	_____

Other

_____   _____

_____   _____

_____   _____

Note. Each employee has a separate record.

EXHIBIT 8.2   In-Service Record for Human Resource Management

DATE:_____ TIME: From _____To _____ PLACE OF TRAINING: _____

GROUP TO BE TRAINED: _____
_____

TOPIC: _____
_____

DISCUSSION LEADER: _____
_____

PURPOSE: _____
_____

OBJECTIVES: At the end of this training period, the participant should be able to: _____
_____

EVALUATION CRITERIA: _____
_____

LESSON PLAN: Attached

VISUALS USED: 1. Overhead projector____ 2. Video _____ 3. Slides ___ 4. Tape __ 5. Poster _____ 6. Food models ____ 7. Chalkboard ___
                       8. Self-paced video ____ 9. Computer games ____ 10. Other: _____.

HANDOUTS: Yes _____ No _____ Attached _____

FOLLOW-UP EVALUATION: Participant comments_____
_____

Evaluation form used: Yes _____ No _____

Form attached:

THOSE ATTENDING:

_____   _____   _____   _____
_____   _____   _____   _____
_____   _____   _____   _____

Source: Developed by Ruby P. Puckett©.

SUMMARY

Human resource management deals with the organization's most important resource—its employees. There are numerous federal, state, and local laws and regulations that are intended to protect the rights of both the employee and the employer.

Human resource management covers many of the functions of management that have been discussed in previous chapters. The employment process must be carefully monitored to ensure that all applicants are treated in a fair, objective manner, all laws are carefully followed, and all applicants are asked the same questions. Orientation and in-service training are required by surveying agencies and some local and state laws. Maintaining accurate records is necessary.

KEY TERMS

401 (k) plan
Behavioral objective
Bona fide occupational qualification (BFOQ)
Closed shop
Glass ceiling
Job bidding
Job sharing

Polygraph
Quotas
Roth plan
Sexual harassment
Task analysis
Union shop
Vesting

1. Why is there a need for so many laws that relate to employer-employee relationship?

2. Discuss three laws that have had the most impact on employers and employees in terms of what is good about them and what may be considered difficult to enforce.

3. What is the importance of keeping excellent personnel records from interviewing through in-service training?

4. Explain how a good orientation to the facility and the department not only helps the employee but also the department management.

5. What are the reasons for conducting a variety of in-service training and development programs for employees?

CHAPTER 9

HUMAN RESOURCE MANAGEMENT
Other Needed Skills

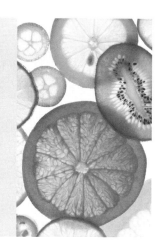

LEARNING OBJECTIVES

- Apply performance evaluations fairly and objectively to appraise the performance of employees.
- Give examples of actual behavior, without judgment, when coaching employees on their performance.
- Present training on diversity in the workplace.
- Follow the steps outlined for corrective action; be fair.
- Implement methods for retaining employees.

THIS CHAPTER AGAIN emphasizes that the most valuable resources within an organization are the employees who do the work to provide the customers quality food and service. In the previous chapter you learned about laws that affect the employer and employee relations, the employment process, orientation, and in-service requirements. In this chapter you learn more about human resources as it applies to:

- Discrimination
- Employee performance evaluation
- Importance of maintaining employee records
- Development of an employee handbook
- Coaching, conflict management
- Methods to handle corrective action—labor relations
- Compensation and benefits
- Employment recognition
- Employee assistance programs

The materials in this chapter also alert you to the importance of following all applicable rules, regulations, and laws.

CULTURAL DIVERSITY OF THE WORKFORCE

An overview of cultural diversity was discussed in Chapter 1. To understand cultural diversity it is necessary to start with a definition. *Diversity* means the way in which people differ from each, their own uniqueness; it also refers to the way people interact on an ongoing basis. People are accepted for who they are regardless of age, sexual orientation, race, religion, gender, body type, and ethnic or social group. *Cultural diversity* can be defined as the representation in one social system of people with distinctly different group affiliations of cultural significance.

Diversity is a challenge for both manager and employees. As the makeup of the population continues to change, the manager will be confronted with ethical and other related challenges. People from different locations have values, customs, religions, traditions, and food habits that are unique to their culture. Managers will need to learn the cultures of their workforce and present training to the department employees about diversity.

It is a known fact that people with like backgrounds and culture are more likely to band together. A culturally diverse workplace can offer a challenge in bringing two or more cultures together to form a harmonized workforce. Another issue is that for the first time in history the workforce is made up of four generations working together. Each of these generations brings its own values, ethics, prejudices, and experiences to the workforce. The manager will need to meld the generational difference with the cultural difference to help each group understand their differences and their likeness.

Yet another concern is that the number of young women (ages 25 to 29) entering the workforce continues to increase but at a substantially lower rate than in 1985. The BLS cites a slower economy and an escalation in the number of births for this age group as reasons for the slowdown. Incentives—benefits, flexible schedules, job sharing, maternity leave, and child care—will need to be available for the women to return to work.

Need for Policies and Procedures

Every organization and department needs to offer diversity training to both managers and employees to help them understand biases and to teach skills and information on "how to" manage diversity. All organizations need clearly defined policies and procedures about diversity, which would include the prohibition of telling ethnic jokes and making derogatory remarks about any cultural group. The policies **must** be enforced. Just because policies are in place *does not* mean rules can be bent or not followed for any one group. All employees need to know and follow their job descriptions, standards, job expectations, outcomes, and the mission of the organization and department.

Barriers to Diversity

When dealing with diverse work groups there will be barriers that will need to be addressed. They include:

- Individual bias—The lack of understanding of groups that may not be included due to differences. Groups are formed based on phenotype and cultural identity.
- Phenotype group—Formed based on physical, visually, observable differences in people. Phenotype affects the way we interact with people. The closer a person's visual appearance is to our own the more we identify with that person.
- Cultural identity group—Members of the same cultural group are individuals who share norms, values, and goal priorities that distinguish one group from another. The group can be based on gender, race, religion, sexual preference, age, social, and so forth.
- Prejudice—A negative attitude toward certain groups and their members.
- Stereotyping—A fixed notion or concept about a person or group.
- Racism/ignorance—Offhand remarks, including jokes that cut or injure another person, which may be made in ignorance and expressed in an inappropriate manner or context.
- Mistrust—We associate with people like us; doing this leads to misunderstanding of those who are different and we mistrust and lack confidence in them.
- Communication problems (the biggest issue)—The problem may be due to misunderstanding, in accuracy, errors, belligerent feelings, especially when various cultures have customs that relate to communication techniques.
- Other—Dress, patterns of behavior, values systems, feelings, attitudes, interaction, and group norms of the members can all have an effect on diversity.

PERFORMANCE EVALUATION SYSTEMS

The level of success attained by a business organization is directly related to the level of performance attained by its employees. Therefore, managers must be thoroughly familiar with the job-related activities and abilities of each employee they supervise. A system for regular and fair evaluation of individual employee performance is instrumental to the success of the department. A performance evaluation is a structured meeting between a supervisor and an employee to provide feedback about the employee's performance over a given period of time; it encourages an exchange about that employee's performance.

- It tracks progress in the development of job skills while identifying and correcting substandard performance.
- It serves as a basis for recognizing and rewarding employee achievements through promotions, salary increases, and other incentives.
- It provides a means of giving verbal and written feedback on individual employee performance.
- It's the overall functioning of the department and the organization.
- It promotes employees' well-being, job satisfaction, and sense of ownership in their work.
- It also identifies needs for improvement and growth and gives employees an opportunity to set personal work goals.
- An equitable and well-prepared evaluation given consistently can improve working relations and communications among employees and between employees and their supervisors. All of these pluses ultimately boost morale and productivity while minimizing costly employee absenteeism and turnover.
- It provides documentation for the employee's personnel record.

In most medium-size and large organizations, the performance evaluation system is administered by the human resource department. However, the foodservice director or manager still has direct responsibility for rating employees according to objective performance standards. The director, who follows procedures established by the human resource department, usually develops these standards. Generally, the performance evaluation process includes two components: a *written evaluation* and a *verbal review*. Regular salary or wage increases are based in large part on their performance evaluations. (Compensation and benefits are discussed later in this chapter.) In addition to determining salary increases, performance reviews can identify areas where training and coaching can improve performance.

Developing and Using the Performance Appraisal Form

Personal appraisals, also known as *performance evaluations*, is a process used by supervisors and managers of formally evaluating performance using established standards for performance of the job and providing feedback to the employee. Written performance appraisals become a part of the permanent employee record. Fair performance standards must be developed before a fair performance appraisal can be made. Performance standards are based on the responsibilities outlined in the job description. Each performance standard should reflect a required work-related behavior and need to be clearly stated in written form. The standard should cite specific task-related activities that can be measured or observed. These standards need to be reliable and valid for the employee/job to be appraised. (See Bibliography for reference for Standards for RDs in Management and Dietary Manager Standards of Performance. See Chapter 2.)

Standards of performance are written and are the basis for the outcomes of the evaluation; they include:

- Quality of work performed
- Quantity of work performed
- Employee's working relationships with coworkers and superiors
- Employee's attendance record
- Employee's work habits
- Employee's personal grooming and hygiene
- Employee's initiative

An employee's attitudes also affect overall performance but are difficult to rate. How an employee behaves toward other employees and how well he or she accepts supervision provide observable attitude indicators that can be rated.

The rating scale for each performance standard should follow the system developed by the human resource department, the food and nutrition department, and from professional associations who have developed and validated them. In most systems, the rating scale is based on descriptive terms that correspond to the points on a scale. These evaluations may be used for future promotions. Any performance to be appraised **must** not be discrimination-based. The appraisal system must ensure that employees who have similar employment situations are treated the same. The legal basis of an appraisal system has appraisals based on job analysis, with written instructions, allowing employees to review the appraisal results and agreement among raters if there is more than one rater, with all supervisors and managers having received "rater" training.

Several errors often occur during the evaluation process. One is the *halo effect*, the tendency on the part of certain supervisors to let very good or very poor performance in one task affect the evaluation of other unrelated tasks. Some supervisors also make the mistake of consistently giving too-lenient or too-severe ratings. Others tend to make the overall evaluation task easier for themselves by giving everyone in similar jobs average ratings instead of ratings based on individual performance. Another common problem is the *recency error*. Here, the supervisor mistakenly judges a whole review period's performance on the basis of the employee's most recent behavior. Because most employees are rated only once or twice a year, much of the employee's work performance could be misevaluated if only recent performance is considered.

To avoid such problems, use of a rating scale based on descriptive gradations. This is referred to as a *graphic rating scale*. Scales based on general terms such as *outstanding, superior, average*, and *poor* should be avoided because they make it too easy to give

average ratings to every employee's performance on every standard. In addition, supervisors can avoid the natural tendency to be influenced by recency error if they make evaluation an ongoing part of everyday department management. Ongoing review is the basis for performance coaching, which is covered later in this section. Notes on individual work performance and coaching sessions could be made regularly—monthly, for example—and then used as the basis for a performance evaluation at the end of the review period.

The human resource department's policy on scheduling regular performance evaluations should be followed. Many organizations have a system of annual review and performance appraisal, whereas others may follow a schedule of quarterly or semiannual reviews. Informal ratings of new employees are sometimes made monthly the training or probationary periods of their employment.

Before the Appraisal

Good preparation for each appraisal session leads to consistency and fairness in the evaluation and ultimately to a more content, motivated, and productive employee. The following suggestions will make the session more meaningful.

1. Review the performance form. Review any *critical* notes that have been collected over the *year*.
2. List any points that need to be discussed. Use measurable objective data that covers the *entire rating period*.
3. List the good points and those that need improvement.
4. Review the last performance appraisal to determine if improvements have been made and goals accomplished.
5. Develop a series of questions that need to be asked about previous goals.
6. Seek input from supervisors or other personnel (such as nursing) that may have had the opportunity to supervise/work with the employee.
7. As appropriate, discuss the appraisal with the next level of supervision.
8. Set an appointment with employee for a specific time and day for the verbal appraisal. Give the employee a copy of his or her last appraisal, job description, performance standards, agreed-on goals, and the appraisal form to be used for the session. Give the employee at least a week to review the materials and to develop comments and questions.

Conducting Verbal Performance Reviews

The second component in the individual evaluation process is the review conference held between the employee and his or her direct supervisor. Individual conferences are scheduled well in advance so that the supervisor and employees have enough time to prepare questions and comments. The reviewer should also schedule enough time for a thorough and unrushed private discussion of each employee's past and future performance. The supervisor needs to prepare for the meeting using a checklist to appraise the work of the employee. Check employee records for attendance at in-service training sessions, corrective action notes, absentee rate, and any commendations.

Conferences are to be conducted in private using a positive and cooperative manner. Be sincere and flexible. Use this opportunity to seek feedback from the employee. Determine what motivates the employee, ask the employee about any work-related problems he or she may have or the need for additional training. This is also a good opportunity to let the employee better understand the relationship between the supervisor and employee. Discuss any standards that were not met. Be specific; give examples based on the entire year. Be objective and calm. Give guidance to assist performance or improve performance. Review standards—are they realistic? *Listen* to the employees and their suggestions. When the problem is behavioral, be specific—such as overuse of sick leave, constant tardiness. If the behavior is major, refer the employee to the human resource employee assistance program. Once areas of good performance have been discussed, the supervisor and employee will need to set realistic goals. Finally, the employee and supervisor can reach agreement as to what steps are needed to improve specific areas of performance, along with a timetable for reaching the desired outcomes. Following up on the mutually agreed-on steps is part of coaching for positive outcomes (discussed in the next section).

It is important that the reviewer remain open-minded throughout the evaluation process by respecting and noting the employee's opinions. The employee also is given an opportunity to provide written responses to the evaluation, to be included with the documents filed in the human resource department. It is the supervisor's responsibility to appraise performance, not personality. Do not show favoritism.

Once the conference is over, both employee and supervisor should sign the evaluation form. In some organizations, the next level of management also may be required to review and approve completed evaluation forms. A copy of the form is made for the supervisor's files and for the employee. The original form, with all the necessary signatures, is placed in the employee's permanent personnel file, which usually is kept in the human resource department. In many organizations, a representative of the human resource department may check the evaluation form for completeness according to accepted personnel policies.

There will be times when employees do not agree with the performance appraisal. When this happens the employee should be allowed to write a rebuttal, to be attached to the appraisal *before* it becomes final. If the issue cannot be resolved a formal appeals process will need to be followed.

Other Methods for Appraisal Performance

There are other methods that can be used in appraising performance of an employee. They include:

Self-evaluations where employees evaluate themselves using the organization appraisal form. This method allows the employees to "honestly" evaluate their job performance. This method also allows the supervisor and employee to compare evaluations and to note any differences in the ranking/opinion and keep open communication.

Peer review is used most often to evaluate higher-level personnel. It is a system where peers at the same level in the organization rate one another—supervisor to supervisor. This method has some pitfalls such as the peer may not understand the scope of the work of the peer, jealousy, or lack of communication.

Subordinate review is a system where employees rate their supervisors. This system also has pitfalls as the subordinate and supervisor may not like each other; the subordinate may have received counseling and need additional training and may use the evaluation as a retaliatory measure.

360° review or *feedback* is a combination of the self, peer, and subordinate reviews, and in some instances, reviews by customers. This type of review is most often used by department heads and other high-level managers. This type of evaluation is time-consuming and expensive. It also can cause some hard feelings toward the person who evaluated the person.

Critical incident is a review of a supervisor's log that details incidents that are both effective and ineffective regarding job performance standards. The incidents are used to evaluate the employee's performance against preestablished standards. For any ineffective incident the employee receives coaching about the observed behavior that may include retraining, corrective action, or demotions. A checklist may be used by the supervisor to rate various performances that could also include the strengths and weaknesses of the employee's performance. The supervisor and the employee sign the form. A space is available where the employee and supervisor list goals with completion dates. A space is also needed for additional comments by the employee and supervisor.

Objective-based performance review is a review based on mutually agreed-on objectives by the employee and supervisor. The basic steps in this type of evaluation are those used by the *management by objectives* (Chapter 5).

Competence

The Joint Commission (TJC) continues to strengthen its human resource standards by addressing competence. The Commission defines *competence* as a "determination of a person's capability to perform up to defined expectations." In a presentation given at a 2000 annual meeting of the Dietary Managers Association, Ruby Puckett defined competence as "improving performance within the organization by employees qualified to perform tasks as outlined in job descriptions/performance outcome descriptions and performance appraisal process through measurable, demonstrated abilities." The Academy of Nutrition and Dietetics (known as the American Dietetic Association until 2012) states that "Competence is the demonstrated ability to perform in one's current practice and specific setting."

The managers or leaders are responsible to ensure that the competence of all staff members is assessed, maintained, demonstrated, and improved continually. Competence begins with the development of competence-based job descriptions and performance standards and proceeds to the employment process (hiring the right person for the job); then to orientation; training, development, and continuing education; performance appraisals; and thus to retention.

A number of methods can be used to check competence:

- Checklist
- Demonstrations
- Observations
- Training records
- Audits
- Peer reviews
- Patient surveys
- Formal assessment
- Quality improvement and problem-solving issues
- Self-assessment using objective criteria
- Assessment against measurable performance standards
- Evaluation on agreed-on objectives for performance
- Counseling records
- Pretesting and posttesting for in-service training
- Level of participation in mandated in-service sessions and committee or team activities

Coaching for Peak Performance

In addition to the regular written and verbal employee reviews, managers should make informal, day-to-day observations of employee performance, accomplishments, or problems. Unlike performance reviews, which are retrospective and infrequent, *coaching* requires concurrent ongoing performance monitoring and feedback for improvement. Regular feedback, or coaching, is basic to effective employee management and can prevent minor work-related problems from becoming major performance problems.

A positive approach to performance improvement, coaching provides individualized direction, information, and support on a daily basis. As a "performance coach," the manager is committed to the employee's development and to helping the employee reach full potential. A participative management style fosters a constructive environment in which coaching can be used to improve individual, team, and department performance. An effective manager provides the opportunity for employees to become involved and the necessary learning through performance coaching. Effective coaching helps people trust their instincts and take responsibility for the organization's success.

The first step in performance coaching is to diagnose performance deficiencies and their causes. Performance gaps exist when employees are not meeting goals, standards, or expectations agreed on with their manager. To identify performance deficiencies, employees must be observed over time. A number of causes may contribute to less-than-satisfactory performance. Some of these are:

- Poor orientation and in-service training
- Lack of ability or knowledge to accomplish assigned tasks
- Lack of interest in doing the job
- Absence of opportunity to grow and advance that creates feelings of helplessness in the employee
- Lack of clearly defined departmental goals
- Employee uncertainty about what is expected of him or her
- Absence of feedback on how well the employee is performing

- No rewards for high performance
- No negative consequences for poor performance
- Lack of resources to do the job
- Limitations or misunderstandings created by cultural differences
- Poor or lack of appropriate supervision

In diagnosing a problem, the first question the manager must ask is whether the employee knows what is expected and has the requisite skills to do the job. If not, the manager as coach must arrange for employee training as outlined earlier in this chapter.

Lack of information or skills is the most common reason for poor performance or goal accomplishment. Causes ascribed to other reasons will make the coaching session even more complex. When coaching, the manager must remain focused on measurable behaviors that can be identified and shared with the employee. *Measurable performance behaviors* are behaviors that can be assessed in comparison to established standards for performance. For example, the supervisor could make a statement like the following in a coaching session: "The standard for preparing and delivering late trays is 15 minutes. However, when you work this station, more than 50 percent of the trays are delivered to patients after 30 minutes. The delay causes a backlog of trays and results in poor customer satisfaction." Coaching can be divided into three segments: creating the game plan, conducting the coaching session, and following up to ensure success and to provide positive feedback.

Create a Game Plan

Coaching takes time because of the preparation involved and the commitment to involve the employee in making performance-related decisions. The following four steps will help create a game plan for discussing performance problems with employees:

1. Identify the behavior or habit that is nonproductive or contrary to policy, quality, or customer service.
2. Decide how the behavior affects the manager, work unit, fellow employees, or customers.
3. Determine why the behavior has this effect on those mentioned.
4. Determine how the behavior should change and the benefits those changes will bring about.

These steps will help the manager stay focused on the behavior in question and keep judgments about the employee from concealing the issue. The game plan must be flexible and capable of being changed as the employee's perceptions and needs change. Flexibility also is necessary for determining what actions should be taken to correct undesirable behavior.

Conduct the Coaching Session

Coaching sessions require the use of effective communication skills on the manager's part. The coaching action plan shown in Exhibit 9.1 may be helpful in providing written documentation of the coaching session. Typically, a coaching session has six steps:

EXHIBIT 9.1   Example of a Coaching Action Plan

Coaching Action Plan		
Employee:		
Job Title:		Date:
Current behavior:		
Expected behavior:		
Action Step	**Completion Date**	**Follow-up**

1. *Describe performance in terms of specific behavior.* Inform the employee of observations of what he or she did or said inappropriately. Describe how the inappropriate behavior affects the manager, the organization, the department, the team, and the employee. Pause to allow feedback from the employee.

2. *Obtain agreement from the employee on information presented in Step 1.* An employee who disagrees with or cannot understand the implications of the offending behavior is less likely to move toward changing it.

3. *Discuss solutions that can be implemented to resolve the performance problem.* Solutions should be mutually agreed on and should involve the employee in the decision-making process to arrive at a resolution.

4. *Agree on an action plan to be implemented for correcting the situation.* Summarize the information shared in the coaching session to ensure that both parties understand the behavior that led to the problem and the agreement on how improvement will occur.

5. *Establish a timeline for the action plan.* Having a time frame in which to assess the employee's progress helps keep the action plan and both parties' efforts focused.

6. *Acknowledge the employee's achievement in correcting the behavior and his or her performance.* The manager should document this improvement for the next performance evaluation.

When describing employee performance, it is important to remain objective and to give examples of actual behaviors. Avoid the following approaches:

- Labeling employee behavior (for example, "unprofessional" or "childish").

- Using absolutes or exaggerations for behavior that was observed only once or twice (for example, "You always do that"). These comments increase the potential for employee resistance.

- Judging the employee as "good," "better," or "worse"; such value judgments imply that the manager is always right and inhibits open discussion of the problem.

- Using someone else's words or implying that the problem is due to another person's observations (for example, "Jim says you often return from lunch late").

Coaching is a positive approach the manager can use continuously to provide information about expectations, observed performance, and skill development and to provide praise and improve self-esteem. Managers and supervisors should have regular meetings with individual employees who report to them. The length of these meetings will depend on the nature of the problem, the complexity of the work, and the responsibility charged to the employee. Coaching should not be confused with discipline, which may be necessary if efforts to improve performance are not successful. (Disciplinary policies and procedures will be covered later in this chapter.) Training and coaching employees to achieve peak performance allows the manager to delegate work effectively.

Follow-Up Coaching Efforts

Consistent follow-up with employees demonstrates the manager's support and commitment to improving their performance and helping them to be successful in their jobs. This step is frequently overlooked by managers, but without follow-up, it is difficult to sustain improvement and assist with future growth. The amount of follow-up should be based on the individual skill levels and needs of the employees. For example, an employee who has difficulty greeting and assisting customers in the cafeteria may need to frequently discuss his or her comfort level with public contact and get suggestions for how to answer customers' questions as well as receive praise for success from the manager. A star performer who is being asked to create a quality control checklist for the first time may need follow-up to ensure that the assignment has been completed successfully.

Mentoring

Mentoring is considered by some human resource managers as a part of training development. Leaders and managers consider mentoring a more formal arrangement between a career employee who is assigned or takes the responsibility to coach, counsel, model, support, encourage, and provide guidance to a newly hired employee or an early career employee. Mentoring is a structured and trusting relationship. A mentor can greatly benefit a new employee, helping the employee understand the organization and providing advice on skills, career progress, and methods to get ahead. The mentor is available after the original orientation to act as a counselor, to help the employee over situations and problems. The mentor is someone who can and is willing to listen and provide guidance to the mentoree. Many institutions have implemented mentoring programs and have found that these programs make a difference in careers. Some professional organizations such as the Academy of Nutrition and Dietetics offer mentoring programs.

Employee Assistance Programs

Many employees at some time during their career develop a personal problem for which they need help in handling. The *employee assistance program (EAP)* is there to provide confidential professional help to employees facing personal problems that might have an impact on their performance, their health and well-being, or the safety or security of other employees.

Problems in the workplace can often be prevented by timely and appropriate response to warning signs or when employees who have trouble handling personal problems ask for help. An employee assistance program is a formal program that provides employees with counseling for family, marital, and relationship problems, gambling, substance abuse, financial difficulty, stress, depression, anxiety disorders, eating disorders, and other mental and emotional problems.

Employees should be encouraged to contact EAP even if their problem is not job related. The supervisor or others assisting will not be informed the employee is receiving counseling. Everything that is said will be confidential. Short-term counseling is available in-house at no cost, while referrals are made to other services or outside professionals for longer-term treatment. When counseled by others, the cost is the responsibility of the employee, but the EAP works to keep it affordable.

If an employee fails to seek help on his or her own, it is the immediate supervisor's responsibility to take appropriate action. The program needs to include:

- *Goals:* short- and long-term goals that are expected to be achieved by the employee and the employer

- *Professional staffing:* the organization should be staffed by professional licensed persons
- *Written purpose:* of program, employee eligibility, role, and responsibility of personnel
- *Confidentiality:* confidential records are maintained
- *Legal requirements:* all legal requirements are known and followed

The manager should never attempt to diagnose a suspected problem, openly accuse an employee, or give advice on sensitive subjects such as alcoholism or chemical dependency. It the organization has no EAP, the manager should strongly recommend that the employee seek qualified professional assistance to identify a possible problem. (For additional information, do a web search for Executive Order 12968 or Employee Assistance program.)

PERSONNEL RECORDS

Every organization is required to keep certain kinds of records on each employee. Official personnel records are usually maintained by the human resource department. Individual departments may keep records on their own employees as well. Generally speaking, department personnel records are less formal than the human resource files. Department records may contain managers' notations on an employee's work performance, coaching action plans, attendance records, copies of vacation requests, notes on scheduling availability, and so forth. The official personnel files should contain the following information for each employee:

- Complete name, home address, telephone number, Social Security number, and name of the nearest relative or person to contact in case of an emergency
- Job title or classification and rate of pay (hourly, weekly, or monthly)
- Reports of initial and periodic physical examinations
- Promotion records (start date, changes in job classification, pay increases)
- All records from the hiring process (application form, interview notes, records of education, references)
- Records on initial training
- Records of attendance (including vacation days, holidays, and sick days)
- Records of regular and overtime hours worked (for hourly employees only)
- Safety records (accident reports, workers' compensation claims)
- Information on benefits (health insurance, life insurance, pension plan, savings plans, and so forth)
- Records of performance evaluations (written evaluation forms signed by employee and supervisor, special awards and notes of commendation, and written comments on performance made outside the formal evaluation process)
- Records of disciplinary actions, grievances, or complaints
- Termination date and acceptability for reemployment, when appropriate

Keeping records of all disciplinary actions and dismissal procedures is absolutely necessary. Complete documentation of work-related problems will be needed if a former employee takes legal action against the organization for any reason. Because of the confidential nature of personnel records, they should be stored in a place that is inaccessible to unauthorized employees. All managers should have a locked drawer or filing cabinet for personnel files kept in the department.

PERSONNEL POLICIES AND PROCEDURES

Most human resource departments in health care organizations develop and administer general *policies* on how employment issues are to be handled. In turn, formal, written personnel *procedures* based on general policies are adopted. Step-by-step procedures are valuable tools for managers' use in administering policies consistently and fairly throughout the organization. Policies and procedures that are understood by all employees and followed by all managers protect everyone from potentially unfair treatment. In addition, they help protect the organization from lawsuits, union and employee grievances, and accusations of illegal discrimination.

Comprehensive organizational policies should cover at least the following basic employment-related topics:

- Mission, vision, and values of organization
- Organizational chart
- Hours of operation, work hours
- Pay periods, overtime pay
- Physical examinations, other health policies, accident and injury reporting
- Performance evaluation
- Promotions and job postings
- Vacations, holidays, and holiday pay
- Confidentiality of information
- Training and educational opportunities
- Personal leaves (maternity, bereavement, family, medical, nonmedical, and military)
- Availability of nonpatient foodservice, hours of operation
- Parking
- Name tags
- Visitors during work hours
- Employee grievances
- Disciplinary and corrective actions, termination
- Tardiness and absenteeism
- Sexual harassment
- Emergency preparedness and safety rules, and workplace violence
- Unions
- Other information applicable to the foodservice department and the organization

The organization's personnel policies usually are written and distributed in an employee handbook, which is given to all new employees and, when updated, copies are provided to all staff. When a personnel policy changes significantly, the change is publicized through memorandums, posters, and other appropriate means. New policies often emerge from topics covered during in-service training sessions.

Every manager is responsible for applying the organization's personnel policies uniformly and consistently to all employees. Personnel policies on employee discipline, promotions, dismissals, and so on must be followed closely to avoid liability risk to the organization because of failure to follow its own policies. For example, an employee who was terminated without warning, even if the termination was justifiable, could sue an organization whose policy on termination stated that an employee would be given a written warning and placed on probation before being dismissed. In addition to legal problems, consistent failure to follow its policies and procedures can expose a facility to charges of favoritism, discrimination, or both. Employee morale problems might be created as well.

Developing a Foodservice Department Employee Handbook

An *employee handbook* that clearly sets the policies and procedures of the department followed in the foodservice department is a useful training and management tool. This handbook is a good source and basis for training new employees and a handy reference for experienced foodservice workers. The handbook, which should be reviewed annually by the department director and updated as necessary, can include at least the following information:

- Welcome letter from director
- Mission, values of department
- Organizational charts
- Patients' rights
- Personal appearance, dress code requirements
- Proper hand-washing procedures and use of gloves
- Universal precautions, infection control standards
- Personal conduct (smoking policy)
- Guest relations with patients and staff
- Personnel policies of food and nutrition service
- Competence evaluations and standards
- Work schedules
- Payroll check distribution
- Food safety and sanitation
- Food and nutrition fire safety and emergency preparedness procedures, right-to-know information on hazardous substances used in the workplace
- In-service training programs
- Relationships between foodservice departments and other departments
- Employee accident report forms and how to fill out
- Employee assistant program
- Incident reports
- Termination procedure
- Other department-specific information
- Table of contents

Employees receive this handbook during departmental orientation. Materials in the handbook are reviewed with the employees by the supervisor. The handbook provides written reference to the policies and procedures of the department. An employee signs that he or she has received the book and that its contents have been reviewed with the employee by the supervisor. The signed form becomes a part of the employee's personnel file.

Maintaining Positive Approach to Corrective Action

Most employees accept policies and procedures as a necessary condition of working, and they expect the rules to be enforced fairly and evenhandedly. Employee morale suffers when certain employees are permitted to violate policies and procedures, which promotes favoritism. More important, employee safety may be at risk if policies and procedures are not followed. For example, violation of safety procedures can cause equipment damage and endanger workers, for which the organization might be held accountable. This is especially the case in the foodservice department, where fire safety and safe food-handling procedures are doubly crucial. For these reasons, prompt and fair disciplinary action is a necessary element of managing employees.

Corrective action is taken in an effort to modify employee behavior. Corrective action can be positive as a way to strengthen employee behavior or improve performance. It does not need to be negative or punitive except in rare cases.

When corrective action must be taken, the appropriate manager should do so immediately. However, the facility's formal written disciplinary procedures must be followed assiduously to ensure that the employees involved are treated fairly and lawfully. Most important, situations requiring disciplinary action should be regarded as teaching opportunities rather than as excuses to impose punishment.

As a form of *discipline*, corrective rather than punitive action is more appropriate for the work setting. With a corrective approach, acceptable behavior is encouraged based on known standards, policies, and procedures whereas unacceptable behavior is discouraged on the basis of its being inefficient, unfair, or potentially dangerous—or all three. Often employees respond reasonably to what should be the first—and, it is hoped, the last—step in disciplinary action: a verbal reprimand. Actual penalties such as fines, suspensions, and dismissals should be rare events.

Although violations of procedure should be dealt with immediately, they should not be addressed hastily or in anger. Before taking action, the manager should thoroughly investigate the situation and determine whether the employee understood that he or she was violating a policy. If it becomes necessary to reprimand the employee (correct the behavior), the manager should do so in private and with diplomacy. The disciplinary action should fit the seriousness of the offense, with the manager having considered fully the circumstance, implication, and effect of the infraction beforehand. An extreme example would be the difference between an employee observed serving himself or herself a meal from the patient tray line versus

FIGURE 9.1 Progressive Corrective Action

Increasing Severity of Offense or Related Offenses

- Informal discussion of the problem (Low-level problems are initially handled in this way. Example: Forgetting to follow standard procedures.)

- Oral reprimand (A more serious or repeated problem. Example: Gambling on the job may draw an oral reprimand as a first step.)

- Written reprimand or warning (This is a very serious step to take. Example: Repeated use of profane or abusive language to others may result in a written reprimand.)

- Disciplinary suspension (An alternative to transfer or demotion, this is the last step before discharge. Example: Fighting.)

- Dismissal (Obviously the most serious step, and usually the last step after others have been tried. In some cases, this may be the first level of disciplinary action. Example: Willful falsification of records.)

an employee discovered loading a box of steaks into a car. The employee who consumed food without paying for it would likely receive a verbal reprimand with an explanation of how his or her actions constitute theft. The employee who stole the steaks, on the other hand, would likely be dismissed.

The primary purpose of a corrective action is to prevent the violation from recurring. For repeated violations, most employers use a system of progressive discipline under which the penalty becomes more severe with each repeated violation (Figure 9.1).

The *first step* in disciplinary action should be a *verbal correction*. A second violation would incur a *written correction* plan to be placed in the employee's permanent personnel record for a predetermined time. With a *third* offense, a *written warning* delineating the potential consequences of future violations would be issued to the offending employee. If the problem is not resolved, the manager might issue another written warning to the effect that a subsequent violation will result in *dismissal or demotion* (the reassignment of an employee to a job with less responsibility and a lower pay scale). Although demotion is sometimes used as a disciplinary action, it has severe drawbacks. For one thing, the demoted employee could become a demoralizing element within the workforce. Also, he or she might do damage to supplies or equipment, otherwise sabotage operations, or do some type of workplace violence. Employee transfers to other work groups as a disciplinary action usually have the same effects.

With few exceptions, dismissal is appropriate only for the most serious or habitual offenses. For example, some personnel policies require the immediate suspension and possible dismissal of any employee who uses or sells illegal drugs anywhere on the work premises.

Whenever dismissal is the only solution to an ongoing personnel problem, such as repeated complaints from other employees or patients, the supervisor must follow the organization's procedures exactly to avoid potential liability consequences for the organization. Employee offenses must be thoroughly documented in writing, as must each step in the progressive chain of disciplinary action (Exhibit 9.2). This evidence must be recorded in the employee's permanent personnel record. The human resource department should be consulted before actual dismissal to make sure that all necessary documentation has been prepared.

The "hot stove" rule applies in these situations. The *hot stove* rule is a method of how disciplinary should be taken. It relates to touching a hot stove:

- Touching a hot stove results in immediate consequences—a burn.
- It is a warning that if you touch a hot stove you will be burned. At this point the disciplinary action is taken to warn the employee that threat is real and pain may occur.
- A hot stove will consistently burn anyone who touches it. Disciplinary rules must be consistently applied to all.

No matter how severe or how minor the department's disciplinary problems, two principles must be kept in mind: consistency of enforcement and objectivity of approach. Every time a violation occurs, disciplinary action must be taken. Without relentless enforcement of policy and procedure in the workplace, employee morale and security can disintegrate, with employees eventually losing respect for their managers. Consistency, however, does not mean rigidity. Each case must be addressed individually and complete information gathered before action is taken.

As for objectivity of approach, disciplinary decisions must be fact-based, not gossip- or rumor-based. That is, an employee must be given opportunity to present his or her side. As mentioned earlier, it cannot be assumed that an employee knowingly violated a policy or procedure. In remaining objective, a manager must exercise unbiased discretion in listening to the employee's side. As shown in the discussion on communication, objectivity is best maintained by separating the message from the messenger; that is, by suppressing personal bias in efforts to resolve a disciplinary problem.

EXHIBIT 9.2   Corrective Action Record

Corrective Action Record

First offense_____

Second offense_____

Third offense_____

Final_____

Name of employee_____

Date of action_____

Reason for action_____

_____

_____

_____

Corrective instruction given_____

_____

_____

_____

Date review will be made to determine effectiveness of instructions

_____

Your signature on this form does not indicate
you agree with the action.

_____		_____
Signature of Employee		Date
_____		_____
Signature of Supervisor		Date
_____		_____
Signature of Department Head		Date

Source: Developed by Ruby P. Puckett©.

Following Grievance Procedures

Employees have the right to register complaints and to have them considered with fairness and objectivity. A *grievance* is a formal complaint about a practice that is regarded as unfair and violates the union contract. A written procedure for conducting grievance hearings should be established whether employees are union members. However, under collective-bargaining agreements between employers and unions, *grievance procedures* are always made part of the labor contract. Usually, the *union steward*, who has been elected by the union members and represents all unionized staff in specific departments, is responsible for helping union members prepare and present grievances to management. Both the union president and union steward have regular jobs, are paid by the employer, and use some time from the job—in addition to personal time—for required union activities. A sound and fair grievance procedure permits union and nonunion employees alike to express their complaints without fear of reprisal or job loss.

Steps in a grievance procedure may vary among organizations, but most follow a pattern. Again, it is vital that managers follow to the letter procedures dictated by organizational policy. In a *nonunionized* health care facility, the procedure typically begins when an employee brings a complaint or employment-related problem to his or her immediate supervisor. The supervisor is usually able to settle the problem at this stage by either granting or denying the grievance. A written record of the decision and of any action taken should be kept in the employee's personnel record (Exhibit 9.3).

When the problem cannot be resolved by the supervisor and employee's joint efforts and the supervisor denies the grievance, the employee can take it to the next level of management. In most cases, the employee's supervisor will have informed his or her own super-visor of the situation so that the grievance will come as no surprise to the next higher authority, usually a department director. If dissatisfied by the decision on this level, the employee may take the grievance higher up, eventually to the topmost authority—in most hospitals, the CEO. Meanwhile, the human resource director may have been consulted at any point for advice on solving the problem. In a nonunion setting, the CEO's decision is final.

In a *unionized* health care facility, a grievance procedure follows similar steps except that a union steward or other union representative would assist the employee through all stages. A union business agent would participate in arriving at a final agreement on the solution if the problem was brought to top-level management. A matter that cannot be settled by the CEO and the union agent may be submitted for arbitration (discussed later in this chapter). *Conciliation*, the act of bringing in a person from outside the organization to reconcile opposing parties, is an alternative to arbitration. The conciliator's role is to help the parties find a common ground for agreeing on a solution to the problem.

The grievance procedure is reviewed at regular intervals by the human resource department to make certain that it is progressing in a satisfactory manner. However, it should be the goal of every manager to handle as many employee grievances as possible within the department. To deal successfully with employee complaints, managers must listen carefully to the facts and deal calmly with the emotions involved. Anger and snap judgments must be avoided, despite pressure to make a decision immediately. The manager should communicate the reasoning behind his or her decision whether to take action on the employee's grievance. Responding to complaints fairly and quickly encourages employees to speak openly about department problems. Productivity and morale may be improved greatly as a result.

EXHIBIT 9.3   Record of Employee Counseling

To be filled out in duplicate

Date: _____

Permanent record of verbal conference with employee (name)

_____

Nature of conference (specify, in detail, event(s) leading to conference)

_____

_____

(Attach additional sheet if more space is needed)

Recommendation_____

_____

_____

_____

_____

_____

_____

_____   _____
Employee's Signature   Date

_____   _____
Supervisor's Signature   Date

_____   _____
Director's Signature   Date

Copy Number 1 will be retained by employee. Copy Number 2 will be sent to the Personnel
Clerk to become part of the employee's permanent record.

Source: Developed by Ruby P. Puckett©.

Dismissal: Nondisciplinary

There are a number of types of dismissal in which the employee makes the decision to leave. These types of dismissal are not disciplinary and they include: (1) *voluntary*, where an employee decides, for personal or professional reasons, to end the job; (2) *discharge, layoff, downsizing, rightsizing* the organization and making this decision based on many factors, including fiscal; (3) *quit*, where an employee may become dissatisfied with the job or a more attractive position in another organization is available; (4) *retirement*, when an employee reaches a certain age years of service or is financially capable to leave a job.

Dismissal for Cause

Dismissal for cause may include:

- *Breach of contract* where both the employer and employee have made a legal binding contract and the employee has not fulfilled his or her obligation.
- *Employment at will* is used by employers to assert their right to end an employment relationship at any time for any cause. This type of employment is usually geared to managers who have no work contract, union contract, or civil service rules.
- *Ethical violations* that could include receiving kickback, unethical conduct on and off the job, providing confidential (all types) information to a competitor, patient rights.
- *Random drug test*: when a random test is made and an employee is found to be using drugs.
- *Fiscal theft*, embezzlement, computer crime, theft of medicines, food, other supplies and equipment, misuse of e-mail and web (searching for porn), and waste of employer's time.
- *Whistleblowing* is the disclosure by an employee of an employer's illegal, immoral, or illegitimate practice to persons or organizations that may be able to take corrective action that may or may not result in dismissal of the employee and possible legal action by the employee against the employer.
- *Last step in progressive discipline.*
- *Workplace violence* such as sexual harassment, hostile workplace, fighting.

The final authority for hiring and firing is usually the responsibility of the department head. However, it is necessary to instruct others on how to carry out this function. Probably, a supervisor's most unpleasant job is having to dismiss an employee. The following are three suggestions to help supervisors handle the situation:

1. Prepare your case.
   Plan your action. Never stand in the middle of the kitchen and yell "You're fired!"
   Be sure the right thing is being done.
   Do not act too hastily; gather all the facts. Do not overlook any detail, no matter how small.
   Follow the health care organization's policies.
   Make sure all obligations have been fulfilled. Was this employee properly oriented? Were the policies explained?
   Make an objective, fact-verified decision and stick to it.
2. After the case has been carefully prepared and in some cases approved by human resources and administration, schedule an interview.
   Ask the employee if he or she wants union representation.
   Have a witness available throughout the discharge action.
   Keep the interview short. Do not keep the employee in suspense.
   Do not use clichés of regret: "This hurts me as much as it does you."
   Use facts to explain why the employee is being dismissed. Do not attack the employee's personality.
   Do not give advice. This is not the time, and it will not be appreciated.
   Be considerate and always fair and consistent to all employees. Do not try to destroy the employee.
   Be positive.
3. Employees should be given the opportunity to appeal, or grieve, any action taken against them.
   Give the employee a copy of the dismissal letter.
   Explain the reason for the action to the employee.
   Explain the loss of benefits to the employee. Be polite, and answer any questions with honesty.
   Explain about the last paycheck.
   If appropriate, inform the employee about the appeal or grievance procedure.

Conducting Exit Interviews

Many human resource departments routinely conduct exit interviews with employees shortly before they leave the organization. During *an exit interview*, the outgoing employee is advised of his or her right to continued medical- and life insurance coverage or to receive vacation or severance pay, as well unemployment insurance benefits and carryover for health insurance. This is also an opportunity to discuss why the employee is leaving the organization, the quality of supervision and training received, the adequacy of advancement opportunities, benefits and incentives, and other related topics.

The information disclosed during exit interviews can be valuable to department managers, including human resource managers (Exhibit 9.4). For example, managers may learn where problems lie in their training programs and management skills. Or light may be shed on shortcomings in the compensation and benefits structure or in working conditions.

Reducing Employee Turnover

It is wise to try to retain valuable employees and to reduce the cost of the employment cycle. Employees like to have interesting work; be involved in decision making, feedback, and training; and receive respect for abilities and differences. They want to work in an environment that is relatively stress-free, to be empowered, and to be part of the department organization. However, some employees still leave jobs for a number of reasons.

Whenever an employee leaves a job—either voluntarily or involuntarily—it costs the organization money, time, goodwill, and other resources. The more skilled the employee, the higher the replacement cost. The rate at which employees leave their jobs—called employee *turnover*—can be determined by using a simple formula. The rate of turnover equals the total number of separations per year divided by the average number of employees on the payroll and multiplied by 100. Or:

$$\text{Turnover rate (\%)} = \frac{\text{Number of separations per year}}{\text{Average number of payroll employees}} \times 100$$

For obvious economic reasons, it is to the organization's advantage to keep the turnover rate as low as possible. Furthermore, because high turnover endangers employee morale and reduces productivity, managers should try to identify the causes of high turnover and, when possible, take action to improve the conditions that have led to the unacceptable levels. It is difficult to define which levels of turnover are acceptable and which are not: turnover rates are affected by the geographical location of the organization as well as by the availability of other employment opportunities in the area. For example, an annual turnover rate of about 10 percent might be acceptable in a large urban area on the West Coast but would be considered unusually high in a rural community in the South.

High rates of turnover frequently are caused by errors in the employment process, specifically, hiring the wrong person for the job. Managers can help correct this situation by taking more time to analyze the employee qualities for specific jobs before screening, interviewing, and selecting employees. Other reasons for high turnover rates include:

- Choosing the wrong person for the job
- Poor employee orientation procedures
- Insufficient training of new employees
- Lack of retraining opportunities for current employees
- Poor supervision and management of employees
- Lack of consistency and objectivity in enforcing policies and procedures, which can lead to favoritism
- Lack of opportunity for professional growth and development
- Failure to appreciate and recognize employee achievements
- Lack of team work
- Ongoing unresolved conflicts
- Quality-of-life issues
- Lack of effective supervision
- Stress
- Politics of department or organization
- Poor recruiting methods
- Poor communication between employee and supervisor
- Boredom
- Lack of job security
- No opportunity for advancement
- Racism
- Sexual harassment
- Lack of respect between employees and management
- Personal reasons
- Low compensation for amount of work
- Poor working conditions and equipment
- Hostile work environment
- Unfair and unequal work assignments
- Lack of recognition by peers, supervisors, or managers
- Insufficient staff, too many supervisors and not enough workers
- Schedule—too rigid
- Low compensation—especially for fringe benefits
- Lack of diversity

EXHIBIT 9.4   Resignation Form

Resignation Form

Instructions: Please fill out this form if you are planning to resign. Present it to the Food and Nutrition Services Personnel Clerk. The clerk will arrange an Exit Interview for you with Personnel, Room H-9, Ground Floor. Comments in the remarks section on your term of employment will assist us in evaluating our services. Thank you.

Date_____   Name_____

Address_____
_____

To Whom It May Concern:

I wish to tender my resignation from the Department of Food and Nutrition Services, XYZ Hospital. Effective date:
_____
_____

Reason for leaving (please be specific):_____
_____
_____
_____

Forwarding address (if not known, give family's address):_____
_____
_____

REMARKS

How would you rate this department? Circle your choices. E = Excellent, G = Good, F = Fair, P = Poor

1.	Salary	E	G	F	P
2.	Job security	E	G	F	P
3.	Chance for promotion	E	G	F	P
4.	Working conditions	E	G	F	P
5	On-the-job training	E	G	F	P
6.	Were the supervisors interested in you	Yes	No	Sometimes	Not at all as a person?
7.	Were you shown appreciation for work done?	Yes	No	Sometimes	Not at all
8.	Was discipline handled in a fair manner?	Yes	No	Sometimes	Not at all
9.	Were you kept informed about changes	Yes	No	Sometimes	Not at all in the department?
10.	Would you recommend this department	Yes	No	Sometimes	Not at all as a good place in which to work?

Comments:

Source: Developed by Ruby P. Puckett©.

Reducing Absenteeism

High levels of employee *absenteeism* often are tied to the same factors that cause high turnover. Although employees miss work for any number of personal reasons (such as illness and family emergencies), unacceptable surges in absenteeism usually signal work-related problems such as poor working conditions (inefficient systems or outdated equipment), slumping morale (due to favorit-ism or lack of incentive, for example), and inadequate supervision (supervisor apathy or poor interpersonal skills). Thus, a manager who notices excessive absenteeism should first look within the environment for clues and then take steps to improve the situation. An employee attitude survey or a culture audit would be a useful tool in this respect (see Chapter 4).

The rate of absenteeism can be determined by using another simple formula. The rate of absenteeism equals the number of workdays lost per pay period divided by the average number of employees, multiplied by the number of days worked, and then multiplied by 100. Or:

$$\text{Absenteeism rate (\%)} = \frac{\text{Number of workdays lost per pay period}}{\begin{array}{c}\text{Average number of employees}\\ \times \text{number of days worked}\end{array}} \times 100$$

COMPENSATION AND BENEFITS ADMINISTRATION

The human resource department is responsible for establishing and maintaining an organization's *compensation* and *benefits program*. An equitable and competitive program is essential to the organization's ability to attract and retain competent and qualified employees. The compensation system is the mechanism by which the human resource department sets salary and wage rates for new employees, approves increases for current employees, maintains and updates wage and salary schedules and job classification schedules, authorizes position changes, and authorizes the creation of new positions.

Managers outside the human resource department play a role in compensation administration when they recommend salary or wage adjustments for individual employees, when they recommend changes in the pay scale for positions under their management, and when they recommend salaries or wages for new or newly promoted employees.

Role of the Human Resource Department in Compensation Administration

Compensation programs of all but the smallest health care organizations are directly administered by the human resource department. Typically, human resource managers develop and maintain programs through a series of ongoing activities, including:

- With input from the department, formulating and regularly updating job descriptions for every position
- Evaluating each position and ranking it according to standard factors such as educational level required, degree of job responsibility, level of skill needed, number of employees supervised, amount of experience required, and a local, state and national comparison of compensation for like positions
- Assigning each position to a wage grade on the basis of the position's rank in comparison to all other positions in the institution
- Establishing a pay scale for each wage grade
- Conducting regular (usually annual) wage surveys of comparable employers in the same geographical area
- Using the results of wage surveys to adjust pay scales of comparable work so that the organization remains competitive in its labor market
- Determining pay system, pay grades, pay policies, and reviewing and approving the salary and wage adjustments recommended by managers on the basis of individual employee performance reviews

- Reviewing and approving the salary and wage adjustments recommended by managers for employees who have been promoted or assigned to newly created positions
- Reviewing and approving salaries or wages recommended by managers for new employees
- Taking part in negotiations to determine compensation agreements for unionized employees

Role of the Foodservice Director in Compensation Administration

The foodservice director must work within the compensation program set up by the organization's human resource department. Although position pay scales within the department are determined by human resources or by a compensation committee, the foodservice director may suggest changes in pay scales when the responsibilities of individual positions are increased or decreased or when the director becomes aware that salaries or wages are no longer competitive.

The foodservice director determines the salaries or wages of individual foodservice workers, within the limits of the compensation system. Most positions are compensated by a range of pay. For example, the position of foodservice assistant might be assigned to job grade C, which has a pay scale that ranges from $7.25 to $9.25 per hour. When a new foodservice assistant is hired, the director decides whether to pay the new employee at the bottom of the range, the middle, or the top. The new employee's starting wage is based on his or her level of experience or training. Therefore, a new employee with three years' experience as a foodservice assistant would be considered well qualified and be offered a salary at least at the middle of the range for that position.

Performance evaluations have a direct influence on the pay increases awarded employees. Generally, the process of performance evaluation culminates in the reviewer's recommendation for a pay increase based on the employee's work performance. Here again, the foodservice director works within the limits of the overall compensation system. In many organizations, the human resource department determines a range of pay increases for current employees. This range is based on the organization's current level of profits (for-profit health care facilities) or current level of assets (not-for-profit facilities) and current economic conditions.

Most employers of nonunionized workers use a system of merit increases for rewarding employee performance as determined during the performance evaluation process. *Merit increases* are intended to reward some employees more than others on the basis of their overall productivity and quality of work. For example, employees who were rated by their supervisors as "outstanding" in all aspects of their work might receive a higher raise (merit increase) than employees who were rated as "acceptable."

The merit increase system is based on the idea that employees will work harder if they know they will be rewarded monetarily for their increased effort. However, as shown in Chapter 2, many other factors play a role in worker motivation, and merit pay increases may or may not result in increased productivity. Effectiveness of the merit increase system is also affected by the fact that because of current economic conditions, health care providers have been forced to limit their compensation spending. As a result, the difference between consistently outstanding performance and acceptable performance might mean a differential of only one or two percentage points in merit increases. For the merit increase system to surely boost employee productivity, pay differences based on performance differences must be more than marginal. Unfortunately, many health care organizations no doubt will be unable to meet this demand in the foreseeable future.

Other methods of compensation include *cost-of-living adjustment (COLA)*. These increases are based on the inflation rates and are used to keep employees' purchasing power intact despite the economic changes over time. When this type of compensation is used, it applies to all employees. This is a permanent increase to the base pay. *Pay for performance* is an incentive-pay program that may be used in combination with other compensation plans. Incentive plans involve accomplishing predetermined goals. This type of compensation is a one-time pay and is not added to the base pay. *Annual bonus* is a type of payment that is given one time a year for outstanding performance. The bonus paid to groups of employees may be the same, whereas management-level personnel receive a larger bonus. This is a one-time payment and does not change the base pay. *Cash award* is a one-time pay for performance for outstanding and significant contributions. It does not change the base. *Improved skills* is a compensation that is added to the base pay when employees increase their skills through education or acquiring additional skills.

Benefits Administration

As shown, monetary compensation is one element of the compensation package. Benefits are the other. A competitive benefits program is key to attracting and retaining qualified employees, but it has little effect on employee performance because the benefits offered are tied to employee status. In other words, all full-time employees are covered by the same benefits, but certain benefits (such as the amount of life insurance coverage) may be linked to salary level.

Large employers may offer a full range of benefits whereas the benefits offered by small employers usually are more modest. Several kinds of benefits may make up a compensation package. One is pay for time not actually worked—vacations, sick leaves, paid holidays, and unemployment compensation. Insurance benefits, extremely important to most employees, include medical coverage for the employee and (sometimes) the employee's spouse and dependents, life insurance, disability insurance, dental insurance, and (sometimes) vision insurance. Retirement benefits may include a private pension plan administered by the employer. Social Security is also considered a retirement benefit because employers make contributions to the fund on behalf of their employees. (Employees are required to make contributions as well.) Another kind of benefit is employee services such as employee credit unions and tuition reimbursement programs.

Benefits provision is costly for U.S. employers, estimated by authorities to equal more than one-third of the average employee's annual salary. Employee benefits have become a major expense

during the past 15 years or so because of rising health insurance premiums, increased Social Security payments, and changes in the way pension plans are administered.

Because of the economic pressures in the health care industry, human resource departments are continually reviewing and revising benefits plans in terms of their cost, relevance, and value. As a result, foodservice directors are often called on to explain benefit changes to foodservice workers.

Recognition and Awards Programs

Many health care organizations have developed recognition and awards programs for the staff. These programs are an acknowledgment of best practice. The rewards may be small or large, for example, if an employee is doing a good job let them know immediately. This could include making them employee for the day, giving out gold stars, and so forth. Another excellent method for recognition is to write a personal letter to the employee or recognition in a staff meeting.

Other methods include:

- Keep a book of remembrance with photos of employees caught doing more than expected.
- Give special privileges such as a free parking space for a month.
- Develop a monthly newsletter and spotlight the employee of the month.
- Give meal tickets or, if approved, movie tickets.
- Customer awards; the employee who receives the most positive comments receives prizes in the form of money or gifts.
- Awards may be given on an organization-wide basis and may include banquets where service awards are given for years of service.
- National week promotion such as Dietitian Week and Pride in Foodservice Week, where food and nutrition personnel may be honored by the department and the organization.
- Have monthly birthday parties with all levels of department management for all employees whose birthdays fall within the month.
- During time of stress (weather conditions, increased census, and shortage of personnel), if appropriate and possible have the director push a beverage/snack cart throughout the department and serve the employees. This is an excellent time to listen to employee concerns.
- Let your imagination come up with other ways to recognize employees. (Be sure to follow organization policies and procedures and, where needed, obtain administration approval.)

Labor Relations

In 1974, health care employees became a class of workers covered by the federal laws that govern collective bargaining between unions and management in the private sector. *Collective bargaining* is the activity engaged in when representatives of an employee's organization, association, or union and representatives of the employer's management negotiate wages, hours, and other conditions of employment. Before 1974, the collective-bargaining activities of health care workers were covered by state law. However, when health care came under federal jurisdiction by authority of the Health Care Amendments to the National Labor Relations Act (the Taft-Hartley Act) in 1974, union organization activities in hospitals increased significantly. Today, it is not uncommon for hospitals to have one or more bargaining units or even for the entire workforce, except for supervisors and administrators, to be unionized.

The human resource department is responsible for interpreting and applying the provisions of a labor contract between the health care organization and the union. Problems with enforcing the contract or with the work of individual employees covered by the contract are handled according to a strict grievance procedure dictated by the terms of the contract. When grievances involving union employees cannot be settled within the organization, a special form of negotiation is required as set forth in the union contract. *Binding arbitration* is the process by which an impartial outside party is called in to settle a labor dispute. The *arbitrator* is an expert in labor law hired by the organization and the union to analyze the labor contract, listen to both sides of the issue, and make a decision on the validity of the grievance. The arbitrator's decision is *binding* in that both the organization and the union must abide by it. The

system of binding arbitration prevents any kind of strike during the period covered by the labor contract.

SUMMARY

Human resource management deals with the organization's most important resource—its workers. Employee performance and productivity are controlled through systematic performance evaluations. Leadership and communication skills are required in every aspect of recruiting, screening, interviewing, and hiring new employees. These skills are also required in handling personnel problems and in making valid employee evaluations based on performance merit. Productivity, leadership, and employee motivation are also required for effective human resource management.

Employees need written information concerning department work rules; this can be accomplished through an employee handbook that has been explained to the employee by the supervisor. There will be occasions when it will become necessary to give correction to an employee. When this happens the action needs to be immediate, objective, and the action taken needs to be fair for the offense. Union and nonunion health care facilities approach correction action according to polices and or union contract. The foodservice director has a role in determining fringe benefits and compensation for the foodservice personnel.

Employees who have problems are to be referred to the employee assistance program. Employees need to be recognized for a job well done. A number of suggestions are provided.

KEY TERMS

360° review

Absenteeism

Administration

Arbitrator

Benefits administration

Coaching

Collective bargaining

Compensation

Competence

Corrective action

Cost-of-living adjustment (COLA)

Dismissal

Employee assistance program (EAP)

Employee handbook

Grievance procedure

Mentoring

Peer review

Performance evaluation

Self-evaluation

Turnover

Union steward

Whistleblowing

DISCUSSION QUESTIONS

1. Employees want to know "How am I doing?" To answer this question performance appraisals and coaching are good methods to use. Choose a method and practice giving an appraisal, using the various methods noted in the text.

2. When it is appropriate to take corrective steps, what steps should be followed, and what records need to be kept?

3. How would a manager handle a grievance filed in a unionized department versus one filed in a nonunion department? Discuss the role of the shop steward.

4. How can you use the results of an exit interview to improve the operation of the foodservice operation?

5. Calculate the turnover and absenteeism rate in your department using the formulas found in the text and determine why the rate is high. Then develop a program to reduce both.

6. Define the role of the foodservice director in the compensation plan for employees.

7. Design an employee recognition program. (You choose the type.)

CHAPTER 10

MANAGEMENT INFORMATION SYSTEMS

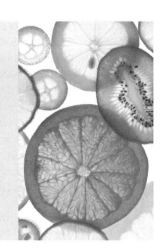

LEARNING OBJECTIVES

- Seek demonstrations of software programs from vendors who specialize in foodservice software.
- Discuss with IT personnel the need for a computerized system for foodservice.

THE COMPLEXITIES FACED by today's health care foodservice managers make it necessary to implement methods for producing precise, sophisticated information. This need has led to the development of the *management information system* (*MIS*), a network of people, procedures, and equipment used to gather and process data to provide routine information to managers and decision makers. Its techniques include selecting, storing, processing, and retrieving operational data. In so doing, the MIS supports the foodservice department's functional units, such as marketing, purchasing, production, menu planning, clinical management, and meal service forecasting, inventory control, food safety, payroll and special reports, and financial management by providing routine reports about these units. The reports are used by management to support decision making, with a focus on operational efficiency.

Learning how to use technology in the slowdown of the economy and high employment rate is necessary for the foodservice operation. The use of e-mail, voice mail, online discussions, video conferencing, virtual or computer media meetings, *Facebook* and other *links* must be closely monitored organization-wide. Organization-wide policies and procedures must be implemented to prevent the loss of productivity. The use of technology to spread information—grapevine as well as relevant information—internally as well as organization-wide can save time and resources (labor,

supplies that reduce most filing cabinets and the landfill). When used properly e-mail and other forms of electronic communication can assist in knowledge sharing, references, and record keeping. The most rapid changes in MIS are communication and collaboration among groups/departments.

A foodservice manager can facilitate the development of an MIS for analyses. The use of computers and programs specific to foodservice is discussed. The foodservice director and staff will need to be aware of the speed with which information is disseminated and the improvement of the tools used. It is your and your staff's responsibility to keep informed.

INFORMATION CONCEPTS

Information is one of a health care foodservice operation's most valuable resources. As foodservice managers we can no longer resist computer *technology*. Current environmental pressures such as cost-containment mandates, changing patient demographics, and workforce diversity require that the department's MIS produce accurate information in a timely manner. It is challenging to stay current in information technology, but it is a necessary job requirement that we become fluent in the language and the application of information technology. Developing, implementing, and operating an MIS are probably among the most time-consuming tasks faced by a foodservice manager. Although the terms *information* and *data* frequently are used interchangeably, they are not to be confused with one another in discussing an MIS.

Distinguishing Data from Information

Data consist of raw facts about the transactions that occur during the course of providing goods and services to customers. The check total for a single cafeteria customer is an example of one unit of data (or datum). If a health care foodservice manager were to sort through all single or unit transactions (that is, all data) generated by the cafeteria, he or she would be unable to carry out other managerial responsibilities. Therefore, data must be transformed into a more accessible form; that form is information. Data are held in a *database*, a computer-based set of information. *Information* is the product that results from sorting, processing, and combining data to produce a collection of facts that has value beyond the value of the individual, separate facts. Thus, a manager would find the total weekly cafeteria sales to be more valuable than individual check totals. Information technology is the use of computer technology in managing, processing, and accessing information.

Measuring the Value of Information

The value of information is directly linked to how it helps a foodservice manager achieve the operation's goals and objectives. That value typically is measured in money or time. In monetary terms, value equals either increased revenues or decreased expenses. In terms of time, the value of information might be measured by how much less time is spent on making a decision. In *Principles of Information Systems: A Managerial Approach*, R. M. Stair says that information should have certain characteristics before it can be deemed valuable to managers. In most cases, it must be accurate, complete, economical, flexible, reliable, simple, timely, and verifiable to qualify as valuable.

Characterizing an Effective MIS

Information, as indicated earlier, can only result from carefully designed systems. Although MIS design varies from operation to operation, certain characteristics are common among effective systems. In *Computer Systems for Foodservice Operations*, Kasavana lists these five features:

1. The MIS provides a means by which to achieve organizational goals and objectives.
2. The MIS treats information as an important resource and is responsible for its proper handling, flow, and distribution.
3. The MIS enables improved integration of operations, communications, and coordination.
4. The MIS interconnects people and equipment in relationships designed to free personnel to fulfill jobs requiring human capabilities.
5. The MIS stores large volumes of transactional data to support planning, decision making, and analytical activities.

INFORMATION MANAGEMENT

A variety of methods can help managers generate information from operational data. In some cases, the manager can process data mentally, for example, by estimating the appropriate menu price based on cost data. Other informal information systems, such as oral communication during training sessions, have been used with some success. Because of the volume of data generated by most health care

foodservice operations, formal systems for data processing and transformation have become commonplace. Information management is the effective production, storage, and dissemination of information in any format and on any medium.

Manual Systems

Originally, a foodservice operation's MIS relied on repetitive manual procedures whereby input was provided for each transaction by means of a source document, usually in paper format. Each transaction was then posted by hand and calculations performed either by hand or by means of a calculator. Reports were handwritten or typed up individually. At best, manual systems could generate elementary outputs on meal equivalents, customer counts and sales, labor hours and costs, food and supply costs, and personnel records.

Computer-Assisted Systems

Although manual systems are still used in some health care foodservice operations, as the complexity of operations increases, so too does the demand for an MIS that can provide more information with more accuracy and within a shorter period than can be generated by traditional manual systems. Undoubtedly, the most important advancement in collecting, maintaining, and processing data has been the development of computers. Once available data are entered (input) into the computer, the data can be stored, retrieved, and processed rapidly and accurately as many times as needed to meet the operation's information needs. More and more facilities that formerly depended on manual systems are now converting to computerized MIS.

Converting from a manual to a computerized system requires a great deal of time and expense. Therefore, the conversion process should yield concrete benefits for a facility's operations. Again, according to Stair, benefits include:

- *A higher degree of accuracy.* With manual systems, because more than one employee might be responsible for reviewing reports for accuracy, inaccurate reporting may occur due to faulty cross-checking. With computerized systems, accuracy can be checked not only by employees but by the computerized system as well.
- *Timeliness of documentation and reporting.* Manual systems can take days, weeks, or months to produce even the most routine reports. Computerized systems can significantly reduce this time. This can prove to be a valuable attribute in data processing for functions such as payroll or nutrient analysis of menus.
- *Service expansion and enhancement.* Manual systems may not afford the rapidity with which operations need to meet their customers' expectations. Computerized systems that link functions (such as customer orders and inventory) can facilitate improved customer service.
- *Labor efficiency.* Manual systems are extremely labor-intensive. Computerized systems can substantially reduce clerical labor requirements. This is the case when data are used for multiple purposes. For instance, after cost data have been entered and stored by the computer, they can be

processed into information for financial statements, variance reports, and menu pricing.

- *Data and information integrity.* Only information that is accurate, current, and relevant can be of value to the operation. Because manual systems have no determinants for information discrimination, systems with inherent check-and-error prompts are a decided advantage.

Note that *computerization* of a manual information system does not guarantee improved MIS performance. If the basis on which the manual system was built is flawed, computerization will only serve to magnify rather than diminish an operation's problems—and those of its MIS. A successful computer-assisted system can evolve only from an effective manual system.

COMPUTERS IN FOODSERVICE OPERATIONS

Every health care institution in the nation makes use of computers in some phases of its operation. Although the computers cannot do any original thinking, they are excellent tools for keeping records, doing computations, and producing reports. The most common use of computer time is to absorb a variety of boring and repetitive tasks, thereby releasing the user for the more important tasks of deciding, planning, and managing.

In foodservice operations, there are many applications for computers and computer programmers. They help to assure quality and variety in foodservice, to reduce costs of operation, to reduce the hours spent doing paperwork, and to produce required documents (such as recommended daily allowance computations, menu plans, food inventories, and purchase orders).

Many people take to using computers so naturally that it seems they have been around them all their life. Others are more hesitant and worry (incorrectly) that computers may be too complex to use or that some embarrassing or costly mistake is sure to occur. Whether one is experienced with or new to computers, virtually all users have two things in common. First, almost every foodservice operator is interested in building computer skills for application on the job. Second, everyone is pleased to discover that commercial packaged programs are available that are simple to operate and do not require technical skills to use.

In a large hospital, computer software is apt to run on a large mainframe computer at some distance from the foodservice department. Instruction must come from manuals or consultants. Usually a computer professional is on hand to instruct on how to use the equipment. It is not unusual to have one or more personal computers (PCs) in the foodservice department. Some of the producers of dietary management computer systems have designed versions of their software that will run on either mainframe computers or PCs, and some provide instructional services to users. Many foodservice software programs are available. Some programs are packaged to cover all of the operations of the foodservice operations; others are stand-alone programs for a specific task such as nutrient analysis. A foodservice manager must know what he or she wants the programs to do and the initial costs, ongoing maintenance fees, telephones, technical support, labor and supply cost, training of personnel, and the motivation of staff.

Below are some common applications for computer software that has been designed for foodservice use. Each permits managers to apply their knowledge from this course while the computer performs the extensive record keeping, computations, and report preparation that make use of this knowledge. Each form listed below contains an instruction sheet that contains *what the report does, the specifics, and notes.*

Purchasing, Inventory, and Receiving

A computer is capable of analyzing planned menus and calculating the quantity of each item needed and when it will be needed. It can take current food inventory into consideration and generate purchase orders or storeroom requisitions in the right form. An example of these forms has been supplied by CBORD: Figures 10.1 and 10.2 are examples of purchasing orders, which can be prepared using different vendors for various products. Figures 10.3 and 10.4 show inventory tally worksheets, which can be used to record physical inventory and help reduce unnecessary investment in inventory. Figures 10.5 and 10.6 show the received variance by order form, which focuses on the difference between what was ordered and what was received. A number of other companies have developed specific programs for foodservice operations.

Ingredient File

The ingredient file is a file that contains all ingredients listed on a recipe (not all systems use this file). Ingredients are identified by code name or code number. The ingredient code name or number should correlate to the purchasing and inventory file. When changes are made in a food item (such as from heavy syrup to light syrup), the change should be input into the computer. Changes in cost should also be input to assure an accurate cost of recipes, food, and the like.

Production-Related

Figure 10.7, Production Distribution Summary, and Figure 10.8, Production Distribution Summary, are forms that provide an overview of the day's production task.

Recipe Filing

All recipes that have previously been standardized can be entered into the computer. Recipes should be given a code number or name, which shift to prepare item, preparation, and cook time; cooking temperature and internal temperature and the number of serving and the total amount of food produced; the number of portions, the portion size, the ingredients, the amount of each ingredient used, the method of handling ingredients to produce the recipe (hazard analysis critical control point [HACCP] format); the cooking time, cooking temperatures, and any other relevant information specified. Recipes may also be cost by inputting recipe ingredients and other data requested by the program. Cost per portion may be calculated. See Figures 10.9, 10.10, 10.11, and 10.12 as examples.

FIGURE 10.1 Purchase Order

What This Report Does:

Provides a printed copy of a purchase order.

Use it to keep a permanent record of orders you have created, or to serve as a hardcopy checklist when verifying the items on the order prior to transmission.

The Specifics:

The report header displays the name, address, and phone number of the unit of your facility that created the order, as well the Account Number, PO Number, PO Date, Delivery Date, Vendor, and Vendor Address with the shipping address and contact name.

Following the header is a list of items included on the order.

For each item, the report shows:

- Item Name ("Description")
- Purchase Unit
- Item ID
- Ordered quantity ("Quantity")
- Unit cost ("Price")
- Extended cost ("Total")

The report also provides totals for the Quantity and Price columns.

If the order includes a Vendor Note, it appears near the end of the report.

Notes:

➢ This report is available through either Ordering Reports or Receiving Reports.
  — Create it through Ordering Reports for an order has not yet been received.
  — Create it through Receiving Reports for a received order.

➢ The report includes a signature line so the driver and receiver can sign and date the delivery and receipt of the order.

Source: Reproduced by permission of The CBORD Group, Inc. ("CBORD").

FIGURE 10.2 Main Kitchen Production Purchase Order

Main Kitchen Production Unit

Purchase Order

PO Number: 1161
PO Date: 11/29/2002
Delivery Date: 12/03/2002

Account #: 4240060

Confirmation: 1201

— Vendor —

Acme Food Wholesalers
143 Foodcentral Drive

Dryden, NY 13053
Phone:607-555-9200 Fax:607-555-9201
Attn: Ann Locksley

— Ship To —

Main Kitchen Production Unit
CBORD Foodservice
61 Brown Rd.

Ithaca, NY 14850
Attn: Receiving Manager

Vendor Phone: 800-555-2345   Vendor Fax: 607-555-9876

Description	Purchase Unit	Item ID	Quantity	Price	Total
MARG REDDI PATS 12# CASE	1 12#/CS	0000890	10	8.28	82.80
EGGS MED 15 DOZ/CS FRESH	15 CS	0003830	3	8.40	25.20
EGGS LIQUID WHL 15-2# CS	15 CS	0004290	3	20.25	60.75
CAKE CHEESE ASSORTED	4 CASE	0005325	7	40.20	281.40
DANISH SM ASSORTED FZ	96 CASE	0006685	2	20.95	41.90
SPINACH CHOPPED FROZEN	12 2.75	0016825	1	9.48	9.48
APPLESAUCE SWEETENED CAN	6 #10/CS	0017300	2	19.28	38.56
TEA DECAFFEINATED	5 100/CS	0029965	2	26.78	53.56
DRESSING ITALIAN DELUXE	4 1 GAL	0031700	2	22.07	44.14
MUSTARD	4 1 GAL	0036450	1	8.90	8.90
SOUP CREAM OF CHICKEN	12 #5/CS	0039750	4	17.60	70.40
SOUP VEGETABLE VEGETARIAN	12 #5/CS	0041000	2	17.20	34.40
MAYONNAISE PC 12 GR	200 CASE	0057300	14	6.40	89.60
SPICE PEPPER PC	3000 CS	0057550	12	6.35	76.20
ONIONS DEHD CHOPPED	1 10# BA	0063400	1	22.09	22.29
SUGAR GRANULATED	1/25 lb	0066250	4	11.00	44.00
SAUCE PICANTE MILD	1 4-1 GA	0084070	1	26.90	26.90
Totals:			71		$1,010.48

Driver _____ Receiver_____ Date _____ Time _____

Vendor Note:

Have delivery sent to main loading dock door B. Produce deliveries must arrive before 9:45 AM.

Source: Reproduced by permission of The CBORD Group, Inc. ("CBORD").

FIGURE 10.3 Inventory Tally Sheet

What This Report Does:

Provides a convenient document on which to record physical inventory counts by hand for later entry into the system using the *Inventory* module's Enter Counts option.

Create a Tally Worksheet before you take physical inventory. The worksheet lists all items to be counted, with a blank box in the Quantity column where you can manually fill in the amount on hand for each item.

The Specifics:

For each item in the worksheet, the report shows:

- Bin number
- Item Key Name
- Item name
- "Linked?" (**blank** = the item is linked to a vendor item; **N** = it is not)
- Stock Unit
- Par level
- Reorder point
- Inventory quantity (if a count has already been entered into the system)
- Order quantity
- Cost/SU (unit cost per stock unit)

Notes:

➢ The report has a separate section for each storage area. Within each storage area, items are grouped by bin location and listed alphabetically within bins.

  If an item has been assigned to two or more storage locations, it appears on the report multiple times, once for each of its storage locations.

➢ If the item has more than one stock-taking unit, there is a separate line for each stock-taking unit, so you can fill in the exact quantity you count (for example, 4 cases and 2 #10 cans).

➢ At the bottom of each page, the report provides blank lines for a signature or initials and the date and time the inventory was taken.

➢ You can immediately see which items are not linked to vendor items, because they have the letter N (for No) as the entry in the column titled "Linked." A blank in the Linked column means that the item is linked to one or more vendor items.

➢ After you print an Inventory Tally Worksheet and fill in the actual counts, return to the Inventory module. Use the Enter Counts option to call up a screen version of the worksheet and type in the counts for all items.

➢ If inventory counts already exist for a given unit and date when the report is run, the report will provide the inventory quantities rather than blank boxes. Therefore, another way to use this report is to create a tally worksheet *after* you have taken inventory and recorded the counts. In that case, the Inventory Tally Worksheet provides a printed record of the results.

Source: Reproduced by permission of The CBORD Group, Inc. ("CBORD").

FIGURE 10.4 Inventory Tally Worksheet

Main Kitchen Production Unit

Inventory Date: 9/30/2002
Description: End of month Sept 2002

Storage Area: *Produce Cooler*

Bin	Key Name	Item Name	Linked	Stock Unit	Par	Reorder	Count	Order	Cost/SU
Back Wall	Applecious	Apples Red Delicious		125/cs					17.20
	Appleeach			Apples					0.14
	Grapwhite	Grapes White		22 Lb Case					19.79
	Lemonfr	Lemon Fresh		1/7#	1				4.30
	MelonCant	Melon Cantaloupe		Melon					0.58
	MelonHone	Melon Honeydew		Melon					1.81
	OrangeNa	Oranges Fresh		113 Ct Case	1				10.53
	Citrusalad	Salad Citrus Orange Grapefruit		8 Lb tub	1				9.48
	Strawberr	Strawberries Fresh		12/1 Pt	2	1			13.10
	Melonwater	Watermelon Fresh		Melon					5.60
Left Wall	BroccoliW	Broccoli Fresh		10 Lb Case					6.94
	Cabbared	Cabbage red		Head					1.57
	CeleryWh	Celery		Head	3	1			0.48
	EggplantLg	Eggplant Fresh		Eggplant					0.63
	LettuceShr	Lettuce Shredded		5 Lb Bag					5.48
	MushrShk	Mushrooms Shiitake		5 Lb Case					8.14
	OnionYel	Onions Yellow Medium		10 Lb Bag	3				7.03
	ParsleyBn	Parsley Bunch		Bunch	4	2			0.23
	PepperGr	Pepper Bell		5 Lb Case	1				3.21
	Radishes	Radishes Cello Pack		6 Oz Bag					0.79
	SpinachLe	Spinach Fresh		2.5 Lb Pkg					1.56
	TomatoFres	Tomatoes Fresh		12 Pt/cs	1				10.20
Right Wall	CabbGreen	Cabbage Green Medium		Head					10.08
	Carrots	Carrots Bulk		25 Lb Case	2	1			0.24
	Cucmburpls	Cucumbers		5 Lb Case	1				5.68
	GarlicClov	Garlic Cloves Fresh		5 Lb Bag	1				2.11
	KaleGrns	Kale fresh	N	Head					9.84
	LettuceClea	Lettuce Cleaned & Cored		24-30/Ct	2	1			0.46

Total Inventory Value for Produce Cooler

Taken By: _____ Date: _____ Time: _____

Source: Reproduced by permission of The CBORD Group, Inc. ("CBORD").

FIGURE 10.5   Received Variance by Order Form

What This Report Does:

Focuses on one received order, highlighting any differences between what was ordered and what was received.

The Specifics:

For each item on the order, the report shows:

- item name, purchase unit, and item ID
- ordered quantity and received quantity, and the variance (difference) between them
- total cost of the ordered quantity, total cost of the received quantity, and the variance between them

The report also provides order totals: number of cases ordered, number received, total ordered cost, total received cost.

The report includes a sign-off line at the bottom.

Notes:

➤ The page heading shows the unit that submitted the order, the vendor, the PO number, the delivery date, and the order's status.

➤ An asterisk (*) following a variance value indicates that the variance is listed as zero because the item has Void as its line status.

➤ Any out-of-stock items are marked with the # symbol.

➤ If you have implemented the Partial Receiving feature, the item's line status is listed in the Item Status column. If you do not have this feature, the only Item Status entry is NONE.

➤ The report is in landscape format.

Source: Reproduced by permission of The CBORD Group, Inc. ("CBORD").

FIGURE 10.6 Received Variance by Order Report

Main Kitchen Production Unit

Vendor: Johnny's Whole Produce			PO Number: 1032			Delivery Date: 12/15/2002				Status: Received		
Vendor Item				Quantities			Item Status			Extended Prices		
Item Name	Purchase Unit	Item ID	Ordered	Received	Variance Received	Received		Ordered	Received	Variance Received
Celery Stalk, Fresh	1/24 CT	2133666	4	4	0	ALL	46.00	45.72	0.28
Parsley, Curly FDSVC Fresh	1/12 CT	1123559	1	1	0	ALL	2.63	2.76	(0.13)
Potato, Baking Fresh	1/50 #	3166789	1	1	0	ALL	11.69	12.32	(0.63)
Potato, Red #1 Fresh	50/SZ A	4131156	1	1	0	ALL	9.61	9.87	(0.26)
Tomato, Bulk Fresh	25/6x7	5399334	1	1	0	ALL	8.44	8.65	(0.21)
Order Total:			8	8				78.37	79.32	

Approved by: _____   Date: _____

# indicates an out of stock item
* **Void orders have zero variance**

Source: Reproduced by permission of The CBORD Group, Inc. ("CBORD").

FIGURE 10.7   Production Distribution Summary Form

What This Report Does:

Provides an overview of the day's production tasks. It lists what to produce for a given day and identifies where to send the produced items.

This report is especially useful for a foodservice operation that has multiple serving units.

The Specifics:

For each date and meal, the report lists the needed recipe items.

For each item, it gives the portion description, the total yield needed, and the number of portions to be distributed to each service unit. It also shows the serving pan to use or, if the recipe is itself an ingredient in another recipe, it names that recipe.

Notes:

> There is separate distribution information for each menu item portion size. Different portions of the same recipe are listed as part of the distribution.

> If you choose to use Recipe Rounding, the extra amounts are listed under "[OVERPRODUCTION]." Rounding is especially useful for items like breads, quiche, and pizza, where you round up to whole yield units.

Source: Reproduced by permission of The CBORD Group, Inc. ("CBORD").

FIGURE 10.8   Production Distribution Summary Report

Main Kitchen Production Unit

			Yield	Portions		Serving Pan/or Recipe
Monday, October 14, 2002						
Hot Food						
Beef Stew			9.00	Gallon		
Jacques Bistro Service	Dinner	02/14/2002	1.17	25	3/4 Cup	Half Pan 6"
Main Cafeteria Service	Dinner	02/14/2002	5.72	12 2	3/4 Cup	Half Pan 6"
Patio Grill Service Unit	Dinner	02/14/2002	1.83	39	3/4 Cup	Half Pan 6"
[OVERPRODUCTION]	Dinner	02/14/2002	0.28	6	3/4 Cup	Half Pan 6"
Chicken Paprika			14.00	F Pan 2"		
Jacques Bistro Service	Dinner	02/14/2002	2.10	10 3	3 oz	Full Pan 2"
Main Cafeteria Service	Dinner	02/14/2002	5.70	28 5	3 oz	Full Pan 2"
Patio Grill Service Unit	Dinner	02/14/2002	5.66	28 3	3 oz	Full Pan 2"
[OVERPRODUCTION]	Dinner	02/14/2002	0.54	27	3 oz	Full Pan 2"
Soup Cream of Broccoli			29.00	Gallon		
Jacques Bistro Service	Dinner	02/15/2002	4.69	75	Cup	Full Pan 4"
Main Cafeteria Service	Dinner	02/15/2002	13.36	28 5	3/4 Cup	Full Pan 4"
Patio Grill Service Unit	Dinner	02/15/2002	10.50	22 4	3/4 Cup	Full Pan 4"
[OVERPRODUCTION]	Dinner	02/15/2002	0.45	10	3/4 Cup	Full Pan 4"

Source: Reproduced by permission of The CBORD Group, Inc. ("CBORD").

FIGURE 10.9   Kitchen Production Recipe

Kitchen Production Recipe
and
Kitchen Production Recipe (Compressed)

What This Report Does:

Provides detailed, scaled recipes for menu items being served at meals during the report period.

Create the Production Recipe report for a given meal in advance of the meal. Distribute it to the kitchen preparation areas to use while preparing the meal.

The sample report shown here is the compact, paper-saving "compressed" version of the report. For most recipes, it is only one page long.

The regular (uncompressed) version has larger print and has blank lines between ingredients and between instructions. It provides plenty of white space for easy reading, and plenty of room for handwritten notes, comments, and highlighting.

The Specifics:

Each recipe includes complete information required to prepare the item, including:

- Yield
- Preparation and cooking time
- Cooking temperature and internal temperature
- Ingredients and ingredient quantities
- Step-by-step instructions

If the recipe yield is to be distributed to more than one serving unit at your facility, the report provides a breakdown at the bottom of the page of how the yield is to be distributed among those units.
The distribution information includes:

- Serving unit
- Day and date
- Meal
- Yield
- Actual yield box
- Portions
- Actual portions box
- Serving pan/utensil

Notes:

➤ The report scales each recipe to accommodate the customer and portion counts forecasted for the service menu in which the item appears.

➤ The recipes include accompanying instructions, which can include HACCP checkpoints.

➤ The report sorts recipes by preparation area, and each recipe appears on a separate page.

➤ If you use the recipe-rounding feature, excess production is listed as "overproduction."

Source: Reproduced by permission of The CBORD Group, Inc. ("CBORD").

FIGURE 10.10 Production Recipe for Swiss Steak

Main Kitchen Production Unit   *Production Recipe*

Steak Swiss
Hot Food   *(0127100338)*
Production Date: Tuesday, 10/1/2002   **Production Shift: Dinner**

Times	Temperatures	Production Amount
Prep Time:20 Min	Cooking Temp: 325*F	Yield: **85 SERVINGS**
Cooking Time: 1-1.5H	Internal Temp: 155*F	

Ingredients and Instructions

Swiss Steak 5 Oz	21 Pound + 4 Ounce	(0045100000)
All Purpose Flour	1 ¼ Quart	(0067300000)
Salt	1 Tablespoon	(0071500000)
Pepper	2 7/8 Teaspoon	(0071000000)
Paprika	3/8 Teaspoon	(0070900000)
Margarine, Melted	6 Ounce	(0193900000)
Onions, Sliced Thin	1 Pound + 11 Ounce	(0038100000)
Carrots, Diced ¼"	1 Pound + 11 Ounce	(0039300000)
Chopped Garlic in Oil	1 3/4 Teaspoon	(0454100000)
Celery, Diced ¼"	1 Pound + 11 Ounce	(0038700000)
Beef-meat Fat-roasted	5 Ounce	(0416000000)
All Purpose Flour	1 ¼ Cup	(0067300000)
Beef Base	3 ½ Ounce	(0008200000)
Water, Hot	3 ¼ Quart + ½ Cup	(0000000000)
Crushed Tomatoes in Puree	1 ½ Quart + 3/4 Cup	(0066500000)
Salt	2 Teaspoon	(0071500000)
Pepper	2 7/8 Teaspoon	(0071000000)
Kitchen Bouquet	3 1/3 Tablespoon	(0038200000)

```
METHOD OF PREPARATION:
1. COMBINE FLOUR, SALT, AND PEPPER.
2. DREDGE STEAKS IN SEASONED FLOUR.
3. ARRANGE ON GREASED SHEET PANS. SPRINKLE WITH PAPRIKA AND MELTED FAT. BROWN IN
400-425F OVEN.
4. TRANSFER STEAKS TO ROASTING PANS. PUT 25 STEAKS PER PAN: DO NOT CROWD.
5. BRAISE VEGETABLES IN DRIPPINGS UNTIL ONIONS ARE GOLDEN. POUR VEGETABLES OVER STEAKS
IN ROASTING PANS.
*** CCP: COOK UNTIL INTERNAL TEMP IS 145 DEGREES F. RECORD TEMPERATURE ON FOOD
PRODUCTION SHEETS.
*** CCP: MAINTAIN COOKING SURFACE AT TEMP GREATER THAN 300 F FOR 15 SECONDS.
RECORD TEMPERATURE AND TIME ON FOOD PRODUCTION SHEETS.
6. MAKE ROUX OF FAT AND FLOUR. WHIP INTO HOT STOCK AND COOK UNTIL SLIGHTLY THICKENED.
7. ADD TOMATOES & SEASONING TO SAUCE AND MIX WELL. POUR OVER STEAKS & VEGETABLES IN
PANS.
8. COVER AND BAKE AT 325F FOR 1 TO 1 ½ HOURS OR UNTIL STEAKS ARE TENDER.
*** CCP: COOK UNTIL AN INTERNAL TEMP. OF 155 DEGREES F IS MAINTAINED FOR 15 SECONDS.
  RECORD TEMPERATURE AND TIME ON FOOD PRODUCTION SHEETS.
*** CCP: HOLD/SERVE AT TEMPERATURE BETWEEN 140 AND 150 F. RECORD TEMPERATURE ON
  TASTE/TEMPERATURE LOG.
```

Distribution

	Yield	[Actual]	Portions	[Actual]	Serving Pan/Utensil
CAFETERIA					
Tuesday, October 01, 2002 Dinner	85 SERVINGS		85 1 STEAK		Full Steam Pan 2 ½" Spatula

FIGURE 10.11   Precost Summary

Preservice Cost Summary

What This Report Does:

Summarizes the expected service menu costs, sales, and profit margin of each meal in the time period you choose.

Use it in general menu planning, when comparing overall food costs for meals, and average food costs over many meals and days, if you do not need details about individual items.

The Specifics:

For each day and meal in the service menu selected, the report shows:

- Customer count forecasted
- Total predicted sales for meal, in dollars
- Total cost of meal, in dollars
- Total profit margin (= sales – costs), in dollars
- Cost, as a percentage of sales
- Sales, cost, and margin on a per-customer basis

In addition, the report provides daily totals, daily weighted averages, and meal averages (for example, the average cost per customer for breakfast over the time period selected for the report).

Notes:

➢ The per-customer figures are obtained by dividing the totals by the customer count for that meal.

Source: Reproduced by permission of The CBORD Group, Inc. ("CBORD").

FIGURE 10.12   Main Cafeteria Service Precost Summary

Main Cafeteria Service Unit

Preservice Cost Summary

Report Period: 10/20/2000 – 10/26/2000

Item Name		Cust Count	Totals			Cost (%)	Per Customer		
			Sales	Cost	Margin		Sales	Cost	Margin
ALL MEALS									
Sun	10/20/2002	880	5,856.75	1,447.47	4,409.28	25%	6.66	1.64	5.01
Mon	10/21/2002	1302	8,537.70	1,961.54	6,576.16	23%	6.56	1.51	5.05
Tue	10/22/2002	868	6,021.55	1,423.79	4,597.76	24%	6.94	1.64	5.30
Wed	10/23/2002	815	5,526.10	1,274.12	4,251.98	23%	6.78	1.56	5.22
Thu	10/24/2002	925	6,312.20	1,354.57	4,957.63	21%	6.82	1.46	5.36
Fri	10/25/2002	1000	6,652.00	1,630.09	5,021.91	25%	6.65	1.63	5.02
Sat	10/26/2002	910	6,350.25	1,509.41	4,840.84	24%	6.98	1.66	5.32
Totals		6700	45,256.55	10,600.99	34,655.56	23%	6.75	1.58	5.17
Daily Wghtd Avg:			6,607.46	1,546.06	5,061.41	23%			
Breakfast									
Sun	10/20/2002	180	1,050.75	233.20	817.55	22%	5.84	1.30	4.54
Mon	10/21/2002	400	2,335.00	454.69	1,880.31	19%	5.84	1.14	4.70
Tue	10/22/2002	188	1,097.45	245.81	851.65	22%	5.84	1.31	4.53
Wed	10/23/2002	180	1,050.75	238.80	811..95	23%	5.84	1.33	4.51
Thu	10/24/2002	190	1,115.00	202.07	912.93	18%	5.87	1.06	4.80
Fri	10/25/2002	240	1,401.00	344.12	1,056.88	25%	5.84	1.43	4.40
Sat	10/26/2002	170	997.50	209.10	788.40	21%	5.87	1.23	4.64
Totals		1548	9,047.45	1,927.79	7,119.66	21%	5.84	1.25	4.60
Daily Wghtd Avg:			1,444.61	303.34	1,141.27	21%			
Lunch									
Sun	10/20/2002	320	2,108.00	534.24	1,573.76	25%	6.59	1.67	4.92
Mon	10/21/2002	422	2,938.70	716.97	2,221.73	24%	6.96	1.70	5.26
Tue	10/22/2002	290	2,253.10	601.89	1,651.21	27%	7.77	2.08	5.69
Wed	10/23/2002	350	2,494.25	569.56	1,924.69	23%	7.13	1.63	5.50
Thu	10/24/2002	310	1,952.25	421.15	1,531.10	22%	6.30	1.36	4.94
Fri	10/25/2002	320	2,072.00	520.13	1,551.87	25%	6.48	1.63	4.85
Sat	10/26/2002	275	1,893.85	463.05	1,430.80	24%	6.89	1.68	5.20
Totals		2287	15,712.15	3,826.99	11,885.16	24%	6.87	1.67	5.20
Daily Wghtd Avg:			2,286.89	556.08	1,730.82	24%			
Dinner									
Sun	10/20/2002	380	2,698.00	680.04	2,017.96	25%	7.10	1.79	5.31
Mon	10/21/2002	480	3,264.00	789.89	2,474.11	24%	6.80	1.65	5.15
Tue	10/22/2002	390	2,671.00	576.09	2,094.91	22%	6.85	1.48	5.37
Wed	10/23/2002	285	1,981.10	465.76	1,515.34	24%	6.95	1.63	5.32
Thu	10/24/2002	425	3,244.95	731.35	2,513.60	23%	7.64	1.72	5.91
Fri	10/25/2002	440	3,179.00	765.84	2,413.16	24%	7.23	1.74	5.48
Sat	10/26/2002	465	3,458.90	837.25	2,621.65	24%	7.44	1.80	5.64
Totals		2865	20,496.95	4,846.22	15,650.73	24%	7.15	1.69	5.46
Daily Wghtd Avg:			2,996.34	709.28	2,287.06	24%			

Source: Reproduced by permission of The CBORD Group, Inc. ("CBORD").

Menu Preparation and Analysis

A computer can maintain a file of many thousands of recipes, which can be modified or added to as needed. After the style of menu has been selected, the computer can print finished menus for every meal. Some computer programs will remind the data-entry clerk if the same recipe has been used within the past few days; this helps to ensure variety in planning. The nutritional values of recipes and menus can be generated to assist the dietitian in assessing the adequacy of diets. Nutrient values can be shown in comparison with recommended daily allowances. Patients' tray cards can be printed showing special diets. Some programs include information on the effects of drugs on nutritional status, and others can produce reports on food-medication interactions. Other programs analyze individual intakes in light of client weight profiles. There are other programs that can *forecast customer counts* based on past trends and historical data. Programs are available that can determine the *popularity of menu items* and the number portions served each time the item was served. Other helpful programs include: sales analysis, the cost of menu item, profit/loss, *menu cost*, which can be determined in advance of a menu that is within budget constraints and acceptable.

Food Safety

Maintenance equipment software programs can be programmed to collect data automatically—temperature logs, for example. Using existing software programs for HACCP, the software program can be modified to meet individual organizational needs.

Human Resources—Labor

Automated timekeeping programs are available. When an employee swipes his or her identification badge through a reader, the information may be sent to the foodservice department and payroll administration. Employee schedules may be created, ensuring that adequate full-time-equivalent employees are on duty for each shift and each day. Other applications may include training records, corrective action reports, performance evaluations, and other information deemed necessary by the organization.

Forecasting

Using historical data, a computer can forecast (project) the number of menu items needed for any meal and the number of menu items that will be sold. The software program an organization chooses for forecasting should meet the needs of its facility.

Nutrient Analysis

Nutrient analysis programs are software programs that will calculate the nutrient value of each food, using data inputted from a menu and recipes. Many commercial programs are available; these vary from relatively inexpensive (hundreds of dollars) to expensive (thousands of dollars). Each foodservice department should choose the one that meets the needs of its facility.

Financial Management

Recipe costs can be calculated by a computer using correct costs from vendors. Using this information, as well as the number of current or forecasted clients, the computer can determine the cost of each menu that has been prepared as well as preference, forecast the popularity of the menu item, and the portions served. Some programs can determine in advance if a menu is within budgetary constraints as well as an acceptable margin of profit. Some software systems are capable of monitoring several thousand food items. Reports of menu costs can be printed for review by the foodservice supervisor or administrator. The computer can generate a daily food cost report and sales records (point-of-sales system), track labor costs, track budget compliance, and calculate new budgets. Sales analysis may be calculated by total sales, the quantity of each item sold, sales dollar amount by menu item, sales by each individual cashier, and an accurate profit/loss statement.

Clinical Management

Software programs have been developed that have replaced calorie counts and nutrient analyses, time-consuming tasks that dietitians at one time performed manually. An experienced data-entry employee can enter the following data and provide reports to the dietitian, dietetic technician, or dietary manager.

- Print, tally, and generate tray cards and sort them for tray line sequence
- Perform nutritive analyses of menus
- Perform nutrition screening and assessments
- Perform drug-nutrient interaction analyses
- Calculate calorie counts
- Develop a consulting schedule and follow-up appointments
- Monitor outpatient return visits
- Meet other specialized needs of the clinical staff
- Other programs that may be applicable to the institution
- Approved diet manual
- Electronic medical records

Menu Planning

Software programs are available that will plan the regular menu, modify for needed diets, complete a nutrient analysis, and determine how often an item is on a menu. When other data have been entered into the menu, each item can be priced. Menus can be printed on a computer screen, and where patients choose from a menu on the screen in their rooms, the program will tally the needed portions for each menu item. Data can be stored for catered events, special holidays, kosher foods, and so forth.

Special Reporting

Minimum data sheets are forms that must be completed for assessment and care screening of residents in skilled-nursing facilities. Foodservice software that is entirely appropriate for an individual department's use may not have all of the features listed earlier, but all are available.

Information from nutrition screening and assessment that has been performed by an interdisciplinary team can be entered and compared with standards to determine the need for additional follow-up. Analysis of drug-nutrient interactions is a dual program between the pharmacy and clinical nutrition services. The pharmacy department sends to the nutrition manager a list of specific drugs that may cause an interaction with certain foods. From this information, the nutrition clinical staff can revise menus as applicable and provide instructions to the patient.

Management Issues

Policies and procedures need to be developed concerning employees' use of computers and computer software while on duty. The foodservice manager needs to monitor how the programs are used. Game playing, excessive web search, nonbusiness e-mail, and pornography will not be allowed. The policy and procedures must be specific in the authorization of computer use. Persons authorized to use a computer should be provided with a password that will need to be changed frequently. Passwords should not be written down or passed on for others to use.

An information systems manager (ISM) should be designated with a specific job description and the authority to oversee all operations. Backup personnel need to be trained to assist the manager and train other users. The ISM should be on the alert for *viruses* or *spam* to the system and devise a system to run virus-detection software at least weekly. Viruses can wipe out programs and damage the computer's *hard drive*.

The ISM will need to back up programs and data. *Backup* provides security in the event of a hard-drive failure, natural disasters, and terrorist activity. All backup data should be stored in a secure container and off-site. Backup should be run regularly according to the organization's policies. The backup data should be tested periodically to determine if the data are viable and if the staff knows how to load and use the data. Another concern that needs to be addressed in policies and procedures is *downtime*. Downtime may be due to power failure, hardware failure, disasters or emergencies, or other problems. If the downtime lasts for an extended time, manual procedures will need to be implemented.

Software Review

Because of the critical role that software plays in a computerized MIS, its performance should be reviewed carefully. For instance, a problem would arise if the system were designed to value inventory by an average cost method and the operation specified the standard cost method. Problems identified during this process may require modification of customized or full-featured programs. Usually this is best done by the program developers. However, in the case of generic software, most problems can be resolved by users.

Hardware and Telecommunications Review

Existing equipment, hardware, and telecommunications systems must be evaluated for their efficiency and effectiveness. Input and output devices (such as bar-code readers and high-speed printers) are commercially available, and their potential benefit to foodservice operations should be assessed. Vendor demonstrations and presentations in house should be encouraged.

Database Review

Database review is critical because this component "houses" the raw facts that feed the computerized MIS. The databases of a foodservice operation should be evaluated for accuracy of data, speed of retrieval, and storage capacity. The product data provided by vendors should be checked for accuracy. Errors for characteristics such as price, size, and packaging need to be corrected before implementation and use of the database.

Personnel

Personnel review, an evaluation of the staff responsible for operating the computerized MIS, should focus on the number of staff and their skill levels. The capability of existing staff to handle a new application program should be determined before additional applications are implemented. This can be accomplished by reviewing continuing education credits and administering written and skill exercises. Ethics is a growing concern in organization where there may be a computer on every desk. Employees should **never** be allowed to seek credit information, health records, police reports, or other personal information on management or fellow employees. Employees must **never** surf the web for pornographic material, send sexual materials to other employees, or send harassing e-mail to fellow employees or supervisors. Management frequently monitors employees' use of the computer and the above violation may lead to termination. Policies and procedures must be developed to protect fellow employees and the organization. When an employee is caught violating the above procedures corrective actions need to be taken immediately.

Procedures

As with any other procedure developed by a health care foodservice operation, procedures that support the computerized MIS should undergo routine review and be revised as necessary. This ensures meeting the changing needs of the department, the health care operation, and regulatory mandates. As new equipment or software is added, procedures must be developed so that they will be operated properly. For example, when a bar-code reader is purchased for inventory control, operational procedures must be developed and implemented.

FINAL WORD

Hardware and software programs are changing so rapidly that foodservice managers must be kept informed. The manager needs to maintain a close working relationship with the IT department. It is also a good idea to frequently check with your provider concerning updates and cost. There are so many software programs on the market that you may find you need to check quarterly with companies for the latest update. Seek information and request a demonstration.

SUMMARY

The health care industry operates in an extremely dynamic business environment. As a result, the operations of all units of a health care facility—including the foodservice department—are affected. There is increased pressure for decision makers in foodservice departments to make not only more decisions but also more qualitative decisions in less time. This environmental mandate has resulted in the implementation of MISs that is designed specifically for health care foodservice operations.

In this chapter, several key concepts related to an MIS were introduced and described. The four basic elements of an MIS (input, processing, output, and feedback) were identified and discussed. Even though many traditional manual systems incorporate all four elements, they have been judged by many foodservice directors to be inadequate for their needs.

To design an effective health care foodservice MIS, a systematic approach must be taken that investigates and analyzes the current manual system. Once problems are identified in the existing system, the new system should be designed to meet the information needs of decision makers in a timelier and more efficient manner. Design considerations encompass specifying software, hardware, database, telecommunications, personnel, and procedure needs. A wide variety of computer software has been developed specifically for health care foodservice operations, among them full-featured and generic software. After the system has been implemented, the system components should be maintained regularly and reviewed routinely, with the development of specific policies and procedures on the use of the system. If these steps are followed, the foodservice department can realize the full potential of a computerized MIS.

KEY TERMS

Backup
Database
Downtime
E-mail
Facebook
Hard drive
Hardware
Link

Listserv
Mainframe
Management Information Systems (MIS)
Software
Spam
Technology
Telecommunications
Viruses

DISCUSSION QUESTIONS

1. What information is needed to operate a foodservice?
2. How can an automatic system save time and labor?

CHAPTER 11

CONTROL FUNCTION AND FINANCIAL MANAGEMENT

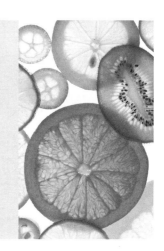

LEARNING OBJECTIVES

- Apply basic business concepts to foodservice operations.
- Define the different kinds of budgets used in foodservice operations and prepare an operational and personnel budget.
- Identify the four types of control.
- Determine productivity statistics.
- Analyze a month's cost for food, labor, and supplies and determine profit and loss.
- Tabulate the productive and nonproductive hours for a one-month period.
- Write a justification request for a major piece of equipment.

CONTROL IS THE fourth basic function of managers in organizations. *Organizational control* is defined as the regulation of the organization's activities with the purpose of helping the organization to reach its goals and fulfill its objectives. In most organizations, the use of four types of resources is controlled: physical resources, human resources, information resources, and financial resources.

The control function is closely linked to the planning function. Planning is the first management activity that takes place. Planning sets the organization's goals and objectives and develops strategies for meeting those goals and objectives. Next, organizational and leadership activities ensure that the work of the organization is actually performed. Then, control activities determine whether the organization's goals and objectives are being carried out as planned. Finally, information gathered during the control process is channeled back to planning. The organization's goals and objectives then are evaluated in relation to the organization's actual performance.

As a result, new strategies are developed to improve the organization's performance. Alternatively, the goals and objectives are revised in light of the organization's real performance.

One essential part of the planning process is the allocation (or distribution for specific purposes) of the organization's financial resources to the units or departments within the organization. (The financial resources of a health care institution include its cash on hand, its supply inventories, the value of the property and equipment it owns, its investments, and the revenue it expects to earn from its current business activities.) The financial control process involves determining how effectively and efficiently the various units and departments have used those resources. The organization's budget is the primary tool used in financial control.

The foodservice director plays a central role in the control process. The director oversees inventory control, quality control, equipment management, human resource management, production control, and financial management for the foodservice department. In this chapter, the general control process and the foodservice director's role in financial management are discussed.

The changing trends and focus within the health care industry have definite implications for health care facilities' individual departments, which are responding in various ways. At the departmental level—including the foodservice department—there is increased emphasis on cost-effectiveness, cost-efficiency, and cost containment. To control costs and adapt to changes, foodservice department managers and their staff must know where and how costs originate. They must be able to predict how costs will be affected by economic conditions and changing levels of service delivery. Executive decisions about resource allocation require skill and insight backed by appropriate *financial information*. *Financial management* is concerned with accessing information that helps managers make financial decisions whose ultimate purpose is to

FIGURE 11.1 Financial Management Systems Model for Health Care Foodservice Operations

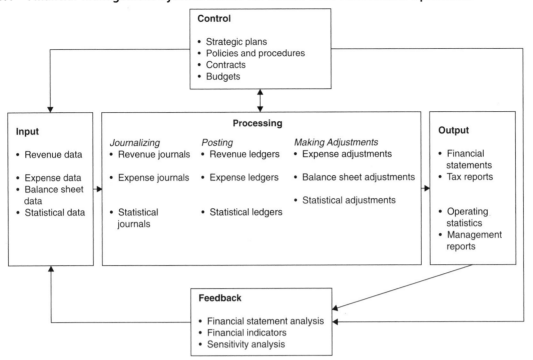

FINANCIAL MANAGEMENT SYSTEMS MODEL FOR HEALTH CARE FOODSERVICE OPERATIONS

provide high-quality nutrition and foodservices while maximizing revenues and minimizing costs.

To assist health care managers in meeting this challenge, their institutions' accounting and finance departments generate and distribute a variety of reports. Although these reports can be useful in directing departmental operations, many times they fail to provide the detail necessary to fully evaluate a department's performance. In some cases, managers may not receive reports soon enough to pinpoint areas where corrective actions are needed. For this reason, a sound system of financial control and management is essential for the operation of an efficient and effective foodservice department.

This chapter discusses control of the system, the budgeting process, and financial management as basic functions of an organization.

FINANCIAL MANAGEMENT SYSTEMS MODEL FOR HEALTH CARE FOODSERVICE OPERATIONS

The ability of an operation's financial management system to satisfy the information needs of foodservice managers and decision makers can be evaluated by analyzing the current manual system (as discussed in Chapter 10). As the basic operating device of systems analysis, the model is effective in representing the elements of an actual system. A model is always less complex than reality, but a good model has sufficient detail to approximate major characteristics of the actual system. Therefore, models that incorporate desirable elements can be useful in systems evaluation.

A financial management system is based on the system management model of a department or organization. Like all systems, the model consists of five essential elements. These same elements are

used by all systems and subsystems within a foodservice operation. They are (1) *control*, (2) *input*, (3) *processing*, (4) *output*, and (5) *feedback*. The model is illustrated in Figure 11.1, which also shows the components of each element. Note that the processing element is further divided into three standard accounting cycle steps: (1) journalizing, (2) posting, and (3) making adjustments. Each element in the model is connected by lines with arrows that depict the flow of financial information within the system.

Types of Control

Control activities are essential parts of the responsibilities of managers at all levels in an organization. *Control* is the management function that ensures that planned goals and objectives are being accomplished with the most efficient and effective use of the organization's resources. The resources concerned determine the types of control.

There are four types of control:

1. *Operational control* deals with the organization's physical resources. These resources include supply inventories, equipment, and physical facilities. Operations control oversees the actual production of goods or services within the organization. Operations control is determining whether the organization's supplies, equipment, and facilities are being used effectively and efficiently to produce a quality product or service.

2. *Human resource control* oversees the organization's use of its employees. The organization's systems for selecting and placing its employees are overseen by the human resource

department. The organization's employee training and development programs, its performance evaluation system, and its compensation and benefits program are examined as well.

3. *Information control* deals with the effectiveness of the organization's sales and marketing activities. A second area covered by information control is the organization's system for forecasting the future demand for its products and services. The organization's information control system also oversees the effectiveness of the organization's public relations program.

4. *Financial control* watches over the organization's financial health. Financial control deals with budgets, revenues, liabilities, and overall assets. (*Revenues* are the payments the organization receives for providing everyday services. *Assets* include all of the items owed to the organization by its customers [accounts receivable], the value of its inventory and supplies, and so forth. *Liabilities* are the counterparts of assets and include the current operating expenses of the organization and its long-term debt. However, financial control extends to the other three areas of control as well. For example, ineffective human resource policies would lead to high levels of employee turnover. High levels of turnover would lead to decreased productivity and higher recruiting and training expenses. For this reason, problems in human resource control also become problems in financial control. Similarly, poor performance in inventory control and production control affect the organization's financial performance. Ineffective sales and marketing decrease the organization's potential revenues, and so on.

Effective Control Systems

Because control is a central function in all organizations, the system of control used must suit the products or services the organization is producing. There are many kinds of control systems. *Cybernetic control* systems (complex electronic systems) perform the control function automatically in that controls are built into the organization's procedures. For example, in some foodservice departments, the inventory control system is set up so that new supplies are ordered when inventories decrease to a certain level. In this way, the department is assured of not running out of the supplies it needs to operate.

Control systems can also be *non-cybernetic.* That is, the control function depends on a monitoring system that is outside the operating system. For example, a foodservice department that relies on a purchasing agent or supply clerk to determine when new supplies need to be ordered has a non-cybernetic inventory control system.

In addition, control systems can be placed into categories according to the timing of the control function. *Preliminary control* determines the appropriateness of the organization's resources before they become part of the operation. The quality and quantity of raw materials are monitored before the materials enter the operating system. *Screening and control* measures the quality of products and services during the production process. Finally, post-action

control evaluates the quality of completed products and services. Most organizations use more than one of these control systems to ensure the quality of their products or services and to monitor the effectiveness of their internal systems.

No matter what type of control system the organization uses, to be effective, control systems should have the following characteristics:

- Most important, control systems should be extensions of the planning process. The organization's actual performance needs to be compared with its planned performance. Goals and objectives are reevaluated to assess where any discrepancies lie. If the original plans are deemed inappropriate, corrective action should be taken to bring about desired results. The planning process may need to be adjusted in consideration of the organization's actual performance as identified in the control process.
- Control systems should be flexible enough to deal with changes in the business environment inside and outside the organization.
- Control systems should provide accurate and up-to-date information.
- Control systems should be objective. They should be based on fair observations of actual data, activities, and conditions and not on the opinions of individuals.

Control Process

To varying degrees, almost all managers take part in the process of control. Managers help establish standards. They measure performance and compare performance with established standards. They take action as necessary to improve the organization's performance or to change the standards. Except for small organizations, most organizations—including most health care institutions—also have managers who specialize in performing the control function. These managers are called *controller* or, in some organizations, *comptrollers.* The role of the controller is to help line managers, such as the foodservice director, handle the control process. The organization's controller is also responsible for organizing the overall control system and for gathering and distributing the information related to the process.

However, the foodservice director in most institutions is directly responsible for conducting control activities in the department. The control process can be broken down into four basic steps:

1. Setting standards
2. Measuring performance
3. Comparing performance with standards
4. Taking corrective action

Step 1: Setting Standards

Standards are the predetermined targets against which future performance will be measured. To be effective, standards must be based—at least in part—on the formal goals of the organization. Standards should also be similar to the organization's objectives in that the objectives and standards for performance need to be stated in measurable terms. For example, in a health care institution, one organizational goal could be to become more competitive in offering services to patients and to aggressively market these services. The foodservice department would then have as one of its objectives providing room service, gourmet meal service, and on-demand meal service. Therefore, the standard would be to offer on-demand meal service, room service, and gourmet meal service within the next six months and without complaints from administrators, physicians, staff, or patients. The interdisciplinary team and the marketing department provide assistance and marketing for the new meal service.

Standards may be classified as tangible and intangible. *Tangible standards* measure the quality and quantity of the organization's output, the cost of producing the output, and the time it takes to produce the output. For example, in the foodservice department, standards can be set for such things as the number of trays assembled per minute, the number of meals prepared and served per labor hour, and the total meal cost per patient. *Intangible standards* are much more difficult to develop. Intangible standards attempt to measure such things as the reputation of the facility with the public, customer satisfaction, and the level of employee morale in the foodservice department.

Standards for the organization and for units and departments within the organization are based on several factors. Standards should be based on the overall goals of the organization, which are identified and developed during the strategic planning process.

However, specific details in the standards—the details that can be objectively measured—involve quantity, quality, and time factors. These factors can be grouped under the term *productivity*. *Productivity standards* are often based on the past performance of the unit or department. More formal productivity standards are sometimes developed for the organization by **industrial engineers**. An *industrial engineer* is an individual who specializes in designing and improving systems for managing an organization's human, material, equipment, and energy resources. (A more detailed discussion of the role of the industrial engineer in setting standards for health care institutions is beyond the scope of this manual on foodservice management.)

In health care institutions, the standards set and followed by individual departments are also directly affected by government regulations such as CMS and OBRA. In addition, most hospitals and many other health care institutions in the United States voluntarily follow the standards published by The Joint Commission.

Step 2: Measuring Performance

To determine whether the standards set in Step 1 are being met, performance must be measured. Step 2 in the control process—measuring performance—is an ongoing process. It depends on observations, verbal and written reports, and quality control tests.

In the foodservice department, observing the various activities that go on simultaneously can be time-consuming. However, identifying strategic control points can make systematic observation a more efficient control system. *Strategic control points* are places in the production and service system that are key indicators of the quality and quantity of work being performed. Strategic control points can be established anywhere from the start of an activity to its completion. One of the main advantages of this type of control system is that corrective action can be taken immediately once a problem has been observed. For example, in the delivery of patient food trays, a strategic control point is the foodservice's implementation of the department's guest relations program. If a nutrition aide is not following program procedures, program corrective action should be taken at once.

Verbal and written reports on the status of work are essential parts of the control system for foodservice departments in large health care institutions. Because employees work in two or three shifts and because they may actually work in different physical locations, the foodservice director cannot rely on personal observations alone. However, the director needs to make sure that the reports he or she receives are clear, concise, accurate, and complete. Such reports would include information on quality control activities and the quality assurance program, nutrition-related problems and solutions, cafeteria and catering service problems and complaints, and safety and sanitation inspections.

Quality control tests can be made at any time, at any location, and for any reason. Spot checks for quality and accuracy in the food production system are a must. The elements of quality in foodservice include the food's sensory characteristics, its nutritional value, and its microbiological safety.

Step 3: Comparing Performance with Standards

Once the performance has been objectively measured, the third step in the control process is to compare the performance with the standards already established in Step 1. There may be many reasons why the performance does not meet the standards. The foodservice director must determine why the standards were not met. Then he or she must decide what, if anything, needs to be done to correct the inconsistency between standards and actual performance. The director would investigate the reasons behind the substandard performance by discussing the situation with foodservice employees. For example, there might be a standard that a registered dietitian should perform 100 nutrition assessments on patients with renal disease, write 100 sets of chart notes, and review the potential for food and drug interactions for all the patients seen during the current month. The registered dietitian assigned to the dialysis unit might have been able to do assessments on only 75 patients and chart notes on 65 patients. The director should ask why the standard was not met and whether the standard was unrealistically high. In such a case, the director might discover that the problem was in neither the standard nor the dietitian's performance. For example, the unit might have been closed for some time during the month because a dialysis machine failed, and the unit's patients were sent to another facility for treatment.

Step 4: Taking Corrective Action

The final step in the control process is taking corrective action when actual performance does not coincide with preestablished standards. Action should be considered only after all of the relevant information has been analyzed. The following actions, or decision not to act, would be appropriate:

- In some cases, the actual performance may be only slightly higher or lower than the standard requires. In such cases, no action would be needed. However, the director must use valid information to determine which differences between performance and standard are significant and which are not and if any action needs to be taken.
- In some cases, it may be found that the standards were unrealistically high or low. In such cases, the appropriate action would be to change the standards to reflect the realistic work situation.
- In other cases, the problem may be in individual work performance. The director should determine whether employees need retraining or counseling. Some employees may need to be counseled for negligence or for safety and sanitation violations.
- In some cases, the shortcoming in work performance may be the result of equipment problems. In such cases, the equipment should be repaired or maintenance procedures should be improved.
- In some cases, inadequate performance may be the result of poor supervision, inefficient procedures, or inadequate staffing. In such cases, the director should take immediate action to correct these management-related problems.

FINANCIAL CONTROL AND MANAGEMENT

Financial responsibility and accountability are a significant part of the function of managers in most organizations. This is particularly true of managers in health care institutions. Health care managers are faced with the challenge of providing high-quality care and at the same time controlling rising costs. For this reason, a sound system of financial control and management is essential for the operation of an efficient and effective foodservice department.

Effective financial management depends on written statements of the organization's goals and of the department's objectives, along with detailed written procedures for reaching those goals and objectives. Furthermore, a system of records and reports is needed for the timely documentation, evaluation, and control of the department's activities and expenses. Although many acceptable systems exist for keeping records, record-keeping procedures should be standardized enough to permit the comparison of the department's actual expenses with the expenses allowable under the operating budget. In addition, standardized record-keeping procedures are valuable for comparing the foodservice department's financial data with those of other departments within and outside the institution. Especially during difficult economic times, the challenge of containing costs while providing needed services requires that all health care managers place a high priority on their function as financial managers and controllers.

Budgets as Tools for Financial Control and Management (This Is Important)

Financial control and management rely on the development and use of one or more plans that estimate the organization's proposed expenses for a given financial period and its proposed means for meeting those expenses. These plans, called *budgets*, are almost always based on dollar values. *Nonmonetary budgets* are expressed in nonfinancial terms, for example, labor hours or units of output. Budgets provide managers with useful tools for allocating resources, setting standards, evaluating performance, and controlling costs. Budgets are the foundation of most control systems (Figure 11.2).

There are no uniformly defined budgetary terms. Some organizations use *master budgets* to include the operating budget, a capital budget, a cash budget, and a budgeted balance sheet. *Cash budgets* deal with cash on hand, accounts receivable, accounts payable, the cost of credit, and cash flow. The *budgeted balance sheet* is a statement of the assets and liabilities of an organization based on budget elements. For this book, two types of budgets are used, the financial budget and the operating budget.

In general, the *financial budget* shows where the organization intends to get its cash for the specified fiscal (or financial) period and how it plans to spend that cash. The financial budget includes the cash-flow budget, the capital budget, and the balance sheet. The *cash-flow budget* represents management's best estimate of cash income and cash expenditures (or outlays) over a specified period. The purpose of the cash-flow budget is to ensure that the organization will have enough cash to meet its financial obligations at the time the obligations come due. The *capital budget* is a plan for making and financing major improvements in or purchases of physical facilities, equipment, or property during the period covered by the budget. The *balance sheet* is a type of control budget that illustrates the organization's financial condition on a particular date. It shows what the organization's *assets* (things of value owned by the organization) are and how they are balanced against its *liabilities* (debts of the organization). All of these financial budgets are used by top-level managers in health care institutions. However, the operating budget is the most important budget in the financial control and management of the foodservice department.

The *operating budget* describes in financial terms the organization or department's plan for operations during a specified period of time—usually a *fiscal year*, or a period of 12 months used for accounting purposes that does not necessarily coincide with the calendar year. It can begin on any date and end on any date but must include 365 days, except for leap year, which is 366 days. Most organizations and state and governmental agencies use fiscal year as the period for a budget year. A *calendar year* is for the 12-month period that begins on January 1 and ends December 31. An *accounting period* is the time period designated by an organization for the purpose of financial reporting; this is usually monthly but in some instances may be quarterly or semiannual. The operating budget includes the revenue budget, the expense budget, and specific project budgets. The *revenue budget* shows all of the income from normal operations that can be expected for the upcoming fiscal year. Similarly, the *expense budget* shows all of the anticipated expenses for the fiscal year. Expense budgets deal with all anticipated costs. This may be a single budget or broken down into sub-budgets such as labor, materials, overhead, and other operating expenses. Often, the revenue and expense budgets are combined on one form. Budgets for special projects (such as extending catering services to the community) are also included in the department's operating budget.

FIGURE 11.2 Development of a Budget for Financial Management

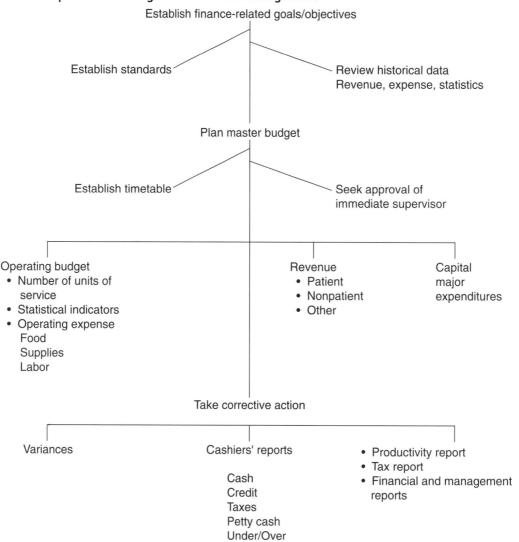

Source: Developed by Ruby P. Puckett©.

The operating budget is more than an operating plan for the upcoming year. It is also a control device for comparing actual operational performance with performance forecasts. When a *variance* (or a significant difference) occurs between the forecasts in the operating budget and the data on actual performance, the manager must follow the steps in the control process (determining the problem, identifying its cause, and taking appropriate corrective action) to correct the inconsistency. This usually means determining the variance by documentation and comparison on a monthly basis.

Preparation of the Operating Budget

The operating budget for the foodservice department is only part of the health care institution's overall operating budget. Other department-level managers in the institution submit operating budgets for their departments, and top-level managers prepare a final operating budget for the whole institution. Often, a financial controller for the institution coordinates the budget preparation

process among department heads and top-level managers to make sure that the final budget reflects the institution's established goals.

In general terms, budget preparation and approval in most organizations—including most health care institutions—follow these nine steps:

1. The heads of the various departments or operating units prepare estimates of revenues and expenses for the upcoming fiscal year and develop budget proposals based on those estimates.
2. The heads of the departments or operating units submit their budget proposals to their immediate superiors for approval. The superior may or may not require the department head to make revisions in the proposed budget.
3. The superior, who is often the head of a division within the organization, combines the various budget proposals from the department heads who report to him or her. For example, in some large hospitals, the foodservice director

receives proposed budgets from the medical nutrition therapy (MNT) manager for nutrition care services and the assistant director for food production. Then, the director combines the proposals to prepare an overall budget for food and nutrition services.

4. The division's proposed budget is submitted to a top-level manager such as the CEO or the chief financial officer (CFO). In some organizations, the proposals are submitted to a budget committee that is made up of top-level managers, including the CEO and the CFO.

5. The top-level manager or the budget committee reviews the budget proposals from every department in the organization, corrects any inconsistencies, and deletes any repeated information.

6. The organization's controller or CFO evaluates the combined proposed budget and prepares the final budget for the organization.

7. The CEO examines the final operating budget. He or she may approve the budget or request further revisions.

8. The organization's board of directors reviews and approves the final operating budget.

9. The final budget is communicated to the various managers of the departments and operating units within the organization.

The annual operating budget for the foodservice department works as a financial plan for the allocation of the department's resources, including labor, food, supplies, and equipment. The budget also serves as an organizational plan for meeting the department's objectives. In addition, the budget represents a forecast of the department's activities for the upcoming year, for example, the number of meals to be served, the number of nutrition assessments to be performed, and the number of patient visits to be made. In preparation for these anticipated activities, the foodservice director draws up employee work schedules, purchases food and supplies, and makes arrangements for the preparation of foods to meet the forecast demand for specific menu items.

The degree of the department-level manager's responsibility and authority in budget preparation varies among the various sizes and types of health care institutions. However, almost all foodservice directors are responsible for preparing proposed operating budgets for the foodservice department.

The 10 basic steps in the preparation of the foodservice department's operating budget are:

1. Setting a timetable for the budget preparation process
2. Examining the department's objectives for the upcoming fiscal year
3. Analyzing the financial feasibility of the department's objectives
4. Asking for information from responsible members of the foodservice staff on factors that may affect the upcoming budget, for example, current food and supply costs
5. Reviewing historical data on units of service (meals served, nutrition assessments made, and so forth) and costs from previous years

6. Estimating the number of units of service for the upcoming fiscal year using past data and the implementation of any new programs
7. Estimating operating expenses for the upcoming fiscal year plus a review of past service plus any proposed new programs
8. Determining statistical indicators for the upcoming fiscal year including any new programs
9. Calculating productivity indicators for the upcoming fiscal year including any new programs
10. Preparing a proposed operating budget that shows all of the financial information required for the upcoming year's financial planning and control

Step 1: Setting a Timetable for Budget Preparation

Because financial planning requires a considerable investment of time and resources, the foodservice director's first step in preparing the department's budget proposal should be to set up a timetable for budget-planning activities that corresponds to the institution's overall timetable as determined by the CFO. Adequate time is allowed for considering and formulating operational decisions that will affect the financial health of the foodservice department and the institution as a whole. This is very important if new programs are being added. A budget developed under the pressure of time may not be accurate enough or insightful enough to adequately guide operational decisions for the upcoming year.

Step 2: Examining the Department Objectives

The second step in preparing the foodservice budget should be examining and finalizing the department's objectives for the upcoming fiscal year. Before the operating budget can be planned, prepared, and submitted for approval, clear and specific objectives covering the extent and quality of service to be provided to patients or residents and other customers must have been established. The setting of goals and objectives is an important part of the planning process that must be performed before control activities such as budget preparation start.

The department's objectives must be compatible with and contribute to the accomplishment of the goals of the institution and the objectives of the other departments within the institution. For example, if the institution's goals were to expand outpatient services and to extend services to the community in other ways, then the foodservice department would need to plan for providing meals to outpatients and for developing educational programs on general nutrition and modified diets.

Step 3: Analyzing the Financial Feasibility of the Objectives

The director's third step should be to analyze the financial feasibility of conducting the specific programs and offering the specific services identified in the department's objectives. The foodservice director must analyze the objectives in consideration of the financial limitations of the department and the institution. The resources needed to provide such services and the costs associated with each kind of service eventually must be allocated to appropriate areas in the operating budget. If the potential revenues that may be gained from the planned services are lower than the anticipated costs of supplying the services, the director will need to reexamine the department's objectives or identify additional sources of financial support (with the help of the administration) for the services before an operating budget for the department can be proposed. This situation applies to services such as the employee cafeteria where administration has given a directive for employee meal discounts and outpatient educational programs to long-term care facilities.

Step 4: Asking for Information from the Foodservice Staff

As the fourth step in the budget preparation process, the director should ask for specific information on foodservice operations from responsible foodservice staff members. Although this step may be unnecessary in small health care institutions, in large health care institutions, managers other than the foodservice director may have the primary responsibility for the MNT care services and food production activities in the department. Responsible staff members could be called on to provide information on labor costs, food costs, supply costs, equipment costs, and other related costs. Staff members also may be able to provide valuable information on potential increases or decreases in the number of units of service forecast for various units within the department (for example, the employee cafeteria).

Step 5: Reviewing Historical Data

In the fifth step of the budget preparation process, the director performs the vital function of reviewing data on the past information of the foodservice department. Most operating budgets are based on the preceding fiscal year's operating budget and a predetermined increment.

This increment may depend on a number of factors such as inflation rate, labor contracts, profitability, operating losses, restructuring, and downsizing changes in operational procedures. Changes in the business environment and the country's economic environment, the preceding year's performance, and proposed changes in service are incorporated into the former budget to arrive at a new proposed budget. To arrive at accurate forecasts of future activities and projected costs, the historical data used in budget preparation must be reliable.

The second budgeting approach, which disregards the previous year's budget completely, is referred to as *zero-based budgeting* also called *project-based budgeting*. Zero-based budgeting does not rely on the previous year's budget as a starting point. It requires the foodservice director to write budgets from scratch and to justify every dollar of proposed spending. Zero-based budgeting is not well suited to all organizations. They are difficult to prepare and consume a great deal of the foodservice director's time and energy. There are some benefits, but they may not justify the additional cost.

There are two exceptions to the practice of basing upcoming budgets solely on the *preceding year's budget* also known as the *traditional budget*. These two approaches are fixed and variable budgets that are a variation of zero-based and incremental budgets.

Fixed budgets are plans for which funds are allocated for the entire fiscal year. They are also known as *static budgets*. Fixed budgets provide managers with goals for financial performance that can be measured each accounting period. Fixed budgets do not have enough flexibility to respond to changes in the volume of service or work that must be completed. If unforeseen changes occur, such as a disaster, then the budget will not be accurate and the foodservice director will be out of compliance or in a variance state.

Variable budgets or flexible budgets are plans in which expenses vary in response to actual production, volume, or revenue. The flexible budget is usually prepared for levels of service both higher and lower than the original estimate. The levels commonly reflected in flexible budgets are 90, 100, and 110 percent of the estimated level of service. Although this budgeting approach requires more preparation and maintenance time, it enables the foodservice manager to adjust expenditures in relation to actual levels of service.

Step 6: Estimating Units of Service

After the preliminary gathering and analysis of background information has been completed, the foodservice director should be ready to start the process of making actual estimates of the units of service the department will be expected to provide during the upcoming year. The number of patient days (for inpatients) expected by the institution determines the number of patient meals the department will need to serve. In an institution that provides outpatient services, the number of clinic visits determines the level of activity in the outpatient nutrition program. Obviously, this information on the expected volume of service (available from the finance department) directly affects the department's expense estimates.

Step 7: Estimating Operating Expense

The seventh step in budgeting preparation involves estimating expenses for the upcoming fiscal year. In most foodservice operations, the department that has an expense budget is considered a *cost center*. Foodservice and other departments that generate revenue are also referred to as a *revenue center*. Departments such as pharmacy may have a profit center, where income exceeds operating cost. Foodservice departments must project income based on sales of products or services rendered, such as outpatient counseling. This is called a **revenue** budget.

To arrive at accurate forecasts of future activities and projected costs, the historical data used in budget preparation must be reliable. The financial record-keeping and reporting system of the institution and the department may be simple or complex, depending on the amount of specific information required. However, the department's records and reports must be as accurate as possible. In addition, they must be based on standardized accounting procedures so that the data from the foodservice department's records can be compared with data from other sources and so that data from previous years can be compared with current and future data on performance.

EXHIBIT 11.1   Cashier's Report

Cashier: _____   Date: _____

1.	Ending		_____
2.	Beginning reading		_____
3.	Total sales plus tax		_____
4.	Less charge sales		_____
5.	Subtotal		_____
6.	Less over rings		_____
7.	Total cash sales		_____
8.	Actual cash turned in		_____
9.	Cash (+) over; (−) under		_____
10.	Receipt number		_____
11.	Cash turned in		_____
	Currency	$1	_____
		$5	_____
		$10	_____
		$20	_____
	Coin		_____
	Other		_____
	Subtotal		_____
	Less cash back		_____
	Total		_____
	Verified by		_____
	Business office cashier		_____

Revenue Budgets   Revenue sources for the foodservice department include patient meal services and nonpatient services. In most health care institutions, the revenue from patient meal service is handled as a noncash transfer of funds to the foodservice department from the institution's operating revenues. The transfer of funds takes place in the accounting department. Revenues from nonpatient sources include cafeteria sales, charges for catering special events and community functions held in the institution, sales from vending machine operations, and revenues from clinical nutrition services to inpatients and outpatients. Nonpatient revenues usually come in the form of cash receipts.

Careful control procedures must be followed for handling cash in the foodservice department. They must ensure honesty and accountability for all personnel who handle cash.

Basic principles of control for handling cash include:

• Sales reports from all revenue centers, both patient and nonpatient, must be kept daily and reported monthly. (Monies are turned into the head cashier on a daily basis). If there is a discrepancy in the report and the funds this must be handled at once. This may mean an audit that could lead to corrective action such as termination or a criminal arrest.

• All cash must be collected frequently from cash registers and from cashiers. These revenues are documented by a cashier's report, which is produced manually or by using a computerized *point-of-sales (POS)* cash register system. The POS is a useful report as it records all transactions and maintains very detailed records of sales. Information may be reported by location, date, meal period, item purchased and what other information that has been programmed into the POS, such as cashier. The cashier's report should include, at least, the number of customers served, total sales, and appropriate sales taxes. Exhibit 11.1 is a report that the cashier and a supervisor would fill out to verify the cash that was returned to the department. It shows the various ways money was acquired and if there were overages or underages in the amount turned in. If a cashier has a constant report of overages or underages, action must be taken that may include retraining, cameras on the cashier, and correction action that may include a police investigation. The cash receipts should be deposited in a safe by a superior designated to have this responsibility.

• The cash receipts should daily be deposited in a bank or picked up by an armored transport system, such as Wells Fargo. (Some smaller institutions have the funds turned in to the business office where a daily record is kept.)

- Cash receipts, as recorded on the cash register, should be matched with the cash on hand at frequent, specified intervals by a person other than the cashier. (It is a good practice to make unannounced audits and not to allow the cashier to see the beginning and ending register readings.)

- An electronic register that provides sales data on specific items or groups of items should be used whenever possible. The greater capacities of electronic registers for providing information for analysis and control make them especially useful for large foodservice operations.

- Catering income should be controlled through appropriate documentation of orders and charges, along with proper handling of receipts. (See also the discussion of catering in Chapter 3.)

Petty cash is a small amount of money that is kept on hand for emergency purchases. Petty cash funds should contain enough money for a month's worth of transactions. A running account should be made of all expenditures, and an invoice should be attached to the ledger. At the end of the month, all invoices should be totaled and the amount subtracted from the petty cash on hand at the beginning of the month. A requisition to the finance office, along with all receipts, should be made to bring the fund up to the established level. Some organizations use a credit card for monthly emergency purchases. Petty cash funds and purchases must be carefully monitored. Item cost must match the product (for example, 4 dozen eggs at $1.00 a dozen—petty cash that is spent must be $4.00).

Some organizations require persons who handle cash to be bonded and fingerprinted. A *bonded employee* signs a binding agreement to pay a certain amount of money (usually a percentage of the loss) on failure to perform or complete a job properly. When an employee is bonded, it ensures the organization against financial loss by an employee.

Security of Cash The cash collected by the retail operation and patient revenue must be secured at all times.

- The money should be placed in a safe until it is transported by an armored transport system or to the finance office. Use security guards to walk with cashier to finance office.

- Combinations to the safe **must** be well guarded, and only those who need to know are provided the combination. The combination will need to be changed at least quarterly and/or when an employee who had access to the combination leaves the employment.

- Use locking drawers. Keep the drawers **closed** when not performing a sales transaction.

- Give each cashier his or her own "bank" at the beginning of the shift.

- Minimize the amount of money in a drawer—have the head cashier or supervisor remove cash from the drawer throughout the meal period.

In some institutions, vending machines are used to provide food and beverage service on a 24-hour basis. Often, the machines are owned and operated by outside contractors. However, vending operations can be profitable and should be considered as an additional source of revenue by the foodservice director. When vending machines are owned by the facility the funds must be removed at least one time per day but more often depending on the traffic and locations. Vending will need to be reported separately on a sales report, regardless of who owns and operates them. Cash from machines should be protected, as described above.

Revenue from all sources must be accounted for by using reporting techniques approved by the institution's financial officer. Revenue and expense data should be prepared so that unit-of-service costs and profit-and-loss figures can be analyzed. This helps determine whether patient revenues are subsidizing nonpatient meals. Medicare reimbursement policies require that revenues from patient services be kept separate from those from nonpatient services. Also, the policies require that patient services do not subsidize nonpatient services.

Profit and Loss The foodservice director and the organization's CFO often work together to develop monthly *profit-and-loss statements*. The reports' degree of sophistication depends on whether the institution is a for-profit or not-for-profit organization and the financial policies of the organization. A simple format for a monthly profit-and-loss statement is shown in Exhibit 11.2. Formal revenue statements and budgets for the facility are prepared by the institution's finance department.

EXHIBIT 11.2   Format for Monthly Profit-and-Loss Statement

Food revenues	$ _____
Cost of food	
Purchases	$ _____
Less: inventory	_____
Net food costs	$ _____
Cost of labor	
Salaries/wages	$ _____
Benefits	
Total labor costs	$ _____
Operating costs	
Office rent	$ _____
Laundry	_____
Maintenance	_____
Telephone	_____
Postage	_____
Utilities	_____
Depreciation	_____
Equipment	_____
Total operating costs	$ _____
Total Expenses	$ _____
Operating Profit (Loss)	$ _____
(Revenues minus total expenses)	

A profit-and-loss statement is a report developed by the finance and accounting departments that lists revenue and expense and the difference between the two. A *profit* is when there is money available after all expenses have been paid from the total revenues. The profit-and-loss statement will vary on a monthly basis because of the fluctuation in cost of purchases, inventory on hand, increase in operating expense, and depreciation. Another source of revenue that may be added to a profit-and-loss statement is *subsidy*. Subsidy is funds received from external sources such as the "free breakfast" program in schools and special meals for interns/residents paid to the department by the medical staff/college. Another control measure is to determine the *breakeven point*. This point is where income and cost are equal and the operation is not making or losing money.

Depreciation is an accounting procedure that spreads the cost of capital equipment or building over the life span of the item. It is calculated by dividing the purchase price of an item by its expected lifetime. Foodservice departments also have assets and liabilities. *Assets* are items of value owned by the department such as inventories and equipment. *Liabilities* are debts that are an obligation of the department such as invoices owed for food and supplies, payroll, and interest payments. There are *fixed assets* such as land, buildings, equipment, and improvements. Fixed assets are capitalized and depreciated over time. *Liquid assets* are items on hand that can be easily converted to cash, such as food and supply inventory. Two other accounting terms that affect the profit-and-loss statement include accounts receivable and accounts payable. *Accounts receivable* is the record of money owed to a business for products that have been received and for which an invoice has been sent. *Accounts payable* is the record of money owed by the organization (foodservice) to a creditor for the purchase of food and supplies, rent, and any other outstanding loan.

Labor Cost Budget   Payroll records are a convenient source of data on labor costs. The hours worked and the costs associated with the work are usually documented by a time-card system. Smaller operations may still use manual systems, in which case the department is involved in collecting labor cost data. However, this is one of the most commonly computerized functions in health care operations. With these types of systems, the foodservice manager may merely need to review the data that will be used by the payroll system to determine labor costs. In addition to the costs of wages and salaries, the cost of providing benefits, both optional and required by law, must also be determined.

A *labor budget* includes all personnel, full- or part-time, and contract employees (if used) who are needed to get the work accomplished; it does not include benefits. (Some organizations include fringe benefit to reflect a more realistic account of labor cost. All merit raises, bonuses, or cost-of-living adjustments [COLA] are also calculated and become a part of the labor budget.) Labor budgets as well as expenses, material, and other operating costs may be allocated to various cost centers such as MNT, administration, catering, production, and retail operations. Labor cost may also be broken down to direct and indirect labor costs. *Direct labor costs* are the costs of labor plus overtime or other pay in lieu of benefits, such as pay to a consultant. *Indirect labor costs* include benefits such as insurance, taxes, and paid time off.

Materials Budget Foodservice also has a materials budget. Materials include raw materials to be used in the production and service of food and meals. Other materials may include office supplies, books, chemicals, computer paper, continuing education, and replaceable small equipment such as knives, china, glasses, and printing costs.

Requisitioning, maintaining inventory, and controlling stock for such supplies are the same as those for food supplies. The costs involved and the quantities used are also determined by calculating beginning inventory, monthly purchases, and closing inventory. Records may also be kept and information reported by type of commodity, such as paper supplies and cleaning supplies.

When possible, all supply costs should be allocated directly to either patient or nonpatient services. The ratio used to determine patient and nonpatient costs for food and labor can be used for supply costs as well. For example, if 51 percent of the meals prepared by the department are served to nonpatients, 51 percent of the supply cost should be allocated to the cost center for nonpatient services.

Food Cost Budget Purchasing, food issues, and transfer records are used to document food costs. Purchasing transactions are documented by means of invoices that accompany deliveries or by bills issued by vendors. The actual food issued to the production units of the foodservice department can be documented by requisition forms prepared by production employees or produced by computerized systems. Other aspects of food costs that should not be overlooked are the cost of food transferred to patient floors and other units of the organization. A count of all food items transferred should be recorded on a form similar to the one illustrated in Exhibit 11.3. Food costs for all areas and events need to be documented and available for auditing.

Overhead Budget Most foodservice operations incur costs for products and services that do not fall in the categories of costs discussed previously. Examples include repairs and maintenance, laundry services, pest control, telephone, postage, breakage, and utilities cost. These costs can be allocated directly back to the foodservice department based on the existence of a variety of source documents. Theft of food and supplies is a separate entity under overhead cost.

Allocated Cost Budget The final cost category is those costs generated by the health care operation or foodservice department but for which no source document exists. For instance, the foodservice department is usually one of the largest consumers of energy. However, unless the department has separate utility meters, the cost data for energy are not available and cannot be collected. These costs may be divided by department and then allocated to that department.

EXHIBIT 11.3 Food Transfers

ABC Foodservice Department
Nourishment Cost Report   1NW Acct: 1626
For the Month of: July   Patient Days: 825

Item Description	Item Cost	1	2	3	4	5	6	7	…	25	26	27	28	29	30	31	Total Count	Total Cost
APPLE JUICE	$0.14	14	15	15	10	10	10	10		14	14	10	10	10	10	8	359	$50.26
CRANBERRY JUICE	$0.34	10						10	0	10					6		81	$27.54
GRAPEFRUIT JUICE	$0.14	14	4	4	10	10		10	15	14	10	10	10	10		10	251	$35.14
PINEAPPLE JUICE	$0.29																0	$0.00
PRUNE JUICE	$0.34						6			10					10		36	$12.24
TOMATO JUICE	$0.21																0	$0.00
NECTARS	$0.33																0	$0.00
ORANGE JUICE	$0.14								5								5	$0.70
ORANGE JUICE (QT)	$1.10	3	4	2		3	2		3	3	3	3	3	2	2		67	$73.70
GATORADE	$1.13																0	$0.00
COKE	$0.35	6			6						12						62	$21.70
DIET COKE	$0.35																0	$0.00
TAB	$0.35																0	$0.00
SEVEN UP	$0.35		3						2				6		2	4	32	$11.20
DIET SEVEN UP	$0.33																0	$0.00
DR. PEPPER	$0.33								6								6	$2.10
DIET DR. PEPPER	$0.35																0	$0.00
GINGERALE	$0.35																0	$0.00
SKIM MILK	$0.15																0	$0.00
WHOLE MILK	$0.15	10			10		8	4	8	10		10	10	6	6	3	146	$21.90
CHOCOLATE MILK	$0.15																3	$0.45
BUTTERMILK	$0.15																0	$0.00
ICE CREAM	$0.12			6			4							6			23	$2.76

TOTAL NOURISHMENT COST	$259.69
NOURISHMENT COST/PD	$0.31
BUDGET	$0.26
VARIANCE	$0.05

Step 8: Determining Statistical Indicators

In Step 8, the foodservice director calculates various statistical indicators and the unit costs per meal. Salary and benefit expenses per meal, food expenses per meal, supply expenses per meal, and other expenses per meal are determined. Total operating expenses per meal, net cost per meal, and net cost per patient day are also calculated.

Step 9: Calculating Productivity Indicators

The calculation of **productivity indicators** for the upcoming fiscal year includes the number of meals served per hour paid to an employee as well as the number of meals served per hour worked by the employee. (The first indicator takes into account actual costs for vacation days, sick days, and holidays.) The number of meals served per patient day is also an indicator of the productivity of the foodservice department.

Labor Hours Data As mentioned earlier, the same system that provides labor cost data usually is capable of providing data about the labor hours that were paid for by the department during a specific period. The system must be capable of providing data about regular productive hours, overtime, and nonproductive hours (hours paid but not worked, as in the case of holiday or sick pay). These data are collected by either a time-card system or tracked by a computerized system. Regardless of the method used, labor hours data are a necessary input so that further analysis of the department's productivity can be performed.

Volume-of-Service Data All health care operations should keep a daily record of the volume of services provided to customers. This includes a count of the number of meals served to patients and nonpatients. The most accurate method of collecting volume data is to count the number of trays prepared for each meal and to keep a record of the total number counted for each day (Figure 11.3.)

FIGURE 11.3 Excerpt from Annual Foodservice Department Operating Budget

	January Total			February Total			Annual Total		
	Patient	Nonpatient	Total	Patient	Nonpatient	Total Patient	Patient	Nonpatient	Total
1. Patient Days									
2. Patient days	2,250		2,250	2,050		2,050	27,500		27,500
3. Clinic visits		4,000	4,000		4,100	4,100		50,000	50,000
4. Meal Count									
5. Patient meals	6,300		6,300	5,740		5,740	77,000		77,000
6. Cafeteria meals		3,500	3,500		3,250	3,250		40,975	40,975
7. Stipend meals		500	500		475	475		6,650	6,650
8. Special-function meals		750	750		700	700		9,000	9,000
9. Other meals		0	0		0	0		0	0
10. Total meals	6,300	4,750	11,050	5,740	4,425	10,165	77,000	56,625	133,625
11. Operating Expenses									
12. Salary and benefit expenses	$6,010	$2,563	$8,573	$5,476	$2,387	$7,863	$73,458	$30,550	$104,008
13. Food expenses	6,151	4,145	10,296	5,604	3,861	9,465	75,175	49,411	124,586
14. Supply expenses	901	669	1,570	821	623	1,444	11,011	7,973	18,984
15. Other expenses	392	161	553	358	150	508	4,797	1,920	6,717
16. Total operating expenses	$13,454	$7,538	$20,992	$12,259	$7,021	$19,280	$164,441	$89,854	$254,295
17. Less: cash receipts	0	8,000	8,000	0	7,400	7,400	0	95,750	95,750
18. Net dietary expenses	$13,454	$(462)	$12,992	$12,259	$(379)	$11,880	$164,441	$(5,896)	$158,545
19. Statistical Indicators/Unit Cost per Meal									
20. Salary and benefit expenses	$0.9540	$0.5396	$0.7758	$0.9540	$0.5394	$0.7735	$0.9540	$0.5395	$0.7784
21. Food expenses	0.9763	0.8726	0.9318	0.9763	0.8726	0.9311	0.9763	0.8726	0.9324
22. Supply expenses	0.1430	0.1408	0.1421	0.1430	0.1408	0.1421	0.1430	0.1408	0.1421
23. Other expenses	0.0623	0.0339	0.0500	0.0624	0.0339	0.0500	0.0623	0.0339	0.0503
24. Total operating expenses	$2.1356	$1.5869	$1.8997	$2.1357	$1.5867	$1.8967	$2.1356	$1.5868	$1.9032
25. Less: cash receipts	0	1.6842	0.7240	0	1.6723	0.7280	0	1.6909	0.7166
26. Net cost per meal	$2.1356	$(0.0973)	$1.1757	$2.1357	$(0.0856)	$1.1687	$2.1356	$(0.1041)	$1.1865
27. Net cost per patient day	$5.98		$5.77	$5.98		$5.80	$5.98		$5.70
28. Productivity Indicators									
29. Meals per hour–paid	5.00	8.80	6.14	4.97	8.30	6.02	4.97	8.78	6.09
30. Meals per hour–worked	4.03	7.09	4.95	4.01	6.69	4.85	4.01	7.08	4.91
31. Meals per patient day	2.8		2.8	2.8		2.8	2.8		2.8

The nonpatient meal count can be broken down into subaccounts, such as meals for staff members, meals for employees, meals for special functions, catered meals, and so forth. The methods used for determining the number of nonpatient meals served each day vary among operations, depending on whether an operation follows a cash payment system or whether employees purchase monthly meal tickets. Stipend meals (meals provided free of charge to special groups—interns, for example) also are taken into account. A common method for determining the number of nonpatient meals requires the operation to track and report total cash sales.

Step 10: Preparing the Proposed Operating Budget

In the final step in budget preparation, the foodservice director uses all of the financial information gathered in the preceding steps to prepare a formal operating budget proposal. The following data are needed to complete the foodservice department's operating budget:

- Forecast number of patient days (information may be secured from financial office) and outpatient clinic visits.
- Forecast number of patient meals, cafeteria meals, stipend meals, meals for special functions, and other nonpatient meals (actual count of patient days, which is an average meals served per day of usually 2.7 meals per patient day—this figure would not be 3.0 due to nothing by mouth (NPO) orders and patients on oral or tube feedings).
- Total wage, salary, and benefit expenses for foodservice employees.
- Total expenses for patient and nonpatient meals.
- Total supply expenses.
- Total of all other direct or allocated expenses (called *other expenses*). These expenses are a percentage of the total cost for each of these other expenses. The CFO makes the determination to what percent to allow to departments.
  Occupancy charges
  Mortgage payments
  Taxes
  Insurance (fire and liability)
  Depreciation
  Security, pest control, waste management
  Administrative overhead (human resources and other nonrevenue departments

After top-level managers within the health care institution have approved the proposed budget, the budget will serve as an invaluable tool in the ongoing management of the department's performance. Table 11.1 shows a section of an annual operating budget for a foodservice department.

The main objective in preparing an operating budget is to formulate a carefully thought-out plan for making management decisions and controlling the activities of the department throughout the upcoming year. For this reason, the annual budget for the foodservice department is broken down into 12 monthly schedules. Having an operating budget that shows monthly estimates of units of service and expenses allows the foodservice director to identify financial problems as they come up. In addition, the director can maintain an accurate record of the department's actual performance for monthly comparisons with the budgeted forecasts of its performance. Monthly budget review also allows the director to determine whether the department's objectives are being met and to take corrective action if they are not.

When performance is analyzed regularly during the actual period, estimates of expected performance for upcoming months can be adjusted as necessary to match actual performance. It should be kept in mind that projections can only be estimates of performance.

The business and economic climate of health care organizations can change relatively quickly. Despite the best projections, many turn out to be too high or too low. Revising the projections for the upcoming months of the fiscal year does not reduce the budget's value as a basis for financial management; rather, it indicates that the foodservice director is keeping track of operational performances and general business trends.

Capital budgeting is the process of planning for major expenditures, called *capital expenditures*. These expenditures involve large sums of money and usually are depreciated over the life of the expenditure. Generally, these criteria specify that the item is not consumable and the cost level and usable time period of the item are defined. Capital expenditures include new or replacement equipment or furnishings, renovation projects, and the purchase of new facilities. When planning the capital budget the need for the expenditure needs to be put into priority order such as *urgent, essential, economically desirable,* and *general.* By listing needs by the most urgent would be desirable. The request will need to include the need for the expenditure and to specify if the requested expenditures is new, additional equipment, or replacement, renovation, and if the new item is salvageable (to be sold or donated to a charitable nonprofit organization). A written justification should accompany the request to include any additional reduction in labor, cost analysis—sales, water, energy, and an increase in revenue—and so forth.

Most departments in a health care facility will be in competition for the limited capital dollars. The CFO and CEO must review the strategic plan and decide which projects can be achieved with the funds available. In emergency situations a department may receive the capital funds two years in a row or if a specialized piece of equipment cost more than had been allocated, part of the capital funds may be used to cover these costs. As part of the budgeting process the foodservice director will need to prepare a capital budget request, especially if the request is urgent, such as a replacement for a burned out stove/oven.

Budgetary Control

Budgetary control is defined as the management and control of an organization or a unit within an organization in accordance with the organization's approved budget. The purpose of budgetary control is to keep expenses within the limits of the organization's available assets and expected revenues.

In the foodservice department, budgetary control starts with menu planning. The menu dictates the varieties, forms, and quality levels of food to be offered. All of these factors affect the amount of

TABLE 11.1 Sample Monthly Operating Statement

	January Total		
	Actual	Budget	Variance, %
1. **Patients Days**			
2. Patient days	2,192	2,250	−2.6
3. Clinic visits	4,132	4,000	3.3
4. **Meal Count**			
5. Patient meals	6,136	6,300	−2.6
6. Cafeteria meals	3,539	3,500	1.1
7. Stipend meals	493	500	−1.5
8. Special-function meals	728	750	−2.9
9. Other meals	0	0	—
10. Total Meals	10,896	11,050	−1.4
11. **Operating Expenses**			
12. Salary and benefit expenses	$ 8,839	$ 8,573	3.1
13. Food expenses	10,698	10,296	3.9
14. Supply expenses	1,606	1,570	2.3
15. Other expenses	533	553	−3.6
16. Total operating expenses	$21,676	$20,992	3.3
17. Less: cash receipts	(8,808)	(8,000)	1.0
18. Net dietary expenses	$13,596	$12,992	4.6
19. **Statistical Indicators/Unit Cost per Meal**			
20. Salary and benefit expenses	$0.81	$0.78	4.6
21. Food expenses	0.98	0.93	5.7
22. Supply expenses	0.15	0.14	6.2
23. Other expenses	0.05	0.05	—
24. Total operating expenses	$1.99	$1.90	4.9
25. Less: cash receipts	(0.74)	(0.72)	2.7
26. Net cost per meal	$1.25	$1.18	6.3
27. Net cost per patient meal	$6.20	$5.77	7.4
28. **Productivity Indicators**			
29. Meals per hour—paid	5.88	6.14	−4.3
30. Meals per hour—worked	4.74	4.95	−4.2
31. Meals per patient day	2.83	2.80	1.2

labor that will be required in meal preparation and the amount of equipment and supplies that will be needed. Food, labor, supplies, and equipment expenses all translate into the average cost per meal. The operating budget gives the foodservice director a target average cost to aim toward in menu planning. Although it is seldom possible to make the cost of every meal match the targeted average cost, the average cost of meals for the menu-planning period should match the budgeted cost per meal as closely as possible. To balance the costs of planned menus, the director should use cost-controlled standard recipes. The costs of the recipes should be kept up to date

with changes in supply and food prices. Menus are also valuable tools in menu planning and control activities.

The cost of food, supplies, and labor must be kept within the limits set by the department's operating budget in other areas as well. Purchasing control procedures depend on good menu planning and meal forecasting to determine the quantities of food needed. Using purchasing specifications and a system of competitive bidding ensures adequate financial control in purchasing. Inventory control depends on careful receiving procedures and requisition practices. Food spoilage during storage can be controlled by following adequate food storage and rotation practices. Financial losses due to ineffective receiving practices and poor storage conditions can be prevented, but they are often overlooked. (Chapters 17 through 20 discuss food purchasing and selection and inventory control, receiving, and storage.)

Food production is another key area for cost control. A common source of increased meal costs is overproduction of menu items. Accurate meal forecasting is vital and is easier to control by the use of cycled menus. Ingredient central systems/areas help reduce overall cost in health care institutions. Policies and procedures are needed to control portion sizes.

The foodservice department's human resources should also be used in a cost-effective manner. Employees should be trained and motivated to follow the procedures that have been established for cost and quality control. In addition, staffing and scheduling patterns that make the best use of labor time are an important means of controlling labor costs.

Operating and maintenance costs also merit attention, particularly in the area of energy conservation. Reducing energy waste in the foodservice department may require retraining employees, rescheduling activities, improving equipment maintenance procedures, or replacing or retrofitting obsolete equipment. Such efforts can result in long-term decreases in energy use.

For the foodservice director, budgetary control also requires that operating expenses be recorded and analyzed on a regular basis throughout the fiscal period. Operating expenses should be recorded on a monthly operating statement that summarizes the cost of providing services to patients and other customers. In addition, monthly expenditures should be compared with the forecast budget, and areas of variance should be noted and acted on when necessary. The preparation of monthly operating statements ensures that budget guidelines are followed and that the department's financial health is maintained. An operating statement, a document prepared by the organization's finance and accounting department, usually monthly, compares actual cost against budget projections and provides a variance between the two.

By preparing monthly operating statements, the foodservice director is able to monitor the overall performance of the department and determine which activities, if any, need to be adjusted to meet budget targets. This aspect of budgetary control involves three steps:

1. Comparing actual operations data with budget forecasts
2. Evaluating actual operations data according to an adjusted operating budget
3. Reviewing operating procedures, standards, and expenses

Table 11.2 shows an example of a monthly operating statement for a foodservice department. The remainder of this section uses Tables 11.1 and 11.2 as bases for a discussion of the monthly operating statement as a control device for a foodservice department.

Step 1: Comparing Operations Data with Budget Forecasts

The five main sections of the monthly operating statements coincide with the sections of the foodservice department's annual operating budget. The sections include patient days, meal count, operating expenses, statistical indicators, and unit cost per meal, and productivity indicators.

The patient days section (Table 11.1, lines 1 through 3) represents the overall level of business activity in the department during the month of January. The operating statement shows that the number of actual patient days was 2.6 percent below the budgeted level. The lower number of patient days indicates that comparably lower expenses for the month are needed to keep costs within the budgetary guidelines for the month and eventually for the entire fiscal year. The number of clinic visits, however, was 3.3 percent above the budgeted level. This slight increase in activity over estimated levels for the month could affect the budgeted expenses associated with the nutrient outpatient clinic if the upward trend continued into later months.

The meal count section (Table 11.1, lines 4 through 10) shows the actual number of meals served in January to all of the department's customers, including patients and nonpatients. The foodservice director should note that the number of patient meals, stipend meals, and special-function meals was lower than budgeted: 2.6 percent, 1.5 percent, and 2.9 percent, respectively. However, the number of cafeteria meals served was 1.1 percent higher than anticipated. If the trend continued into later months, an adjustment in the budget for later months in the fiscal year would be called for.

The section on statistical indicators of unit cost per meal (Table 11.1, lines 19 through 27) also shows that expenses and unit costs were significantly over budget. In addition, the section on productivity indicators (lines 23 through 31) suggests that the department's performance was below the targeted level. However, the number of meals served per patient day was slightly higher than budgeted.

The preceding step in the financial review of January's operations highlights the variances between actual performance and budgeted performance. The variance analysis is a report made each accounting period by the foodservice director to explain and justify any deviations from the budget. Next, the foodservice director needs to perform a deeper analysis of the financial data to determine strengths and weaknesses in the department's performance.

Step 2: Evaluating Operations Data According to a Revised Budget

To evaluate the performance of the foodservice department for the month of January, the budget must be adjusted to show the estimated cost at the actual level of patient days and the actual level of patient and nonpatient meals served. To accomplish this evaluation, the number of patient days and the number of total meals served are adjusted on the budget to respond to the actual data for the month. These two indicators are recorded in the revised budget (Table 11.2). To determine the amount of budgeted resources needed to supply the services listed under operating expenses, the revised budget column is determined according to the method shown in Table 11.3.

The revised budget amounts are recorded in the revised budget column of Table 11.3. Because the revised budget and the actual levels of expenses and statistical indicators are now based on the same financial data, the foodservice director can make more

TABLE 11.2 Sample Monthly Operating Statement and Revised Budget

	Actual	Revised Budget	Variance	Percentage of Total Operating Expense Variance	Cash Receipts Variance Applied on Basis of Percentage Variance	Adjusted Variance
			January Total			
2. Patient days	2,192	2,192	0			
10. Total meals	10,896	10,896	0			
11. Operating Expenses						
12. Salary and benefit expenses	$ 8,839	$ 8,499	+$340	4.0%	+35%	$82	$258
13. Food expenses	10,698	10,133	+565	5.6%	+58%	136	429
14. Supply expenses	1,606	1,525	+81	5.3%	+8%	19	62
15. Other expenses	533	545	−12	−2.2%	−1%	(2)	(10)
16. Total operating expenses	$21,676	$20,702	+$974	4.7%	100%	$235	$739
17. Less: cash receipts	(8,080)	(7,845)	+235	3.0%			
18. Net dietary expenses	$13,596	$12,857	+$739	5.7%			
26. Net cost per meal	$1.25	$1.18	+$0.07	5.9%			
27. Net cost per patient day	$6.20	$5.87	+$0.33	5.6%			
28. Productivity Indicators						
29. Meals per hour—paid	5.88	6.14	−0.26	−4.3%			
30. Meals per hour—worked	4.74	4.95	−0.21	−4.2%			
31. Meals per patient day	2.83	2.80	+0.03	1.2%			

Notes: Lines 11 through 18 of the tables indicate the operating expenses for salaries and benefits, food, supplies, and other expenses. In January, the actual expenses for salaries and benefits were 3.1 percent higher than allowed for in the budget. Actual food expenses were 3.9 percent higher. And supply expenses were 2.3 percent higher than anticipated. The "other expenses" category showed a 3.6 percent decrease over budgeted figures. Total operating expenses were 3.23 percent higher than budgeted. In addition, higher-than-budgeted cash receipts can be credited to improved cafeteria sales. Overall, the net expenses for the foodservice department in the month of January were 4.6 percent over budget.

TABLE 11.3 Method for Calculating Revised Operating Expenses

Meals Operating Expenses	Budget Unit Served		Revised Cost, $		Budget, $
12. Salary and benefit expenses	10,896	x	0.78	+	8,499
13. Food expenses	10,896	x	0.93	=	10,133
14. Supply expenses	10,896	x	0.14	=	1,525
15. Other expenses	10,896	x	0.05	=	545
16. Total operating expenses	20,702				
17. Less: cash receipts	10,896	x	0.72	=	(7,845)
18. Net dietary expenses	12,857				
26. Net cost per meal	12,857	x	10,896	=	$1.18
27. Net cost per patient day	12,857	x	2,192	=	$5.87

meaningful comparisons. The variance column shows that actual expenses were higher than budgeted expenses in every category. From this evaluation, the variance in the actual net cost per patient meal from the budgeted net cost is significant at 5.9 percent. In addition, the productivity indicators demonstrate that more labor hours than budgeted were used to produce fewer meals than budgeted.

The evaluation has made it clear that the foodservice department's operating expenses are above the levels authorized in the operating budget. The level of productivity is also clearly lower than is required by the operating budget. Variances occurred in several categories of the operating expenses: salary and benefits, food, supply, and other expenses. The foodservice director at this point must identify the reasons for the unacceptably high operating costs and prepare a plan for taking corrective action.

Step 3: Reviewing Operating Procedures, Standards, and Expenses

To identify the problems in foodservice operations that may be behind the unacceptable expense levels, the foodservice director needs to review the department's operating procedures and standards. In the category of food and supply costs, the following factors (discussed in detail in later chapters) should be examined:

- Physical inventory
- Invoice records
- Invoice payments
- Receiving and storage procedures
- Purchasing specifications
- Production requisitions
- Menu plans

The factors to be considered in the category of labor cost include labor time and work schedules. The category called other expenses should also be examined. However, other expenses include fixed payments that are made periodically without regard to the level of activity. The variance between the actual other expenses and the budgeted other expenses may reflect an error in the original budget.

In large part, the foodservice director's ability to perform such operational reviews depends on adequate financial record keeping and reporting. This subject is the topic of the next section.

Financial Records and Reports

Successful financial management requires a system of records and reports that presents financial information in the most efficient and usable way possible. Few health care institutions can afford to prepare more financial records and reports than they need to keep managers informed of the institutions' fiscal status. For this reason, the foodservice department's financial record-keeping system should concentrate on providing information valuable for evaluating, allocating, and controlling the department's expenses.

The types and number of records needed for determining foodservice costs and the methods used for allocating the costs to the various services provided by the department are dictated by the institution's financial policies and procedures. Systems vary among health care institutions.

Records must be compiled on daily, weekly, monthly, and annual bases. These data are used as the basis for the department's monthly performance report, which is part of the institution's overall financial control system. In some institutions, the foodservice director may develop monthly performance reports as required by the organization. In others, the accounting department prepares the actual monthly performance report. In the latter case, however, the foodservice director is responsible for the accuracy of the report. The following records are needed for completing the monthly performance report:

- Records of meals (or equivalent) served to patients and nonpatients, including the daily census of meals served
- Records of purchasing, receiving, inventory, and issuance activities, including the monthly raw food costs
- Production forecasts and records
- Labor records, including monthly labor costs
- Records of overhead costs, supply costs, and miscellaneous costs
- Records of revenues from patient and nonpatient sources

Daily Census of Meals Served

All health care institutions should keep a daily census (or count) of the number of meals served to patients and nonpatients (Exhibit 11.4). The nonpatient meal count can be broken down into subaccounts, such as meals for staff members, meals for employees, meals for special functions, catered meals, and so forth. The most accurate method of determining the number of patient meals served is to count the number of trays actually prepared for each meal and to keep a record of the total number counted for each day. A disadvantage of this method is that it can be time-consuming. An alternative method that can be used in hospitals is to survey the number of trays served over a week or so to determine the average number of trays served per day. This average can then be multiplied by the midnight census of inpatients (less newborns) to find the total number of patient meals served for a particular day. The average factor is 2.7 meals per patient day. The averaging method is not accurate enough to be used for cost allocation. However, it may be used for budget preparation.

The methods used for determining the number of nonpatient meals served each day vary from institution to institution. The method used depends on whether the institution follows a cash-payment system or whether employees purchase monthly meal tickets. Stipend meals (meals provided free of charge to special groups—for example, interns) are also taken into account. The method most often used for determining the number of meals served in a cash-payment cafeteria requires calculating the average selling price for a full noon meal (including meat, potato, vegetable, salad, beverage, and dessert). When a selective menu is offered, the average price of each meal component (for example, the entrée, vegetable, salad, or dessert) should be used in the calculation of the average number of meals. Once the average selling price of a meal has been determined, the total cash sales can be divided by the average price per meal to determine the *daily meal equivalent*, or the average number of meals served per day for record-keeping purposes. Health care foodservice systems still disagree on what is the "best" way to determine meal counts.

Monthly Raw Food Costs

Purchasing, receiving, inventory, and issuance records are used to determine monthly raw food costs. The data needed for these records are the total cost of the foods purchased during the month and the value of physical inventories at the beginning and end of the month. The total cost of purchases for the month can be calculated by adding up all of the purchasing invoices paid to suppliers during the month (Figure 11.4).

The physical inventory figures are used to determine the amount of food actually consumed during the month (versus the amount purchased during the month). The following three steps represent one method of calculating the total cost of food used during the month:

1. Start with the value of the beginning inventory (including food in storage and food being used in the kitchen).
2. Add the total value of purchases made during the month (the total of invoices paid during the month).
3. Subtract the value of the inventory at the end of the month (total of the physical inventory and the stock in the kitchen) to arrive at the total cost of the food used during the month.

FIGURE 11.4 Food Purchases Register

ABC Foodservice Department
Food Purchases Register   Supplier: XYZ Foods
For the Month of: July

Invoice Date	Invoice Number	Meat/Fish Poultry	Egg/Milk Frozen	Produce	Dairy	Bakery	Grocery	Beverage	Invoice Total
7–02-XX	32448	$185.97	$156.12				$606.70		$606.70
7–08-XX	32575	$93.79					$274.05		$523.96
7–11-XX	2560						$238.98		$238.98
7–16-XX	32507					$674.86	$248.12		$922.98
7–23-XX	32542	$201.31					$218.41		$419.72
7–30-XX	32634		$104.21				$249.26		$353.47
Vendor category total		$481.07	$260.33	$0.00	$0.00	$674.86	$1,835.52	$0.00	$3,251.78
Tot Purchase/Category		$25,997.00	$8,092.00	$5,450.00	$10,912.00	$1,592.00	$20,705.00	$5,705.00	$78,453.00
% of Tot Purchase/Category:		1.85%	3.22%	0.00%	0.00%	42.39%	8.87%	0.00%	4.14%

Department of Nutrition and Foodservice
Daily Meal Count
Month of _____

Date	Patient Meals			Totals	Guest trays	Cafeteria Meals			Special Function	Totals
	C	Tray line	Late trays			B	L	D		
01										
02										
03										
04										
05										
06										
07										
08										
09										
10										
11										
12										
13										
14										
15										
16										
17										
18										
19										
20										
21										
22										
23										
24										
25										
26										
27										
28										
29										
30										
31										
Total:										

The value of the kitchen inventory may be deleted from the calculation if the amount is small or has high turnover or if calculating its value is too time-consuming. Other methods of determining raw food costs can be used. However, the time involved in using other methods as well as their accuracy should be considered.

Once the total raw food cost for the month has been determined, it can be expressed as **food cost per meal equivalent** (as calculated by the method already described). However, this figure only indicates the average cost of all meals served. The director should also be concerned with the cost per meal for each group served, whether patient or nonpatient. Therefore, a method is needed to allocate costs efficiently and accurately. The simplest method is based on patient and nonpatient meal counts. A ratio of the two types of meals served should be determined and the costs assigned accordingly.

In addition to total food costs, the director may want to break down costs into categories according to food group, such as meat, fish, poultry, and eggs; dairy products; fresh produce; frozen goods; bakery goods; and groceries. Cost breakdowns are useful for evaluating the nutritional contributions of various foods and for detecting month-to-month fluctuations that may require the manager to take corrective action. For example, a decrease in the average amount spent for meat, fish, poultry, and eggs may indicate that the meals served during the month were lower in protein content than those served during the preceding month. A considerable increase might reflect increasing market prices, over which the director has no control, or the inappropriately frequent use of expensive meat items. Small month-to-month variations are normal, but wide variations may point to the need for corrective action.

Sometimes it is desirable to calculate food costs more frequently than once a month. If day-to-day figures are needed, the form shown in Exhibit 11.5 can be used. However, the value of these data should be considered in relation to the time and effort required to record and report them. The fact that daily cost calculations are even less accurate than weekly or monthly cost figures because of variations in purchasing and use patterns should also be taken into account. However, the daily food cost record does reflect the approximate cost per day. In addition, it provides data for calculating monthly total purchase and cost figures that can be used in preparing the monthly performance report. The monthly performance report can then be compared with the operating budget. Computer-assisted inventory and accounting systems are able to provide weekly or even daily food cost data with relative ease and at reasonable expense.

Other food costs that should not be overlooked are the cost of food stocked on patient floors and the cost of supplementary nourishments served from the kitchen. Periodically, a count of all food items sent to patient floors should be recorded, and the costs should be assigned. The total cost of these items is then divided by the number of patient days for that period to determine the average cost of floor-stocked food per patient day. The costs of other nourishments not stocked on patient floors are usually considered a part of the patient food cost and are not treated separately in the accounting process.

EXHIBIT 11.5 Daily Food Costs

Daily Food Costs

Month:_____Year:_____

To Day (1)	Total Purchases					Net Food Cost To Date		
	To Kitchen (2)	Cost Storeroom (3)	Cost Today (4)	Cost to Date (5)	Issues from Storeroom (6)	Today (2 + 6) (7)	Actual (8)	Budgeted (9)
1								
2								
3								
4								
5								
6								
7								
8								
9								
10								
11								
12								
13								
14								
15								
16								
17								
18								
19								
20								
.								
.								
.								
31								
Total								

Example of food cost for one month:

Beginning Inventory	$12,000
Purchases	$10,000
Subtotal	$22,000
Ending inventory	$9,000
Monthly Labor Costs	
Total cost	**$13,000**
($12,000 + $10,000 − $9,000)	**$13,000**
To determine the percent of food cost	**$13,000/$34,000 (allocated for food cost) = 38%**

FIGURE 11.5 Labor Cost Analysis

Labor Time and Cost Record

Date: _____

Number of working Dates: _____

Employee Classification and Number	Total Hours					Total Pay ($)			
	Productive[a]		Nonproductive[b]			Productive			
	Regular	Overtime	Sick	Vacation	Holiday	Regular	Overtime	Nonproductive	Fringe Benefits[c]
Tray line employees (701)									
Smith	112	11	8		8	346.00	53.00	52.00	91.00
Johnson	104	—	4		8	338.00	—	39.00	84.50
First cook (900)									
Jensen	160	—	—	12	—	880.00	—	66.00	220.00
Monthly total									
Daily Average									

[a]Productive hours are those hours worked, including overtime.

[b]Nonproductive hours are hours paid (sick, vacation, holiday, and so on) but not worked.

[c]Fringe benefits vary from 10 to 34 percent of total pay and may include unemployment insurance, other insurance (such as health, life, dental), meals, uniforms, education and recreation pay, parking fees, and employer's share of Social Security.

Payroll records are a convenient source of data on labor costs. A form such as the one shown in Figure 11.5 can be used to record labor hours worked and paid on a monthly basis. In some cases, institutions may prefer reporting by week or by pay period. Either of these alternative reporting periods offers the advantage of supplying data based on a fixed number of days. This simplifies the comparison of labor hours and costs. However, monthly reporting has the advantage of relating labor costs to other expenses reported and summarized by the month. The form shown in Figure 11.5 also provides a convenient record of overtime worked, sick days taken, and vacation days used.

Labor costs must be allocated to patient and nonpatient meals. In most cases, the ratio used to allocate food costs is also used to allocate labor costs. The hours and labor costs of some employees can be allocated directly if their work time is spent exclusively in either the patient or nonpatient area. Periodic time studies can be used to confirm the accuracy of the ratio of patient-to-nonpatient labor costs in combined patient and nonpatient functions.

Analyzing labor costs is necessary to determine total cost per meal and total cost per patient day. In addition, analyzing labor costs identifies operational areas that need improvement. The efficiency of labor use can be evaluated more precisely by calculating productivity statistics each month and by comparing them with those for past months or with statistics from other institutions.

Productivity is the relationship of the amount of resources used to the amount of products or services produced, or the relationship between inputs and outputs. Productivity can be simply calculated by dividing the amount of input by the amount of output. For example, dividing the number of labor hours worked (input) by the number of meals served (output) provides a meaningful indicator of productivity in the foodservice department. Overall, productivity is a valuable index of the department's efficiency and performance. Productivity statistics include the following types of data:

- The number of patient trays (or the equivalent) served per patient day
- The number of labor minutes per patient meal
- The number of labor minutes per nonpatient meal equivalent
- The amount of revenue produced per full-time-equivalent employee assigned to nonpatient meal service
- The number of customer transactions performed per each full-time-equivalent employee assigned to nonpatient meal service
- The total number of foodservice employee work hours per patient day
- The total number of foodservice employee work minutes per unit of service

Changes in productivity statistics may indicate the need to change operating procedures or staffing levels. Indicators are calculated on a regular monthly basis and analyzed promptly; the director can make appropriate changes before the department's long-term financial goals are negatively affected.

Monthly Supply Costs

To some extent, expenses can be controlled for such nonfood supplies as dishware, glassware, service ware, kitchen utensils, disposable paper products, cleaning compounds and equipment, printed forms and other office supplies, and small equipment. Procedures for all tasks, such as purchasing, requisitioning, maintaining inventory, and controlling stock for supplies, are the same as for food supplies. The costs involved and the quantities used are also determined by calculating beginning inventory, monthly purchases, and closing inventory. Records may also be kept and information reported by the type of commodity, such as paper and cleaning supplies.

Monthly Performance Report and Other Control Reports

The kinds of other control reports that need to be maintained in the foodservice department vary from institution to institution. Some examples include monthly performance reports, budget variance reports, quality control reports, productivity reports, and in-service education and orientation reports. Only the monthly performance report is discussed in this chapter.

After all the individual cost categories have been determined for the month, it is helpful for the foodservice director to prepare a summary form that includes all of the important operational data for the department. The foodservice performance report shown in Exhibit 11.6 is an example of a comprehensive and useful monthly summary. It provides a means for comparing current costs against budget targets from one month to the next. If cost allocations have been made properly, the true costs of patient and nonpatient meals will be indicated.

An analysis by the foodservice director that relates to variances in month-to-month costs and revenues should be carefully performed. Differences that cannot be explained by similar changes in patient census or nonpatient meal counts should be carefully reviewed. Some differences can be controlled, while others cannot be. For example, if fewer patient meals were served with no change in labor hours, labor costs per meal would be higher. This might be an uncontrollable cost difference over the short run. However, if this situation persists, the foodservice manager needs to seek ways to decrease the number of labor hours.

The following methods are useful in controlling expenses:

- Avoid overtime, schedule enough employees to meet the needs of the department.
- Orient all new employees to the department and the task, provide education and training as needed.
- Use more ready-to-eat foods, especially foods that are labor-intensive to prepare on site.
- Maintain equipment.
- Use technology for menu planning, issuing, purchasing, nutrition, and so forth.
- Monitor energy and water use—repair all leaking faucets, maintain a comfortable temperature, do not heat ovens to 500°F when a lower temperature would work, keep walking refrigerator and freezer doors closed, check insulation, have engineering do a walk-through to check insulation on doors and windows, check all doors for fit. Turn off lights and appliances when not in use.
- Control disposables, individual packets of condiments, napkins, straws, especially in the cafeteria.
- In food production, use standardized recipes and follow up on use.
- Control portion sizes no over- or undersizes.
- Constantly check receiving procedures, first-in, first-out (FIFO), monitor temperatures, eating in the kitchen, plate waste.
- Use foods in season.
- When there are leftovers utilize them within the allotted time.
- If the organizations approves establish an incentive plan based on reduced cost and increased revenue.

EXHIBIT 11.6   Example of a Monthly Performance Report Form

Hospital: _____

Period: _____

Prepared by: _____

Meal Count		Current Week	Percentage of Total (7)	YTD Meals		Labor Cost		Patient Service	Nonpatient Service	Total Labor	YTD Labor
Patient meals	(1)		%			Patient service direct	(8)	$	$	$	$
Cafeteria meals	(2)		%			Nonpatient service direct	(9)				
Free meals	(3)		%		Total full-time equivalents	Allocated labor	(10)				
Special-function meals	(4)		%			Total labor cost	(11)	$	$	$	$
Other meals	(5)		%			Total labor hours	(12)				
Total meals	(6)		%								

Food and Supply Costs

		Food Costs										Supply Costs				
		Meat, Fish, and Poultry	Fresh Produce	Frozen	Groceries	Milk and Dairy	Bakery	Total Food	YTD Food	Dis-posables	Cleaning Supplies	China, Silver, and Utensils	Other	Total Supplies	YTD Supplies
Beginning inventory	(13)	$	$	$	$	$	$	$	$	$	$	$	$	$	$
Purchases	(14)														
Ending inventory	(15)														
Gross cost	(16)	$	$	$	$	$	$	$	$	$	$	$	$	$	$
Percentage	(17)	%	%	%	%	%	%	%	%	%	%	%	%	%	%

Less nourishments	(18)	
Less transfers	(19)	
Net food cost	(20)	$

Less transfers	(19a)	
Net supply cost	(21)	$

Exhibit 11.6 *(Continued)*

Net food cost × ___% Patient meals and nourishments = Patient food cost = (22) $___ Net supply cost × ___% Patient meals = Patient supply cost (23) $___

Remarks			Recap									
			Patient Costs					**Nonpatient Costs**				
			This Period	Cost per Meal	Budget Cost per Meal	YTD Total	YTD Cost per Meal	This Period	Cost per Meal	Budget Cost per Meal	YTD Total	YTD Cost per Meal
	Labor	(24)	$	$	$	$	$	$	$	$	$	$
	Food	(25)		·								
	Supplies	(26)										
	Total	(27)	$	$	$	$	$	$	$	$	$	$
	Less revenue received	(28)										
	Net cost	(29)	$	$	$	$	$	$	$	$	$	$
			Patient meals/labor hour_____(30)					Nonpatient meals/labor hour_____(31)				
	Balance Sheet Data											

A *balance sheet* is a financial report that illustrates the foodservice operation's financial condition on a particular date. It shows what the operation's assets are and how they are balanced against its liabilities. Assets include all items owned by the organization that have financial value. These items include actual cash on hand, accounts receivable, the value of inventory and supplies, and so forth. Liabilities, the opposite of assets, include the organization's current operating expenses and its long-term debt.

Because the balance sheet may not be as valuable to a department manager as the revenue expense statement, it may not be generated on a routine basis by the financial departments. However, when it is generated, the required asset data include cash on hand, beginning inventory, accounts receivable, value of equipment and furnishings, and accumulated depreciation. Data about the operation's liabilities include accounts payable, wages payable, and taxes payable. These data are used by the processing element to generate the balance sheet.

Statistical Data

Statistical data are necessary for the production of nonfinancial reports, which are components of the output of the financial management system that generally focus on the foodservice operation's productivity. Productivity is the relationship of the amount of resources used to the amount of products or services produced, or the relationship between inputs and outputs of the foodservice department. Overall, productivity is a valuable index of the department's efficiency and performance. To determine the department's level of productivity, labor hours data (the input) and volume-of-service data (the output) must be provided.

PROCESSING ELEMENT

All the data collected during the accounting period focus on the process of managerial accounting. Although the function of financial accounting to provide historical information according to strict accounting procedures is important, usually this function is the responsibility of the accounting department. The foodservice director is more likely to need and use information that results from managerial accounting processes. This approach to accounting focuses on providing information on which future decisions may be made. Although both approaches to accounting generally use the same data, managerial accounting is much more flexible in its approach to the handling and processing of data than is the structured approach of financial accounting.

Characteristics of Processing

The processing element of a foodservice operation may be simple or complex, depending on the amount of specific information required. However, this element must produce accurate and timely reports. To accomplish this objective, the actions of this element must be based on standardized managerial accounting procedures as defined by the operation, so that the information from the foodservice department's reports can be compared with current and future performance.

Although manual systems can be designed to provide basic information, this is best accomplished on either a full-featured computer system or a specific type of generic software such as an electronic spreadsheet. Accuracy of information can be increased and the time required to process data decreased with computerized systems. In addition, once data are entered, they are available to be used in an infinite number of reports.

Activities of Processing

Three classes of data (revenue, expense, and statistical) must first be processed by means of journalizing, a process that records each transaction in the journal designated for that specific class of data. At the end of the accounting period, each journal must be totaled and the information recorded in the appropriate ledger. The final process, making adjustments, includes the end-of-period mathematical matching of revenues and expenses, recording changes in balances of assets and liabilities, and calculating and matching statistical information such as labor hours and volume of services.

Essential Components of Processing

Financial management requires that revenues, expenses, and operating statistics be recorded and analyzed on a regular basis throughout the fiscal period. These factors should be reported on a monthly operating statement that describes the outputs of the department (labor hours, number of meals, and the like) and summarizes the cost of providing services to patients and other customers. Journalizing, posting, and making adjustments are the processes by which this is accomplished.

Journalizing

Journalizing is the process of recording in chronological order each activity or transaction that occurs during an accounting period. Data about each activity should be recorded in the appropriate transaction journal. Transaction journals consist of either manual worksheets or electronic spreadsheets designed for a specific type of data. The transaction journals typically maintained by a health care foodservice operation to record revenues include a cash receipts journal and a sales journal. In general, expenses are recorded in purchase registers, and operating statistics are recorded in journals reserved for labor hours and volume of service. A departmental payroll journal is optional based on whether this function is centralized for the entire health care operation.

Revenue Journals

Revenue generated by the foodservice department generally results in the collection of cash from the customer at the point of service or charges made to the customer. The amount of cash collected and its source (patients, nonpatients, staff, and so on) should be recorded in the cash receipts journal. For example, the amount of daily cafeteria and vending sales should be recorded separately based on appropriate source documents. Source documents for other types of cash transactions should be collected and recorded by type of transaction in the cash receipts journal. This separation by type of transaction allows the foodservice manager to monitor not only cash sales but also the level of cash generated by each type of service.

A record should be made in the sales journal of any sales transaction for which the customer will be billed. Again, the specific source of this type of revenue should be identified to allow for tracking and analysis.

Expense Journals

Expenses of the foodservice operation are generally composed of consumables such as food and supplies, services that are generally classified as other expenses, and labor. The purpose of the purchase register is to monitor all purchases for food, supplies, and other expenses purchased on account. In addition to recording total costs, it is advisable to break down food costs into categories according to food group (described earlier in this chapter). Supply costs also might be kept and information reported by type of commodity, such as paper supplies and cleaning supplies. Cost breakdowns such as these enable the manager, during the course of the feedback processes, to further scrutinize costs for month-to-month fluctuations that may require corrective action.

Posting

At the end of the accounting period, the transactions recorded in the journals must be summarized, a process usually accomplished by totaling the transactions for each journal maintained by the operation. For manual financial management systems, this involves adding up all transactions to determine the total for a journal. If the journal has been maintained on an electronic spreadsheet, the total is available as soon as the last entry has been completed.

Each revenue, expense, and statistical journal must be summarized as described above. For instance, the cash revenue generated by the operation during the accounting period is determined by adding up all the cash revenue–producing transactions that have been recorded in the cash receipts journal. The total cost of food purchases for the month can be calculated by adding up all food-purchasing transactions, based on invoices from suppliers, during the accounting period. The two journals for operating statistics (labor hours and volume of services) also must be summarized similarly. At the end of this process, the transaction journal totals are transferred to the *general ledger*, which contains a separate section for each type of transaction monitored by the operation.

Ratios

Most foodservice operations may not ever need to use ratios; however, ratios need to be briefly described. *Ratios* are the relationship of one number to another. There are a number of ratios that are used to make up a ratio analysis. A *ratio analysis* is any analysis of financial data from different classifications such as liquidity and profitability. *Liquidity ratios* show how an organization's ability to meet short-term obligations. *Quick ratios* is cash accounts receivable and marketable securities divided by current liabilities. *Solvency ratios* indicate how well the organization can meet long-term debt. *Operating ratios* use data from income statements. *Profitability ratios* help evaluate an organization's ability to make a profit. There are other ratios used by financial and business organizations.

SUMMARY

Under the current health care environment, informed financial management is critical to the viability of health care organizations. The current health care financial management focus is on predicting costs before they are incurred. This proactive management approach requires departmental information, including foodservice information.

In the midst of changes that will continue to occur in the health care industry, the foodservice manager has emerged as the controller of significant and valuable resources, accountable for their efficient allocation. Thus, financial management has become one of the primary responsibilities of the foodservice manager. To meet the departmental and organizational needs for financial information, foodservice managers may find it necessary to develop and implement comprehensive financial management systems, such as the model described in this chapter.

KEY TERMS

Accounting period
Accounts payable
Accounts receivable
Assets
Balance sheet
Budget
Budgeted balance sheet
Capital outlay
Cash-flow budget
Control
Controller
Cybernetic control
Daily meal equivalent
Depreciation
Expense budget
Financial control
Fiscal year
Fixed and liquid assets

Fixed budget
Human resource control
Information control
Journalizing
Liabilities
Operating budget
Operations control
Petty cash
Point-of-sales (POS)
Productivity
Profit-and-loss statements
Ratios
Revenue budget
Standards
Traditional budget
Variable budget
Variance
Zero-based budget

DISCUSSION QUESTIONS

1. Describe the four types of control.
2. How do you calculate the productive and nonproductive hours for a department for one month?
3. Outline financial standards, methods to use to measure the result of the standards, compare the outcome—internally as well as externally—and the actions to be taken if standards are not met.
4. How do you develop an operational budget?
5. Design a labor budget, using FTE, part-time, and contractual personnel.
6. Determine the daily patient and nonpatient meals served.
7. Compare the planned budget to actual budget and, as applicable, write a variance.
8. Justify the urgent need for a major piece of equipment when capital funds are limited.

PART TWO

OPERATION OF THE FOODSERVICE DEPARTMENT

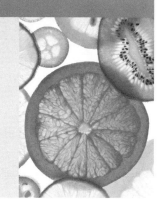

PART TWO OF this book deals with foodservice operations. The following chapters are subsystems of the major system, which is composed of inputs → transformation → outputs. These chapters are referred to as functional subsystems and include environmental waste, food safety and sanitation, menu planning, the procurement subsystem (purchasing receiving, issuing, and inventory), production, distribution, and service, and facility design. The system also contains controls and feedback.

Chapter 12 deals with waste management, sustainability and the impact on the environment, the need for clean air and potable water. Chapter 13 is important because the discussion centers on microbial, chemical, physical hazards, and temperature control. Chapter 14 details hazard analysis critical control point, federal, state and local regulations, environment sanitation, health inspections, and pest control. Chapter 15 presents information on safety, security and emergency preparedness; it also alerts the foodservice director on how to train employees on fire safety, security and workplace violence. Chapter 16 helps the foodservice director prepare menus and gives steps to help in modification of the menu for medical nutrition therapy. Menu planning is the beginning of the transformation subsystem, which is the major control system. Chapters 17, 18, and 19 make up procurement, which is the next step in transformation. Chapter 20 shows how to transform raw materials into edible food. Chapters 16 to 20 describe the transformation subsystem. Once the transformation has taken place, the products

will need to be distributed and served as outlined in Chapter 21. Chapters 16 to 20 complete the interlocking or linking process of the transformation. (Linking process is where the menu as a control links procurement, production, sanitation, safety, distribution, and service together to produce the output.) Chapter 21's distribution and service are outputs and complete the system.

Chapter 22 provides details on the role of the foodservice director or designee and the foodservice consultant in the construction of a new facility, a renovation, or an existing facility. The role of the team is explained, along with the responsibilities of various members. Equipment needs, justification for equipment, cleaning methods, and maintenance of equipment are also outlined.

All systems must have controls, such as plans, regulations, and laws; records must be maintained and feedback improvement is used to keep the system working. The output is the provision of quality meals and services that meet the perception, wants, and needs of the customers while maintaining the budget and providing attractive, well-planned, and nutritious meals.

Even though sanitation, safety, and security are usually considered after the procurement and production interlocking (linking) system, the author has chosen to present this information first because it has a major effect on the total system. The facility must be safe, secure, and sanitary to produce safe-quality food. Energy and waste disposal are major environmental concerns that affect the operation.

CHAPTER 12

ENVIRONMENTAL ISSUES AND SUSTAINABILITY

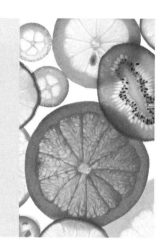

LEARNING OBJECTIVES

- Explain the concept of zero waste.
- Describe how the 4Rs are a major component of sustainability.
- Devise methods to reduce the landfill.
- Implement a program to conserve energy and water consumption.
- Complete a study on the use of disposable supplies versus reusable.
- Determine the best method to become a sustainable operation.

FOODSERVICE DIRECTORS or managers are expected to know about issues that will affect the cost and efficiency of their operations. Environmental issues such as the disposal of solid biological waste and hazardous waste (including medical waste and hazardous chemicals), air pollution, energy conservation, water and air quality and quantity, and the cost and availability of natural resources are some of the issues predicted to influence health care foodservice operations during the next several decades. Hospitals are challenged by the public to take a more active role in addressing environmental concerns within the community. As a result, many hospitals now provide leadership in developing strategic environmental programs that extend into the community.

This chapter presents an overview of environmental issues, suggests waste management strategies that can be implemented in health care foodservice departments, emphasizes the importance of top-management support and employee involvement in developing and implementing programs to become a more sustainable opera-

tion. Two methods of identifying a facility's waste stream, waste-stream analysis and waste auditing, are described. Next, hazardous waste management in a nutrition and foodservice operation is examined, with specific emphasis on hazardous chemicals waste, storage, and disposal.

Using a five-step model, guidelines for energy use and conservation through an energy management program are presented. Air pollution and water conservation are examined in light of current legislation. All these are tied into comprehensive environmental issues as they affect a foodservice department director's responsibilities.

SUSTAINABILITY

Sustainability has been defined in various ways depending on what "group" is defining it. In 1970 the U.S. National Environmental Protection Agency (NEPA) formally established as a national goal and the creation and maintenance of conditions under which human and nature "can exist in productive harmony, and fulfill the social and economic and other requirements of present and future generations of Americans."

In 1987 the U.N. Brundtland Commission defined sustainability as "meeting the needs of the present without compromising the ability of future generations to meet their own needs." The Report of World Commission on Environment and Development has adopted this definition and published it as a part of The Report of World Commission on Environment. The House of Delegates of the American Dietetic Association appointed a task force on sustainability and defined *sustainability* as "the capacity of being maintained over long term in order to meet the needs of the present without jeopardizing the ability of future generations to meet their needs." These definitions are to inspire us to become better stewards of the environment along with growth and social goals of conservation.

The 4Rs are the foundation of sustainability. The most accepted 4Rs are:

Reduce
Reuse
Recycle
Rethink

Everyone uses the first three Rs. Other organizations/businesses have changed the last R to describe their own particular business. These Rs include Renew, Repair, Refine, Redesign, Refuse, Rebuy, and Respect. Regardless of the Rs used, they all mean "protect our environment for the future." Each of the Rs is discussed later in this chapter.

All organizations find *waste management* as a major problem and one that has the greatest impact on the environment. For those reasons, waste management will be discussed first.

Solid Waste Management

The U.S. Environmental Protection Agency (EPA) defines *solid waste* as the products and materials discarded after use in homes, commercial establishments, and industrial facilities. Anywhere we look—highways, parking lots, or yards—waste can be found; it is everywhere. Solid waste disposal is currently one of the most costly environmental problems, affecting not only the foodservice department but also every department in a health care facility.

The EPA defines *municipal solid waste* as "waste such as durable goods, containers and packaging, food scraps, yard trimmings, and miscellaneous inorganic waste from residential, commercial, institutional, and industrial sources." Thus, all the waste generated in foodservice operations, excluding chemicals, is municipal solid waste. Increased disposal fees, landfill shortages, government regulations, and consumer demands for a safer environment are cited as priorities that require immediate action on the part of health care foodservice facilities.

In recent years and still increasing is the cost of placing waste materials in a landfill, called a *tipping fee*, more than tripled in some localities. Tipping fees (the costs of transporting and discarding municipal solid waste at transfer stations or landfills) increased about 5.9 percent during the past decade. They are expected to continue to escalate as stricter government regulations have been passed that are associated with Subtitle D of the Resource Conservation and Recovery Act (42 USC, Chapter 82), federal legislation that was adopted in 1976 and amended in 1984 by the Hazardous and Solid Waste Amendments. This act is the statutory basis the EPA used to establish a comprehensive program to control hazardous waste from generation to its final disposal. Because the amendments are enforced, local and state governments must develop solid waste management plans at the same time that the cost and difficulties of siting new landfills are increasing. Methane gas from landfills can pollute the area. Toxic leachates can contaminate water supply.

Approximately 50 to 65 percent of the waste (weight and volume) generated in commercial and noncommercial foodservice

TABLE 12.1 Percentage Volume of Materials Disposed of by Two Noncommercial Foodservice Operations

Material	College or University Study, %[a]	School Study, %[b]
Cardboard	44.6	27.5
Food waste from production and service	21.3	22.9
Paper	13.1	8.4
Paperboard	8.6	23.4[c]
Plastic (including film)	7.5	4.0
Metal (including tin and aluminum)	4.3	6.8
Miscellaneous (including wood, glass, and so on)	0.6	7.0

[a]University foodservice operation is a centralized conventional food production system serving an average of 3,300 meals per day. Data are based on a fourteen-day waste-stream analysis, excluding liquid waste.
[b]School data are based on analysis of average waste generated for ten days in six schools serving an average of 4,500 lunches per day.
[c]Gable-top milk cartons made up greatest percentage of waste.
Note: Volume is uncollapsed because facility had no compactor.

operations is food waste. Paperboard and corrugated cardboard are two materials that contribute most to the volume of packaging waste. Other packaging materials found in health care foodservice waste include tin, plastic, aluminum, glass, and Styrofoam. Some factors influencing the volume of each type of material disposed of include the type of service ware (reusable or disposable) used for the service of patient and nonpatient meals; type of production system; availability of volume reduction equipment such as compactors, pulpers, and disposals; accuracy of forecasts and production and service controls, such as use or disposal of leftover food; portion control; and reuse of plastic and glass containers after sanitization. The waste management industry estimates that from 0.5 to 1.5 pounds of total waste is generated per meal served, depending on the type of foodservice operation. Research at noncommercial foodservice facilities found an average of 0.39 to 0.61 pound per meal, or 0.002 to 0.03 cubic yard per meal of total waste (production, service, and packaging). Table 12.1 compares the composition of waste generated in two noncommercial operations.

The volume of packaging waste can be reduced by about 50 percent if corrugated cardboard boxes are collapsed and tin cans are crushed. Because most health care operations pay on the basis of dumpster capacity and waste disposal pickup frequency, their waste disposal costs would be reduced if waste volume were decreased. However, the cost of waste management equipment (such as compactors and balers) and labor costs must be analyzed and compared with waste-hauling expenses.

An integrated waste management system designed to decrease the quantity of waste to be disposed of is recommended. About 80

FIGURE 12.1 Integrated Solid Waste Management System

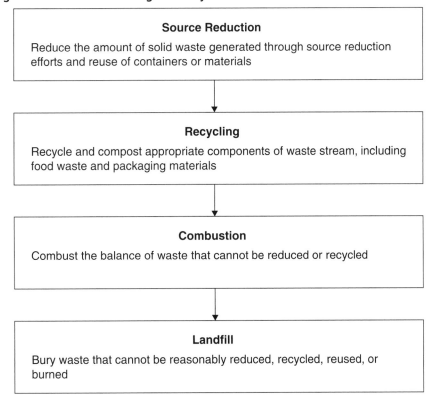

Source Reduction

Reduce the amount of solid waste generated through source reduction efforts and reuse of containers or materials

Recycling

Recycle and compost appropriate components of waste stream, including food waste and packaging materials

Combustion

Combust the balance of waste that cannot be reduced or recycled

Landfill

Bury waste that cannot be reasonably reduced, recycled, reused, or burned

percent of municipal solid waste is landfilled, 10 percent incinerated, and 10 percent recycled. According to the EPA, the term *integrated system* refers to "complementary uses of a variety of waste management practices to safely and effectively handle the municipal solid waste stream with the least adverse impact on human health and the environment."

In such a system, renewable natural resources are not disposed of as waste but are reused, recycled, and composted. Incineration is one option for reducing the volume of waste while capturing energy. In an integrated system, burying waste in landfills should be the last alternative. Figure 12.1 illustrates the components and order of preference of an integrated solid waste management system.

Lean Path, the experts in food waste tracking, say that foodservice operations should strive for *zero waste*. Zero waste is defined as a method to minimize waste, reduce consumption, maximize recycling and diversion, and ensure that products are produced to be reused, repaired, or recycled back into nature or the marketplace. In other words, zero waste aims to eliminate rather than manage waste. The zero waste program is based on tracking. Tracking allows the foodservice director to measure the amount of waste produced by the department and make decisions where waste can be reduced. To reduce waste the director will need to focus on the area where most of the waste is generated and develop methods to reduce. Information on how to implement this program is found at www.leanpath.com.

The foodservice director and *all* employees have an ongoing responsibility to protect the environment. One method that all businesses, especially foodservice can do this is by the *4Rs—Reduce,*

Reuse, Recycle, and Rethink. A brief discussion and examples of source reduction and reuse (recycling and composting) are presented in the following sections because these are options that foodservice directors can implement. The foodservice director needs to assess the feasibility of combusting packaging materials if the health care facility has an incinerator. Because of its water content, food waste usually is not combusted.

Reduce/Reuse

Foodservice operations account for approximately 40 percent of the landfill. If at least one pound or more of the 4.6 pounds of waste produced per person per day were reduced, there would be a profound effect on the environment. Landfill can reduce tipping fees, when less garbage is generated in the foodservice operation that usually goes to the landfill. Reducing the amount of waste generated, or *source reduction*, is a preventive approach that eliminates the need to determine the most cost-effective method of waste disposal. Source reduction also conserves natural resources and preserves the environment. The first thing the foodservice director needs to do is a complete review of products presently used. Determine what products are necessary for the operation of the department and do not order any more of the "unneeded" products. (This audit may also help reduce overall expenses.) If there is a large "grab and go" audience, charge a fee for the reusable container then exchange it each time the customer takes a meal to go. The following are other examples of reduce-and-source reduction efforts that have been beneficial in health care foodservice operations:

- Working cooperatively with manufacturers and distributors to reduce packaging materials
- Purchasing reusable products or products packaged in reusable containers or having products delivered in reusable containers rather than in cardboard boxes, specify packing products as free as possible of toxins, purchase durable, long-lasting products/goods
- Purchasing cleaning products in more concentrated form
- Purchasing products in bulk form rather than in smaller packages
- Reducing the quantity of disposables used or purchase the newer disposables that are biodegradable, or wood fibers and bamboo that can be composted, to help reduce landfill
- Evaluating which packaging material generated the largest volume of waste (for example, products such as sauces and salad dressings in individual portion packages rather than in bulk containers, such as polyethylene pouches or tin cans)
- Using sanitized glass or plastic containers for product storage
- Evaluating the accuracy of production forecast to minimize quantity of leftovers
- Serving condiments and beverages from dispensers rather than in single-service containers
- Minimizing waste potential through careful menu planning
- Introducing a program in cash operations where discounts are given to employees who use a reusable mug when purchasing beverages, use alternatives to bottle water, avoid polystyrene products
- Donating unused food from catered events to homeless shelters, schools, long-term care facilities, or other social programs (foodservice directors must obtain approval from health departments to ensure compliance with sanitation codes and must consult their organizations' legal counsel to avoid risk liability)
- Determine the recyclable content of products:
  a. Reduce the use of plastic by using recycled paper, bamboo, and wood that can be composted.
  b. Reduce the landfill.
- Constantly monitoring the forecasting and production methods, make changes as appropriate
- Planning menus to reduce waste, for example, purchase precut vegetables

How effective each of these approaches is depends on several factors. Some of these are the organizational culture; the extent of commitment and involvement on the part of managers, employees, and customers or recipients; and the education, training, and motivation of foodservice providers.

Recycling

Recycling is the second method for decreasing waste. The Foodservice and Packaging Institute defines *recycling* as "the act of removing materials from the solid waste stream for reprocessing into valuable new materials and useful products." For example, recycling efforts have not been successful in areas where markets for recyclable materials are limited or nonexistent. Before initiating a recycling program, a foodservice manager must contact a local waste hauler to learn whether the company offers its customers a recycling option. Many major waste management companies have developed programs whereby they provide special dumpsters for recyclable materials. When this type of recycling program is used it will be necessary to separate materials such as glass, paper, and metal into the proper dumpster. Some haulers are agreeable to commingling recyclables, while others may require that materials be separated and stored in a separate dumpster. If commingling is an option, foodservice directors should work to negotiate a new contract with the hauler. Training employees on what types of materials to separate and how to separate them will need to be in the new contract. If plastics are placed in recycling bins, the employees must determine what is recyclable. (To determine the recyclability check the icon or logo on the bottom of the container.) If an operation is located in an area where recycling is not available, the next option is to identify buyback centers that accept or purchase recyclable materials. Choosing disposable products that are compostable or recycled is another option. Buying recycled content products keeps the cyclical nature of the recycling economy healthy.

Recycling of equipment by either selling or donating to another user or to a metal recycling company helps provide valuable raw materials for future use. Each time something is recycled it means less products that go to a landfill. Recycle fats, oils, and grease for converting to biodiesel fuel, reducing fossil fuel use. All of these efforts help stimulate the development of greener technology and reduce the need for new landfills and incinerators.

Even though recycling has increased, collecting recyclable material and developing a market for these products is a challenge. The process can be expensive.

Rethink

To save our planet and reduce landfills foodservice director and **all** employees must rethink waste management and its total effect on the environment. There are many programs and organizations that have reduced their waste management by 80 percent. These people worked together as a team and found various ways to reduce and recycle.

Composting

Composting, as it relates to foodservice waste management, is the process of separating organic waste (that is, food and other organic waste from production and service areas, including plate waste, napkins, paper, paperboard, and cardboard) from other waste so that the organic waste is stored and eventually used as fertilizer or land conditioner. Composting has been implemented successfully in operations located in close proximity to a commercial compost facility. The foodservice director must first assess the financial feasibility of composting and the availability of storage space for holding waste before pickup. About 50 to 60 percent of waste generated in foodservice operations is organic (or biological). Removal of organic waste from trash sent to landfills could significantly decrease waste-hauling expenses.

The methods described above are the major component of a sustainability program. To complete a sustainable plan an *audit* can help the department to focus on both internal as well as external areas.

Perhaps looking at the *location* of the department in relationships to loading dock, trash/waste removal, parking for employees/vendors will help determine the amount of travel time for employees assigned these tasks. Once this is determined complete an audit on the big users of resources:

- Water and energy; for example, thawing foods in the refrigerator rather than under running water will save from *50* to *150 gallons* of water per month.
- Running the dish machine when there is only a full load can save *400* to *800* gallons of water monthly.
- Repairing a leaky faucet can save *20 gallons* daily for every leak stopped.

This is just an example of how water can be saved, thereby reducing the overall consumption and cost for water. As you perform the audit you will find many examples of saving resources and becoming more sustainable.

Waste-Stream Analysis

If recycling appears to be a feasible option, the next step is to become familiar with the *waste stream*, that is, the type and quantity of waste generated throughout the foodservice operation. Two methods can help make this determination: waste-stream analysis and waste auditing. A *waste-stream analysis* involves the simultaneous collection, separation, and determination of volume and weight of all waste generated and disposed of in all production and service areas for a certain period (such as five days or one week). Wastes are sorted by type of packaging material (corrugated cardboard, plastic [high-density polyethylene, low-density polyethylene, film], paper, or food-soiled). The weight and volume of each material collected are recorded at different times throughout the day. The total weight and volume are then computed per day and per week.

A *waste audit*, whose data (although similar to those obtained from a waste-stream analysis) are not as detailed, is easier and less labor-intensive and can provide the essential information for planning a recycling program. Conducting a waste audit involves assessing the type of waste generated (including hazardous waste, discussed later in this chapter) in each area of the operation (receiving, food production, service areas, dishwashing, sanitation and pest control, office, and so on). Information is recorded on a recycling form, such as the one shown in Exhibit 12.1, or on similar forms developed by foodservice suppliers. When conducting a waste audit, department managers must use a separate sheet for each major category of waste (cardboard, plastic, and so on).

A practical way to collect this information is to investigate waste generated in a given area or during a specific activity. For example, to assess quantity and type of waste generated in the production area, an employee would collect the waste containers, sort the waste, and record its weight and volume throughout an entire day. The number of days this information is collected will depend on variability in menu offerings, type of production system, market form of food, product acceptability, and effectiveness of control measures.

Information collected should result in a profile of food waste and an identification of major reasons for waste. The director can use the profile to identify alternatives for decreasing and disposing of waste and determining which materials can be recycled.

The information also may be used to evaluate the economics of recycling, that is, disposal costs and savings to be realized vis-à-vis waste volume. Costs of labor, supplies, and equipment must be included in the evaluation. All local and state codes must be followed (Figure 12.2). Other worksheets can facilitate planning a recycling program that includes selection of materials storage containers, materials transportation options, and baler or crusher options (Exhibits 12.2, 12.3, and 12.4, respectively). In addition, the logistics of how recyclable materials will be collected, sorted (if required by hauler or buyback center), and stored must be well delineated. Again, the need for waste reduction and processing equipment—compactors, balers, pulpers, crushers, and the like—should be evaluated. Sanitation remains an issue throughout the process, including waste storage. If other departments in the health care facility have implemented recycling programs, consult their managers to learn from their experience and then coordinate efforts where feasible. Volunteer to participate or invite a foodservice representative to work on the institution's recycling or waste management team.

EXHIBIT 12.1   Recycling Materials Flow Plan Worksheet

Department_____

Instructions

Complete a recycling flow plan(s) for each area of the foodservice department. Identify location(s) of the recyclables in each area at location 1. Move the materials from location 1 to location 2, 3, and so on until it is picked up by the recycler or waste hauler. At each location in the flow procedure, identify the container(s) to be used and who will be handling the materials. Handle materials as few times as possible.

<table>
<tr>
<td>

Location 1

Source of Materials

</td>
<td>

List recyclables to be collected at this location. Move recyclables to storage locations 2 and 3.

A._____
B._____
C._____
D._____
E._____
F._____

</td>
<td></td>
</tr>
<tr>
<td>

Collection Container(s)

A._____
B._____
C._____
D._____
E._____
F._____

</td>
<td>

Instructions

A._____
B._____
C._____
D._____
E._____
F._____

</td>
<td>

List employees collecting material.

A._____
B._____
C._____
D._____
E._____
F._____

</td>
</tr>
<tr>
<td>

Location 2

Temporary Storage

</td>
<td>

List containers to be used for storage or moving of each recyclable listed above.

A._____
B._____
C._____
D._____
E._____
F._____

</td>
<td>

List employees picking up materials.

A._____
B._____
C._____
D._____
E._____
F._____

</td>
</tr>
<tr>
<td>

Location 3

Recycling Center or Roll-Off Unit

</td>
<td>

List containers to be used for storage or moving of each recyclable listed above.

A._____
B._____
C._____
D._____
E._____
F._____

</td>
<td>

List employees picking up materials.

A._____
B._____
C._____
D._____
E._____
F._____

</td>
</tr>
</table>

Source: Used by permission of the Florida Extension Service, University of Florida.

FIGURE 12.2 Economics of Recycling: A Worksheet

Volume Data

What type of waste disposal container is in use? _____

How many refuse containers are being used? _____

1. Determine the present volume of waste that you are disposing of.
   How many pickups per month do you have? _____
   Estimate the number of tons per month from waste volume. _____
   (Calculate this by multiplying the waste capacity of the container by a factor
   that corresponds to the number of tons that container typically holds.)

2. Estimate the potential volume of recyclable materials.
   Estimate percentage of extractable recyclables. _____%
   Estimate the tons per month. _____ tons of _____ (material 1)
   Estimate the tons per month. _____ tons of _____ (material 2)

3. Calculate the waste volume left after recycling.
   Estimate the number of tons per month left after recycling. _____
      (Subtract line 2 from line 1.)
   How many pickups per month will you have? _____
      (This will be reduced in proportion to the percentage of material recycled.)

Waste Disposal Cost Data

4. Determine your present monthly waste removal costs.
   (If no invoice is available, you can estimate.)
   What is the pickup charge each time? $_____
   Multiply the pickup charge by the number of pickups per month (#1). $_____
   What is the landfill "tipping" fee per ton? $_____
   Multiply the tipping fee times the estimated number of tons per month. $_____
   Are you paying monthly container rental or lease fees? $_____
   Add up your total current monthly waste disposal costs. $_____

5. Determine your waste removal cost per ton (#4 divided by #1). $_____

6. Estimate your waste removal costs after recycling. $_____
   Pickup charges $ _____ times number of pickups _____ = $_____
   Tipping fee $ _____ times number of tons _____ = $_____
   Monthly equipment rental or lease fee = $_____
   Add up your total current monthly disposal costs after recycling. $_____

7. Monthly waste disposal costs you avoided (#4 minus #6). $_____
   (Calculate your savings by subtracting your disposal costs after recycling
   from your total current waste disposal costs.)

8. Annual avoided waste disposal costs (#7 times 12). $_____

9. Calculate the recycling program start-up investments.
   Recycling containers, boxes, or carts. $_____
   Recycling equipment, balers, compactors. $_____
   Cost of training program or internal publicity. $_____
   Other. $_____
   Total start-up investment for recycling program. $_____

10. Estimated revenues from recyclables. $_____
    From your estimate of the volume of recyclable materials (#2)
    _____ tons of _____ (material 1) times $_____ /ton = $_____
    _____ tons of _____ (material 2) times $_____ /ton = $_____
    (We recommend you use a conservative market price for these recyclables.)
    Your total monthly revenues from sale of recyclables. $_____
    Your total annual revenues from sale of recyclables. $_____
       (Multiply the monthly revenues by 12 to get annual revenues.)

Summary of Savings

11. Annual avoided waste disposal costs (from line #8). $ +_____
    Your total annual revenues from sale of recyclables. $ +_____
    Total annual savings. = $_____
    Total 5-year savings (multiply annual savings by five). = $_____
    Total start-up investment for recycling program (line #9). = $_____

12. Net estimated 5-year profit on recycling program. $_____

Source: Adapted from "How Your Business Can Profit from a Recycling Program," by D. Strathman and B. Drake. Provided by the Public Utilities Department, City of Jacksonville, Florida, 1991. More information can be found on the web at www.econedlinkorg/lessons/index.cfm?lesson=EM218. Accessed August 9, 2003. This data is similar to the zero waste program. This may seem like a lot of work but savings can be as much as $3,000/year upward, depending on the total reduction.

EXHIBIT 12.2   Selection of Waste Materials Storage Containers: A Worksheet

Company	Cost of Purchasing Roll-Off Containers	Cost of Leasing Roll-Off Containers	Length of Lease	Size of Compartments	Choice of Container Color?	Are Compartments Labeled?	Who Is Responsible for Repairs?	Who Is Responsible for Cleaning Containers?	Location Requirements Concrete or Pavement
1. Phone #									
2. Phone #									
3. Phone #									
4. Phone #									
5. Phone #									
6. Phone #									
7. Phone #									

Source: Used by permission of the Florida Extension Service, University of Florida.

EXHIBIT 12.3 Selection of Waste Materials Transportation Options: A Worksheet

Transporting recyclable materials to an intermediate processor or materials recovery center is usually done by a waste hauler or recycling center. Careful research needs to be done before signing contracts.

Company	Charges for Transporting a Leased or Purchased Roll-off	Fees for Picking up Materials in Smaller Containers	Add-on Charges such as Franchise Fees or Gas Surcharges?	Hours of Pickup	How Often Are Materials Picked Up?	How Much Notice Is Required for Pickup?	Length of Contract	Provide Weight Records	How Often Are Containers Cleaned?
1. Phone #									
2. Phone #									
3. Phone #									
4. Phone #									
5. Phone #									

Source: Used by permission of the Florida Extension Service, University of Florida.

EXHIBIT 12.4 Selection of Waste Baler or Crusher Options: A Worksheet

Company Name	Model #	Bale Size	Cost	Delivery and Installation	Warranty	Equipment Features
1. Phone #						
2. Phone #						
3. Phone #						
4. Phone #						
5. Phone #						

Source: Used by permission of the Florida Extension Service, University of Florida.

The completions of Exhibit 12.1, 12.2, 12.3, and 12.4 may appear as unnecessary and a waste of time. As a foodservice director you can only guess at what waste is being generated, in what area of the department and best methods to reduce the materials going to a landfill. In smaller institutions Exhibit forms 12.1 and 12.2 would provide you objective information to make decisions concerning waste management. This system is similar to the newer zero waste system.

Factors Influencing Success

Several factors affect the success of a recycling program. Probably the two most critical internal factors are management support and motivated, educated employees and guests. Management should initiate recycling education and incentive programs that stress the role played by employees in a program's success. Employee involvement and feedback, along with a team approach throughout program planning and implementation, are essential. External factors that influence the long-term success of recycling as a cost-effective component of waste management include a continuous source of supply of recyclable materials, a significant volume of recyclable materials, and adequate end-use markets for recycled products that support sufficient market value for such materials. Foodservice operators should purchase as many products made from recycled material as is economically feasible.

Waste Removal

Timely waste removal in a foodservice operation is a must. Food, garbage, and trash must be handled carefully to avoid the potential of contaminating food, equipment, and utensils and attracting insects and other pests. Standards for most surveying agencies state that a garbage can must be lined with an impervious bag and have a tight-fitting lid. Policies and procedures for waste removal must be written and followed.

Local government or private contractors may handle waste removal. In making the decision, these factors need to be analyzed:

- Cost of services
- Frequency of service
- Need to separate trash into food waste, plastic and cans, and paper
- Storage containers such as dumpsters and location of dumpsters
- Quality of service of companies; check with other users
- Security
- Cash for recycling of cans and plastic

After the decision has been made, policies and procedures need to be implemented for trash and garbage removal from the foodservice operation. These policies and procedures need to meet local health regulations and accreditation standards. The policies and procedures should include:

- Types of garbage and trash containers that are impervious, pest-proof, with tight-fitting lids
- Use of plastic liners
- How often garbage and trash should be removed from various areas of the department
- Storage area for garbage and trash bins
- Can-washing area that is located away from food production and storage area
- Procedure for can and trash containers sanitation

When mechanical devices such as garbage disposals and pulpers are used in the department, policies and procedures need to be posted above the equipment. When disposals and pulpers are used, the solid waste can be reduced by 75 to 85 percent. Pulpers are expensive, and employees will need to be trained how to use, clean, and maintain them. They require a lot of maintenance; therefore, a contract for maintenance needs to be drawn up and signed before employees actually use them. They must be cleaned daily to remove wads of garbage that have collected. This "wad" can harden like a rock and ruin the machine. Before a pulper is purchased, the engineering department will need to check local codes for the disposal of waste.

The cost of disposing of food waste varies depending on the method used. The most economical method is by food waste disposals and wastewater treatment plants. The most expensive is incineration. Many landfills are banning food waste. Landfill is the least desirable destination for food waste. Food waste decomposes faster than other organic materials and releases methane gas into the air. Some companies are experimenting with the use of the released methane gas for heating fuel.

HAZARDOUS WASTE MANAGEMENT

Handling and disposing of *hazardous waste* present unique challenges to the health care industry. Even though hazardous materials make up only 10 to 15 percent of hospital waste, waste management procedures have become more complex and costly following enactment of the Medical Waste Track Act of 1988, an amendment to the Resource Conservation and Recovery Act. The cost of hazardous waste disposal is three to five times more per ton than for other types of waste generated. Hazardous materials include infectious waste; diagnostic equipment batteries; laboratory solvents and acids; therapeutic radioactive chemicals; and chemicals used for cleaning and sanitizing equipment, mercury, surfaces, service ware, utensils, and so on.

Medical waste disposal has been a sensitive public issue since 1987 when hypodermic syringes, containers of blood, and other medical effluvia washed ashore on East Coast beaches. After enactment of the Medical Waste Track Act, the EPA issued "Standards for the Tracking and Management of Medical Waste" (codified at 40 CFR § 259). These standards provide health care facilities and other operations generating medical waste with definitions and procedures for disposal, transportation, incineration, and management of this type of waste. In general, the foodservice department is not directly affected by these regulations, what with its limited (if any) contact with medical waste. Nonetheless, managers should be familiar with their organization's policies and procedures regarding medical waste. Either the foodservice director or a department representative should participate on the facility's infection control committee or continuous quality improvement team and provide input regarding service of meals to patients in isolation and the handling of soiled service ware and leftover food (in most instances, isolation trays are handled the same as other medical waste). The director should see to it that policies and procedures for handling and disposing of infectious waste are communicated to all foodservice employees.

Hazardous chemicals, as defined by the Occupational Safety and Health Administration (OSHA), "any chemical [that] is a physical hazard or health hazard," influence foodservice departments more. Hazardous chemicals require the director to implement specific policies and procedures for purchasing, storing, handling, and disposing of all chemical compounds used in the operation. In addition, OSHA standards (known as *hazardous communication standards*; also referred to as the *right to know*) mandate that all employers provide information to their employees concerning hazardous chemicals through an established hazardous communication program. In turn, manufacturers and importers of chemicals are mandated to assess the hazard potential of the chemicals they produce or import, information that is communicated to end users on material safety data sheets (MSDSs). (See Chapter 15 for more information.) Part of a sample MSDS is shown in Exhibit 12.5.

When ordering chemicals (for example, detergents and other cleaning compounds), the purchasing agent should request MSDSs for products for which none are already on file at the facility. Multiple copies of each MSDS are helpful so that a copy is available in the work area where the chemical is used as well as being on hand for use in developing training materials and instructional guides for using a particular chemical. (The recommended content of a training program and the foodservice director's responsibilities related to OSHA's hazardous communication are discussed in Chapter 15.) Some distributors of cleaning supplies have developed training materials and MSDS manuals for their products. In addition to cleaning and sanitizing chemicals, the foodservice director should be familiar with and have on file MSDSs for chemicals used by exterminators.

The foodservice manager will need to work with facility maintenance or the waste hauler to determine how to dispose of empty chemical containers. In most instances, these should be disposed of following the same procedure as for other hazardous waste. Chemical containers **must never** be rinsed and used to store food.

EXHIBIT 12.5   Material Safety Data Sheet (Excerpt)

Material Safety Data Sheet May be used to comply with OSHA's Hazard Communication Standard, 29 CFR 1910.1200. Standard must be consulted for specific requirements.	U.S. Department of Labor Occupational Safety and Health Administration (Non-Mandatory Form) Form Approved OMB No. 1218-0072
IDENTITY *(As Used on Label and List)* Extra Strong Degreaser / High Alkline Oven Cleaner/Degreaser	*Note: Blank spaces are not permitted. If any item is not applicable, or no information is available, the space must be marked to indicate that.*

Section I

Manufacturer's Name Chemicals Unlimited	Emergency Telephone Number 1-800-000-1234
Address *(Number, Street, City, State, and ZIP Code)* Tanktown, USA, 00001	Telephone Number for Information 1-123-000-4567
	Date Prepared February 31, 1989
	Signature of Preparer *(optional)*

Section II — Hazardous Ingredients/Identity Information

Hazardous Components (Specific Chemical Identity; Common Name(s))	OSHA PEL	ACGIH TLV	Other Limits Recommended	% (optional)
Sodium Hydroxide (Caustic Soda) 1310-73-2	2		2 C	5
Butoxyethanol (Butyl Cellosolve) 111-76-2	240		120	10

(Skin) — This product contains no other component considerd

　　　hazardous according to the criteria of 29 CFR

　　　1910.1200.

Section III — Physical/Chemical Characteristics

Boiling Point 212°F		Specific Gravity (H$_2$O = 1) 1.05-1.08	
Vapor Pressure (mm Hg.) N/A		Melting Point N/A	
Vapor Density (AIR = 1) N/A		Evaporation Rate (Butyl Acetate = 1) N/A	
Solubility in Water 99%			
Appearance and Odor 　Opaque red/purple liquid: slight glycol ether odor.			

Section IV — Fire and Explosion Hazard Data

Flash Point (Method Used) N/A	Flammable Limits N/A	LEL N/A	UEL N/A
Extinguishing Media N/A			
Special Fire Fighting Procedures 　Product does not support combustion.			

Unusual Fire and Explosion Hazards 　　　None

(Reproduce locally)　　　　　　　　　　　　　　　　　　　　　OSHA 174, Sept. 1985

Source: U.S. Department of Labor, Occupational Safety and Health Administration, 1985.

ENERGY UTILIZATION AND CONSERVATION

Despite legislation and consumer pressure, energy conservation programs have not been a priority among foodservice directors. Even though the energy crisis of 2000 is a fading memory for most directors, the United States still faces serious energy problems, not the least of which is increasing energy cost.

Foodservice operations are a major user of resources, and as we just learned, a major contributor to food waste. The Energy Information Administration states that "foodservice operations are the most energy-intense users of electricity [in the commercial sector] due to the long hours of operation and specialized equipment." Foodservice operations comprise 7 percent of all commercial building energy use in the United States. According to Green Seal Energy the typical energy use composition for restaurants and foodservice operations is:

Cooking equipment 35%
Heating/cooling 28%
Dishwashing 18%
Lighting 13%
Refrigeration 6%

No discussion of energy can be made without discussing where this energy comes from and its total impact on the environment. Power plants product this energy through the burning of coal, biomass, fossil fuels, and the use of nuclear products in specially designed nuclear plants. Alternative sources of energy, such as solar, wind, and waste materials, are options for filling the demand for energy. These options are being studied and tested by scientists. To date these methods show promise but are expensive. Therefore, electricity is an important portion of the consumer's carbon footprint. All forms of electricity generation have some level of environmental impact. The foodservice department is a high user of electricity and it is important to learn to use electricity more efficiently.

Effective energy management practices can eliminate wasteful energy used in several key areas, including the design of the operation and the selection, use, and maintenance of foodservice equipment. Furthermore, proper equipment operation and ventilation systems can reduce energy costs and improve employee productivity and comfort.

Energy Measurement and Rates

The unit of measurement for heat is the British thermal unit (BTU). A *BTU* is the amount of heat required to raise one pound of water 1°F. Electrical rates are based on the amount of electricity actually used and the demand charge, which is the price the utility charges for being able to supply the maximum of electricity an operation might require during its peak demand periods. To control energy costs, the foodservice manager needs to evaluate what the cost is for various types of operations within the department, determine what operation has the highest use, and develop and, where possible, implement a plan to reduce the area of highest use.

Energy Management Program

Five key steps dictate the design of an *energy management* program, as delineated in Figure 12.3. The energy management will involve **all** of the foodservice employees, housekeeping, and engineering. All of these employees can serve as a team to conserve energy. As a team, representatives from each of these departments can work together to develop an energy conservation plan. The team leader should be someone whose knowledge of and commitment to conserving energy is outstanding. The first thing the team members will do is make a "walkaround" to determine how energy is being used. They will record their finding on a preprinted audit sheet highlighting areas in the department that are wasting energy. Working with engineering they can determine the cost of energy. (See Figure 12.4.) Once the team knows the cost of energy and how it is being used, the team will develop goals and objectives to conserve energy. All objectives should be measurable in cost and the reduction of energy. The objectives and strategies need a cost per strategy to be achievable. Next the team drafts a plan and discusses with the foodservice director and engineering as to the feasibility of implementation, what problems may be encountered, other ideas, and suggestions. Once they all agree, the foodservice director meets with employees to train them on new procedures/strategies. When the plan is implemented the director seeks employee input and suggestions, being flexible as appropriate, and if necessary, makes any needed changes. To know if the plan is working, all results (bad and good) are measured. The plan may still need some modification, so continue to involve employees and seek their input. Keep the employees informed. Continue to monitor the program.

Energy Conservation

Natural Gas

Natural gas is used in some foodservice operations, but it is also wasted. The Pacific Gas and Electric Company (www.fishnick.com) offers 10 ways to save on gas. I have listed the 10 steps. The full content of the paper is available at the web address listed above.

1. Turn it off, turn it down, keep it clean.
2. Specify ENERGY STAR steamers and fryers.
3. Pay attention to the thermostat.
4. Check the ductwork for leaks.
5. Set heated make-up air duct thermostats to 55°F.
6. Install low-flow pre-rinse spray valves.
7. Repair water leaks.
8. Maintain dishwasher and use it wisely.
9. Set the water heater thermostat at 140°F.
10. Use patio heaters wisely.

For each of these 10 points the handout lists cost savings in dollars and resources.

Air Pollution

For decades now, concerns about air pollution have commanded national and international attention. *Air pollution* is the presence of substances in the air in an amount sufficient to interfere directly or indirectly with human comfort, safety, and health. Most pollutants emerge from activities associated with human comfort and a life-

FIGURE 12.3   Energy Management Program

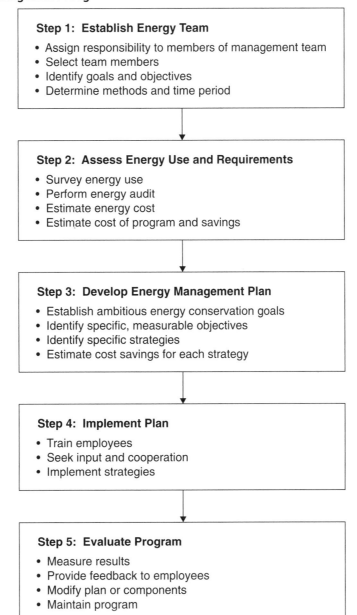

Step 1: Establish Energy Team
- Assign responsibility to members of management team
- Select team members
- Identify goals and objectives
- Determine methods and time period

Step 2: Assess Energy Use and Requirements
- Survey energy use
- Perform energy audit
- Estimate energy cost
- Estimate cost of program and savings

Step 3: Develop Energy Management Plan
- Establish ambitious energy conservation goals
- Identify specific, measurable objectives
- Identify specific strategies
- Estimate cost savings for each strategy

Step 4: Implement Plan
- Train employees
- Seek input and cooperation
- Implement strategies

Step 5: Evaluate Program
- Measure results
- Provide feedback to employees
- Modify plan or components
- Maintain program

style oriented to conveniences and possessions. Widely recognized pollutants are products of combustion and include carbon monoxide, sulfur, and nitrogen oxides, hydrocarbons, and other particulates. These pollutants have been linked to environmental concerns such as global warming (the greenhouse effect), ozone depletion, and acid rain.

Clean Air Legislation

The first *Clean Air Act* (Public Law 88–206) is a U.S. federal law enacted by Congress to control air pollution on a national level, and passed in 1963, that established a national program to control community air pollution. Subsequent legislation has included the Air Quality Act of 1967, which identified geographical areas with significant problems and designated air quality control regions, and the 1970, 1977, and most recently, 1990 amendments to the Clean Air Act (42 U.S.C.§ 7401) to improve the quality of the air we breathe. The goal of the 1990 amendments was to remove two-thirds of U.S. air pollutants by 2005. The act also contains regulations that will directly affect foodservice operations, in that it contains mandates affecting the production and use of chlorofluorocarbons (CFCs) and hydrochlorofluorocarbons (HCFCs). These gases are commonly used as refrigerants in air conditioners, dehumidifiers, freezers, and refrigerators. They cause little harm when contained in appliances, but scientists fear that they may contribute to the growing depletion of the earth's ozone layer when released in the atmosphere. In an

FIGURE 12.4   Foodservice Energy Management Survey

Instructions:

Questions have been divided into seven categories and points assigned to each question. Circle the points for each question if you can answer "yes" at least 90% of the time. Do not circle point value for a question answered with "no" or "not applicable."

At end of each section, total the circled points and record on the survey summary sheet. Record the points in each section that were not applicable for specific design of your operation.

Question	Points if Yes	Not Applicable
Category 1—Lighting		
1. Has a lighting survey been completed?	2	
2. Is sunlight used (and overhead lights turned off) during the day?	1	
3. Has lighting in storerooms and aisles been reduced to one-half of the tray line?	2	
4. Are lights turned off in the cafeterias when not in use?	2	
5. Have iridescent bulbs been replaced with fluorescent?	2	
6. Have rheostats been placed in large lighting-usage areas?	1	
7. Are lights cleaned at least monthly?	1	
8. Are timing mechanisms, dimmers, or automatic photocells used?	2	
Total Points for Category		

Category 2—Heating, Ventilation, Air Conditioning

(Thermostats save 5% off energy bills, for every degree you lower the thermostat below 70° in winter when occupied and 62° and when unoccupied; in the summer when occupied 79°–80° and unoccupied to 85°. The purchase of ENERGY STAR equipment may save money on energy over a period of time.)

Question	Points if Yes	Not Applicable
1. Can heat requirements be controlled by each area of the kitchen?	3	
2. Is heat-generating equipment placed so that heat can provide employee comfort?	2	
3. Are ventilation hoods designed to recirculate heat?	5	
4. Are filter hood screens cleaned weekly?	2	
5. Are hoods thermostatically controlled?	4	
6. Are hoods covering all ovens, grills, dishwashers, kettles, and steamers?	2	
7. Can air conditioning be adjusted for the kitchen?	3	
Total Points for Category		

Question	Points if Yes	Not Applicable
Category 3—Serving Area		
1. Are serving wells individually controlled?	1	
2. Are all serving wells covered when on?	3	
3. Is water in the serving wells (up to 50% saving over dry)?	3	
4. Is warm-up time for all hot wells, plate warmers, etc., controlled to 15 min. or less? (Follow manufacturer's recommendation)	3	
5. Are serving wells turned off 5 min. before the end of the serving period?	1	
6. Are compressor filters on carbonated beverage and juice machines cleaned weekly?	1	
7. Are warmers individually controlled?	1	
8. Are refrigeration units cleaned and free of ice?	2	
Total Points for Category		

Question	Points if Yes	Not Applicable
Category 4—Refrigeration		
1. Are compressor and condenser clean, maintained and serviced according to manufacturer's guide?	1	
2. Are thermostats set at maximum acceptable temperatures?	1	
3. Do all walk-in doors have automatic closers?	1	
4. Are food items unboxed before storage so energy is not used to cool cardboard boxes?	2	
5. Are issues designed so that all items needed for a meal are collected at the same time to reduce door openings?	4	
6. Do all items being refrigerated require refrigeration?	3	
7. Are frozen items defrosted in the refrigerator?	1	
8. Are hot foods cooled according to Food Code 2009 *before* placing in refrigerator?	4	
9. Are plastic airstrips curtains installed in all walk-in and freezer doors?	2	
10. Are hot uncovered liquids put in refrigerator?	1	
11. Are all door gaskets in good repair?	2	
Total Points for Category		

Note: This survey was developed by the Research and Development Committee of the American Society of Healthcare Food Service Administrators (ASHFSA) in 1979. Although this survey may be outdated and is no longer available from ASHFSA, it remains a helpful model for designing foodservice energy management surveys. Revised by Ruby P. Puckett 2010.

FIGURE 12.4   (*Continued*)

Question	Points if Yes	Not Applicable
Category 5—Sanitation		
1. Has dish machine temperature been lowered to the minimum 140°F wash, 180°F rinse (160°F if chlorine booster)? Or is the machine a machine with an internal vent, or one that uses final rinse water—recycled to the wash cycle?	4	
2. Are machines operated at least at 80 percent capacity?	4	
3. Is a chemical rinse used in pot washing instead of 180°F?	3	
4. Are the number of dishes rewashed below 1%?	3	
5. Are drain valves, overflow valves, and wash arms clear and leak free?	2	
6. Is the machine turned off between batches?	2	
7. Is a steam instead of electric booster being used?	2	
8. Are dishes being done in 2 hours per meal or less?	2	

Total Points for Category

Category 6—Production		
Steam		
1. Are all steam lines insulated?	2	
2. Are covers used when steam kettles are in use?	2	
3. Are gaskets and seals tight to prevent steam losses?	2	
4. Are kettles or steamers filled at least 60% before start?	2	
5. Are steam lines delimed at least every 6 months?	2	
6. Is hot water added to kettles to reduce energy demand?	1	
7. Are pressure steamers used in place of pressureless ones?	2	
8. Are small kettles available for sauce making instead of using the stovetop?	1	
Ovens		
1. Are preheat times limited to maximum of 15 min.?	3	
2. Are ovens loaded during warm-up where food quality is not affected?	2	
3. Are ovens used at full capacity?	3	
4. Are ovens turned off between meals?	3	
5. Is a thermometer with external gauge used to check roasts?	2	
6. Are oven timers used?	1	
7. Is the fuel–air ratio on gas ovens checked and/or adjusted at least monthly?	2	
8. Are ovens used at night (for roasting meat) at lower temperatures to take advantage of nonpeak energy charges?	5	
9. Are oven doors left closed during baking and roasting?	4	
10. Are ovens not used to hold food after preparation?	2	
11. Are oven thermostats checked weekly?	2	
12. Are sheet pans double-stacked where possible (e.g., bacon) to increase capacity?	2	
13. Are potatoes baked without foil wrapping?	2	
14. Are casserole dishes baked uncovered?	2	
15. Are microwave ovens used? (Microwaves use 85% less energy than a conventional oven and one-third the energy of a toaster oven)	2	
Grills and Griddles		
1. Are preheat times limited to 15 min.?	3	
2. Are charbroilers turned to medium after briquettes are hot?	2	
3. Are briquettes clean?	1	
4. Are griddles cleaned after every use?	2	
5. Are grills turned off during employee breaks?	3	
6. Are the lowest cooking temperatures possible used?	3	
7. Is maximum surface area used to decrease heat loss to air?	1	
8. Are ovens used instead of grills where possible?	1	
9. Is only that portion of the grill being used heated?	2	
10. On gas units, does the flame tip touch the heating plate?	1	

FIGURE 12.4 (*Continued*)

Question	Points if Yes	Not Applicable
Stoves		
1. Are preheat times limited to a maximum of 15 min.?	3	
2. Are kettles and pots larger than burners?	1	
3. Has foil been placed under range burners to reflect heat?	1	
4. Are only the units being used on?	3	
5. Are kettles covered with tight-fitting lids?	2	
6. Are ranges banked together to allow better insulation?	2	
Total Points for Category		

Category 7—Management of Facility		
1. Are all external doors closed when heating or air conditioners are being used?	3	
2. Are all windows closed when heat or air-conditioning is on?	3	
3. Has gas pressure been checked and compared with equipment demand?	2	
4. Does steam line provide the correct equipment steam pressure?	3	
5. Has a schedule of preheat times, cooking temperatures, and turnoff times been developed and implemented?	4	
6. Are energy areas balanced so that energy demands are constant (ovens turned off when dish machine is operating, etc.)?	4	
7. Have the foodservice energy demands been balanced with those of other departments so when the peak demand for the hospital is high, the energy demands by foodservice are low?	4	
8. Has your push on energy control been scheduled to coincide with the hospital's peak month of energy usage?	4	
9. Do the foodservice administrator and all supervisors know when the hospital's peak demand for energy is?	2	
10. Are new equipment purchases evaluated for reducing energy?	2	
11. Is there a routine maintenance program in place that follows the manufacturer's recommendation on maintaining the equipment?	4	
Total Points for Category		

Energy Management Survey Summary

Category	Possible Points (A)	Points Earned (B)	Points Not Appl. (C)	Percentage (A or B – C) × 100
1	13			
2	21			
3	15			
4	22			
5	22			
6	82			
7	35			
TOTAL	200			

Interpreting the Results:
Scores below 50 indicate a high potential for cost savings through effective energy management. Scores above 140 indicate that additional effort to conserve energy may not produce a high return on time spent. Initial energy management efforts should focus on the area(s) in which you scored less than 50 percent.

TABLE 12.2   Energy Conservation Practices

Area	Conservation Practice
Food preparation	<ul><li>Cook in largest volume possible.</li><li>Cook at lowest temperature that still gives satisfactory results and food is maintained in the safe zone.</li><li>Reduce excess heat loss by carefully monitoring preheat times, cooking temperatures, and maintenance checks, turn off when cooking task is complete.</li><li>Reduce peak loading. Examples: Use high-energy-demand equipment sequentially rather than simultaneously, if possible. Schedule energy-intense cooking, such as baking and roasting, during nonpeak demand time.</li><li>Heat only portion of griddle to be used.</li><li>Use hot tap water for cooking, whenever possible, except in localities where water contains concentrates of heavy metals.</li><li>Do not turn oven to highest temperature for preheating.</li><li>Do not turn oven until needed and turn off immediately when cooking process is complete.</li></ul>
Refrigeration	<ul><li>Open doors as seldom as possible.</li><li>Allow hot foods to cool briefly in accordance with safe food-handling practices [see Chapter 14].</li><li>Clean condenser frequently.</li><li>Keep thermometers properly calibrated.</li></ul>
Lighting	<ul><li>Turn off lights when not in use.</li><li>Install timing mechanisms, dimmers, or automatic photocell devices.</li><li>Color-code light control panels and switches according to a predetermined schedule of when lights should be turned on or off.</li><li>Compare the efficiencies of various types of lamps in terms of wattage, lifetime, and illumination when replacing lightbulbs.</li><li>Replace incandescent lamps with high intensity.</li></ul>
HVAC	<ul><li>Lower thermostat to 68°F in winter; raise to 79°F in summer. (These temperatures are for occupied buildings.)</li><li>Adjust duct registers to give the most efficient airflow within a room and balanced airflow between kitchen and service area if located adjacent to each other.</li><li>Stagger start-up time for individual HVAC unit to reduce demand for kilowatt-hour usage on your system and to eliminate unnecessary cooling or heating during hours before operation opens.</li></ul>
Sanitation	<ul><li>Turn off exhaust fan when not required.</li><li>Fill dishwasher to capacity with dishes, flatware. Do not wash dishes when there is not a full load. (Check out the new dishwashers that use recycled final rinse water for washing.)</li><li>Hot water booster should be within 5 feet of a dishwasher to avoid heat loss in the pipes.</li><li>Install a spring-operated valve on your kitchen and restroom faucets to save water.</li><li>Repair leaking faucets.</li><li>Implement effective maintenance program.</li></ul>

Abbreviation: HVAC, heating, ventilation, and air-conditioning.

Source: Federal Energy Administration, Office of Energy Conservation and the Environment, 1997. Additions made by Ruby P. Puckett 2010.

effort to control the release of refrigerated gases, section 608 of the Clean Air Act addresses the problem of recycling gases contained in home appliances such as freezers, refrigerators, and air-conditioning units. In 1992 this section of the Act was implemented. The law prohibits anyone from "knowingly venting ozone-depleting compounds used in refrigerators into the atmosphere while servicing, repairing, or disposing of air conditioners or refrigeration equipment." Violators may be fined up to $25,000 a day for noncompliance. The control provisions of the act are to be superseded by those of an amended Montreal Protocol (which lists ozone-depleting substances to be phased out) wherever the protocol is more restrictive. Studies indicate that some of the new substances are being used as replacements for the banned ones, and this may have the potential to change the ozone layer. Under the Montreal Protocol, 96 damaging chemicals have been banned and are being phased out. HCFCs will be fully phased out by 2030, and CFC12 was banned in 1996.

An increased cost of coolants, investment in recovery systems, service contracts, and replacement of older refrigerators will affect foodservice budgets. When selecting new refrigeration equipment, foodservice directors must determine the type of refrigerant used, its efficiency, and the expected date it is scheduled to be phased out. Maintenance of refrigeration equipment will become more critical as refrigerant replacement cost increases. Stricter emission standards have been adopted for selected pieces of production equipment (such as char broilers and fryers) in metropolitan areas that fail to meet EPA's air quality standards. When renovating production areas, it is important to check with the state and local air quality office to identify specific regulations that would dictate the type and quality of emissions allowed from an operation.

An alternative fuel such as biodiesel is a cleaner-burning, natural, renewable diesel fuel alternative. This alternative fuel is 20 percent biodiesel, made from soy oil or recycled cooking oil, combined with 80 percent regular petroleum diesel. The EPA has approved the mix to lower emissions of unburned hydrocarbons, carbon monoxide, sulfates, and other particulate matters that reduce air quality and harm the environment. The EPA completed a recent study on B20 biodiesel that shows the reduction of emissions of unburned hydrocarbons by 20 to 30 percent, carbon monoxide by 12 to 20 percent, and particulate matter by 12 to 22 percent compared with petroleum-based diesel. In addition to being cleaner burning, these alternative fuels are nontoxic, biodegradable, and be produced domestically. This lowers the U.S. dependence on foreign imports. Even though biodiesel is slightly more expensive than regular petroleum-based diesel fuel, the benefits of its use outweigh the cost.

The EPA and Congress are continuing to work on the quality of the air we breathe. In 2009, they made some changes in the "greenhouse" gases of the Clean Air Act under section 202(a). There is still much that needs to be accomplished—on a worldwide basis—and world leaders are struggling to develop a plan—hopefully before it is too late.

Tips to Save on Fuel Costs

Overall fuel cost may be reduced when a schedule is developed, followed, and carefully monitored for maintenance and cleaning of equipment. The foodservice manager should work with the facility engineer to develop an ongoing maintenance plan. Follow manufacturers' directions for cleaning the ventilation systems. The fire department should annually check the system to detect grease buildup. On a daily basis all faucets should be checked, and if a leak is found, it should be repaired immediately. As needed, water softeners may be added to the system to reduce cost for soap and detergents. All lights need to be turned off when leaving a room.

WATER CONSERVATION

Another valuable natural resource too often taken for granted by foodservice employees and consumers is water. The contamination of groundwater due to the approximately 60,000 industrial wastes and chemicals, rocket fuel found in many states, human and animal feces, medications and other wastes, landfill leachates (ash), and fertilizer and pesticides is even more prevalent today. In addition, excessive levels of lead and other heavy metals have been found in municipal water supplies.

Clean Water Legislation

The Clean Water Act was originally enacted in 1972 as the federal Water Pollution Control Act. Amendments to the original act were passed in 1977, 1981, and 1987 (the 1987 amendment is formally referred to as the Water Quality Act of 1987). In 1974 the Safe Drinking Water Act was passed to protect water sources. The act gives the Environmental Protection Agency (EPA) to set standards for drinking water. EPA works with public water sources to ensure that standards are met and the water Act (ACCWA) is followed. ACCWA has the same basic goal to protect all of the nation's water. There are some key changes in this bill. The Clean Water Act was implemented to improve the quality of water for human consumption through the elimination of pollution discharges into navigable rivers and to assist in the establishment of public water treatment facilities. Two separate standards were made to facilitate attainment of the goals of the act. These standards are receiving water quality standards and effluent standards. (Effluent means a stream flowing out of a body of water; water that flows out or forth.)

Selected foodservice operations have been affected by these standards as providers that exceed effluent standards are subject to fines. In most cases the operator has been forced to stop the use of garbage disposals. Also, where strainers have been added to pipes discharging water from ware-washing equipment, operations have had to identify alternative methods for collecting and disposing of food waste and scraps and trimmings from food preparation. Consultation with representatives from local wastewater (sewage) treatment plants or the director of facilities management will assist in determining local *water conservation* regulations.

The availability of safe water (*potable water*), in sufficient quantity to meet competing demands in health care operations and within the community will significantly influence operational decisions. Foodservice department areas that require large quantities of water include ware washing, ice machines, food preparation, drinking water, sanitation, and cooling and heating. Water conservation programs patterned after the energy management plan described earlier should identify specific strategies for each of the above areas. Following are some simple commonsense suggestions:

- Repair leaking faucets.
- Do not leave water dripping from faucets.
- Thaw frozen foods in the refrigerator rather than under running water.
- Wash only full loads of dishes.
- Evaluate water consumption requirements when selecting ware-washing equipment.
- Serve water only on request at catered meals.
- Evaluate feasibility of installing water saving devices in sinks and toilets.

The goal of a water conservation program is to preserve the water supply for the most critical needs within the health care operation and the larger community.

The need for clean potable water is a medical concern when patients with blood clots, heart disease, kidney stones, cancer, mental fuzziness, and fatigue do not have potable water to drink.

Patients need to be properly hydrated to meet the daily need for water.

Bottled Water

The International Bottled Water Association states that more than **8 billion gallons of bottled water** was consumed in the United States in 2009 and continues to increase. FDA regulates bottled water to ensure that bottled water is safe. Bottled water must meet these regulations:

- "Standard of identity" regulations that define different types of bottled water
- "Standards of quality" regulations that set maximum levels of contamination—including chemicals, physical, microbial and radiological contamination—allowed in bottled water
- "Current good manufacturing practices" (CGMP) regulations that require bottled water to be safe and produced under sanitary conditions

Types of Bottled Water

FDA describes bottled water as water that's intended for human consumption and sealed in bottles or other containers with no added ingredients except that it may contain salt and suitable antimicrobial agents. (Fluoride may also be added within the limits set by FDA.)

Common types of bottled water:

- Artesian well water
- Mineral water
- Spring water
- Well water
- Tap water

Bottled water may be used as an ingredient in beverages such as diluted juices or flavored bottle water. However beverages labeled as containing "sparkling water," "seltzer water," "soda water," "tonic water," or "club soda," aren't included as bottled water under FDA regulations. The beverages are considered be soft drinks. Bottled water comes under various labels with many different claims for health. If you drink bottled water check the list of the ingredients and cost.

The worldwide disposal of these bottles continues to be a major problem. Bottles have been found in all lakes, rivers, and oceans; beaches, woods, highways, and roads; and in the landfill. Some manufacturers have reduced the type and amount of plastic used in bottles to make them more biodegradable.

Ice

Foodservice operations use many tons of ice daily. Contamination of ice can occur by a variety ways. To protect the ice and the customers the following suggestions should be followed:

- Use only potable water to make ice.
- Store ice in a covered ice bin; keep covered when not in use.
- Wash hands **before** scooping or dispensing ice.
- Never use a glass to scoop; use only a nonbreakable scoop.
- Store scoop on outside of bin with handle up.
- Do not store in bin. (Check local regulations.)
- Clean and sanitize scoop daily by running it through the dishwasher.
- Do not store drinks or other food products in the bin.
- If any glass is broken in the area of the ice machine and the bin is open, remove and discard the ice. Clean thoroughly to ensure no glass is in machine.
- Frequently clean the ice bin.
- Drain. Use caution with chemicals used to clean—do not leave a residue.
- Follow manufacturer's instructions especially if deliming.

SUMMARY

Each of the environmental issues—sustainability, solid waste, hazardous waste, air pollution, energy conservation, and water quality—affects not only operational practices but also the costs of providing high-quality products and services to guests. Each waste management alternative carries with it pros and cons that must be assessed in terms of costs, effectiveness, storage capacity, and environmental effects. Because no one strategy will work for all foodservice operations, managers must look to the long term in selecting viable, cost-effective alternatives to waste management for their foodservice operations. Otherwise, the quality of life valued by most Americans will be threatened. For more information on federal laws, go to www.epa.gov.

KEY TERMS

4Rs (reduce, reuse, recycle, and rethink)
Air pollution
Clean Air Act
Composting
Energy management
Hazardous waste
Natural gas

Solid waste
Sustainability
Tipping fee
Waste audit
Waste stream analysis
Water conservation

1. What is the impact of sustainability on a foodservice operation?

2. Review the literature (see references at end of book) and discuss methods for reducing, reusing, recycling, and rethinking waste management and energy and water conservation.

3. Add other ways to save energy to Figure 12.4, the energy management survey.

4. Review the latest laws relating to clean air and discuss what method you can use to reduce the CO_2 in the air we breathe.

5. Make a list of all the bottled water on the market; compare ingredients and cost. What are the differences?

CHAPTER 13

MICROBIAL, CHEMICAL, AND PHYSICAL HAZARDS; TEMPERATURE CONTROL

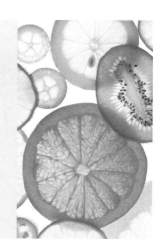

LEARNING OBJECTIVES

- Apply all regulations, rules, standards, and laws in providing safe food to customers.
- Know the pathogens that cause food-borne illness.
- Incorporate changes as printed in the latest issue of the *Food Code*.
- Use the most appropriate thermometers in food production and service.
- Conduct in-service educational programs on the various hazards found in a foodservice operation.
- Distinguish between biological, chemical, and physical hazards.
- Differentiate between food illness, food-borne infections, and food-borne intoxications.

FOODSERVICE DIRECTORS HAVE a responsibility to ensure that their operations serve food that is safe and free of contamination. There are three main causes of foodborne illnesses: improper temperature in storage (dry, refrigerated, and freezer defrosting), cooking (hot-holding, improper cooling) and reheating; second, poor personal hygiene (improper hand washing and use of gloves, infected persons handling food); and third, cross-contamination (contaminated prepared food and raw ingredients and contaminated food preparation surfaces). FDA estimates that 2 to 3 percent of all food-borne diseases can lead to secondary long-term illnesses. For example *E. coli* 0157:H7 can cause hearing failure in young children and infants. These causes illustrate that most food-borne illness can be prevented if food sanitation practices and temperature controls are an integral component of a continuous quality improvement program (Table 13.1).

In a study recently conducted by the Centers for Disease Control and Prevention (CDC), food-borne illness is a major economic and health problem costing $8 billion to $75 billion annually. Hospitalization is estimated to cost $3 billion annually, and lost-production costs are estimated to range between $20 billion and $80 billion per year. It is estimated that one case may cost more than $1 million; the average cost is $250,000. This cost includes medical care, lost wages, legal action, lost business, long-term disability, increased insurance cost, adverse publication for the organization, and investigation of food-borne outbreaks. The CDC estimates that the number of food-borne illnesses in the United States ranges from 24 million to 81 million, with 325,000 hospitalizations, and 5,000 cases of death per year. Research data from the CDC have shown a 23 percent overall drop for seven bacterial food-borne illnesses since 1996. The four major bacterial food-borne illnesses—those caused by *Campylobacter jejuni* (estimated annual number of cases 5,000,000 in 2009, estimated cost unknown); Salmonella species, all sources (estimated annual number of cases 1,397,187 in 2009, estimated cost $2,649,413,401); *Shigella toxin*–producing *E. coli* 0157 (STEC 0157) all sources (estimated annual number of cases 73,480 in 2009, estimated cost $478,381,766); *Listeria momocytogenes* (estimated annual number of cases 2,797, no cost information available) and non-0157 shigella toxin–producing *E. coli* (non-STEC 0157—all sources (estimated annual number of cases 31,229, no cost figures available). These numbers are staggering, as only 2 percent of all the cases are reported to CDC.

Health care foodservice operations should take particular caution to prevent food-borne illness caused by microbial (biological), chemical, or physical hazards. Highly *susceptible populations* are those consumers who are among the high-risk populations for contracting food-borne illness, and the symptoms are more server than the normal population who are at less risk. *At-risk*

TABLE 13.1 Estimates of Leading Causes of Food-Borne Illness

Pathogen	Percentage Testing Pathogen as Top Three Causes	Estimated Percentage of Food-Borne Illness Caused by Pathogen
Salmonella species	90	9.7
Escherichia coli 0157:H7	56	1.3
Staphylococci	36	1.3
Shigella species	32	0.6
Campylobacter jejuni	18	14.2
Listeria monocytogenes	16	<0.1
Hepatitis A virus	8	<0.1
Clostridium perfringens	8	1.8
Norwalk-like virus	5	66.7
Other viruses	4	67.2
Giardia lamblia	3	1.4
Streptococci	2	0.4

Source: Jones and Gerber, 2001.

groups—immune-compromised persons who cannot tolerate even small levels of microorganisms—include infants, fragile elderly, pregnant women, inpatients, malnourished individuals, those with controlled physical and metabolic disorders such as diabetes mellitus and high blood pressure, and persons with immune disorders. FDA stipulates that greater care must be taken when serving this population as their symptoms are greater, which leads to dehydration and malabsorption of nutrients and more difficult recovery.

Controls must be established throughout an operation. Employees should be trained in proper food-handling and sanitation practices. The importance of monitoring food-handling practices must be stressed to all supervisors. Purchasing food from reputable suppliers is essential in controlling food contamination and providing high-quality products. During production food must be handled safely, kept either hot or cold, and personnel must be free from infections.

The foodservice director's responsibilities include:

- Provide clean, properly equipped, and temperature-controlled storage and work areas that meet state and local health department standards.
- Purchase wholesome food from sources that meet the standards developed by regulatory agencies
- Receive and store such foods under conditions that maintain their wholesomeness and minimize the risk of contamination by microorganisms, insects, rodents, and toxic substances.
- Develop written policies and procedures for maintaining staff personal hygiene and for preparing and serving food safely on a daily basis.

- Develop written policies and procedures for cleaning and sanitizing equipment, utensils, and work areas.
- Dispose waste materials according to accepted sanitation principles and local health department regulations.
- Develop programs for training and supervising employees to ensure implementation of policies and procedures established by the department and approved by the facility's administration.
- Ensure that the person in charge (director) demonstrates knowledge of food-borne disease prevention, and the requirements of latest issue of the *Food Code* are followed.

To implement an effective sanitation program, all managers and employees must understand causes and preventive methods for protecting food from biological, chemical, and physical hazards that can result in food-borne illness. Each operation should have established procedures that minimize risk, monitor time and temperature and cross-contamination, and initiate hazard analysis critical control points (HACCP) practices. Maintaining a clean physical plant and conducting frequent self-inspections are essential components of this effort.

This chapter addresses how foodservice directors can help their operations protect workers and consumers against food-borne illness due to contaminated food, equipment, or work surfaces that come into contact with food. In addition, this chapter provides information for establishing and maintaining a sanitation program for training employees.

Food-borne pathogens that cause illness will be described so that managers can help guard against food-borne infections (for example, salmonellosis), food-borne intoxication (for example, staphylococcal contamination), and food-borne toxin-mediated infections (for example, gas gangrene caused by *Clostridium perfringens*). Other common pathogens in the United States are described, along with safeguards for suppressing them.

Hazards—chemical, physical—are discussed. The use of thermometers is outlined.

It is highly recommended that the foodservice department maintain a copy of the latest edition of the *Food Code, The Joint Commission Standards, OSHA regulations, OBRA Standards,* and CMS regulation, local and state regulations, department policy and procedure manuals and know and practice the rules, laws, regulations, and policies found in these regulations. A major part of the director's job is to employ and properly train employees on food safety.

CONTAMINATION BY MICROBIAL HAZARDS

Contamination is the presence of substances or conditions in food that can be harmful to humans. There are four sources of microbial contaminants that include: bacteria, viruses, parasites, and fungi. Bacteria and viruses pose the greatest safety challenges for all food establishments. Contaminants cannot be seen with the naked eye. Many types of food contamination can cause illness without a change in appearance, odor, or taste of the food. *Cross-contamination* happens when germs are transferred from one food item to the other, usually from raw food to ready-to-eat foods, by contaminated hands, equipment, utensils, unclean and unsanitized work surfaces, and unsanitized cleaning cloths used to wipe work surfaces. Microbial (biological) hazards cause the greatest number of outbreaks of food-borne illness and are the most difficult to control because they involve microorganisms. *Microorganisms* are microscopically small living creatures that multiply rapidly given the right environment and are the most common type of food contamination. Some microorganisms serve a useful purpose while others cause food-borne illness and are called *pathogens*. These microorganisms are classified into four major groups: bacteria, viruses, parasites, and fungi (specifically, yeasts and molds). Familiarity with each of these organisms and how they can lead to food-borne illness is essential to a foodservice director and the staff.

Bacteria

Of all microorganisms in a foodservice, bacteria are most abundant and are the most common cause of approximately 90 percent of food-borne illness. A *bacterium* is a small single-cell organism that, like all living organisms, requires nutrients and other environmental factors such as proper pH and temperature to survive. *Anaerobic* bacteria grow in an environment with little or no oxygen. These bacteria may grow in the center of a large quantity of food, such as dressing/stuffing. *Aerobic* bacteria require air to grow. Other bacteria that cause food-borne illness that can grow with or without oxygen are called *facultative*. Bacteria can exist in a *vegetative state*; during this phase all cells grow and reproduce, producing waste or *toxins* while other bacteria may produce *spores*. Spores are helpful to bacteria survival especially when the environment is too hot, dry, cold, acidic, or when food is limited, however spores cannot grow or reproduce. When food that contains vegetative cells and spores are heated to 165°F (74°C) the spores will survive (resist heat) and may change to vegetative when the food is not properly stored at the proper temperature or when not cooked properly.

Bacteria cause food-borne illness in one of two ways: as pathogens or as toxins released by the bacteria. Not all bacteria produce toxins. Some bacteria cause infectious diseases. *Pathogens* obtain their nutrients from potentially hazardous foods—meat, eggs, dairy—and reproduce rapidly in favorable temperatures. Other bacteria in and of themselves do not cause food-borne illness, but the toxins they release as waste and decomposed material into food products cause illness when eaten by humans. Examples of bacteria that produce toxins are *Salmonella* species, *L. monocytogenes, C. perfringens, Bacillus cereus, Clostridium botulinum, C. jejuni, E. coli* 0157:H7, *Staphylococcus aureus,* and *Vibro parahaemolyticus. Salmonella* species, *L. monocytogenes, C. jejuni,* and *E. coli* are most often linked to death from the illness. Features of bacteria are described in the following subsections.

Mobility

Bacteria have been described as "notorious hitchhikers" because of their attachment to humans. Bacteria are found in the hair; on the skin; on scars; under fingernails; on clothing; and in the mucous membranes of the nose, mouth, and throat of every individual. They are present in the intestinal tracts of humans and animals and are transported from place to place by the air, other human beings, water, food products, rodents, insects, and other animals. Because bacteria are everywhere, they frequently end up on human hands and, if proper hygiene and food-handling practices are not followed, end up in food products served to an operation's clients, employees, and visitors.

Growth and Reproduction

Bacteria grow by increasing their number through cell division rather than by increasing the size of individual cells. Thus, one cell becomes two, two become four, four become eight, and so forth. Bacterial growth follows a regular pattern on four phases. The first phase is the *lag phase* in which they increase little or not at all, and last a few hours at room temperature if the temperature is not kept below 40°F. The second phase is the *log phase*. At this phase bacteria grow very rapidly, doubling in numbers every few minutes. This is a critical phase and must be closely monitored. The third phase is the *stationary phase*, in which the number of new organisms being produced equals the number dying. The fourth and last is the *decline phase*. At this phase the bacteria began to die off due to the lack of nutrients and poisoning by their own toxins. The rate at which growth occurs varies among different kinds of bacteria. In approximately five hours one cell can produce 1 million cells. The rate of growth is affected by environmental temperature, moisture levels, available food sources, oxygen levels, acidity or alkalinity of the environment, presence or absence of inhibitors, and the length of time available for reproduction (Table 13.2).

The six conditions needed for bacteria to grow are **F**ood, **O**xygen, **T**emperature, **T**ime, **W**ater, and **A**cidity (often referred to by the mnemonics *FOTTWA* and *FAT TOM*).

Temperature

Temperature and time are the most critical factors affecting the growth of bacteria in foods. Bacteria grow over a wide range of temperatures. Even though most grow best between 60°F and 120°F (15°C and 49°C), some grow at even higher temperatures—from 110°F to 150°F (43°C to 65°C). Most disease-causing bacteria can grow within a temperature range of 41°F to 135°F (5°C to 57°C). This range is referred to as the *temperature danger zone*. Others live and multiply under refrigeration. By varying the temperature of the environment, bacterial growth can be increased, inhibited, or stopped altogether. Therefore, the growth of most bacteria can be inhibited—although not totally stopped—by reducing the temperature of foods to 41°F (5°C) or lower. This fact makes quick cooling and adequate refrigeration an important means of preventing food-borne illness caused by bacteria. Bacterial growth can be stopped completely by raising food temperature to a point at which pathogenic (disease-causing) bacteria are reduced through a process called *pasteurization*. This process heats the foods just long enough to destroy the pathogenic microorganisms; pasteurized foods still contain nonpathogenic microorganisms and spores. *Sterilization* is another process that uses heat to a point at which all pathogenic, spoilage, spore-forming, and toxin-forming organisms have been destroyed. At temperatures above 120°F (49°C)

FIGURE 13.1 Route of Food Contamination

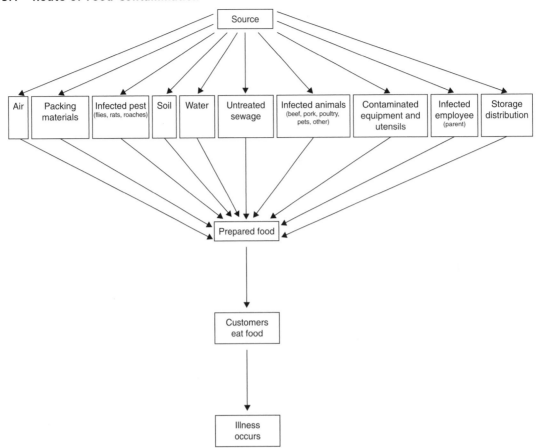

Note. Some causes of food contamination: (1) growing use of unapproved herbicides and pesticides; (2) use of water that contains a high amount of fecal matter; (3) sewage from septic tanks that leaked in water, floods, and the like; (4) employees with infectious disease; (5) infested with pest droppings, larvae, and possible metal or glass in products.

Source: Ruby P. Puckett 2010.

TABLE 13.2 Bacterial Growth Needs

Needs	Description
Food	Especially protein-rich food (such as meat, dairy, eggs, seafood), cut melons, garlic and oil mixtures, canned vegetables, unwashed fruits and vegetables, foods with a high moisture content (such as cooked rice, beans, and potatoes)
Acid	Most bacteria prefer a neutral environment of pH 7.0 but are capable of growing in food that has a pH range of 4.6 to 7.5
Temperature	Time and temperature are the most critical factors affecting the growth of bacteria in foods. Bacteria grow slowly at temperatures below 41° F (5°C) They begin to die at 135°F (57°C). Grow most rapidly in foods at 60°F to 120°F—keep it hot or keep it cold
Time	Bacteria go through a lag phase of little growth and continue to multiply until they reach a stationary phase and then decline; most bacteria multiply and increase in number by simple cell division. Bacteria need about 4 hours to grow high numbers to cause illness This is the total time food is between 40°F to 135°F Less than 2 hours refrigerate or use immediately. Between 2 and 4 hours use immediately. More than 4 hours throw it out. (There is some disagreement concerning the danger zone temperature: The *FDA Food Code* has identified the danger zone as 41°F-135°F)
Oxygen	Most bacteria (except *Clostridium botulinum*) need air
Water activity	Water activity (Aw) is the amount of water available for favorable growth of bacteria; (moisture) salt and sugar use the available water and can reduce microbial growth rate; Aw is the ratio of the vapor pressure of a food to that of pure water. Disease-causing bacteria can only grow in foods that have water activity higher than 0.85, for example, mayonnaise, raw bacon, American cheese, steamed rice, raw beef, halibut, egg yolks, egg whites. Water activity is a measure of how much water is available to the bacteria.

many bacteria begin to die or are injured; more are killed as food temperatures are increased. Because most bacteria are destroyed at 140°F (60°C), that temperature is recommended as a minimum temperature for cooking and holding foods. Figure 13.2 illustrates the effect of temperature on bacterial growth in food. Contamination usually occurs between preparation and serving, so it is important that the total time between preparation and service be limited to two hours. Food held longer than two hours must be immediately refrigerated at 41°F or below or heated to at least 165°F for 15 seconds. Otherwise, the food must be discarded. Some bacteria develop a heat-resistant form as they grow, posing another hazard. In this form, called a *spore*, the organism's capacity to survive under unfavorable conditions is increased. Spores are so resistant to the effects of heat that very high temperatures, such as those used for canning low-acid foods (240°F [115°C]), are required for their destruction.

Moisture

In general, bacteria need water to grow. The amount of water available to bacteria is decreased in the presence of high concentrations of sugar or salt. This fact explains some of the preservative effects of sugar and salt solutions. Similarly, when foods are frozen, no water is available to support bacterial growth. The drying of food also reduces the moisture content to levels that cannot support the growth of most bacteria, although spores may survive the drying process (Figure 13.3).

Bacteria cannot take their food in solid form. They must receive their nutrients in some kind of water solution. *Water activity* is a measure of the amount of water that is not bound to the food and is therefore available for bacterial growth. Water measures from 0 to 1.0. Disease-causing bacteria can grow only in foods that have a water activity higher than 0.85. Typical water activity limits

FIGURE 13.2 Effect of Temperature on Bacterial Growth in Food

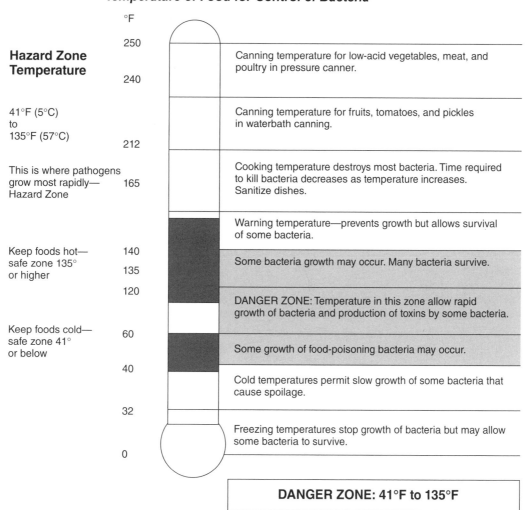

Temperature of Food for Control of Bacteria

Hazard Zone Temperature

41°F (5°C)
to
135°F (57°C)

This is where pathogens grow most rapidly—Hazard Zone

Keep foods hot—safe zone 135° or higher

Keep foods cold—safe zone 41° or below

°F
250
240
212
165
140
135
120
60
40
32
0

Canning temperature for low-acid vegetables, meat, and poultry in pressure canner.

Canning temperature for fruits, tomatoes, and pickles in waterbath canning.

Cooking temperature destroys most bacteria. Time required to kill bacteria decreases as temperature increases. Sanitize dishes.

Warning temperature—prevents growth but allows survival of some bacteria.

Some bacteria growth may occur. Many bacteria survive.

DANGER ZONE: Temperature in this zone allow rapid growth of bacteria and production of toxins by some bacteria.

Some growth of food-poisoning bacteria may occur.

Cold temperatures permit slow growth of some bacteria that cause spoilage.

Freezing temperatures stop growth of bacteria but may allow some bacteria to survive.

DANGER ZONE: 41°F to 135°F

Note. Temperature danger zone of bacterial growth is from 41°F to 135°F. Refrigerators must be cooler to facilitate this temperature. Within this range, growth of food-poisoning bacteria is possible. Food temperature should be within safe temperatures at which microbial growth is slow or nil: below 41°F and above 135°F.

FIGURE 13.3   Water Activity (A_w) or Moisture of Various Foods

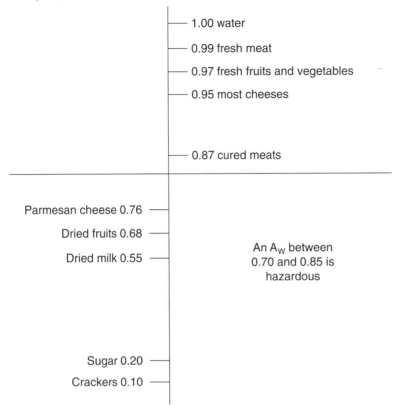

microbiological growth. Moisture and activity vary depending on the organism. Some bacteria can exist indefinitely in dry, powdered foods.

Food

Like all living organisms, bacteria need food to fulfill their energy needs and to provide the building blocks of their physical structure. Various bacteria have markedly different food requirements: Some can grow on glucose, ammonium salts, water, and certain mineral ions. Others require complex foods including vitamins, minerals, and proteins. The bacteria that cause food-borne illnesses thrive in many of the foods humans eat, especially in foods that contain proteins such as milk, milk products, eggs, meat, poultry, fish, and shellfish.

Acidity and Alkalinity

The *pH* symbol is used to designate the acidity or alkalinity of food. The pH is measured on a scale ranging from 0 to 14. Pure distilled water has a pH of 7.0. Slightly acidic (sour) foods have a pH of less than 7.0; neutral foods have a pH between 4.6 and 9.0; and slightly alkaline (bitter) foods have a pH above 7.0, which can support the growth of bacteria that cause food-borne illnesses. Such food materials include those of animal origin (such as meat, poultry, seafood, eggs, and milk) and low-acid vegetables (such as corn, peas, beets, and beans). Acids such as vinegar are used in food preserva-

tion to slow down bacterial growth and, in some cases, can be used in food preparation to inhibit bacterial growth. For example, commercial mayonnaise is acidic enough to suppress bacterial growth in salad mixtures when it is added early in the preparation process. Acidity also increases the sensitivity of bacteria to heat. For example, low-acid vegetables must be treated at a higher temperature and for a longer time in the canning process than is required for high-acid fruits.

Many bacteria prefer a neutral environment (pH of 7.0) but are capable of growing in foods that have a pH range of 4.6 to 9.0. Disease-causing bacteria grow best when the food they live on has a pH of 4.6 to 7.0; such foods include milk, fish, and meat. As the pH increases or decreases, the organisms adjust to their surroundings and then start growing again but more slowly. Some foods are naturally acidic (vinegar, pickles, fruits). At a pH of 4.6 (acidic) or below, organisms grow slowly or not at all.

Inhibitors

Many naturally occurring or manufactured chemicals, called *inhibitors*, can be used to prevent or slow down bacterial growth. For example, sodium nitrite (which is used in the curing of bacon, ham, and sausage) is effective in preventing the growth of *C. botulinum* (the organism that causes botulism) even at low levels of concentration; lactic acid and/or citric acid make more acidic food; salt, sugar, and alcohol lower water activity; and vacuum packing removes oxygen.

Time

Bacterial multiplication takes place over time. How rapidly bacteria grow depends on environmental conditions, including those factors already described. In foodservice operations, the objective is to keep foods at the recommended temperatures and under sanitary conditions for the recommended periods to prevent bacterial growth. Foods requiring refrigeration after preparation must be cooled rapidly to an internal temperature of 41°F (5°C) or lower. Large quantities of such foods need to be cooled in shallow pans, under quick-chilling refrigeration, or by cold-water circulation around the food container. The cooling time needed to reach 41°F (5°C) should be no more than four hours (140°F to 70°F, two hours, and to 41°F, four hours). On the other hand, cold foods should be heated as rapidly as possible to an internal temperature of 165°F (74°C) for 15 seconds or higher and should be held at that temperature for no more than two hours.

To reduce and/or prevent food-borne illness caused by bacteria, implement food safety policies:

- Promote good personal hygiene—only healthy workers should handle food, frequent hand washing, and proper use of gloves.
- Prevent cross-contamination—use clean utensils, keep all work spaces clean/sanitized, store foods properly.
- Use proper cooking methods.
- Keep hot food hot, keep cold foods cold—cook to proper internal temperature and hold at proper temperatures.
- Separate raw and cooked foods.
- Store foods in refrigerators where enough space will allow cold air circulation.
- Use proper *thawing techniques*—**never** thaw food on a counter because this allows food to be in the "hazard" zone for a length of time for bacteria to grow.
- Thaw food in a refrigerator at a temperature no greater than **41°F**.
- Food may also be thawed in an airtight, watertight bag submerged in **cold water that is changed every 20 minutes** or under running cold water.
- Foods may be thawed in a microwave, providing the food is cooked entirely after thawing.

Viruses

Viruses, another type of microorganism, are defined as noncellular organisms consisting of nucleic acids and protein that reproduce in host cells. They are the smallest and perhaps the simplest form of life and are a concern of foodservice managers because, unlike bacteria, viruses do not grow in food. Once viruses enter a living cell, they force the cell to stop its life processes and to assist in producing more viruses.

Sources of food-borne outbreak or water-borne viral disease include contaminated water supply, food handled by an infected employee who failed to follow correct personal hygiene practices, and, if eaten raw, molluscan shellfish (oysters, mussels, and clams) harvested from polluted water, iced drinks, water, salads, and ready-to-eat foods are the most sources of viral food-borne illnesses. The virus is found in urine and feces of infected persons and in contaminated water, cooked in polluted water, such as food from salad bars; and raw or slightly cooked shellfish, mussels, and oysters that live in polluted water. Any food not cooked before serving and handled by an infected person who practices poor personal hygiene can cause food-borne illness. To help control outbreaks, management should insist that all employees wash their hands thoroughly and often with hot water and soap, especially after toileting. As further assurance, shellfish should be purchased only from safe, certified sources, and potable water should be used to clean and cook foods. Use potable (safe) water for preparation and cleaning.

Parasites

Parasites are organisms that must live in or on a specific host to survive. They do not grow in food. Parasites can be either *invasive* or *noninvasive*. In the noninvasive stage a person may cough up the food parasite. In the invasive stage the parasite penetrates the lining of the stomach and small intestine and must be surgically removed. There are basically four types of parasites of importance to foodservice. They are nematodes (roundworms), trematodes (flukes), cestodes (tapeworms), and protozoa (one-celled parasites). Some food-borne parasites may be transmitted through contaminated water and food when these products are ingested by humans. Some live in food animals and are not digested. The parasites may contaminate drinking water, foods handled by infected persons, or vegetables and fruits grown on soils fertilized with feces.

Parasites are naturally present in many animals, such as pigs, cats, rodents, and fish. Pork and fish must be cooked to the proper temperature or food-borne illness could result.

Trichinosis, anisakiasis, giardiasis, and crytosporidosis are four major food-borne illnesses caused by parasites, while it is also important to recognize two other parasites—*Toxplasma gonndii* and *Cryptosporidiossis*. Trichinosis is caused by ingesting undercooked pork or wild game infested with the larvae of *Trichinella spiralis*. When humans eat undercooked, infected meat, trichinosis can result and in its severest form can be fatal. Hogs contract the disease by consuming infested uncooked garbage. Because most commercial pork producers no longer feed garbage to hogs, trichinosis is much less prevalent today than earlier in the 20th century.

Heating pork to an internal temperature of 137°F (58°C) destroys the parasite, although at this temperature pork is rare and pink and is not palatable. Current recommendations for cooking pork—chops, tenderloin medallions to an internal temperature of 145°F for 15 seconds (USDA recommends safe internal temperature for pork to be 160°F, newer technology suggest 145°). Pork cooked in a microwave should be cooked to 170°F. Processing at the temperatures used for ready-to-eat hams and canned hams also renders the meat free from potential contamination. Frozen storage at 5°F (−15°C) or lower for 20 days also destroys the organism that causes trichinosis. The FDA has approved the irradiation of pork to control *Trichibella spiralis*.

Another potential source of larvae is cross-contamination from equipment used first to grind pork infested with the parasite and then to grind other raw meat. Equipment used to grind raw pork should be thoroughly washed, rinsed, and sanitized before it is used for grinding additional ingredients. The larvae can be killed if pork products less than 6 inches thick are stored at 5°F (−15°C) for 30 days, −10°F (−23.3°C) for 20 days, or −30°F (−34.4°C) for 12 days.

Anisakiasis is caused by an *Anisakis* roundworm, which is found in some finfish bottom feeders, such as herring, cod, mackerel, and Pacific salmon. It can be invasive or noninvasive. Foods that potentially could contain this parasite include raw fish such as sushi, ceviche, salmon, herring, lightly cooked fish fillets, and some seafood salads.

Control measures include purchasing all fish products from reliable suppliers, obtaining guarantees that products have been properly frozen (−31°F [−25°C] or lower for 15 hours), and cooking fish to an internal temperature of 145°F (63°C). (Parasites in fish products can survive the acidity of marinades.)

Cyclospora cayetanensis is a parasite that is found in contaminated water, such as that used for irrigation, and can be transferred to food washed in contaminated water. Fresh fruits (raspberries, strawberries, blackberries) and vegetables can be contaminated at the farm. Cyclospora is passed from person to person by fecal-oral transmission. Contact with fecal-contaminated water or a contaminated food worker contaminates the food. Good sanitation and purchasing ready-to-eat foods from an inspected supplier are important.

Giardia lambia is a single-celled protozoan that causes giardiasis in humans. Human giardiasis may involve diarrhea within a week after ingestion of the organism. Other symptoms include abdominal cramps, fatigue, nausea, flatulence, and weight loss. The illness may last for one or two weeks, but the chronic infection may last from months to years. *G. lamblia* is shed in the feces of an infected individual and is transmitted by the fecal-oral route. Giardiasis is most frequently caused by the consumption of water contaminated by humans or domestic or wild animal feces. Infected food handlers and contaminated vegetables and fruits that are eaten raw have also caused giardiasis. Cool, moist conditions favor the survival of the organism. The use of potable water that has been properly treated and the education of employees about personal hygiene are a must. Thorough cooking of food destroys *G. lambia*.

Toxoplasma gonndii, a parasite found in cats, rats, mice, pigs, cows, sheep, chicken, and birds, can cause toxoplasmosis in humans. The parasites are found in red meat, especially pork, lamb, venison, and beef. Fruits and vegetables can be contaminated with feces.

Domestic cats appear to be the major source for transmitting the parasite to humans and other animals. Unborn babies can catch the parasite from their mothers if the mother is infected during pregnancy. Infestation with *T. gonndii* can result in the fetus being born with complications such as mental retardation, blindness, and epilepsy. To avoid infestation with the parasite, raw and undercooked meat should not be eaten. All fruits and vegetables should be washed before eating, and hands should be washed after handling raw meat and vegetables. Cross-contamination should be prevented.

Cryptosporidiosis is a parasite found in food that has been irrigated with contaminated water, feces from cows and other herd animals, and feces of people infected. The parasite can be spread from person to person in health care facilities and day-care facilities. Proper hand washing is a must as well as purchasing food from reputable suppliers.

Fungi

Fungi are plants that have no roots, stems, flowers, or leaves and do not contain chlorophyll. They obtain their food from nonliving organic matter or as parasites on living hosts. They need nutrients, warmth, and moisture to grow and grow best at temperatures between 80°F (27°C) and 90°F (32°C). They are identified by their velvety, colorful growth. They are destroyed by heat, a highly acidic environment, sunlight, ultraviolet light, or fumigation with ethylene oxide. Proper temperature in cooking and storage prevent the growth of fungi.

Yeast, single-celled organisms that reproduce by budding, is another group of organisms that are present on plants, fruits, grains, and other foods containing sugar. They are present in soil, in the air, in humans, and in food spoilage. (However, yeasts are also useful in the fermentation of wines and the leavening of bakery products.) *Budding* is the process by which a small part of the parent breaks off to form a new organism that is exactly like the parent. Because yeasts cause spoilage of many types of food, their growth should be controlled. Yeast does not cause food-borne illness.

Most yeasts grow best at room temperature, but some grow at the freezing point. Yeast growth is retarded or stopped at temperatures above 100°F (38°C). Yeasts require moisture and food sources such as sugars and acids for growth, which explains the abundant growth of yeasts in carbohydrate foods and in acidic liquids such as vinegar and wine. Yeast-based spoilage can be controlled by following adequate cleaning and sanitizing procedures that kill the cells readily at temperatures above the boiling point of water (212°F [100°C]).

Molds are microscopic fungi that can live on plants and animals. Most molds spoil foods. They are multicelled organisms that usually reproduce by spore formation. Mold spores are extremely small and light and most spoil food. Unlike bacteria, mold can grow in foods that are high acid and low moisture. They also need air to grow. They have branches and roots that look like very thin threads. The roots are difficult to see when mold is growing and may have penetrated deeply into the food. If you see mold on food, all of the product—not just the moldy portion—must be discarded.

The spores of mold can be transported by air currents, insects, water, and animals. Molds form spores when dry that float through the air and find suitable conditions to start growing again. Under favorable conditions, spores actively produce a fuzzy, filamentous growth on the surface of foods and other substances. While most molds like warm temperatures, however, they can grow in refrigerators temperatures—41°F (5°C) or colder. Molds also tolerate salt and sugar so they can grow in open jars of jam and jelly, on cured, salty meats such as ham, bacon, salami, and bologna. Some molds are useful in the manufacture of foods, such as Brie, Gorgonzola, and Stilton cheeses. Many molds spoil foods and, under some conditions, can develop highly poisonous by-products called **mycotoxins**, which can make a person sick.

Some molds produce toxins that can cause allergic reactions and respiratory problems, nervous system disorders, kidney and liver damage. Foods such as corn products, peanuts and peanut products, cottonseed, milk, tree nuts have been caused by **aflatoxin**, produced by molds.

Mold spores and vegetative growth can be destroyed easily by heat. Freezing prevents or reduces the growth of molds but will not destroy them. However, constant care is needed to keep work surfaces, containers, and equipment free from mold to prevent contamination of food products.

Natural Toxins in Food

There are at least 10 natural toxins in food. Four toxins will be discussed in this chapter: two fish toxins (Scombroid and Ciguatera), shellfish toxins, and mushroom toxin, the best known of the plant toxins. The other plant toxins will be listed. *Scombroid toxin* is found in scombroid fish, such as tuna, mackerel, bluefish, mahimahi, and amber jack when the fish begins to spoil. Most of these fish are found in temperate or tropical regions. *Scombroid poisoning* is caused by eating scombroid and other fish high in histamine. Histamine is produced when appropriate temperatures are not maintained, causing spoiling or decomposing, thereby releasing fish toxins that cannot be destroyed by freezing, smoking, cooking, canning, or drying. Fish must be purchased from approved sources.

Symptoms occur in minutes to two hours after eating and from four to six hours to one or two days. Symptoms include redness of face, sweating, burning feeling in tongue and mouth, dizziness, nausea, and headache, followed by rash, hives, and diarrhea.

Ciguatera is caused by the consumption of subtropical and tropical marine finfish and is more common in the Pacific area, and throughout the Caribbean and Indian Oceans, where small fish feed on toxic algae; larger fish eat the smaller fish and the toxin collects. The common fish indicated in *Ciguatera poisoning* are grouper, barracudas, snappers, jack mackerel, and triggerfish. When humans consume the larger fish, they can become ill with a combination of gastrointestinal, neurological, and cardiovascular disorders that may last months or years depending on the severity of the illness. Fish from these waters must be purchased from approved suppliers.

Shellfish associated with toxins include clams, oysters, mussels, scallops, especially shellfish harvested along the Florida coast and the Gulf of Mexico. Shellfish come from many different waters (oceans). Above all, never buy shellfish unless you know the kind, where it was harvested, and the reputation of the supplier. Always seek a vendor certification.

Plant Toxins

There are some *mushrooms* that are toxic. Cooking and freezing of toxic mushrooms will not kill the toxin. When purchasing mushrooms specify by name the type you are ordering. When receiving the product check it to determine if it what you received was what you ordered (check www.mushroomcouncil.org, who will provide information on all types of mushrooms, how to cook, store). When wild mushroom species are picked in the wild the foodservice director must assure that the mushrooms were individually inspected and found safe by an approved mushroom identification expert.

Other Plant Food Toxins

Plant food toxins may be found in:

Honey from bees that gathered nectar from mountain laurel and rhododendrons	Milk from cows that have eaten snake root
	Crocus seeds
	Raw cassava roots
Apricot kernels	Sun-burned green potato skins
Fava beans	Raw castor beans
Jimson weed	Hemlock flowers and leaves
Rhubarb leaves and roots	

POTENTIALLY HAZARDOUS FOODS

Potentially hazardous foods (PHFs) are those that are usually high in protein or carbohydrates and have a pH above 4.6 and water activity above 8.5 and require time and temperature to prevent the growth of microorganisms and produce toxins. The 2009 Food Code of the Food and Drug Administration (FDA) includes the following foods as PHFs:

- Food of animal origin that is raw or heat treated, raw poultry, raw eggs, unpasteurized milk and milk products, raw shellfish and crustaceans, fish, raw ground meats—beef, lamb, pork
- Food of plant origin that is heat-treated or consists of raw seed sprouts, cut melons, and garlic-and-oil mixtures that are not modified to inhibit the growth of microorganisms, baked potatoes, cantaloupe (melons), heat treated rice, beans, vegetables, and tofu or other soy-protein foods
- Cut greens must meet the time and temperature control for safety of foods as outlined in Food Code 2009 Chapter 3 Standards 3.501.17 and 3.501.18 and recommendations to Food Establishments for Serving Cut Leafy Greens is summarized in Annex 2
- Food Code prohibits food prepared in a private home to be used for human consumption in a food establishment
- Juice must be pasteurized or otherwise treated to obtain a 5-log reduction, which is equal to a 99.99% reduction of the most resistant microorganism or be obtained from a processor with a HACCP system. When not processed as described above, a label that states, "This product has not been pasteurized and therefore, may contain harmful bacteria that can cause serious illness in children, the elderly, and persons with weakened immune systems" must be added to the container.

PHFs always require special handling because they have been associated with most food-borne illnesses.

FOOD-BORNE ILLNESSES

Thousands of cases of food-borne illness are reported to the U.S. Public Health Service annually. *Food-borne illness* is a disease carried or transmitted to people by food. Factors that contribute to food-borne illnesses include:

- Improper cooling
- Lapse of 12 or more hours between preparation and consumption
- Improper holding
- Infected persons, poor personal hygiene
- Inadequate heating
- Improper cleaning/sanitizing of equipment
- The remaining factors include: use of leftovers, cross-contamination from raw to cooked food; inadequate cooking; using containers that add toxic chemicals; intentional chemical additives; and food from an unsafe source (the three main sources include bacteria, poor temperature control, and cross-contamination)

The symptoms of food-borne illness vary from "flulike" symptoms to death. In addition, many thousands of cases go unreported. Food-borne illnesses are identified by various degrees of upset stomach, nausea, vomiting, diarrhea, intestinal cramps, dehydration, fatigue, and fever. In more life-threatening types of infections, symptoms can include headaches, anorexia, mucosal congestion, malaise, and bloody diarrhea. Certain members of the population are highly susceptible to food-borne illness. They include infants and young children; the elderly; pregnant women; those with suppressed immune systems, cancer, or diabetes; and people taking certain medications. For these individuals, the symptoms and duration of the illness can be much more severe, even life-threatening. These illnesses are classified as food-borne infections; food-borne intoxications; or food-borne, toxin-mediated infections. Physical and chemical hazards also can cause food-borne illnesses.

Food-Borne Infections

Food-borne infections are diseases resulting from eating foods contaminated with toxic chemicals or pathogenic organisms. *Food-borne disease outbreak* is an incident when two or more people experience a similar illness after eating a common food and a laboratory analysis confirms that the food came from the same source. The growth and activity of the infectious agent itself—bacterium, virus, or parasitic organism—in the human digestive tract causes them. Because illness results from the activity of a large number of cells, the time lapse between ingestion of the contaminated food and onset of symptoms may be 1 to 48 hours. During the hours before symptoms appear, the organisms actively multiply in the digestive tract.

Salmonella (more than 200 types) is the most frequently occurring food-borne infection; Salmonella bacteria of several different types cause salmonellosis. The bacteria are common in the intestinal tracts and feces of humans, animals, poultry, and shellfish from polluted waters. *Salmonella* contamination occurs in a continuous cycle: animals, rodents, and birds that excrete the bacteria and humans who have had the illness and who may remain carriers for some time. The microorganisms are discharged into sewage and manure and can be found in contaminated soil and sewage-polluted waters. During the slaughter of food animals, equipment and employees in the packing plant can become contaminated. In addition, the food animals themselves often are contaminated during processing. Frequently, waste products from the slaughterhouse are made into animal feeds, and viable. *Salmonella* may be transmitted back to farm animals and pets when animal feeds are improperly processed. Thus, bacteria can be found on fresh meat, poultry, shelled or cracked eggs, cheese, contaminated fresh fruits and vegetables, and shellfish from contaminated waters. Bacteria also can be found in foods made from these products and contaminated during preparation. The presence of *Salmonella* bacteria in food is unnoticeable because the appearance, flavor, and odor of the food usually are not changed.

Symptoms of salmonellosis vary in severity, depending on an individual's susceptibility to the infection, the total number of cells ingested, and the bacterial strains involved. Symptoms include nausea, vomiting, abdominal pain, diarrhea, headache, chills, weakness, drowsiness, and possibly fever that usually appear 8 to 72 hours after eating and may last four to seven days, but it may linger. A serious illness can occur if the infection spreads from the intestine to the bloodstream. Without treatment, death may result. *Salmonella* may be found in the feces of personnel who are in the recovery stage, as it may take weeks to recover. Employees who have recently been diagnosed and been off work should have a physician's release to report back to work.

Salmonellosis can be avoided by reducing the possibility of food contamination during handling and processing by adequately cooking vulnerable foods (which can be contaminated even under the best processing conditions), and by preventing the cross-contamination of foods during the preparation process. Therefore, preparation surfaces and cutting boards should be sanitized after each use. Employees should wash their hands thoroughly with soap and hot running water before handling any other food products. Use meat and eggs that have been irradiated. Avoid eating raw or undercooked eggs and other fresh poultry and beef. Employees who have been diagnosed with *Salmonella* should not be allowed to work until released by a physician. *Salmonella* infection may also be acquired from pets, particularly chicks, ducklings, and turtles.

Food-Borne Intoxications and Toxin-Mediated Infections

Food-borne intoxication is caused by eating food that contains a harmful chemical or toxin produced by bacteria or other sources. Toxin-mediated infections are caused by eating a food that contains harmful microorganisms that will produce a toxin once inside of the body. A toxin-mediated infection is different from an intoxication because the toxin is produced inside the body.

The toxins cause food intoxication from living organisms. When food has been contaminated with toxin-producing microorganisms, the toxins may cause disease even after the microorganisms have been killed. These poisonous substances are not destroyed at normal cooking temperatures nor do they change the flavor, appearance, or odor of the food they permeate.

Staphyloccus aureus bacteria are responsible for frequent outbreaks of food-borne illness. The most common source of staphylococcal contamination is the human body, where organisms are found on the skin and in the mouth, nasal passages, and throat of healthy people. Infected pimples, sinuses, and cuts also are reservoirs for the organism. Food supplies and household pets also can be sources of *S. aureus*. Toxins are produced when foods that support the growth of staphylococci are contaminated with the organism and are allowed to stand for a sufficient period at temperatures favorable for bacterial growth. Although the bacteria are killed when subjected to temperatures as low as 140°F (60°C) for 10 minutes, toxins are highly resistant to heat, cold, and chemicals. Freezing, refrigerating, or heating foods to serving temperatures does not significantly reduce the amount of toxin. The more toxins a person ingests, the greater the reaction of the body.

Foods high in protein readily support the growth of staphylococci and have been involved in many outbreaks of food poisoning. Such foods include custards; meat sauces and gravies; fresh meats; cured meats; meat products; roasted poultry and dressing; poultry, egg, and fish salads and mixtures; raw milk; puddings; and cream-filled pastries. Any food that requires a considerable amount of handling during preparation is a possible source of food poisoning, particularly if it is not kept at safe temperatures during or after preparation.

Symptoms of staphylococcal infection usually occur two or three hours after consumption of the toxin-containing food. However, the time may vary from 30 minutes to 6 hours. Specific symptoms of staphylococcal food intoxication include nausea, vomiting, diarrhea, dehydration, cramps, and prostration. Symptoms typically last one to three days; the young and the elderly have a more severe illness.

C. perfringes bacteria have been identified as the cause of numerous cases of food-borne, toxin-mediated infections in recent years. The reasons for this may be better identification techniques and increased reporting of food-borne illnesses rather than actual increases in the occurrence of contamination and illness. The foods most often involved in outbreaks of illness are meat and poultry products that have been cooked and held for long periods or that have undergone prolonged slow cooling followed by reheating to improper temperatures and further holding.

C. perfringens bacteria are commonly found in the intestinal tracts of healthy humans and animals and in soil, water, and dust. The bacteria are able to form spores that are difficult to destroy by heating alone. The growing cells in food are destroyed through cooking. However, because cooking does not kill spores, cooking cannot be relied on to remove the threat of poisoning from these bacteria. The organisms can grow over a wide range of temperatures and are so widespread that it is impossible to reduce their incidence. Consequently, either the spore or the vegetative form should be assumed to be present in foods.

In relatively little time, under anaerobic (oxygen-free) conditions at temperatures of 60°F to 120°F (15°C to 49°C), a large number of these bacteria can develop. An anaerobic condition is produced in meat or meat-containing liquids after air has been eliminated from the food by heating. This condition allows the surviving spores to germinate and multiply rapidly in warm foods.

Large quantities of meat broths, gravies, and meat mixtures that are permitted to cool slowly provide an ideal medium for growth.

The symptoms of *C. perfringens* illness are relatively mild but include the following: abdominal cramps, diarrhea, nausea (occasionally), and fever or vomiting (rarely). Symptoms usually begin between 8 and 22 hours after eating the contaminated food, but they have been observed as early as 2 hours after eating. Symptoms usually last 24 hours. In the elderly the symptoms may last one to two weeks. Complication and death occur only rarely.

Preventing food-borne, toxin-mediated infection from *C. perfringens* requires cooking high-protein foods, particularly meat and poultry, well enough to kill the vegetative forms of the organism. Prevention also involves keeping foods hot (above 140°F [60°C]) until they are eaten. In addition, promptly refrigerating foods in shallow containers for quick temperature reduction slows down multiplication of the vegetative forms of the bacteria.

Other Food-Borne Illnesses

Although the major causes of food-borne illnesses are *Salmonella, Listeria* and *Campylobacter* and *E. coli*, many other microorganisms can cause serious and even life-threatening food-borne illness. Some pathogens that have resulted in food-borne illness are discussed in the following section on emerging pathogens. Other illnesses caused by microorganisms include typhoid fever; paratyphoid fever; streptococcal, shigellosis, or bacterial dysentery; and amebic dysentery.

Prevention of *Bacillus cereus* illnesses requires high standards of personal cleanliness, good work habits, safe water supplies, and exclusion of disease carriers from food preparation jobs. Prevention also requires that foods be cooked, chilled, and held at appropriate temperatures.

Botulism is a type of food-borne intoxication that is almost always fatal. It is rarely a problem when commercially canned foods are used but a serious threat to consumers of home-canned foods. The spores are heat resistant and can survive foods that are incorrectly or minimally processed. Most outbreaks are due to inadequately processing home canned foods, such as sausage, meat products, canned vegetables, and seafood.

A toxin produced by various strains of *C. botulinum* causes botulism. These bacteria grow in low-acid foods that have not been processed at temperatures high enough to destroy the bacterial spores. Only commercially processed vegetables, meats, and other low-acid foods should be purchased. Foodservice employees should never open or use a canned food when the can is bulging, severely dented, or leaky. Such canned goods must be discarded immediately.

CDC states that potatoes or any crop that come in direct contact with soil can easily be contaminated with *C. botulinum,* though cooking usually kills the organism's spores the source of the toxin. Foil-wrapped potatoes hold in moisture that prevents the surface from reaching a high enough temperature to kill the spores. The heat kills off other bacteria, which makes it easier for *C. botulinum* to grow. At room temperature foil-wrapped potatoes provide an oxygen-free environment needed for the toxins to form. Eat within **two hours** of cooking or unwrap and place in refrigerator. Do **not** leave at room temperature for more than **two hours**.

EMERGING PATHOGENS

Until recently, food-borne illnesses in the United States were linked to four well-known pathogens: *S. aureus*, *Salmonella* species, *C. perfringens*, and *Bacillus cereus*. Several other pathogens often referred to as *emerging pathogens* have been identified as important causes of food-borne illness and even death. Examples of emerging pathogens of particular concern to foodservice operations include *C. jejuni*, *L. moncytogenes*, Norwalk virus, and enterohemorrhagic *E. coli* 0157:H7. These pathogens are often transmitted to the food supply through contaminated water or raw manure, carried by humans, or transferred to food products during processing.

Campylobacter Jejuni

Campylobacteriosis is a food-borne infection caused by the pathogen *C. jejuni*. The bacterium is a nonforming anaerobic pathogen widely found in nature. The organism is carried in the intestinal tracts of cows, pigs, sheep, and poultry and frequently contaminates foods of animal sources. Other foods such raw milk, fresh mushrooms, and raw hamburger may be contaminated with *C. jejuni*.

Raw milk or contaminated water causes most outbreaks of campylobacteriosis. Food-borne outbreaks have been linked to raw or undercooked meat, poultry or seafood or being recontaminated after cooking by contact with *C. jejuni*–contaminated materials such as cutting boards.

C. jejuni is sensitive to heat and temperatures below 86°F (30°C) and may be easily destroyed through proper food-handling practices. The growth of this bacterium quickly declines at room temperature and more slowly at refrigerated temperature. The organism also is sensitive to acidic conditions.

Symptoms include fever, headache, and muscle pain followed by diarrhea (sometimes bloody), abdominal pain, and nausea. Onset is two to five days after eating and may last 7 to 10 days. It may spread to the bloodstream and cause serious life-threatening infection.

Listeria Monocytogenes

Although *Listeria*, a related group of bacteria, has been classified as a human pathogen for more than 60 years, the importance of food as a transmission vehicle has been identified only in recent years. *L. monocytogenes* is the species of bacteria that can cause listeriosis. The source of the bacteria is most often contaminated food.

Cross-contamination can pose serious health risks. For example, if certain cheeses that have been contaminated with *L. moncytogenes* come in contact with raw food such as meats, poultry, fish, or raw vegetables, including cantaloupe after the package is opened, the result may be significant growth of the organism at refrigerated temperature.

Individuals most susceptible to listeriosis are persons older than 60, newborns, and patients whose immune systems are compromised by cancer, acquired immunodeficiency syndrome (AIDS), or immunosuppressive medications such as steroids. Individuals suffering from cirrhosis, diabetes mellitus, and ulcerative colitis are more at risk. One-third of all cases of *L. moncytogenes* occur during pregnancy. Complications including miscarriage, meningitis, septicemia, pneumonia, and endocarditis can result from serious cases of listeriosis.

Individuals in these high-risk populations are advised not to consume pâté or low-acid soft cheeses such as Mexican-style cheese, Brie, feta, bleu cheese, Camembert, and chitterlings. These foods have been associated with greater incidences of listeriosis. Other foods that have been found contaminated with these bacteria include raw soil-grown vegetables such as cabbage, celery, and lettuce; unpasteurized milk; raw meat; and poultry.

L. monocytogenes is particularly problematic in foodservice operations because the bacteria grow slowly at refrigeration temperatures (32°F to 34°F [0°C to 1°C]) and on moist surfaces. Procedures to avoid cross-contamination during preparation and service should be followed by all food handlers. Because *L. monocytogenes* can grow on wet floors, on sponges, and in drains, foodservice managers should insist on clean, dry facilities and the avoidance of the use of sponges in the department.

Public health officials recommend that food-processing plants and foodservice operations implement the HACCP system to control transmission of *L. monocytogenes* during processing. Listed below are some specific recommendations for consumers and foodservice employees to consider in efforts to decrease the risk of listeriosis and other food-borne illness.

- Wash hands often in hot soapy water.
- Monitor the temperature of food products and the length of time they are exposed at room temperature.
- Clean and wash **all** raw fruits and vegetables thoroughly.
- Quickly chill products.
- Thoroughly cook all food of animal origin, including eggs, to recommended internal temperature, and reheat leftovers thoroughly—to the recommended internal temperature and time.
- Avoid cross-contamination between raw and cooked products especially when using cutting boards.
- Never purchase raw or unpasteurized milk.
- Thoroughly heat refrigerated foods, including ready-to-eat meats and minimally processed foods such as sous vide products.
- Use hot soapy water and clean mops and brooms to clean up liquid spills in refrigerators.
- Discard any food past "use by date" or expiration date.
- Compounds proved to be particularly effective in inhibiting or inactivating *L. monocytogenes* include iodine (25 parts per million [ppm]), acid sanitizers (130 to 200 ppm), and quaternary ammonium compounds (200 ppm). Also effective is chlorine at different concentrations such as 20 ppm for water treatment and 200 ppm for cleaning walls, stainless steel equipment, and nonporous surfaces. Follow the policies and procedures of your facility and manufacturer's recommendation.

Bacillus cereus is a spore-forming bacterium that can survive without oxygen. There are two types of *B. cereus* illnesses, diarrheal and vomiting. *B. cereus diarrheal* type of food poisoning has an onset of watery diarrhea, abdominal cramps, pain occurs 6 to 15 hours after eating the contaminated food. Symptoms persist for approximately 24 hours. *B. cereus vomiting* is characterized by nausea and vomiting within 30 minutes to 6 hours of eating the contaminated food. Symptoms last less than 24 hours. Foods that cause the diarrheal type include a wide variety of foods, including meat, milk, vegetables, and fish. The vomiting type of illness is usually associated with rice products, and other starchy foods such as pasta, potatoes, corn, cornstarch, soybeans, tofu, flour, and cheese products. Food mixtures such as sauces, puddings, soups, casseroles, pastries, and salads have also caused the vomiting type of *B. cereus*. (Most of the products contain cornstarch or flour.) Improperly stored food (hot-held, cooled) that allows the spores to become vegetative cells may cause the disease. Foods must be cooked and if not immediately eaten held at 140°F (60°C) or above. Foods must be cooled rapidly to 41°F (5°C) prior to storage.

Shigellosis are facultative anaerobic bacteria that cause about 10 percent of the food-borne illnesses in the U.S. Shigellosis is a gastrointestinal disease. The organism is found in the intestines and feces of humans and warm-blooded animals. The bacterium produces a toxin that causes watery diarrhea. Shigellosis is transmitted through the fecal route. A person may contract shigellosis by ingesting fecal material–contaminated food and water, by utensils handled by workers who are carriers of the bacteria, and by fruit and vegetables washed in contaminated water. The most common symptoms are bloody diarrhea, fever, abdominal cramps, chills, fatigue, and dehydration. Onset is one to seven days. This is an extremely contagious disease. The best prevention method is proper and through hand washing especially after using the toilet. Cook foods to appropriate temperatures, avoid cross-contamination, and carefully and thoroughly wash **all** fruits and vegetables in potable water.

Vibrio

Vibrio infections are bacterial in nature, resistant to salt, and are common in seafood. This group of bacteria includes *Vibrio parahaemolyticus* (moderate hazard), *Vibrio cholerae* (severe hazard), and *Vibrio vulnificus* (severe hazard). *V. parahaemolyticus* is natural in certain species of saltwater fish and seafood. *V. cholerae* is spread by fecal contamination, especially in seafood harvested from polluted waters.

These bacteria are natural to certain saltwater species, not a result of pollution, and can kill at-risk individuals who have liver damage. They are associated with the ingestion of raw, improperly cooked, or cooked recontaminated fish, shellfish, or crustaceans. The main problem is from oysters harvested between Texas and Florida from April to October, when *V. vulnificus* thrives in warm Gulf Coast waters. During these months 85 percent of illness occurs. *V. vulnificus* is the leading cause of reported deaths from food-borne illness in Florida. In 1992 11 persons were infected from raw oysters and 9 died. The Florida Administration Code 64D-3,013(6)(a) states that establishments serving raw oysters are required to display "either on menus, table tops or elsewhere in *plain view of all patrons* the following notice:

Consumer Information:

There is a risk associated with consuming raw oysters.

If you have a chronic illness of the liver, stomach, or blood or have an immune disorder, you are at greater risk of serious illness from raw oysters, and should eat oysters fully cooked.

If unsure of your risk, consult a physician.

(Department of Business and Professional Regulations State of Florida Administrative Code)

Molluscan shellfish should be obtained from sources according to law and the requirements specified by the U.S. Department of Health and Human Services, Public Health, FDA, and the National Shellfish Sanitation Program Guide for Control of Molluscan Shellfish. When molluscan shellfish are received via interstate commerce it shall be from sources that are listed in the Interstate Certified Shellfish Shippers List (Food Code 2009).

Cooking to the required internal temperature easily kills *V. vulnificus*, and most healthy people who eat oysters raw are not threatened. To be protected purchase oysters from an approved reputable dealer.

The FDA states that the people at risk of *V. vulnificus* infection are those with:

- Liver disease, including hepatitis, cirrhosis and cancer of the liver
- Diabetes mellitus
- Cancer, especially those undergoing treatment
- Immune disorder, including human immunodeficiency virus (HIV) infection
- Long-term steroid use for asthma or arthritis
- Hemochromatosis, an iron disorder
- Elderly age
- Stomach problems, including previous stomach surgery and low stomach acid from antacid use
- Regular alcohol consumption

Symptoms include diarrhea, abdominal cramps, fever, chills, skin rashes/lesions that may develop quickly and erode into necrotic ulcers, and sometimes vomiting and nausea or blood or mucus in stools. Diarrhea may be severe, and death may occur due to a sharp drop in blood pressure with possible intractable shock.

Viruses

Viruses are the smallest of the microbial contamination. Viruses do not multiply in foods, but once inside a human cell, they will produce more viruses. Viruses may be transmitted to food by the fecal-oral route, either directly or indirectly. The direct route is through an infected employee who has contaminated the food. The indirect route is when food has been contaminated in waters infected by untreated sewage. Viruses are classified as an infection. Good personal hygiene and health of the food handler are a must. Purchasing food from a certified source is required to ensure safety. In addition to the major pathogens listed earlier, the following are causing increasing concern for producing food-borne illnesses: The

Norwalk virus family is considered an emerging pathogen and a moderate hazard with potentially extensive spread. *Norwalk (Norovirus)* is a viral illness that has as its source human carriers; raw vegetables fertilized with manure or contaminated from fecal materials; water supplies (from municipal supplies, wells, recreational lakes, swimming pools, and water stored aboard cruise ships); manufactured ice cubes; shellfish (especially clams and oysters when eaten raw or insufficiently cooked); and prepared salads, especially coleslaw and eggs. The symptoms of the virus include nausea, vomiting, diarrhea, abdominal pain, 24 to 48 hours after ingestion. The illness lasts 24 to 48 hours, but may be found in feces for days after the symptoms end. Because it is a virus, it does not reproduce in food but remains active until the food is eaten. The following methods should be used to control this pathogen:

- Use potable water (water safe to drink).
- Follow all sanitary procedures to avoid fecal contamination from food handlers.
- Purchase shellfish from a certified supplier.
- Thoroughly wash all foods in potable water, and thoroughly cook them.
- Do not let a food handler work if he or she has diarrhea or has been diagnosed with a Norwalk disease.
- Wash hands using appropriate technique, using potable water.

The virus can withstand freezing temperatures and chlorine sanitizing agents. It is susceptible to high temperatures, and cross-contamination should be avoided.

Hepatitis A is another viral infection. The chief sources are shellfish harvested from contaminated water, raw vegetables that have been irrigated or washed with polluted water, and human carriers with poor personal hygiene who handle food that will be eaten raw or equipment that has been used by an employee with feces on hands. The onset is 15 to 50 days after eating the product. A person who develops *hepatitis A* is infectious 14 days before becoming ill. Mild cases last up to two weeks, and more severe cases may last for several months. Symptoms include fever, anorexia, fatigue, jaundice, and in severe cases, liver damage and death. Dark urine and clay-color stools may be present. To prevent *hepatitis A*:

- Exclude employees from working who have jaundice or been exposed to *hepatitis A*.
- Purchase shellfish from approved, certified sources.
- Use potable safe water in preparation, hand washing, and cleanup.
- Cook food to the recommended temperatures.
- Avoid raw shellfish.
- Avoid food contaminated by food handlers who practice poor hygiene.
- Avoid bare-hand contact with ready-to-eat food.
- Wash hands often using appropriate methods.

Another virus of note is the rotavirus. Rotaviruses can cause acute gastroenteritis, which is a moderate illness. The illness may be mild to severe and includes vomiting, watery diarrhea, and low-grade fever. Rotaviruses are transmitted by the fecal-oral route, sewage, and contaminated water. Infected food handlers may contaminate food that required handling and no further cooking, such as salads, fruit, and appetizers, raw seafood. Poor personal hygiene and lack of proper hand washing and food handling practices can also contaminate food.

Enterohemorrhagic *Escherichia coli* 0157:H7

E. coli 0157:H7 is a non-spore-forming facultative bacterium, and many food-related outbreaks have been reported since the pathogen was first identified in 1982. A sudden onset can cause hemorrhagic colitis (bloody diarrhea) and renal failure (hemolytic uremic symptoms). There is an incubation period of one to eight days from the time contaminated food is ingested until the onset of illness, an average of three to four days. The illness may last eight to ten days. *E. coli* illness is caused by ingesting food contaminated with cattle feces and the consumption of undercooked or raw ground beef and red meat (lamb and pork) and unpasteurized milk and juice, sprouts, lettuce, and salami. Contact with cattle may also be a cause, occasionally, waterborne transmission occurs through swimming in contaminated lakes and pools, and drinking inadequately chlorinated water.

E. coli 0157:H7, which has also been found in prepared foods (such as mashed potatoes, cream pies, finfish, and imported cheese), differs from other strains of *E. coli* because the organism is found in the intestinal tracts of animals used as food. Fecal contamination can occur during slaughtering. Important control measures include:

- Good food-manufacturing practices (such as avoiding cross-contamination and maintaining sanitized equipment in processing plants).
- Proper heating of meats; for example, ground beef products should be cooked to 158°F to 160°F (70°C to 71°C); other meats should be cooked to 160°F (for well done) **and** held at this temperature for at least two hours or undergo thorough cooking. Leftover red meat should be reheated to at least 165°F (74°C) for 15 seconds.
- Employees following good hand washing and personal hygiene practices at all times.

Other emerging pathogens include *Salmonella enteritidis* (ovary-infecting), *V. parahemolyticus*, and *Yersinia entercolitica*. The incidence of food-borne illness caused by these organisms is reported less frequently. If food handlers practiced the proper food-handling and sanitation procedures as discussed, the incidences of food-borne illness caused by these organisms would be reduced.

A possible new threat and emerging problem in the United States is bovine spongiform encephalopathy (BSE; mad cow disease), which is a fatal disease that affects the brain and central nervous system of an adult cow. BSE affects only cows, but a person can contract the human form known as Creutzfeldt-Jakob disease (CJD), which is caused by eating prion-infected brains or nerve tissue from a sick cow. (A **prion** is a **pro**teinaceous **in**fectious agent. This means a protein can cause a particular disease, it can be given to another individual, and they can get the same disease.) The risk of contracting this disease is small and death is the ultimate result.

The infectious proteins called *prions* that cause the disease have been found in abundance only in the brain stem, spinal cord, and

TABLE 13.3 Major Known Pathogens to Cause Disease/Death

Bacterial	Parasitic	Viral
Bacillus cereus	*Cryptosporidum*	Norwalk-like
Clostridum botulism	*parvum*	viruses
Campylobacter spp.	*Cyclospora*	Rotavirus
C. perfringers cayetanensis	Astrovirus	
Escherichia coli 0157:H7	*Giardia lamblia*	Hepatitis A
E. Coli non-0157 STEC	*Toxoplasma gondii*	
Other types of *E. coli*	*Trichinella spiralis*	
Listeria monocytogenes		
Salmonella typhi		
Salmonella nontyphoidal		
Shigella spp.		
Staphylococcus food poisoning and food-borne illness		
Vibrio cholerae		
V. vulnificus		
Vibrio, other		
Yersinia enterocolitica		

Source: The Centers for Disease Control and Prevention.

small intestine of infected cows. In the United States, these parts of the cow are not usually eaten by humans. However, these animal parts have been used in the feed that is fed to cattle and thereby has the potential of infecting a healthy cow. The U.S. government has taken steps to provide more inspections, to limit the importation of cows from various countries and to provide surveillance programs that tests "downer cows" for BSE. A *downer cow* is one that is suspected to be too sick to stand unassisted.

A person can have CJD for years before showing the first symptoms. Even though BSE is not common in the United States, a recent outbreak in the West and exporting beef is a major concern (In 2012 a case was reported in California, and there may be others.) The USDA forbids imports of cows, sheep, and meat from countries where animals are infected with BSE. There may be a chance of contacting this disease from eating beef overseas.

Food Additives, Food Preservatives, and Food Allergens

A *food additive* is any substance added to food that changes its characteristics. There are two types of food additives: direct and indirect. Direct additives are added to food for a specific purpose and include such items as salt and sugar. Indirect additions are food additives that become part of the food in trace amounts due to package, storing, and other handling. The Food and Drug Administration maintains a list of thousands of ingredients in food additive data.

Additives are added to food to improve, taste, texture, and appearance; improve/maintain nutrient value, and improve safety. On rare occasions individuals may react to an additive. The two most common ones are FD&C Yellow 5 that causes itching and hives and Monosodium glutamate (MSG) that causes bold tingling or warmth and chest pains; symptoms are mild and usually last less than an hour. Persons with the genetic disease known as phenylketouria (PKU) should avoid foods sweetened with aspartame; if consumed it can cause serious side effects.

Beside the three additives listed earlier some people have concerns especially with sulfides and nitrates. In some states, a notice of the use of either of these chemicals must be printed on the menu or posted in a visible place within the facility. FDA and industry standards prohibit the use of sulfides by foodservice establishments. Sulfides used in food processing are highly regulated. Products that contain sulfides or nitrates must list it on the label.

There are about nine other additives to be aware of. They include BHA and BHT, potassium bromate, acesulfame-K Olestra, sodium nitrite (sodium nitrate), hydrogenated vegetable oil, Blue 1 and Blue 2, Red 3, and Yellow 6. Foodservice employees may not apply sulfiting agents to fresh fruit and vegetables intended for raw consumption or to a food considered to be a good source of vitamin B1.

Reading labels will help persons who may have a reaction to an additive.

Food preservatives are chemicals that help keep food fresh. There are three types of preservatives: (1) antimicrobial, which inhibits growth of bacteria, yeast, or molds; (2) antioxidants, which slow air oxidation of fats and lipids (oxidation leads to rancidity); and (3) preservatives, which target enzymes in food. Sulfides may be used in all three types. Benzoates are used as an antifungal and nitrates are usually found in packaged meats to fight botulism. The second group are *antioxidants* and are found in many foods as a food additive. The most recognized ones are BHA and BHT. The third group is usually citric and ascorbic acid used to keep potatoes and apples from turning brown when cut. Many scientists are researching for preservatives in natural products rather than chemicals.

Food Allergens

A *food allergen* is the body's negative reaction to certain foods that involves the immune system. Depending on the person and the food ingested a "reaction" may occur immediately after the food is eaten to several hours later. When the body detects an allergen it begins to fight it by producing *antibodies*. Antibodies are a type of a protein produce by the immune system in response to a "foreign" substance that has invaded the body. These antibodies act in the same way when fighting an infectious disease. The body realizes that there is a foreign substance in it and reacts by trying to destroying it.

The most common symptoms are hives, swelling of the tongue, lips and mouth; itching in and around of the mouth, face and scalp; difficulty breathing or wheezing; swelling of face eyes, hands or feet; and vomiting, diarrhea, and cramps, loss of consciousness and death. These life-threatening reactions are called ***anaphylaxis***. Anaphylaxis is sudden and can involve all the symptoms listed above.

About 90% of all allergies are caused by eight foods:

Milk and dairy products	Eggs and egg products
Wheat protein	Peanuts
Fish	Shellfish
Soy and soy products	Tree nuts

For some individuals citrus, chocolate, corn, tomatoes, strawberries, and banana have caused severe reaction.

Allergies are serious. It is vital, as a foodservice director and a medical nutrition therapist, to know which foods used in the foodservice department may contain one or more of the allergens. It may be wise to include a note on menus that certain foods may contain an allergen or food was prepared in an area where allergens were present. All foodservice hostesses who interact directly with patients must be taught what foods may be a problem for patients and the signs and symptoms of a food allergy reaction. The FDA requires ingredients be listed on the label of packaged foods. Check TJC standards that relate to food allergens and develop a policy and procedure to protect the customer and the organization.

CRISIS MANAGEMENT

When a foodservice director receives a complaint of food-borne illness, the policy and procedure on "what to do" must be implemented at once. Each foodservice operation needs to develop its own policies and procedures that dovetail with its organizational risk management program and with individual state and local regulations. In addition, foodservice operators designate the forms or format to be used to collect data and the individual responsible for communicating with the media is usually designated by administration with input from the foodservice director.

The following steps are suggested:

- Graciously accept the complaint.
- Obtain all pertinent data, such as name, address, date, time, meal, contents of meal, when and where the food was purchased or served, if food was eaten when purchased or refrigerated, when symptoms occurred, the names of any others who ate the same food, whether medical attention was sought, and if so, the name of the physician.
- Take a food history from the complainant, if possible, of all meals and snacks eaten before and after the suspected meal.
- Listen carefully to the complaint. Do not admit liability or offer medical advice. Do not diagnose or suggest symptoms. Do not introduce symptoms. Record only what the person says. Note the time the symptoms started. Remain polite and concerned (Exhibit 13.1).
- Try to preserve a sample of the suspected food for later microbiological testing. Label and store (refrigerate or freeze). Remove suspected food from sales or service.
- Evaluate the complaint. Is it only one person, or are there multiple complainants? Does it describe a legitimate illness? What is the attitude of the complainant?
- Contact the appropriate people: the owner, general manager, hospital administration, infection control and risk management, and so forth.
- Contact the local health department (follow the regulations for the individual state). Deal positively with all regulatory agencies. Allow inspectors to inspect the property. Provide requested data. Be cooperative.
- Review the information and start an internal investigation to include the following (see Exhibit 13.1):
  All temperature charts
  All employees on duty at time of incident; was anyone ill?
  Check for complaints from the entire staff
  Compare notes
  What is new or different, such as new food items on menu, new supplier, new employee?
  Environmental sanitation
  Date of pest control
  New chemicals being used?
- If only one or two customers complain, offer refunds or gift certificates. If more complaints are received, follow the established local health regulations.
- Arrange for medical services (in health care establishment with nursing, infection control, and employee health facilities).
- Have food tested by an outside laboratory that microbiologically tests food.
- Deal with the media positively. Provide accurate data. Answer only the questions they ask. Avoid jargon. Remain calm and professional. Tell the truth. Do not try to bluff or give out misinformation.
- Continue to investigate.
- Take corrective action, as appropriate.
- Review outcome with all managers and staff. Change policies and procedures and make corrections, as appropriate.
- As appropriate, file findings for future reference.

The CDC defines an *outbreak* as "an incident in which two or more persons experience a similar illness after ingestion of a common food and epidemiological analysis implicates the food as the source of the illness." When laboratory evidence meeting established criteria confirms the presence of a toxic agent, the CDC classifies the outbreak as being of known etiology. Otherwise, it is classified as being of unknown etiology. The CDC reports that for outbreaks of unknown etiology, the following are the probable toxic agents:

Symptoms within one hour of eating indicate probable chemical poisoning; symptoms from one to seven hours after eating indicate probable staphylococcal food poisoning; symptoms from 8 to 14 hours after eating indicate probable *C. perfringens* food poisoning; symptoms more than 14 hours later indicate other infectious or toxic agents.

EXHIBIT 13.1. Food-Borne Illness Record of Complainant

Date:	Time of Interview:

Name of Interviewer:

Address of Interviewer:

Phone No. of Interviewer:

Name of Complainant:

Address of Complainant:

Phone No. of Complainant: (H)	(O)

Date and time of incident:

Complaint:

Nature of problem:

   Illness:

   Unsanitary conditions:

   Spoiled food:

   Other:

What are the three most predominant symptoms?

   1.

   2.

   3.

What was the date and time of the last meal?

What time did your first symptoms appear?

Are you still sick?

Did you seek medical care?	Did you go to a hospital?

Name and Phone No. of Physician:

Name and Phone No. of Hospital:

Did you provide a specimen of foods or fluids to the hospital or to the physician?

What did you eat at our meal?

   Beverages

   Ice

   Soup

   Salad (Salad bar or predished)

   Entrée

   Vegetables

   Desserts

   Condiments

Did you eat any food that you brought from home?

Did you eat any food provided by someone else?

Source: R. P. Puckett©. Used by permission.

CHEMICAL HAZARDS

Chemical hazards can be found in health care facilities, especially in housekeeping and foodservice. Employees need to be taught how to safely use chemicals and what to do if an accident occurs or if food is contaminated. The foodservice director needs to know where the food was grown, under what conditions, and how it was processed, delivered, and stored. Specifications need to include a statement concerning the addition of food additives, agricultural, housekeeping products, and toxins.

Chemical Contamination

The government has set standards on the chemicals that are not allowed in food, and have established "safe" limits. There are two types of *chemical hazards*, those occurring naturally in food and those added during the processing of food. Chemicals that occur naturally in foods can cause illness. *Mycolaxin*, an aflatoxin, is a harmful chemical produced by fungi growing on such foods as grains, nuts, and milk. Aflatoxins may be found in corn, tree nuts, peanuts, cottonseed, and milk. When eaten in large amounts, they can cause abnormalities in digestion and absorption, hemorrhage, liver damage, edema, and in some cases, death.

The most commonly "added" chemicals include food additives, which are used to enhance flavor and to keep products fresh longer. These have previously been described.

Naturally Occurring Chemical Hazards

Better-known naturally occurring chemical hazards include shellfish and mushroom toxins, undercooked red beans, and honey made from rhododendron nectar, which was mentioned earlier.

Added chemical hazards are chemicals that have been added to food from planting to consumption. Most chemicals are not hazardous if added in safe amounts and proper instructions are followed. Added chemical hazards included food additives, pesticides, toxic metals, and toxic housekeeping products. Harmful chemicals at high levels can cause severe poisoning and allergic reactions.

Chemicals and Pesticides

Agricultural chemicals include pesticides, fungicides, fertilizers, antibiotics, hormones, insecticides, and herbicides. The Environmental Protection Agency (EPA), which states how the chemical can be used and the maximum allowable residue, regulates most of these chemicals. Products from unapproved sources may contain a higher-than-accepted level of residue.

Foodservice facilities use *pesticides* to control insects and rodents. An improper or wrong use can contaminate food. Always follow manufacturers' directions when using. For best protection a licensed professional pest control agency should be employed. Foodservice management should make certain that the chemicals being used by the pest control company are safe to use in a foodservice establishment.

All chemicals need to be stored away from food, utensils, and equipment used for food. Chemicals need to be stored in a sepa-rate area and in original containers. When transferring chemicals from a larger container to a smaller container **label** the smaller container and store appropriately. **NEVER mix** chemicals as this may cause an explosion or fire. Follow all OSHA Material Safety Data Sheets (MSDS) when using chemicals. Train all employees in the proper use.

Toxic Metals

Metal poisoning includes contamination by copper, lead, zinc, cadmium, tin, arsenic, and mercury. Lead is the most common contaminant. Ceramic containers that are glazed with a lead-based paint can be hazardous for food storage if the glaze becomes chipped or deteriorates during dish washing. Lead poisoning in some areas is high, especially in drinking water (from pipes). Mercury may be used in fungicides to protect seed grains during storage. Plants can absorb mercury when the soil contains a high level of mercury. High levels of mercury in water (lakes, rivers, oceans) can contaminate seafood, especially fish (Table 13.4). Pregnant women, women of childbearing age, nursing women, and young children should not eat shark, swordfish, king mackerel, or tilefish because they contain high levels of mercury.

Housekeeping Products

Cleaning chemicals, pot and pan, dishwashing compounds, and other cleaning and sanitizing products can result in chemical food poisoning when these chemicals are not properly labeled, stored, and used. Chemicals should never be stored with food; they should especially never be stored in the food production area because many of the chemicals are white granules that have the same appearance as sugar and salt. Food handlers should **always** read labels and follow the material safety data sheets for proper use and storage of all chemicals.

Physical Hazards

Physical hazards include objects such as stones, thorns, small animal bones, wood, clothes, insects, insulation, plastic, bullets or BB shots, needles, human and animal hair, dirt, glass, metal, fingernails, bandages, toothpicks, and jewelry and may be found in food products. Finding these objects in food may cause a psychological trauma or a physical illness or injury to the person. Poor ventilation, poorly maintained facilities, and the use of broken or worn-out utensils and equipment can also contribute to physical contamination. Improperly cleaned vents can blow debris onto food. Leaking overhead pipes can drop moisture, metal, paint, or dirt into food. Unguarded light fixtures can break, and glass can fall into the food. Artificial nails and nail polish can come off in food. Gems from bracelets, earrings, and rings can fall into food. Foreign material contamination resulting from employee sabotage is difficult to monitor. Unscrupulous employees have placed a wide variety of foreign objects in containers in the past. Because of terrorist threats and quality control, foodservice personnel, from the farm to the table, must be diligent in their monitoring as poor food handling practices can occur at various points in the chain from harvest to table.

TABLE 13.4. Nonbacterial Illnesses of Infrequent or Rare Occurrence

Name of Illness	Causative Agent	Foods Usually Involved	How Introduced into Food	Preventive or Corrective Procedures
Arsenic, fluoride, lead poisoning	Insecticides Rodenticides	Any foods accidentally contaminated	Either during growing period or accidentally in kitchen	Thoroughly wash all fruits and vegetables when received, store insecticides and pesticides away from food, properly label containers, follow use instructions, use carefully, guard food from chemical contamination
Copper poisoning	Copper food contact surfaces	Acid foods and carbonated liquids	Contact between metal and acid food or carbonated beverages	Prevent acid foods or carbonated liquids from coming into contact with exposed copper
Cadmium and zinc poisoning	Metal plating on food containers	Fruit juices, fruit gelatin, and other acid foods stored in metal-plated containers	Acid foods dissolve cadmium and zinc from containers in which they are stored	Discontinue use of cadmium-plated utensils as food containers; prohibit use of zinc-coated utensils for preparation, storage, and serving of acid fruits and other foods or beverages
Cyanide poisoning	Silver polish	Any foods accidentally contaminated	Failure to wash and rinse polished silverware thoroughly	Discontinue use of cyanide-based silver polish or wash and rinse silverware thoroughly

Physical materials in food may cause cuts, bleeding, infection, choking, broken teeth, trauma (especially psychological), and in some instances surgery to remove the object. Much of the physical material may come from broken dishes, machinery, packaging, improper processing, nonsharp can openers, pallets, and employee carelessness.

According to the FDA, of all the thousands of complaints of foreign objects in food, 25 percent were related to foreign materials; about 6 percent resulted in illness or injury, with glass, metal, and plastic being the most common foreign objects found.

Food handlers must be trained at all steps of food-handling processes. The equipment and environment should always be clean. There should be strict policies and procedures concerning the use of hair restraints and wearing of jewelry, artificial nails, and nail polish. Ongoing monitoring is essential; immediate corrective action must be taken when policies and procedures, regulations, rules and standards are not followed. (Check Food Code 2009, U.S. Public Health Service, and FDA for a more detailed list.)

Employees who are jaundiced or diagnosed with an infection from Norovirus, *Shigella* spp., enterohemorrhagic, or Shiga toxin-produced *E. coli* must report the condition to the supervisor. Employees may be restricted or excluded from working in food preparation or service. A medical note is required which states the infection is not caused by *hepatitis A* or *other fecal-orally transmitted infection.*

Exclude an employee from working who is diagnosed with an infection from *Salmonella typhi* or a previous infection with *Salmonella typhi* in the past three months. If employee has been diagnosed with *Shigella* spp., enterohemorrhagic, or Shiga toxin and is asymptomatic, the employee should be excluded from serving a highly susceptible population. If an employee is infected with a skin lesion containing pus such as a boil or infected wound that is open or draining and not properly covered the employee must be restricted from handling or serving food. Employees must report any of the above problems to the director and comply with the decision to restrict or exclude the employee from work. The director will exclude or restrict the employee from working. In some cases the employee may be sent to employee health for an evaluation and permission to work. The person in charge has the responsibility to notify regulatory agents concerning the above illness.

Sick employees are also a concern in food-borne illness. Table 13.5 presents guidelines that should be used in deciding whether to allow sick personnel to work in direct contact with food (preparation or service). See additional information later in chapter and the Food Code 2009.

New Concerns

There are four "superbugs" that all health care employees need to know about. These bugs are not related to food but do cause illness and hospitalization and one is highly contagious. The newest superbug, *New Delhi Metallo-beta-lactamase-1* or NDM-1, is named for New Delhi. It was first found in patients who had traveled to New Delhi for surgical procedures. The "bug" has been found in bacteria that cause gut or urinary infections. There are few new antibodies in developing countries to treat the problem. Some infection control physicians are concerned that the gene will spread from person to person, perhaps all over the world. CDC suggests that if a case(s) appears in your facility place the patient on medical isolation. Learn all you can.

Clostridium difficile colitis, better known as *C. diff*, is a bacteria in the intestine that is considered a "bad" or dangerous bacteria. C. diff is found throughout the environment, but is most common in hospitals and other health care facilities. C. diff is passed in the feces

TABLE 13.5 Sick Employees (2009 Food Code)

Disease or Illness	Allowed to Work in Direct Customer Contact	Foodservice Preparation and Service	Establishment's Duration of Restriction
AIDS	Yes	Yes	No restriction for foodservice personnel
Diarrhea/vomiting	No	No	Until symptoms disappear
Strep throat/fever	No	No	Until 24 hours after effective treatment is started
Hepatitis	No	No	Until 7 days after onset of jaundice
Laceration, noninfected	Yes[a]	Yes[a]	
Laceration, infected	No	No	Restricted from food preparation until infection is healed
Respiratory tract infection	No/yes	No/yes	If temperature 100°F or higher, may not work; if temperature less than 100°F, a mask should be worn
Conjunctivitis "pink eye"	No	No	Until eye is clear
Pandemic events	No	No	Until Public Health and Homeland Security gives clearance

[a]Must wear protective covering.

Source: U.S. Public Health Service, Food and Drug Administration, 2009, Chapter 2 Management and Personnel. Constantly check the web for any additions to this list, especially as it relates to any possible pandemic.

and spreads to food, surfaces, and objects. When infected people don't **wash** their hands thoroughly, remove gloves when soiled, or maintain a clean and sanitized environment, a major problem may result. The bacterium produces spores that may stay in a room or on its contents for weeks or months. If the room and or objects have not been cleaned and a person touches the contaminated surface they may ingest the bacteria. People in good health don't usually get sick from C. diff. When antibodies are given to treat the infection they can destroy some of the good bacteria and without enough good bacteria C. diff can grow out of control. When there is an imbalance of bacteria C. diff takes over creating two main types of toxins that affect the body, giving the symptoms of the actual disease. The toxins attack the intestinal wall and left untreated may cause ulceration. To avoid spreading, keep bathrooms, locker rooms, utensils, and all fixtures clean, avoid cross-contamination and **use proper hand-washing procedures**. This is a dangerous infection and highly contagious; if left untreated it can cause death.

Methicillin-resistent *Staphyloccus aureus*, called MRSA, is a drug-resistant bacterial infection causing the deaths of tens of thousands of Americans each year. Infections may be acquired in the community—playgrounds and health clubs—as well as in health care environments. In 2006, health care acquired infections killed 48,000 Americans and cost more than $8 billion to treat. The most common route of infection in health care facilities include: central line–related bloodstream infections, urinary catheter–induced infections, ventilator-related pneumonia, and surgical infections. Patients with MSRA should be on isolation. Health care personnel must use proper hand-washing techniques.

The latest superbug is called *carbapenem-resistant Klebsiella pneumoniae* or CRKP. Fifty-three percent of the infections come from acute hospitals, 41 percent from long-term acute care hospitals and 6 percent from nursing homes. The bacterium tends to strike elderly patients who stay in facilities for an extended period. It is spread primarily from person to person, mostly in the elderly. This

is a serious infection, complicated by the fact that there are so few treatment options.

Although new drugs are developed, germs evolve and the drugs eventually have little to no effect. The mortality rate is high.

THERMOMETERS

There are many different types of and uses for thermometers. In the production area, thermometers are used in ovens, combination steamers, cook-chill equipment, deep-fat fryers, and broilers. Thermometers are also necessary in refrigerators, freezers, dry storage areas, and the general work and service areas.

A number of different types of thermometers can be used to measure temperature on equipment: recording thermometers, bulb thermometers, and remote-reading thermometers. *Recording thermometers* are mounted on the outside of refrigerators and freezers and continuously record the internal temperature. Recording thermometers are also used with cook-chill equipment. *Bulb thermometers* are the most common type to use when there is no built-in thermometer in the door of the refrigerator or freezer. A bulb thermometer should be placed in the warmest area of the unit. (Check the local public health rules and regulations.) *Remote-reading thermometers* are placed outside of refrigerators and freezers and may be monitored in a central control engineering area. These show the temperature within the refrigerator or freezer.

When manual thermometers are used, the temperature of refrigerators and freezers should be recorded at least twice daily by checking in the morning and in the evening.

Other thermometers can be used to test the temperature of food. The most common is called a *bimetal probe* or *dial-instant read* with a dial that can be used to measure temperatures that range from 0°F to 220°F. This type of probe is made up of two metals in a strip with different expansion coefficients that move a pointer on a dial display. This type of thermometer is destroyed if it is dropped, bent, or abused. It is small and may be easily lost or stolen. It is also somewhat difficult to read. The dial-instant thermometer is inexpensive, has a high loss rate, but is easy to use. To ensure that calibration is accurate, the bimetal probe needs to be recalibrated frequently. To ensure that the readings are accurate, the probe should be tested against the temperature of a known substance (such as boiling water at 212°F or a slushy mix of ice water mixed with a small amount of salt to get a 32°F reading). This type of thermometer may be used to measure temperature in roast, soups, and casseroles. It can be place at 2 inches to 2½ inches in the thickest part of food. It is not to be used to measure thin foods unless inserted sideways. The digital instant-read is not designed to remain in food while cooking; check the temperature of food near the end of cooking time.

Thermocouple thermometers are commercially available. A handheld thermocouple thermometer uses various electronic probes that can probe food and provide a digital display in two to five seconds. This handheld unit records time, temperature, and location and has alarms that can be activated for high- or low-temperature variances. It runs on nine volts and can be used for 2,000 hours of operation. Nine different probes are available for the measurement of insertion or immersion temperatures: surface temperatures, ambient air, coolers, and other air temperatures (as well as a bare-tip probe for general-purpose temperature measurement). All four probes can be used to measure up to 500°F and have a 24-inch silicon-jacketed Kevlar-reinforced cable.

Cost varies depending on the probe type because each probe is priced separately. Accuracy is plus or minus 1°F. This type of thermometer is also the most economical in the long run. Recalibration is needed when it is dropped or bent. It produces the fastest response time and highest range accuracy combination and can be used to measure both hot and cold food. This thermometer is made of two conductors of dissimilar metals. As temperatures change, multi-voltage differences change.

Another type of thermometer is a *probe with a digital display* also referred to as a *thermistor*. It is made of two conductors embedded in an electrolytic material with varying resistance as the temperature at the juncture changes. The response time is slower than with the thermocouple probe. It is easily overheated and distorted, but it has a high level of accuracy over a limited range. The sensors are larger and can be used to probe larger masses. Probe selections are limited, and cost is moderate. Temperature calibration is set at the factory. When a digital thermometer is out of calibration, it needs to be standardized to a calibrated thermometer or discarded. It is best used for probing food during various stages of cooking. It is made of ceramic semiconductors to penetrate food; a digital display is ready within seconds.

The latest and most improved thermometer is the thermocouple thermometer, which is recommended by the FDA and the USDA. The increased use of the thermocouple thermometer in the food industry is due to its overall range and accuracy combinations, its quick response times, and because it is available for a wide variety of uses (for example, product surface and air temperature).

Probes are available for specific needs, such as inserting into small, thin pieces of food such as fish, shrimp, and meat patties; immersing in liquids such as soups; and for solid foods such as mashed potatoes and casseroles and frozen products such as ice cream. They can also be used for surface equipment such as cold or hot tops and surface shelves in coolers or freezers. This type of thermometer meets HACCP requirements, complies with public health regulations, and ensures food safety by providing accurate temperature readings. A *noncontact infrared thermometer* measures temperatures anywhere food is subject to a variance in temperature. It is handheld, ergonomically designed, and eliminates cross-contamination during temperature checks.

Other thermometers are programmable by setting the temperature display and intervals to best meet the applications of the facility. The database can scroll forward and backward, it provides degree and time calculations, and it has a memory capacity of 4,096 temperature readings. These thermometers are referred to as recording thermometers.

The latest measuring device is called *The Sure Check (iQuality) Handheld PDA Inspection System*. It is an excellent system to be used with an HACCP program. More information may be gathered at: www.24-7pressrelease.com/press-release/presenting-the-sure-check-iquality-haccp-pda-inspection-system-for-school-food-services-160111.php.

Food Code 2009 defines and specifies the following information concerning temperature-measuring devices:

"Temperature-measuring device" means a thermometer, thermocouple, thermistor, or other device that indicates the temperature of food, air, or water. Food temperature–measuring devices may not have sensors or stems constructed of glass, except for glass sensors or stems that are encased in shatterproof coating, such as candy thermometers, which may be used. Ambient air and water temperature measuring devices shall be designed to be easily readable and accurate if scaled in Fahrenheit to +/– 3°F in the intended range or use and +/– 1.5°C. These measuring devices shall be maintained and in good repair and be accurate with the intended use. Food temperature measuring devices shall be calibrated in accordance with the manufacturers' specifications as necessary to ensure their accuracy. Ambient air temperature, water pressure, and water temperature measuring devices shall be maintained in good repair and be accurate within the intended range of use.

How to Calibrate a Thermometer

The following is one method for calibrating a thermometer such as a bimetal. Other measuring devices should be calibrated in accordance with manufacturers' specifications.

- Fill an insulated container (a foam cup may be used) full of potable crushed ice.
- Add cold water.
- Allow 4 to 5 minutes for mixture to reach 32°F (0°C).
- Insert a bimetal-stemmed thermometer into the center of the cup, keeping it away from the bottom and sides.
- Hold the thermometer until the temperature stabilizes. Record reading. Repeat at least two more times, recording the temperature each time.
- If the thermometer does not read 32°F, use pliers on the nut under the top of the thermometer to adjust to 32°F.

A new electrical 90 volts, 130VAC, 50/60 Hz stainless steel housing "check-tempcalibrator" will calibrate probes of all sizes and has a built-in circuitry to warn if the unit is more than 1°F out of calibration. The unit is simple to set up—just plug in and turn on. The calibrator has a carrying case and can be used in various locations. See more information at www.telre.com.

Conversion Factor

To convert a Fahrenheit temperature to Centigrade, do the following:

1. Subtract 32
2. Multiply by 5
3. Divide by 9

To convert Centigrade to Fahrenheit, do the following:

1. Multiply by 9
2. Divide by 5
3. Add 32

How to Use a Food Thermometer

Food thermometers are one of the most valuable tools used in a foodservice operation. When a thermometer is used correctly, it can reduce food cost, ensure food safety, and improve food quality. Thermometers measure temperature in degrees Fahrenheit (°F) or degrees Celsius (°C) or both. When using a thermometer, know which temperature scale is being used.

- Keep thermometers and storage cases clean.
- Insert into center or into thickest portion (for example, insert into high area of the breast of whole turkey, taking care not to touch bone). Take at least two readings in two different locations (usually the center of the piece of meat).
- Do not touch the sides or bottom of the food container.
- For pork, beef, lamb, veal, ham roasts, chops, or steaks, insert into the center of the thickest part, away from the bone, fat, or gristle.
- Insert sideways into thin items such as meat patties, thin fish, and other thin foods.
- Place between frozen packages of food.
- Wait at least 15 seconds before recording temperature from the time the thermometer stem or probe is inserted into the food.
- When measuring the temperature of liquids, do not let the sensing area of the stem or probe touch the container.
- Sanitize thermometer after each use with alcohol wipes or other appropriate method.
- Sanitize before replacing in holder.

Other Temperature-Measuring Devices

The placement of the temperature-measuring device is important, especially in refrigerators and freezers. If the device is placed in the coldest location in the refrigerator or freezer, it may not record the actual temperature of the unit. Food could be stored in areas of the unit that exceed food code requirements. Therefore, a temperature-measuring device must be placed in a location that is representative of the actual storage temperature of the unit to ensure that all PHFs are stored at least at the minimum temperature. A permanent temperature-measuring device is required in any refrigerant unit storing PHFs because of the possible growth of pathogenic microorganisms should the temperature of the unit exceed Food Code requirements. To facilitate routine monitoring of the unit, the device must be clearly visible and should be located on the outside door of the unit.

The exception to requiring a temperature-measuring device for some types of equipment is primarily related to equipment design and function. It would be difficult and impractical to permanently mount a temperature-measuring device on some equipment. The futility of attempting to measure the temperature of unconfined air as under heat lamps and, in some cases, because the brief period of time the equipment is used for a given food negates the usefulness of ambient temperature monitoring. In such cases, it is more practical and accurate to measure the internal temperature of the food.

The importance of maintaining PHFs at the specified temperature requires that temperature-measuring devices be easily readable. The inability to accurately read a thermometer could result in food being held at unsafe temperatures.

Temperature-measuring devices must be appropriately scaled per *Food Code* requirements to ensure accurate readings. All probes should be sanitized with an approved sanitizer after each use, such as a sanitizer approved for food contact surfaces.

The required incremental gradations are more precise for food-measuring devices than for those used to measure ambient temperature because of the significance at a given point in time, that is, the potential for pathogenic growth, versus the unit's temperature. The food temperature will not necessarily match the ambient temperature of the storage unit; it will depend on many variables, including the temperature of the food when it is placed in the unit, the temperature at which the unit is maintained, and the length of time the food is stored in the unit.

There are a number of other temperature-measuring devices on the market, including:

- Time and temperature indicator strips are liquid crystals that change color when food enters the hazardous zone. The strips change color with the temperature, signaling damage to food in transit, temperatures in storage, or cooking. Strips "change" colors when the temperature rises above a certain point.
- Color-change alarm labels are self-adhesive labels that change from white to black when a threshold temperature is reached. They are used for testing the dishwasher water temperature for 160°F to 190°F (71°C to 88°C), depending

TABLE 13.6. Internal Cooking Temperatures of Food

Product	°F	Product	°F
Eggs & egg dishes		Poultry	
Eggs	Cook until yolk and white are firm	Chicken, turkey—whole	165
Egg casseroles	160	Chicken, turkey—dark meat	165
Egg sauces, custards	160	Poultry—breast	165
		Duck & goose	165
Ground meat & meat mixtures			
Turkey, chicken	165	Stuffing	
Beef, veal, lamb, pork	160	Cooked alone or in bird	165
		Sauces, soups, gravies, marinades	
Fresh beef, veal, lamb		Used with raw meat, poultry, or fish	Bring to a boil
Medium rare	145		
Medium	160	Seafood	
Well done	170	Finfish	Cook until opaque and flakes easily with a fork
Fresh pork	160	Shrimp, lobster, crab	Should turn red and flesh should become pearly opaque
Ham			
Fresh (raw)	160	Scallops	Should turn milky white or opaque and firm
Fully cooked (to reheat)	140		
		Clams, mussels, oysters	Cook until shells open
Roast beef			
Cooked commercially, vacuum sealed, and ready-to-eat	140		

Source: U.S. Department of Agriculture Food and Inspection Service, 2008.

on the equipment and the sanitizers used. A self-adhesive label attaches to the inside or outside of a container to provide a visual assurance of the quality of the product. The liquid in the bulb changes colors to alert staff that the temperature has changed.

- A time-over-temperature alarm point is a small adhesive label containing three windows that change colors in various windows, depending on the time that the product temperature was higher than the alarm temperature.
- Pop-up timers are commonly used in turkey and chicken roasting. The pop-up device is constructed from a food-approved nylon. The inside contains a stainless steel spring and firing material. The firing material is made of an organic salt compound or an alloy of metals commonly used in other thermal sensing devices. The tip of the stem is embedded in the firing material until it melts, releasing the stem, which is then "popped up" by means of the spring. This indicates that the food has reached the final temperature for safety and doneness.
- Oven thermometers can be left in an oven to verify that the oven is heating to the desired temperature. These

bimetallic-coil thermometers can measure temperatures from 100°F to 600°F (38°C to 316°C). Table 13.6 provides the internal cooking temperatures suggested by the USDA Food Safety and Inspection Service (www.fsis.usda.gov).

- T-Stick™ disposal thermometers are single-use, cardboard thermometers that indicate a temperature of 160°F (71°C). The white indicator on the stick changes to black when the product reaches 160°F. T-Stick™ is used in measuring the internal temperature of hamburgers and other foods and eliminates cross-contamination.

Temperature Logs

The temperature of food, equipment, ambient air, water, and equipment should be recorded as outlined in the foodservice operation procedure manual. This is a standard of TJC, CMS, and most health departments. Logs should be filed for the time specified by the local health departments or policies and procedures of the facility. Any deviations in temperature from the standard and how the problem was resolved should be noted on the log.

SUMMARY

Foodservice must adhere to prescribed guidelines that guard against food-borne illness due to food contamination. Common causes of food-borne illness and the bacterial agents that serve as transport vehicles have been described. The items that are needed for bacteria to grow and the lag time it takes are well defined. The definition for food-borne illness and food-borne intoxication is given. The importance of using a variety of thermometers to determine whether food is meeting the proper temperature is discussed.

KEY TERMS

Additives
Aflatoxin
Allergens
Anaphylaxia
Bacterium
C. diff
Contamination
FAT TOM
Food-borne illness
Food-borne infection
Food-borne intoxication
Fungi
Microorganisms
Mold Hazard

MRSA
New Delhi Metallo-Beta-lactamase
Parasite
pH
Potentially hazardous food (PHF)
Preservatives
Spores
Thermocouple
Toxins
Vegetative state
Viruses
Water activity
Yeast

DISCUSSION QUESTIONS

1. Determine methods to reduce the spread of food-borne illness, reducing customer illness and reduce cost.
2. Identify biological, physical, and chemicals hazards and establish methods to protect customers.
3. A customer has claimed he has a food-borne illness from eating cream of mushroom soup—how would you handle a crisis?
4. Evaluate and demonstrate the use of various thermometers.
5. Review the causes of bacteria, fungus, and virus that cause food-borne illness, develop policies and procedures for a foodservice department, to include hand washing and procedures for handling sick employees.

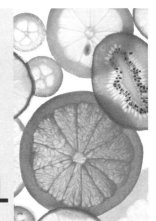

CHAPTER 14

HACCP, HEALTH INSPECTIONS, ENVIRONMENTAL SANITATION, FOOD CODE, AND PEST CONTROL

LEARNING OBJECTIVES

- Successfully implement the HACCP process in a foodservice operation.
- Participate in health inspections and other surveying agencies programs.
- Develop an environmental sanitation program.
- Explain the difference in cleaning and sanitizing.
- Implement standards according to the Food Code.
- Establish a pest control program.

THIS CHAPTER EXPLAINS the HACCP principles and process and its two functions of controlling of food-borne illness and monitoring of food for time-temperature abuse. Adherence to HACCP principles should result in a decreased incidence of food-borne illness and improved quality.

Each operation should have implemented procedures that minimize risk, monitor time and temperature and cross-contamination, and initiate HACCP principles. Maintaining a clean physical plant and conducting frequent self-inspections are essential components to safe food handling

Sanitary food handling—including a recommended technique for hand washing by foodservice personnel—is outlined. Environmental sanitation is stressed and methods to control pests are outlined.

HAZARD ANALYSIS CRITICAL CONTROL POINT (HACCP)

HACCP is a process or system for control of food safety. The process can be used to control any point in the food production process or

system where a hazard or critical situation may occur. These hazards or critical situations may result from pathogenic microorganisms; chemical residue; physical objects; employees; or adulteration or cross-contamination at any point during the distribution, storage, or preparation system.

In 1960 NASA and the U.S. Army Natick Research Laboratories developed the HACCP process. In 1971, the Pillsbury Company, in cooperation with NASA and Natick Research Laboratories, improved the process as Pillsbury was developing food for the space program. It was vital that the food be pure, wholesome, and non-crumbling. (Crumbling could contaminate the atmosphere in the zero gravity inside the space capsule.) After extensive evaluation, Pillsbury concluded that the only way to develop food as nearly as possible 100 percent free of pathogens, toxins, or other hazards was to have control over the entire process—the raw materials, the environment, and the people.

Pillsbury continued to refine this process and, in cooperation with other agencies, recommended and endorsed the HACCP process or system as a "rational and effective approach to ensuring food safety."

The increased focus on providing safe food to customers and the prevention of factors that cause food-related diseases have placed an increased emphasis on the regulators and facilities to implement the HACCP process or system. The HACCP process involves more than concerns over the sanitary conditions and taking food temperatures.

Implementing HACCP

To successfully implement the HACCP process, the foodservice director and higher administration must be committed to the program. The foodservice director has the responsibility of being aware of the benefits and possible cost savings and providing that information to administration. The administration has the responsibility to provide resources for education and training of the staff in safe food handling.

The foodservice management staff has the basic responsibility to orient and educate higher administration in the principles of the HACCP process. The foodservice personnel must ensure that higher administration understands the need for HACCP and will support the implementation of the process by providing any needed funds. The foodservice management staff has the responsibility to implement and be committed to the process.

The foodservice director and administrator have the responsibility to maintain and market sanitation both internally and externally in their organization. They must lead by example at all times while developing job assignments and providing ongoing supervision and training. They also have a major role in providing adequate resources, including machines, money, and sufficient labor. The foodservice director also has the following responsibilities:

- Appoint an internal foodservice team to develop, implement, and monitor the HACCP process.
- Provide in-service training to the entire foodservice staff on "what is HACCP and why it is important."
- Use flow charts and other materials to clearly define HACCP and its seven principles.
- Seek consultation from the infection control committee on infectious diseases, isolation, and employee health.
- Maintain accurate records of meetings, monitoring, and corrective action.
- Use flow charts and recipe updates to follow the HACCP principles.
- Include HACCP as part of the department's continuous quality improvement plan.
- Adhere to all rules, regulations, and standards of inspection/surveying agencies.

To assist the foodservice professionals in their sanitation and safety responsibilities, an HACCP program is currently being supported, monitored, and inspected by many local and state health departments as well as The Joint Commission (TJC). The FDA and the National Restaurant Association have both been instrumental in the support and development of HACCP guidelines and HACCP programs.

The HACCP program includes *seven principles*:

1. List all potential hazards and control measures.
2. Determine critical control points (CCPs).
3. Establish critical limits for each CCP.
4. Establish a monitoring system for each CCP.
5. Establish a corrective action plan.
6. Establish verification procedure.
7. Establish documentation and record keeping.

HACCP is an evaluation system that prevents rather than inspects, identifies potential chemical and biological hazards, establishes controls or preventative measures, continuously monitors

systems, and is designed to ensure food safety by reducing the likelihood of food-borne illness. It is the process of measuring the flow of potential hazards from procurement and receiving to the point of consumption. The goal of HACCP is to protect food and water from physical, chemical, and biological hazards that can cause food-borne illness at any stage of food production and preparation

Upper management's long-term commitment to provide resources and to enforce food-safety policies, procedures, and standards is a primary requirement. With the current ability to determine the cause of death of at-risk patients, coupled with the readiness for legal action, today's foodservice professional cannot afford the risk that comes from not supporting an HACCP program.

ISO 22000 2005 and HACCP

ISO is the International Organization for Standardization. ISO 22000 is a generic food safety management system. It defines a set of general food safety requirements that apply to all organizations in the food chain. ISO 22000 uses HACCP. ISO shows organizations how to combine HACCP and ISO to improve conditions that must be established throughout the entire food chain and the activities and practices that must be performed in order to establish a hygienic environment, this is known as *perquisite programs* (PRPs). PRPs must be suitable and capable of providing food that is safe for human consumption. *Operational prerequisite programs* (OPRPs) are essential to control hazards throughout the food chain.

What Is Hazard Analysis Critical Control Point—HACCP?

In foodservice management, HACCP focuses on the flow of food through the operation, beginning with the decision where to secure food → what foods to include on the menu → continuing with recipe development → food procurement → delivery and storage → preparation → holding or displaying → service → cooling → storage → reheating. Because the potential for contamination exists at each step, the chance that a specific condition or set of conditions will lead to a hazard is a considerable risk.

The plan for the system must be written specifically for each *individual* organization as it relates to procurement, menus, equipment, personnel, process, and operations. Before an HACCP process is implemented, a food safety program needs to be in place. Success relies on the identification of critical control points. Implementing an HACCP system involves seven steps.

Principle 1. List All Potential Hazards and Control Measures

Hazard analysis needs to consider biological, chemical, and physical hazards associated with growing and harvesting raw materials; processing, manufacturing where a hazard could be introduced from the environment, equipment, or personnel; distribution, ingredients, preparation where improper methods are used that may contribute to the growth/survival of microorganisms; marketing and consumption of food. The best method to determine the hazards is by a flow diagram that lists the hazards that may occur and identifies available control measures. *Control measures* are actions and activities that can be used to prevent hazards, eliminate them, or reduce their impact or occurrence to acceptable levels. More than one control measure may be required to control the identified hazard and more than one hazard may be a control measure. Control measures need to be detailed procedures and specifications to ensure their effective implementation.

The hazard analysis is performed with three purposes:

First, identify any hazard of significance.

Second, provide a risk basis for selecting likely hazards.

Third, identify the hazards that can be used to develop the preventive measure for process or product to ensure or improve food safety of the process or product.

Issues to consider during hazard analysis are the intended use of the product and details concerning ingredients to be used in preparation or processing, packaging, sanitation, employee health and hygiene, training of staff, service variables, and preventive measures. By reviewing each recipe and developing a recipe flowchart such as the one shown in Table 14.1, managers and food handlers can learn what microorganisms are likely to cause food-borne illness. Sources of particular concern include raw food of animal origin (raw poultry, shell eggs, fresh seafood, dairy products, cooked rice, gravies and sauces, potato and protein salads, and raw meat) and surfaces of raw vegetables and spices and herbs. Refrigerated food and sous vide products also should be considered potentially hazardous as these foods may be contaminated by bacteria, virus, parasites, cleaning compounds, and by employees who are ill or have failed to use proper hygienic measures, such as proper hand washing. In addition to recipe ingredients, other sources of potential contamination are food handlers, temperature of refrigerated and frozen storage, and food contact surfaces, including equipment and utensils. It is especially important to observe food-handling practices, heating and cooling times, and temperatures. Table 14.2 provides examples of common hazardous practices in foodservice operations.

Figure 14.1 identifies the components of food hazards analysis by defining the CCPs and the process to be used for each. Figure 14.2 depicts a "decision tree" that can be applied to each step in food preparation where a hazard has been identified.

Principle 2. Determine Critical Control Points

According to the USDA, critical control points (CCPs) are "any point or procedure in a specific food system where loss of control may result in an unacceptable health risk." These include any operational practice or procedure at which prevention of hazard could occur and food hazards could be identified or eliminated.

The identification of CCP for the control of a hazard requires a methodical approach. The decision tree in Figure 14.2 can be used as well as those established by the organization. When using the decision tree answer each question in sequence and at each identified hazard. When using the decision tree be flexible and *avoid* unnecessary CCPs.

The following CCPs should be monitored for microbial contamination or time or temperature abuses:

- Cooking, reheating, and hot holding
- Chilling, chilled storage, and chilled display
- Receiving, thawing, mixing ingredients, and other food-handling procedures
- Food procurement, including source of supply and condition of food on receipt
- Food distribution
- Food display
- Employee health, hygiene, and education

Foodservice Systems and HACCP

Depending on the system used in the foodservice operation, the HACCP process would differ. A conventional foodservice system (receive, prepare, cook, hold, and serve) would entail the largest number of CCPs. CCPs need to be developed for each step. Constantly monitor for correct temperatures for both hot and cold systems. Some bacteria will continue to grow and reproduce if safe temperatures are not maintained. A CCP is needed for (1) personal hygiene, (2) utensil, (3) handling, (4) replenishing food, and (5) contamination by customers. (Bare-hand contact of food needs to be considered and individual state laws followed.)

Ready Prepared Foods

A foodservice organization purchases menu items that are produced by others, usually outside of the facility, and held chilled or frozen until heated for service. The CCP for this system must include procedures for receiving a completely nonthawed item and suppliers' certificates. Items must immediately be stored in a freezer once received. The CCP for reheating must include time and temperature for hot foods to avoid any hazard that may have occurred during preparation and reheating. Service would be the same as for conventional foodservice.

Cook-chill or cook-and-freeze procedures would be to receive, prepare, cook, cool (freeze), reheat, hold, and serve. Concerns are the control of time and temperature after cooking and then the rapid cooling or freezing process, during which cross-contamination is possible. Employees must use good personal hygiene and **all** equipment must be completely sanitized before and after use. A good practice is to freeze samples of the food and have it microbiologically tested for pathogens.

Figures 14.3 and 14.4 provide guidelines for cook-and-chill and cook-and-serve procedures with examples of CCPs, monitoring procedures, and the action to take if the monitoring procedure is not followed.

Principle 3. Establish Critical Limits for Each CCP

The procedures to prevent, reduce, or eliminate hazards are determined in this step, and the quality and safety limits are established. The requirements to be met must be observable and measurable.

TABLE 14.1   HACCP Recipe Flowchart

Critical Control	Hazard if standard not met	Standards	Corrective action
		Receiving	
Receiving beef	Contamination and spoilage with thermometer	Accept beef at 45°F (7.2°C) or lower; verify	Reject delivery
		Packaging intact	Reject delivery
		No off odor or stickiness, and so on	Reject delivery
Receiving vegetables	Contamination and spoilage	Packaging intact	Reject delivery
		No cross-contamination from other foods on the truck	Reject delivery
		No signs of insect or rodent activity	Reject delivery
		Storage	
Storing raw beef	Cross-contamination of other foods	Store on lower shelf away from other foods	Move to lower shelf
	Bacterial growth and spoilage	Label, date, and use first-in, first-out (FIFO) rotation	Use first; discard if maximum time is exceeded or suspected
		Beef temperature must remain below 45°F (7.2°C)	Discard if time and temperature abused
Storing vegetables	Cross-contamination from raw potentially hazardous foods	Label, date, and use FIFO rotation	Discard product held past rotation date
		Keep above raw potentially hazardous foods	Discard contaminated, damaged, or spoiled products
		Preparation	
Trimming and cubing beef	Contamination, cross-contamination, and bacteria increase	Wash hands	Wash hands
		Clean and sanitize utensils	Wash, rinse, and sanitize utensils and cutting board
		Pull and cube one roast at a time, then refrigerate	Return excess amount to refrigerator
Washing and cutting vegetables	Contamination and cross-contamination	Wash hands	Wash hands
		Use clean and sanitized cutting board, knives, utensils	Wash, rinse, and sanitize utensils and cutting board
		Wash vegetables in clean and sanitized vegetable sink	Clean and sanitize vegetable sink before washing vegetables
		Cooking	
Cooking stew	Bacterial survival	Cook all ingredients to minimum internal temperature of 165°F (73.9°C)	Continue cooking to 165°F (73.9°C)
		Verify final temperature with thermometer	Continue cooking to 165°F (73.9°C)
	Physical contamination during cooking	Keep covered, stir often	Cover
	Contamination by herbs and spices	Add spices early in cooking procedure	Continue cooking at least one-half hour after spices are added
		Measure all spices, flavor enhancers, and additives and read labels carefully	

TABLE 14.1 (*Continued*)

Critical Control	Hazard if standard not met	Standards	Corrective action
	Contamination of utensils	Use clean and sanitized utensils	Wash, rinse, and sanitize all utensils before use
	Contamination from cook's hands or mouth	Use proper tasting procedures	Discard product
		Holding and Service	
Hot holding and serving	Contamination, bacterial growth	Use clean and sanitary equipment to transfer and hold product	Wash, rinse, and sanitize equipment before transferring food product to it
		Hold stew above 140°F (60°C) in preheated holding unit, stir to maintain even temperature	Return to stove and reheat to 165°F (73.9°C)
		Keep covered	Cover
		Clean and sanitize serving equipment and utensils	Wash, rinse, and sanitize serving utensils and equipment
		Cooling	
Cooling for storage	Bacterial survival and growth	Cool rapidly in ice water bath and/or shallow pans (<4″ deep)	Move to shallow pans
		Stirring food placed in an ice bath	
		Adding ice to the ingredients	
		Using containers that facilitate heat transfer	
		Cool rapidly from 140°F (60°C) to 40°F (7.2°C) in four hours or less	Discard, or reheat to 5°F (73.9°C) and cool one time only
		Verify final temperature with a thermometer; record temperatures and times before product reaches 40°F (7.2°C) or less	If temperature is not reached in less than four hours, discard; or reheat product to 165°F (60°C) and recool one time only
	Cross-contamination	Place on top shelf	Move to top shelf
		Cover immediately after cooling	Cover
		Use clean and sanitized pans	Wash, rinse, and sanitize pans before filling them with product
		Do not stack pans	Separate pans by shelves
	Bacterial growth in time or after prolonged storage time	Label with date and time	Label with date and time or discard
		Reheating	
Reheat for service	Survival of bacterial contaminants	Heat rapidly on stove top or in oven to 165°F (73.9°C)	Reheat to 165°F (73.9°C) within two hours
		Maintain temperature at 140°F (60°C) or above; verify temperature with a thermometer	Transfer to preheated hot-holding unit to maintain 140°F (60°C) or above
		Do not mix new product into old product	Discard product
		Do not reheat or serve leftovers more than once	Discard product if any remains after being reheated

TABLE 14.2. Hazardous Practices Observed in Foodservice Operations

Condition/Area	Hazardous Practices
Preparation and display of potentially hazardous foods with either bare hands or the same pair of gloves (raw poultry, raw meat, raw seafood, dairy products)	▪ Setting up and taking down raw and cooked items for display ▪ Reusing the same kale, lemon, lettuce, or other vegetable garnish or decorative plastic dividers or color enhancers indiscriminately for raw or cooked foods ▪ Displaying cooked foods in the same case as raw seafood, poultry, and/or meat: As to be in physical contact with one another So that drippings from raw items can flow through ice or along garnish and reach the cooked items below Without separation by baffles or in separate cases ▪ Infrequent hand washing by persons who handle these foods ▪ Refrigerators and cases not kept at temperatures between 30° and 34°F (1°C)
Preparation and display of salads	▪ Handling salad ingredients with bare hands during preparation ▪ Soaking vegetables in a sink previously used for thawing or washing raw poultry ▪ Ingredients not prechilled ▪ Slicing, chopping, and grating equipment and utensils not properly cleaned ▪ Foods on display, particularly near top surfaces, not at temperatures of 45°F (7.1°C) or below ▪ Refrigerator temperatures higher than 40°F (4.4°C) ▪ Infrequent hand washing
Preparation of entrées, soups, sauces, stews, and other viscous products	▪ Cooked food left at room temperature for several hours ▪ Inadequate cooking of poultry, pork, and other foods that are likely to be contaminated with vegetative forms of food-borne pathogens ▪ Temperatures of batches of meat, poultry, items containing ground meat, and stuffed items not monitored at the completion of cooking ▪ Insufficient thawing of foods before cooking, which may contribute to inadequate cooking ▪ Leftovers reheated to insufficiently high temperatures ▪ Kitchen personnel handling or otherwise touching cooked foods with their bare hands ▪ Kitchen personnel handling raw foods or eggshells either with their hands or gloves and then handling cooked foods ▪ Table surfaces or cutting boards used for raw meat, raw poultry, raw seafood, and then (without washing or disinfecting) used for either cooked foods or foods that will not be heated subsequently ▪ Cloths and sponges used to wipe raw-food areas or equipment
Holding of hot food	▪ Foods held warm, but not hot, for 8 hours or longer ▪ Foods not held at temperatures of 130°F (54.4°C); (140°F [60°C] to satisfy requirements in many codes) or higher, sometimes in the temperature range of 70°F to 120°F (21.1°C to 48.9°C) within which bacterial growth can be very rapid (Continue to check the *Food Code* and policies and procedures of the facility and local health department regulations) ▪ Hot-holding units not used as designed, for example: Foods on display in baking pans or baskets that are tilted up by objects under the back end of the pans or baskets Foods in bowls while displayed in steam tables Packaged foods on edges of heating elements and on the side framing of the units Items stacked on top of other items ▪ Hot-holding units not operated as intended, for example: Thermostats turned lower than recommended or necessary to hold foods at temperatures of 130°F (140°F to satisfy requirements in many codes) or higher Fans in units not turned on Glass walls removed from units Steam-table water not in
Cooling of products for storage	▪ Storing foods while they are being cooled in large containers, such as: 5-gallon (22.7 L) plastic buckets Stockpots Soup-kettle inserts Pans (plastic or metal) that have heights greater than 4 inches (10 cm) ▪ Tightly covered containers of hot foods during initial cooling ▪ Containers of foods being "cooled" while stacked on top of others ▪ Refrigerator temperatures higher than 40°F (4.4°C) ▪ Inadequate number of racks in refrigerators to adequately store shallow pans of foods ▪ Shelf spacing in refrigerators too great to facilitate the storage of the needed number of shallow pans

FIGURE 14.1 Components of Food Hazard Analysis

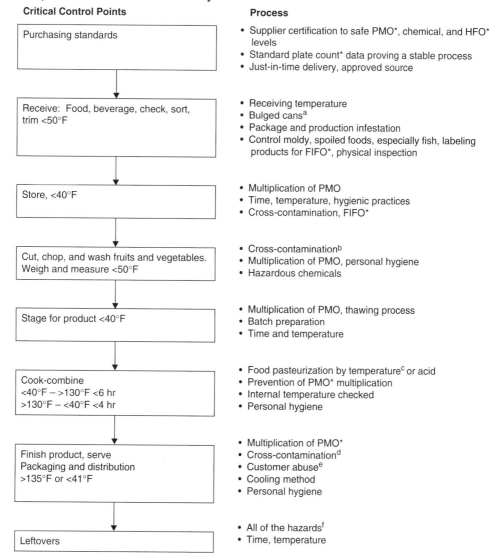

Critical Control Points

| Purchasing standards |

Process
- Supplier certification to safe PMO*, chemical, and HFO* levels
- Standard plate count* data proving a stable process
- Just-in-time delivery, approved source

| Receive: Food, beverage, check, sort, trim <50°F |

- Receiving temperature
- Bulged cans[a]
- Package and production infestation
- Control moldy, spoiled foods, especially fish, labeling products for FIFO*, physical inspection

| Store, <40°F |

- Multiplication of PMO
- Time, temperature, hygienic practices
- Cross-contamination, FIFO*

| Cut, chop, and wash fruits and vegetables. Weigh and measure <50°F |

- Cross-contamination[b]
- Multiplication of PMO, personal hygiene
- Hazardous chemicals

| Stage for product <40°F |

- Multiplication of PMO, thawing process
- Batch preparation
- Time and temperature

| Cook-combine <40°F – >130°F <6 hr >130°F – <40°F <4 hr |

- Food pasteurization by temperature[c] or acid
- Prevention of PMO* multiplication
- Internal temperature checked
- Personal hygiene

| Finish product, serve Packaging and distribution >135°F or <41°F |

- Multiplication of PMO*
- Cross-contamination[d]
- Customer abuse[e]
- Cooling method
- Personal hygiene

| Leftovers |

- All of the hazards[f]
- Time, temperature

Note: Critical control points are indicated by an asterisk. At all steps, hands should be washed and nonlatex gloves changed and disposed of as appropriate.
Abbreviations: HFO, hard foreign objects; PMO, pathogenic microorganisms; FIFO, first-in, first-out.
[a]Return all bulged cans to supplier.
[b]Use clean sink and appropriate cutting boards.
[c]Use correct cooking method, either cold or hot.
[d]Avoid contamination of raw and cooked foods.
[e]Improper handling after purchase.
[f]Proper storage and utilization.
Source: Adapted from P. Snyder, Hospitality Institute of Technology and Management, Inc., St. Paul, Minn., 1991. Adapted by Ruby P. Puckett 2010.

FIGURE 14.2   Decision Tree for Critical Control Points

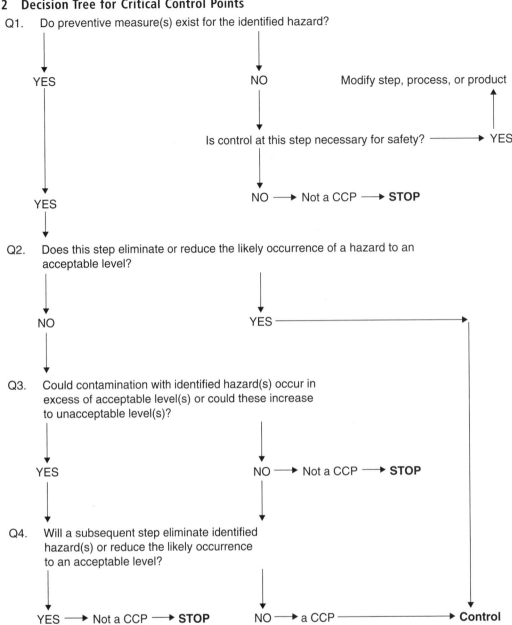

Q1.   Do preventive measure(s) exist for the identified hazard?

Note. Apply at each step in food preparation that has an identified hazard.
Source: *Food Code 2009.* Public Health Service, U.S. Department of Health and Human Services.

FIGURE 14.3 HACCPs for Cook-and-Chill Procedures

	Critical Control Points	Monitoring Procedures	Action If Monitoring Procedure Is Not Met
Receive ingredients	Approved source Raw/cooked separated in storage Refrigerate 41°F or below	Documentation of source Approved temperature of food or storage Separation of raw and cooked foods	Discard food Return food to supplier Separate raw and cooked foods
Prepare ingredients	Wash hands, wash and sanitize equipment Minimize hand contact with products that will not be cooked Prechill all ingredients, including vegetables	Observe quantity of food at room temperature Observe time food is held at room temperature Observe hand-washing procedures Observe sanitizing of equipment	Discard food
Cook	Cook products containing poultry to 180°F, pork to 150°F, and other potentially hazardous foods to 150°F	Ensure food reaches proper internal temperature	Continue cooking until food product reaches proper temperature
Cool	Rapidly cool from 140°F to 70°F in two hours or less and from 70°F to 41°F in four hours or less; cooling methods may include shallow pans, rapid chill refrigeration, ice bath, or blast freezing	Measure temperature during cooling Food depth, food iced Food stirred, food size Food placed in rapid chill refrigerator Food uncovered	Discard food
Combine ingredients	Avoid direct hand contact; use properly washed and sanitized equipment and utensils; hand washing	Observe worker Measure food temperature Observe hand washing	Discard food
Cold hold	Maintain product temperature at 41°F or below; minimize time between heating and service	Observe worker Measure food temperature	Discard food
Rethermalize	Wash hands, wash and sanitize equipment; minimize hand contact with products that will not be cooked; Cook to proper temperature: Beef—145°F Poultry—180°F Pork—150°F Other potentially hazardous foods—140°F	Ensure food reaches proper temperature	Continue cooking until the food product reaches proper temperature
Serve	Food temperature: Hot—145°F or above Cold—41° or below	Ensure food temperatures are maintained for entire period of service	Check equipment for proper working condition Chill/heat to correct temperatures

Note. A hazard may occur at any step of the process. Also, temperature requirements vary from one governmental agency to another.

FIGURE 14.4 HACCPs for Cook-and-Serve Procedures

	Critical Control Points	Monitoring Procedures	Action If Monitoring Procedure Is Not Met
Receive ingredients	Approved source Raw/cooked separated in storage Refrigerate 41°F or below	Documentation of source Approved temperature of food or storage Separation of raw and cooked foods	Discard food Return food to supplier Separate raw and cooked foods
Rethermalize	Wash hands, wash and sanitize equipment; minimize hand contact with products that will not be cooked Cook to proper temperature: Beef—145°F to 170°F Poultry—180°F Pork—160°F to 170°F Other potentially hazardous foods—145°F	Ensure food reaches proper temperature	Continue cooking until the food product reaches proper temperature
Serve	Food temperature: Hot—145°F or above Cold—41°F or below	Ensure food temperatures are maintained Note time not kept at proper temperature	Check equipment for proper working condition Chill/heat to correct temperatures

Note. Temperature requirements vary from one governmental agency to another.

Critical limits are criteria that must be met for each preventable measure associated with a CCP. Each CCP has one or more preventive measures that must be properly controlled to ensure prevention, elimination, or reduction of hazard to acceptable levels.

The goals and objectives for food safety assurance are now developed. The clearly stated plan for meeting the goals and objectives promotes safe and sanitary working conditions. To assist in the process, the following components of hazards analysis are beneficial.

CCPs include time; humidity; water activity; pH; preservation; salt concentration; available chlorine viscosity; hand washing; illness of personnel; storage; preparation and service; temperatures for preparation, holding, and service; appropriate use of leftovers; and rethermalization.

The following is an application example to use in establishing the critical limits for the preventable measures:

- Process step: Cooking
- CCP: Yes
- Critical limits:
  Minimum internal temperature of beef roast: 145°F (63°C)
  Oven temperature: 325°F to 350°F
  Roast weight: 22 to 26 lb (10 to 12 kg)
  Roast thickness: 6 to 8 inches
  Oven humidity

Figure 14.5 provides a flowchart for CCPs.

Principle 4: Establish a Monitoring System for Each CCP

Monitoring is a planned sequence of observations or measurements to assess whether a CCP is under control and to produce an accurate record for use in the future verification procedures. The main purpose of monitoring is:

- Make observations on a continuous basis or at scheduled intervals, to gather objective information.

- Describe methods used, type of measurements (temperature), and if method was visual or microbiologically tested.
- To track the operation, to monitor any trend, correct any action, and to bring the process back into control.
- To determine if a deviation has occurred and to take corrective action.
- To provide written *documentation for verification* of the plan and the person responsible for the monitoring.

The monitoring program should describe the methods, the frequency of observation or measurement, and the recording procedure.

A flowchart should be developed for recipe group CCPs. The *flowchart* can be used to check all steps to be observed and measured. A loss of control or deviation that has actually occurred should be documented. Flowcharts can also be developed for the methods used for cooking, such as roasting, baking, frying, and so forth. At this step, temperature monitoring is critical. Other key areas to monitor are time, pH level, employee performance, records, and documentation. Preventive measures include personal hygiene (especially hand washing), separating raw and cooked products (cross-contamination), and methods for *cleaning* and *sanitizing* the environment and equipment.

The monitoring procedures track the system or process of operation. The monitoring indicates when loss of control and deviation have occurred. Exhibit 14.1 is an example that can be used to monitor CCPs for employee behavior, equipment, food, hot holding, and transporting. The supervisor would fill out this form and initial, noting any needed correction and what measures were taken to correct any problem. This form is verification of documentation. The form should reside with the product throughout the process and then be filed for a specified period of time.

The written documentation is provided. When establishing the monitoring procedures, the team must establish the interval of

FIGURE 14.5 Flowchart for Critical Control Points

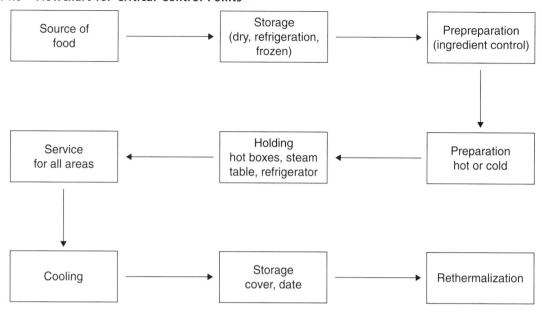

Source of food	→ Storage (dry, refrigeration, frozen)	→ Prepreparation (ingredient control)
Service for all areas	← Holding hot boxes, steam table, refrigerator	← Preparation hot or cold
Cooling	→ Storage cover, date	→ Rethermalization

Source of food: Check for condition of products on delivery

Storage: Store products in an appropriate area (dry, refrigerated, frozen)

Prepreparation: Thaw food using an approved method; clean any raw products under cool water and use a vegetable brush as needed

Preparation: Cook according to recipe directions; when an oven is used, preheat it

Holding: Maintain temperature; avoid cross-contaminiation during preparation and service

Service: Stir the product, keep it covered, and keep the serving utensil in the food; do not add old product to new product

Cooling: Cool product rapidly in an ice bath, blast chiller, and the like; use a shallow pan as appropriate, cut larger pieces into smaller pieces, and so forth

Storage: Keep product covered, dated, and stored in the refrigerator or freezer

Rethermalization: Reheat to temperature (165°F [74°C] for 15 seconds) to kill acquired pathogens

the monitoring. Care should be taken to do the monitoring rapidly with an assignment of responsibility.

Continuous monitoring is preferred when feasible. However, continuous monitoring is not always feasible due to cost, lack of labor, and the like. The team should establish a monitoring interval that is reliable enough to indicate that the hazard is under control. The foodservice manager should assign responsibility for monitoring, train staff, and do random sampling.

Principle 5: Establish a Corrective Action

Each area in the food production process must be examined for deficiencies. The workplace is to be reviewed, monitored, and analyzed through food safety audits, environmental monitoring, identification of the person(s) responsible for implementation and monitoring of the process and self-inspections to identify CCPs that could lead to a food-borne illness. The first step is to determine what went wrong, what action was taken to correct the problem, what to do with the product that has been compromised, and then appropriate action should be chosen, applied and recorded. Specific corrective action must be developed for each CCP. When there is a deviation it may be necessary to take appropriate corrective action to regain control at the CCP.

A continuous review of the flowcharts, recipes, and procedure manuals will indicate steps for correction. As the corrections are identified, they should be added to the appropriate documents.

All control points should be reviewed from source to serving. A corrective action plan for each CCP is then developed. The CCP should be shown to be brought under control as documented in the HACCP plan. The responsible person should check for breaks in employee health policies, cross-contamination, temperature controls, thawing, cooling, and reheating. Whether food should be discarded should be determined. If appropriate, an outside laboratory can be used to test for microorganisms. Methods should be devised that can be implemented to immediately correct the problem.

Foodservice professionals must demonstrate that the problem is under control. An account of steps taken and follow-up must be documented. The corrections are added to the flowcharts, procedures, and manuals.

The most important task is to communicate the change(s) to employees. The training process is ongoing with an HACCP program. Employees must be encouraged to bring hazardous food operating conditions to the supervisor or manager's attention for correction.

Principle 6: Establish Verification Procedures

A verification procedure for individual CCPs needs to be developed. Verification and auditing methods, any test, random sampling and analysis can be used to determine whether the HACCP system is working correctly and achieving the desired results. The team should specify methods and procedures to be used. The critical limits that have been established for the CCPs should be verified that they will prevent, eliminate, or reduce hazards to an acceptable level. The overall effectiveness of the HACCP plan should be verified.

Verification procedures may include: inspection of the operation to check that CCPs are kept under control and monitoring is effective; validation of critical limits, review of deviations, correction action and measures taken, and self checking audits. Check the system when changes such as new products, new procedures, new vendors supplying products, and any other changes occur.

Principle 7: Establish Documentation and Record Keeping

Setting up a record-keeping system is essential to providing documentation that proves that HACCP is being used. Foodservice professionals may consider the record-keeping phase burdensome, but not keeping records is the same as not having an HACCP program.

Records need to be reviewed (some daily) to make sure that the controls are effective, the correct data are collected, and the employees are completing their duties. When the records are reviewed on a daily basis, problems can be immediately identified, investigation made, and corrective action taken. All records should be filed, and any action taken should be documented.

Record keeping makes the HACCP system work. Records should validate that the HACCP plan is based on current evidence-based science and technical knowledge concerning product and the process. The sophistication depends on each individual operation, but the simplest form of record keeping is the best.

EXHIBIT 14.1. HACCP Documentation

Items to Be Initialed by Shift Leader	Date	Initial
Critical Control Point (CCP)/Control Point (CP)		
Employee Behavior CCPs		
Proper hand washing		
Ill employees not working		
Proper uniform		
Hair covered		
Processing CCPs		
Equipment and utensils sanitized		
Avoid direct contact with hands		
Production CCPs		
Use appropriate cutting board for raw and cooked products		
Food cooked to proper temperature		
Avoid cross-contamination		
Hot Holding CCPs		
Avoid mixing leftovers with new		
Discard unused cooked product		
Food protected from contamination		
Transporting CCPs		
Food protected from contamination		

Essential records to maintain are:

- All items relating to the development of the HACCP plan
- Validation of the plan
- Clearly identified CCPs and critical limits
- Inspection sheets
- Flowcharts
- CCP monitoring and recording procedures
- Review of deviations and their resolutions, including the disposition of food
- Implementation strategy
- Visual inspection to determine if CCPs are under control
- A list of teams and responsibilities, training, and competency
- Description of product and intended use
- The monitoring of temperatures on all equipment and deficiencies corrected
- Random sample collection and analysis
- Periodic monitoring of room temperature and humidity (a kitchen that is too hot will promote the use of fans that can stir up microorganisms)
- The monitoring of temperature throughout the food storage, preparation, and service cycle
- Monitoring requirements for finished product and distribution
- All data on equipment repairs
- The monitoring of the frequency of pest control and the use of all chemicals (material safety data sheets must be made available, and personnel must know the hazards of chemicals and be well trained in their use)
- Flowcharts (include as part of the procedure manuals)
- Records
  Flowcharts from receiving to consumption
  CCPs for each step as appropriate
  Hazards associated with each CCP and the preventive measures
  Critical limits
  Monitoring system
  Corrective action plans for deviation from critical limits
  Record-keeping procedures
  Procedures for verification for HACCP system

It is suggested that all records be kept for a minimum of six months. These records can be reviewed by inspectors or surveyors. The documentation allows for validation of the HACCP plan development, changes in processes, changes in equipment, changes in food supply problems that occur, and any new information. An example of the HACCP plan documentation for the cooling step is provided in Figure 14.6.

FIGURE 14.6   HACCP Cooling Plan Documentation

Process Step	Cooling
CCP	**Critical Point # XXX**
Criteria or critical limit	Cool food rapidly in small quantities to 41°F (5°C) cool for 2 hours to 70°F (21°C) plus 4 hours to 41°F
Establish monitoring	Department personnel break down food into small quantities and monitor cooling process
Corrective or preventive action	Modify cooling procedures or discard
HACCP records	Blast chiller cooling log
HACCP system verification	Safety audit by shift leader

Briefly, HACCP is a program used to identify potential food safety hazards so Critical Control Action can be taken to reduce or eliminate the hazard before it happens. The system is used in all phases—from the source to consumption. Securing the food → food receiving → food storage (storeroom, refrigerators, freezers) → food preparation (hot and cold) → serving lines (patients, others) → safety and sanitation → review CCPs → monitor system (employees, work areas, use checklist) → if necessary, take corrective action (use problem-solving method to get problem under control) → verify (the system is working, needs some modifications, keep staff informed) → maintain records (keep files of problems and solution and other pertinent information) → verify the systems are working.

FIGURE 14.7   HACCP Action Plan for Implementation

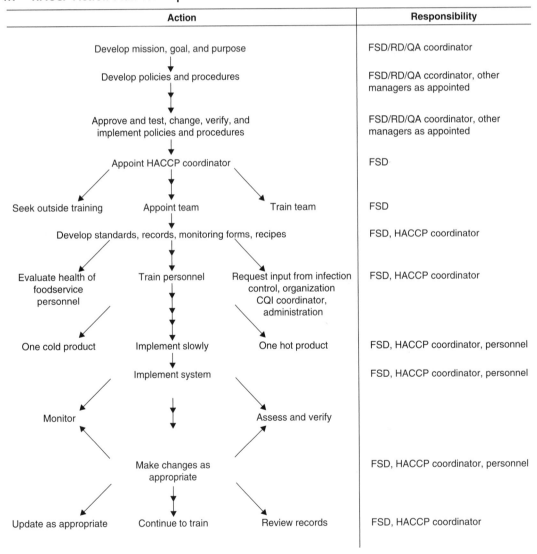

Action	Responsibility
Develop mission, goal, and purpose	FSD/RD/QA coordinator
Develop policies and procedures	FSD/RD/QA ccordinator, other managers as appointed
Approve and test, change, verify, and implement policies and procedures	FSD/RD/QA coordinator, other managers as appointed
Appoint HACCP coordinator	FSD
Seek outside training / Appoint team / Train team	FSD
Develop standards, records, monitoring forms, recipes	FSD, HACCP coordinator
Evaluate health of foodservice personnel / Train personnel / Request input from infection control, organization CQI coordinator, administration	FSD, HACCP coordinator
One cold product / Implement slowly / One hot product	FSD, HACCP coordinator, personnel
Implement system	FSD, HACCP coordinator, personnel
Monitor / Assess and verify	
Make changes as appropriate	FSD, HACCP coordinator, personnel
Update as appropriate / Continue to train / Review records	FSD, HACCP coordinator

Note. Abbreviations: FSD, foodservice director; QA, quality assurance; CQI, continuous quality improvement; RD, registered dietitian.

Source: Ruby P. Puckett©. Used by permission.

HACCP Inspections

Establishments operating under a variance requiring an HACCP plan will be inspected differently. HACCP plans have critical limits that must be routinely monitored and recorded by the establishment. Monitoring and other elements of the plan must be verified by the inspector. Most states, through their Division of Business and Professional Regulations, and in some instances through the state extension service, developed HACCP inspection forms that are used by the state for inspection of hotels and restaurants. To secure copies for individual states check with local health departments or state professional regulation departments.

FEDERAL, STATE, AND LOCAL RULES AND REGULATIONS

The purpose of governmental regulations in the food industry is to protect the food served to the public. Because there are many opportunities for food to be contaminated from the farm to the consumer, the government (local, state, and federal) monitor both the process and producers to ensure the safety of food.

Federal Regulatory Agencies

FDA (www.fda.gov) activities are directed toward protecting the health of the nation against impure and unsafe foods, drugs, cosmetics, and other potential hazards.

The USDA (www.usda.gov) works to improve food production and strives to cure poverty, hunger, and malnutrition. It also works to protect soil, water, forest, and natural resources and, through its inspection and grading services, it safeguards and ensures standards of quality in the food supply.

The CDC (www.cdc.gov) is a federal agency charged with protecting the public health through prevention and control and through response to public health emergencies.

The EPA (www.epa.gov) protects and enhances the environment today and for the future. The agency's mission is to control and battle pollution related to air, water, solid waste, pesticides, radiation, and toxic substances.

The National Marine Fisheries Service (NMFS, www.nmfs.gov) of the U.S. Department of Commerce develops voluntary standards for the sanitary quality of fishing waters and processing methods.

The Occupational Safety and Health Administration (OSHA, www.osha.gov) develops and promotes occupational safety and health standards, develops and ensures regulations, conducts investigations and inspections, and issues citations and proposes penalties for noncompliance with safety and health standards and regulations.

Other Organizations

The following professional organizations offer assistance to consumers and professional members in food safety. Most of these organizations have websites that contain valuable help as well as references.

Information and assistance with specific food safety questions may be obtained from the following organizations.

- Academy of Nutrition and Dietetics (new name for American Dietetic Association)
- American Public Health Association
- Association of Food and Drug Officials
- Association of Nutrition and Food Professionals (new name for Dietary Managers Association)
- Food Marketing Institute
- Food Safety and Inspection Service
- Meat and Poultry Hot Line
- Ednet: e-mail
- International Classification of Diseases, 9th revision (ICD-9)
- Food Safety Educator
- National Environmental Health Association
- National Restaurant Association Education Foundation
- National Science Foundation International NSF
- Underwriters Laboratories (UL)

Surveys by Governing Agencies

A health care foodservice department may be surveyed by TJC, Center for Medicare and Medicaid Services (CMC) state licensing agencies, Omnibus Budget Reconciliation Act (OBRA) county public health departments, and other agencies. The agency surveyors follow standards that have been established under federal and state laws or by various state, county, and municipal agencies. The purpose of these surveys is to protect the health of the public by preventing or correcting unhealthy sanitation practices.

Health Inspections

Environmental health specialists monitor the conditions of individual establishments to determine whether they are in compliance with state and local laws. These specialists are registered sanitarians. The local registered sanitarian conducts the inspection. It is the responsibility of the foodservice manager to be aware of the purpose and function of the local inspection. It is also the foodservice manager's responsibility to secure copies of rules and regulations concerning the inspection, to follow the rules and to ensure that foodservice employees adhere to the rules. Performing self-audits and surveys should be routine, and when a deficiency is found, action needs to be taken to correct it. Self-audits help maintain a safe and sanitary department. Self-audits also help in being prepared for visits from the health inspector, state surveyor, or TJC.

It is also the responsibility of the foodservice manager to be available to answer questions, tour the facility with the inspector, and have all necessary records well documented. When a violation is cited, a report will be given to the foodservice manager with a date by which the violation must be corrected. Fines and possible closure of the department can result when warnings are not taken seriously. If the foodservice manager does not understand the violation or needs more information about the problem, he or she should ask the inspector for additional resources.

The health inspectors are looking for what is on the checklist. The following are among the categories that will be inspected. (Inspections vary from locale to locale.)

- *Supervision.* Knowledge—some states require the person in charge to have passed a state approved safety and sanitation exam or ServSafe.
- *Food.* From an approved source, free from spoilage; no **home-processed foods**; **no food brought in from the outside for a patient**; no dented or damaged cans; washing of fruits and vegetables; foods are labeled and all food in all areas are free from contamination by pests, chemicals, and physical hazards.
- *Food protection.* PHFs meet temperature requirements; food properly thawed; thermometers provide; handling of food minimized; food protected during storage, preparation, display, and transportation.
- *Personnel.* With infection restricted, when and where hands are washed, fingernail maintenance, prohibition of certain jewelry, uniforms are clean, and hair restraints are used, places for eating and drinking and tobacco use. (Some states also have regulations on body piercing and perfume.)
- *Food equipment and utensils.* Dishwashing facilities provided with accurate thermometers; pressure gauge and chemical test kit; clean equipment and utensils properly stored and handled to prevent contamination; food contact surfaces of cutting boards, meat slicers, can openers, work counter, and the liked washed, rinsed, and sanitized; and surfaces free of abrasive and detergents.
- *Safety.* Fire extinguishers, proper sprinkler system, and sufficient, well-lighted exits; electrical wiring is in good repair; gas appliances are properly installed and maintained.
- *Plumbing.* Properly installed and maintained, there are no cross-connections between potable and wastewater, and backflow devices are in place.
- *Insect, rodent animal control.* No insects, rodents, or other animals are present; outer openings are protected; and pest control management is in place.
- *Garbage and refuse disposal.* Garbage containers are sanitarily maintained and covered, and outside area is maintained and clean.
- *Toilets and hand-washing facilities.* Hand-washing sinks are accessible, hand sinks are provided with soap and single-service towels; toilet rooms are clean and in good repair; doors are self-closing; trash receptacles are available.
- *Other.* Toxic cleaning agents are stored away from food preparation and utensil washing areas; toxics are labeled; the premises is clean and maintained; there are no unnecessary articles; cleaning maintenance equipment is properly stored; only authorized personnel have access.
- *Lighting, ventilation, floors, walls, and ceiling meet all applicable codes.*
- *Water.* Safe; hot and cold are under pressure including bottled water.
- *License.* Current and properly displayed; food management certification is valid.

There may be other requirements set up by individual states. It is your responsibility to know and follow the rules/regulations for your geographic location.

Health, Hygiene, and Clean Work Habits

Providing safe and sanitary foodservice obviously relies on the employment of healthy workers who are thoroughly trained in safe food-handling procedures, practice good personal hygiene, and perform their duties without undue fatigue. Humans can trace many cases of food-borne illness to contamination, so the ongoing training and supervision of foodservice employees should stress good health, careful personal grooming, and good work habits. All foodservice employees should observe the following procedures:

- Check *Food Code*: Chapter 2–2 Employee Health that outlines the following:

1. Reportable symptoms	2–201.12 Exclusions and Restrictions
2. Reportable diagnosis	Nine points are included here.
3. Reportable past illness	2–201.13 Removal, adjustments to and retention of exclusions and restrictions
4. Reportable history of exposure	
5. Reportable history of exposure	Twenty-two points under this title.
6. Responsibility of person in charge to notify the regulatory authority	As of September 29, 2011, a Supplement to *Food Code* became effective.
7. Responsibility of the person in charge to prohibit a conditional employee from becoming a food employee	There are other changes that need to be added to employee training and policies procedures.
8. Responsibility of the person in charge to exclude or restrict	
9. Responsibility of food employees and conditional employees to report	
10. Responsibility of food employees to comply	

The foodservice director will need to review the *Food Code* to ensure that policies and procedures are developed in compliance with employee health.

- **NEW**—In a verifiable manner, the employees are required to report information about their health and activities as they relate to diseases transmissible through food.

- Employees must report any illnesses that cause diarrhea, vomiting, sore throat with a fever, jaundice, infected cut, or open wound and drainage, or lesions containing pus on hand, wrist, or exposed part of the body that is not properly covered. All food handlers should undergo a health examination by a physician designated by the organization before beginning employment and at intervals specified by public health agencies or the institution. The medical records of employees should be maintained in a separate file from their personnel file. The history should include a history of exposure to a foodborne illness such as Norovirus, *E. coli* 0157:H7, hepatitis, typhoid fever, shigellosis, salmonella, and others as designated by the organization and local and state public health department. (A written release may be needed from employee to the foodservice director to review the health record.) The manager or the organization's infection control representative must notify public health of jaundice and other communicable diseases.
- All foodservice employees should be clean and well groomed. Clean uniforms and aprons are essential. If employees are permitted to wear street clothes while on duty, the clothing should be made of washable fabric. Appropriate hair restraints (nets, hairpins, and surgical caps) must be worn.
- *Clean hands and fingernails are a must.* Foodservice employees should thoroughly wash their hands before and after handling food, after smoking, after using the toilet, and after using a handkerchief or tissue. Thorough and frequent hand washing is the best defense in the control of hepatitis A outbreaks. Hand sinks with hot running water must be located at the entrance to the kitchen, production area, or workstation. No other sinks (such as food preparation or three-compartment sinks) should be used for hand washing. The following seven-step, double-hand-wash method is recommended for use by all employees involved in food-handling activities:

Step 1: Turn on hot, flowing water (110°F to 120°F) and wet hands in a hand-washing sink that is equipped with single-use towels, soap dispenser, hot and cold water, and a waste receptacle. (Note: Sufficient pressure and volume of flowing potable water are important in reducing high levels of organisms such as Shigella dysenteriae.)

Step 2: Apply an antibacterial soap to hands and onto fingers in sufficient quantity to produce a good lather. Hands and arms should be lathered up to sleeve or as far up arm as necessary to clean any exposed area, including surrogate prosthetic devices for hand or arms. Rub vigorously for at least 20 seconds—the time it takes to sing Happy Birthday twice.

Step 3: Thoroughly rinse hands in hot (110°F to 120°F) flowing potable water.

Step 4: Repeat Steps 1 and 2 to ensure that all pathogens have been removed.

Step 5: Rinse hands and arms in hot flowing potable water.

Step 6: Use single-use towel to turn off faucet. Secure another towel and dry hands with single-use paper towels or a warm air blower. In some locales, health departments require the use of warm *air* blowers rather than single-use paper towels.

Step 7: Use hand towel to open door and discard hand towel in receptacle outside of door.

If approved and capable of removing the types of soils encountered in the food operations involved, an automatic hand-washing facility may be used by food employees to wash their hands or surrogate prosthetic devices.

Hand antiseptic must meet the conditions as outlined in *Food Code* 2009.

Hands should be washed:

After touching bare human parts other than clean hands and clean exposed portions of arms

After using the toilet

After coughing, sneezing, using a handkerchief or disposable tissue, using tobacco, eating, or drinking

After handling salad equipment or utensils

During food preparation, as often as necessary to remove soil and contamination and to prevent cross-contamination when changing task

When switching between working with raw food and working with ready-to-eat food

Before putting on and after removing gloves

After engaging in other activities that contaminate hands:
Handling chemicals
Taking out garbage
Cleaning tables and equipment

The CDC and TJC have approved the use of special hand-washing wipes for use in some areas in health care facilities.

Other Employee Restrictions

The FDA and USDA in the Food Code recommend:

- Employees who have persistent sneezing, coughing, or runny nose that causes a discharge from the eyes, nose, or mouth may not work with food, service ware, utensils, or preparation equipment or serve food to any customer.
- Foodservice personnel should have trimmed, filed, and maintained nails and edges and surfaces that are cleanable and not rough.
- When preparing food, foodservice employees may not wear jewelry on arms and hands except a plain ring such as a wedding band.
- Unless wearing gloves, fingernail polish or artificial nails are prohibited when working with exposed food.
- Hats, hair restraints, or nets should restrain hair (including beards) and clothing that covers body hair and are designed and worn effectively keep hair from contacting exposed food; clean equipment, utensils, and linens; and unwrapped single-service and single-use articles. All other body hair is to be covered by clothing. This does not apply to food employees such as counter staff who may serve beverages, wrapped or packaged foods, hostesses, and waitstaff.
- The use of excessive perfume should be discouraged.

- Avoid sweat dropping into food; wear proper uniform and shoes, no open-toed shoes.
- Keep uniform and underclothes clean and in good repair. When aprons are worn, they must be clean and changed often during food preparation and service.
- Bathe daily using soap, water, and deodorant.
- An employee may drink from a closed beverage container if the container is handled to prevent contamination of the employee's hand, the container, and exposed food, equipment, utensils, linens, and unwrapped single-service and single-use articles.
- In areas of the country that require it by law, employees should wear disposable gloves when preparing and serving food. The foodservice department should provide a variety of sizes of gloves. Disposable gloves should never be washed and reused. Wearing gloves does not prevent cross-contamination of food and food-borne pathogens because gloved hands touch as many contaminated surfaces and ingredients as do ungloved hands. Nonetheless, when gloves are mandated, employees should change them if they become punctured or soiled and between handling raw and processed ingredients and food products, before beginning a different task, changed at least every four hours or more often as needed. Employees should wash their hands after removing gloves. Nonlatex gloves should be used. Cloth gloves may not be used in direct contact with food **unless** the food is subsequently cooked as required for frozen food or primal cut of meat. Bare-hand contact with food is prohibited under the Food Code.
- Use of tobacco products should not be permitted. Most health care organizations and university campuses have banned smoking anywhere on the grounds/campus.
- Employees should avoid contact between their hands and fingers and food, and they should pick up serving and eating utensils only by their bases or handles.
- Spoons or other utensils used in food preparation should not be used for tasting; only separate spoons and forks (washed after each use) or disposable utensils should be used. The two-spoon method is best: take one spoon to take a sample of the food, transfer the sample to another spoon and taste. Use two clean spoons each time a new food is sampled.
- Employees should consume their meals only in designated dining areas.
- Personal belongings should be kept out of food preparation and service areas and stored in lockers located outside the foodservice department.
- Only authorized persons should enter the kitchen. Once entering the kitchen, they need to cover their hair with a hair cover.
- All cuts should be bandaged with waterproof protectors, and employees with cuts on their hands should wear watertight disposable gloves.
- The foodservice department must implement and enforce procedures for ensuring that employees are protected against on-the-job injuries or diseases that could result in food contamination. Employees with open lesions, infected wounds, sore throats, or communicable diseases should not be permitted to work in food preparation and service areas. The facility's designated physician should clear an employee known to have suffered a respiratory tract infection before being allowed to return to work.
- A tuberculin (purified protein derivative) skin test should be used to screen employees for tuberculosis on a yearly basis if required by the local health department or health care organization.
- There is no scientific evidence that AIDS or HIV infection can be transmitted through food. It cannot be spread through casual contact that occurs between employees or customers or through contaminated food. Managers should know the legal ramifications of firing or transferring an employee who has AIDS or an employee who has tested HIV positive from the foodservice department simply because the individual handles food. AIDS is covered by the Americans with Disabilities Act, which provides civil rights protection to infected employees.

ENVIRONMENTAL SANITATION

A clean working environment is vital to good sanitation practices. Whether it is part of a new suburban facility or an older inner-city hospital, every foodservice department can meet basic standards of cleanliness through careful planning and management. Modern foodservice equipment, materials, and furnishings should be designed to be cleaned easily with hot water, detergents, and sanitizing agents. Floors should be constructed of materials that resist absorption of grease and moisture. Good sanitation also depends on having an adequate number of conveniently located sinks and floor drains to facilitate washing. Walls, ceilings, and ventilation equipment should be designed and constructed to accommodate frequent thorough cleaning. Sanitation is a must for any surface that comes in contact with food, which includes all dishes, utensils, pots, and pans.

Sanitary features should be a major consideration in the purchase and placement of new equipment, which should be installed so that soil, food particles, and other debris that collect between pieces of equipment and surrounding walls and floors can be removed easily. Equipment cleaning must be scheduled regularly to prevent accumulation of dirt and spilled food, which reduces the possibility of contamination of food by microorganisms and helps in pest control.

- High standards of environmental sanitation can be maintained in both modern and older facilities by meeting certain basic requirements: All work and storage areas are kept clean, dry, well lighted, and in good order.
- Overhead pipes have either been removed or are covered by a false ceiling. Because they collect dust and might leak, such pipes are a hazard in food preparation areas and could lead to food contamination. (State and local sanitation and building codes should be complied with.)

- The walls, floors, and ceilings in all areas should be cleaned routinely.
- Ventilation hoods prevent grease buildup and moisture condensation, which can collect on walls and ceilings and drip into food or onto food preparation areas. Filters and other grease-extracting equipment are removed regularly for cleaning or replaced if they were not designed for easy cleaning in place.
- To prevent cross-contamination, kitchenware and food preparation areas are washed, rinsed, and sanitized after every use and after any interruption of operations during which contamination could occur. Manufacturers' instructions are followed for the cleaning of all equipment.
- The food-contact surfaces of grills, griddles, and similar cooking equipment and the cavities and door seals of microwave ovens are cleaned at least once a day. Deep-fat cooking equipment and filtering systems need not be cleaned daily. Surfaces that do not come into contact with food should be cleaned as often as necessary to keep the equipment free from accumulations of dust, dirt, food particles, and other debris.
- A ready supply of safe potable hot water (120°F to 140°F [49°C to 60°C]) is always available, and the temperature of the hot water meets the minimum requirements of state and local codes.
- Adequate lighting (at least 20 foot-candles) is provided for all food-preparation areas and at equipment and utensil-washing stations. All lighting fixtures located over, by, or within food storage, preparation, service, and display areas are equipped with protective shields that keep broken glass from falling into food. Areas where equipment and utensils are washed and stored are also protected from glass falling from broken lightbulbs.
- Effective rodent, pest, and insect control is carried out routinely. Openings to the outdoors are protected by tight-fitting and self-closing doors, tightly closed windows, and adequate screening or controlled air currents or by other means.
- An adequate number of insect-proof, rodent-proof, and fireproof containers for garbage and refuse disposal are available, kept covered, and cleaned frequently. (Disposal of such materials should be in accord with local ordinances.)
- Plumbing is properly installed and maintained with no **cross connection**, which is a dangerous link between an outlet of drinkable (potable) water system and unsafe water. There is no **backflow**, preventing contaminated water from flowing into potable water. The backflow or backsiphonage prevention device installed on a water system needs to meet American Society of Sanitary Engineering (ASSE) standards for construction, installation, maintenance, inspection, and testing for that specific application and type of device. **Backsiphonage** occurs after a loss in pressure in the water supply; water is siphoned back into the potable water. An **air gap** is an unobstructed air space between an outlet of potable water and the flood rim of a fixture or equipment. The air gap between the water supply inlet and the flood level rim of the plumbing fixture, equipment, or nonfood equipment is to be at least twice the diameter of the water supply inlet and may not be less than one inch (25mm) The foodservice such be aware of leaks, drips, and leakage that might contaminate food or food preparation areas.
- Toilets and hand-washing facilities are accessible, provided with soap, hot water, single-service towels and in those states that approve, an air dryer for drying hands. Lined garbage cans are placed just outside of the door for discarding towels. All toilet rooms should be clean (as often as necessary) in good repair, and have self-closing doors.

It is the foodservice manager's responsibility to see that all equipment is clean, that all employees wash their hands, and that good housekeeping methods are rigidly followed. The food consumed by customers must be safe. Employees must be taught to clean as they go, to keep everything in its place, and to put away all supplies before leaving duty. Good work habits should be taught.

Cleaning schedules should be posted and include what is to be cleaned, who is to do the cleaning, when the cleaning is to be done (frequency), and how the cleaning is to be done (for example, using cleanser and its proportions or sanitizer and its proportions). Every employee should have some cleaning responsibility. Inspections by the director and the supervisor should be made periodically using an inspection check sheet. Figure 14.8 is a proposed schedule for cleaning equipment. The results of inspections should be posted and areas that need attention should have follow-through.

The foodservice director and supervisors identify cleaning needs and seek input from employees who are the main users of the equipment by conducting a survey of the department. Once all survey and input data has been collected a master cleaning schedule can be developed that outlines *what, when, who,* and *how* procedures for each task. The schedule should be objective and fair in assigning the task. Once implemented seek feedback from the employees. Be flexible; make adjustments as needed.

Using Cleaning Compounds

The foodservice department uses cleaning and sanitizing compounds. *Cleaning* is the process of removing soil and food from a surface such as a coffee cup or dusting a desk through the use of chemicals. Cleaning is a step in sanitation process. *Sanitizing* is the process of removing/reducing the number of harmful microorganisms, on any surface, to a safe level, using chemicals or heat. Even when something is "clean" it still may pose a threat for illness if not properly sanitized. Cleaning and rinsing needs to be accomplished before sanitizing as this is a two-step operation.

Detergents are most often used for cleaning. A *detergent* is a cleaning agent, solvent, or any other substance that will remove foreign material from surfaces. Detergents are designed to loosen grease and oil, deposits of minerals, protein-based stains caused by eggs or meat, and dirt that has been baked onto contact surfaces. Manufacturers' instructions need to be followed, such as accurately measuring the amount of detergent to be used.

Synthetic detergents are used in water to break down the dirt. All detergents contain agents called *surfactants* that dissolve in water

FIGURE 14.8   Schedule for Cleaning of Equipment

Daily
1. Ranges and stoves washed
2. Can opener
3. Coffee urns
4. Coffee and tea dispensers
5. Garbage cans emptied after each meal and washed
6. Garbage disposals after each meal
7. Floors in kitchen and dining room after each meal
8. Clean outside of steam kettles
9. Refrigerators and freezers wiped and washed
10. Ovens wiped out and washed
11. Stainless-steel shelves, counters, and tables
12. Steam food warmers
13. Dining tables, chairs, stools, and counter after each meal
14. Food carts after each meal
15. Dish machine after each meal
16. Cart-washing area
17. Sweep and mop storeroom

After Each Meal
1. Cutting boards
2. Drain boards
3. Potato peeler
4. Food chopper
5. Meat and food slicer
6. Steam jacketed kettle
7. Griddle
8. Broiler
9. Steamer
10. Food mixer, small and large
11. Toaster
12. Deep-fat fryers (filter grease)
13. Food grinders

Weekly
Clean sides of oven
Refrigerators
Clean drawers in tables
Legs and undershelves of all tables
Can-washing room
1. Remove and clean filters of hood over stove
2. Thoroughly clean ovens inside and outside
3. Thoroughly clean ranges inside and out, jets of burners, etc.
4. Defrost and clean freezers and refrigerators
5. Thoroughly clean coffee urn—remove and clean gauges
6. Ice machine
7. Thoroughly clean dish machine using a sanitizer
8. Clean vents in refrigerators
Cleaning schedules may also include the person/title who is to do the cleaning, the procedures for cleaning, including the cleaning compounds and if necessary if protective clothing is to worn/used.

Monthly
Ice-cream cabinet
Ice-making machines
Walls
Floor—clean completely, scrubbing, etc.
Janitor's closet—clean completely
Flush out floor drains

and spread by means of suds. Detergents are usually inexpensive. They are the most cost-effective, all-purpose cleaning products. When rinsed properly, they do not leave a soapy residue, work well with chemical sanitizers, and are safe to use to clean food surfaces.

The foodservice department uses four general types of cleaning compounds: *acidic*, *alkaline*, *neutral*, and *solvent/degreaser*. It is important to use the correct cleaning compound to avoid harming food preparation surfaces or equipment. The following are recommendations:

- **Acidic** compounds are used sparingly to remove lime deposits, rust, and tarnish. Use with caution as acid cleansers may cause skin irritation.
- **Alkaline detergents** compounds are used to neutralize and dissolve most food deposits. These compounds can also be used for heavy cleaning such as oven doors, and in dish machines.

- **Neutral (can be called abrasive)** compounds are neither acidic nor alkaline. They are used frequently to clean floors, metal surfaces such as tabletops, and pots and pans. When these products are used to scourge surfaces they should be used with caution as they may scratch the surface, which may increase contamination as scratches may harbor bacteria and promote growth.
- **Solvents cleaners/degreasers** used to break down and remove grease build-up.

All cleaning compounds must be used as directed by their manufacturers. They should be stored separately from food, insecticides, rodenticides, and other poisons. All foodservice employees should be trained in the proper use of various compounds, and managers should check periodically to ensure that cleaning compounds are used appropriately. All cleaning compounds should have material safety data sheets (MSDSs) on file, accessible to all employees.

Using Germicides and Sanitizers

The sanitation regulations of all state and local governments specify that any surface that comes into contact with food must be cleaned after every use. This requirement applies to nearly all areas in the foodservice department.

Germicides and *sanitizers* are chemicals that kill or retard the growth of bacteria and other microorganisms on environmental surfaces. This type of product must be registered with the USDA to be called a germicide or sanitizer. The three most common chemicals used are *chlorine, quaternary*, and *iodine*. Chlorine is frequently combined with other chemicals and used for dish washing. A detergent is sometimes combined with a sanitizer and is called a *detergent sanitizer*. (With the concern with protecting the environment new products are available in some markets, check with your chemical supplier. Make sure that any new product purchased is safe to use around food and that the supplier furnishes an MSDS.)

Manufacturers' directions for using these potentially harmful chemicals must be closely monitored. Only compounds approved by the FDA for use around food should be allowed in the department. They should be stored away from food supplies. Instructions for mixing these chemicals with water before use should be posted and carefully followed.

An enclosed separate storage space, away from food and food preparation, should include:

- Space for storage of cleaning supplies
- Equipment for cleaning (buckets, cleaning cloths, brooms, mops, brushes, and any other supplies)
- Area will need to be well lighted
- A floor drain to dump dirty water
- A utility sink with running hot and cold water
- A towel rack for drying towels
- A space for personal protective equipment (PPE)
- A policies and procedures manual outlining for cleaning procedures
- A posted cleaning schedule
- An MSDS notebook that contains all chemicals used in the department. (All chemicals and cleaning supplies **must be clearly labeled**).

According to *Food Code*, wiping cloths (3–304.14):

A. Cloths in-use for wiping food spills from tableware and carry-out containers that occur as food is being served shall be:
   1. Maintained dry.
   2. Used for no other purpose.
B. Cloths in-use for wiping counters and other equipment surfaces shall be:
   1. Held between use in a chemical sanitizer solution at a concentration (see § 4–501.114) shall be free of food debris and visible soil, shall be stored on the floor and used In such a manner that prevents contamination of food, equipment, utensils, single-service, or single-use article.
   2. Laundered daily.

Single-use disposable sanitizer wipes must meet EPA-approved manufacturer's labels and used as instructed.

Cleaning Equipment

Equipment should be cleaned after every use and according to manufacturers' directions, which should be posted along with schedules and work assignments for routine cleaning. Managers should conduct weekly department inspections and take immediate action to correct any problems that interfere with meeting sanitary standards.

When cleaning stationary equipment, disassemble, clean, and sanitize it according to the manufacturer's instructions. The following cleaning method can be used for almost any large electrical equipment:

- Disconnect the power.
- Disassemble the equipment, wash, rinse, and sanitize the individual parts. Immerse them in a sink if possible. Be careful not to place any sharp materials in the sink.
- Wash and rinse remaining surface.
- Sanitize all food-contact surfaces with approved sanitizing solution.
- Wipe down all other surfaces with sanitizing solution.
- Air dry before putting equipment back together.
- Resanitize any food-contact surfaces that were touched when equipment was reassembled.

Stationary equipment too large to place in a sink should be washed by hand or cleaned through pressure.

Cleaning and Sanitizing Utensils and Service Ware

The most effective food protection program is wasted if the dishes, equipment, and utensils that come into contact with food are improperly cleaned and sanitized. Therefore, effective cleaning procedures must be established, employees must be trained in their application, and equipment must be operated properly to achieve adequate sanitation of food-production equipment and service ware.

Mechanical Ware Washing

Ware washing is the process of washing and sanitizing dishes, glassware, utensils, and pots and pans either manually or mechanically. Three-compartment sinks and dish and pot machines are the most common equipment for this process. There are many new and innovative changes that have been made to "new" ware washing machines. Several changes include reusing the final rinse for washing dishes using cold water, and machines that are self-vented. More data is available from equipment suppliers, but the following information is appropriate for most models. Dish machines come in various sizes and shapes and cost. Regardless, the same principles apply for cleaning and sanitizing dishes.

Spray or immersion dishwashers must be installed properly and maintained in good repair and operated according to manufacturer's instructions. Likewise, automatic dispensers for detergents, wetting agents, and liquid sanitizers must be properly installed and maintained. Utensils and equipment placed in the machine must be exposed to all cycles. The following procedures should be observed for cleaning and sanitizing all dishes and utensils that come into contact with food:

- The pressure of the final rinse water must be at least 15 pounds per square inch (psi) but no more than 25 psi in the water line immediately adjacent to the final rinse control valve. The data plate is affixed to the machine by the manufacturer and includes the temperature required for washing, rinsing, and sanitizing; conveyor speed for conveyor machines; or cycle time for stationary rack machines. (The data plate attached to the machine states the pressure recommended for that particular dishwasher.)
- Machine- or water line–mounted indicating thermometers must have a numerical scale, printed record, or digital readout in increments no greater than 1°F or 2°F in the intended range and must be provided to show the water temperature of each tank in the dishwasher and the temperature of the final rinse water.
- Baffles, curtains, or some other means to minimize entry of wash water into the rinse tank must protect rinse-water tanks. Conveyors need to be timed to ensure adequate exposure times in wash, rinse, and drying cycles.
- Equipment and utensils should be placed in racks, trays, or baskets or on conveyors in such a way that food-contact surfaces are exposed to an unobstructed application of detergent and wash and clean rinse waters and in such a way that the water can drain freely.
- When hot water is used for sanitizing, the following temperatures must be maintained:
  Single-tank, stationary-rack, dual temperature machine: wash temperature, 165°F (74°C), and final rinse temperature, 180°F (82°C)
  Single-tank, stationary-rack, single-temperature machine: wash temperature and final rinse temperature, 160°F (71°C)
  Single-tank conveyor machine: wash temperature, 165°F (74°C), and final rinse temperature, 180°F (82°C)
  Multi-tank conveyor machine: wash temperature, 150°F (65°C); pumped rinse, 160°F (71°C); and final rinse, 180°F (82°C)
  Single-tank pot, pan and utensil washer (stationary or moving rack): wash temperature, 140°F (60°C), and final rinse, 180°F (82°C)
- When chemicals are used for sanitizing in a single-tank, stationary-rack spray machine and glass washer, the following minimum temperatures should be maintained: wash temperature, 120°F (49°C), and final rinse with chemical sanitizer, 75°F (24°C), or no less than the temperature specified by the machine's manufacturer.

- All dish-washing machines must be thoroughly cleaned after each meal, broken down, and thoroughly cleaned after the last meal of the day.
- When chemicals are used for sanitizing, they should be of a type approved by the local or state health authority. They should also be automatically dispensed in a high-enough concentration and for a long-enough period to provide effective bactericidal treatment (according to the manufacturer's specifications).
- After sanitization, all equipment and utensils must be air dried. Drain boards of adequate size for handling soiled and clean tableware should be provided. Mobile dish tables can be used for these tasks. **Never** towel dry dishes.
- Temperatures for dish washing and pot washing should be taken each time the machine is used. Temperatures should be recorded on a chart posted in the area. The temperature for wash and rinse should be recorded. Any variance should be noted on the chart, along with the action taken to correct it.
- In areas where hard water is a problem, the machine should be delimed as needed.

There are a number of new machines on the market; one uses the final rinse water, recycled to wash dishes, another has a self-vent. Due to the concern over the environment many new and innovative machines and methods are coming to the market. Check advertisements in trade magazines and with equipment suppliers for the latest trend.

Some organizations have a policy that the employee on "dirty end" of the dish machine wears disposable gloves. The employee on the "dirty end" should **not** remove clean dishes without removing gloves and washing hands.

Seven steps to follow in mechanical ware washing

1. *Separate.* Separate any items that will need special attention such as heavily soiled items, like items together.
2. *Prescrape or preflush.* Remove all food particles, napkins, tray covers, and so forth from trays.
3. *Rinse and stack like items together.*
4. *Rack.* Rack like items together, don't overfill racks, don't mix items.
5. *Wash.* Move racks into machine that has been checked for correct temperate and detergent (see above).
6. *Sanitize.* Check temperature gauge to ensure the temperature is 180°F. Check level of drying agent.
7. *Air dry.* Air dry the dishes on the racks.

After cleaning and sanitizing, all dishes and utensils must be stored in an area to prevent contamination.

Manual Ware Washing

The following standards should be observed for manual cleaning and sanitizing:

- A sink with at least three compartments must be used for the manual washing, rinsing, and sanitizing of utensils and equipment. The compartments should be large enough to accommodate the largest equipment and utensils. Hot and cold water sources should be provided for each compartment.
- Drain boards or easily movable dish tables of adequate size should be provided for handling soiled utensils before washing and cleaning utensils after sanitizing.
- Equipment and utensils should be preflushed or prescraped and, when necessary, presoaked to remove gross food particles. (Note: A fourth sink compartment equipped with a garbage disposal is useful for this purpose and could be easily included in plans for facilities being renovated and for new construction.)
- Except for fixed equipment and utensils too large to be cleaned in sink compartments, the following work sequence should be followed.
- If needed rinse, scrape, and/or soak:
  Wash equipment and utensils in the first sink compartment at a maintained temperature 110°F (43°C) or higher with a hot detergent solution that is changed frequently to keep the compartment free from soil and grease.
  Rinse equipment and utensils with clean 120°F (49°C) water in the second compartment and change the water frequently.
  Sanitize equipment and utensils in the third compartment, using one of the following four methods: (1) Immerse the equipment and utensils for at least 30 seconds in clean hot water maintained at 120°F (49°C). A heating device is needed to maintain this temperature, and a thermometer should be used to check the temperature frequently. Dish baskets should be used to immerse utensils completely. (2) Immerse the equipment and utensils for at least one minute in a clean solution that contains at least 50 parts per million (ppm) available chlorine as a hypochlorite or iodine or quaternary ammonium at a temperature of at least 75°F (24°C). (3) Immerse the equipment and utensils for at least one minute in a clean solution that contains at least 12.5 ppm available iodine and has a pH no higher than 5.0 at a temperature of at least 75°F (24°C). (4) Immerse the equipment and utensils in a clean solution that contains any other chemical sanitizer approved by local and state health authorities that will provide the equivalent bactericidal effect of a 50-ppm chlorine solution at 75°F (24°C) for one minute.
  All utensils and equipment should be air dried after sanitizing.
- Equipment that is too large to immerse can be sanitized by treatment with clean steam, provided that the steam can be confined within the equipment. An alternative method is to rinse, spray, or swab the equipment with a chemical sanitizing solution mixed to at least twice the strength required for immersion sanitization.

Storing Equipment and Utensils

Cleaned and sanitized equipment and utensils must be stored properly to protect against contamination. The following standards should be maintained:

- Store them at least six inches above the floor in a dry, clean location in a way that protects them from contamination by splashes and dust. Stationary equipment should also be protected from contamination.
- Glasses and cups should be stored in an inverted position. Other utensils should be stored covered or inverted whenever practical. Storage containers for tableware should be designed so that only their handles are presented to the employee or consumer.
- Pots and pans are to be stored upside down.
- Air dry utensils before putting them away.
- Store items so they can be picked up without touching the food-contact surface.
- Do not store in restrooms or other areas where possible contamination may occur.

SELF-EVALUATION OF SANITARY CONDITIONS AND PRACTICES

Ongoing self-evaluation of the foodservice department's sanitary conditions and practices is necessary to ensure day-to-day protection of all employees and all customers served. The primary benefit of self-monitoring is that managers and employees remain aware of the advantages of maintaining a safe and sanitary operation and avoiding a serious health hazard. The checklist given above in Health Inspections can be used as a guide for developing a sanitation self-evaluation program. Local health departments also can be consulted on questions concerning food sanitation standards for specific localities.

TJC dietetic standards include standards for infection control that can be incorporated into the institution's program. These standards also include certain provisions for the institution's policies and procedures and for communicating them to all employees. The Center for Medical Services (CMS) also has standards that must be met concerning sanitation and food safety.

As part of the sanitation evaluation and control program, a department representative usually serves on the facility's overall infection control committee. The committee also reviews the foodservice department's policies and procedures, along with those of every other department in the facility.

PEST CONTROL

The most common and dangerous pests likely to invade kitchens are rats, mice, flies, roaches, birds, and ants (Table 14.3). They walk and feed on garbage or other waste matter, thus picking up germs and carrying them on or inside their bodies. Rodents, in particular, are great carriers of disease.

It is important to protect food against pollution from these pests. By careful control measures, insects and rodents may be

TABLE 14.3 Some Common Kitchen Pests

Pest	Habits	Disease Transmission	Control
Flies	Lay 100–250 eggs in any kind of excrement, fermenting wastes, rotting fruits or vegetables, garbage, or human wastes; eggs hatch in 1 or 2 days and go through two stages (maggot and pupae); in 4 days an adult fly emerges	They cover their legs, bodies, and wings with filthy material and deposit it on the next surface; disease germs are picked up and deposited on food and utensils	Eliminate breeding places; place screens on doors and windows; keep garbage cans tightly covered; provide clean, ventilated toilets; keep food protected; kill by spraying, poisoning, or using an electric bug zapper; be sure to read labels; do not use chemicals around foods when labels prohibit it
Roaches	Lay 25–30 eggs, live 5 years, eat anything, are always thirsty, have a disagreeable odor; come out at night and spend days in cracks and crevices, often near steam pipes; live in drain areas, waste sinks and toilet bowls, furnace areas, and rubbish pits	Their offensive odor clings to the dishes they run over; they carry disease on their bodies and feet	Keep sinks and areas around pipes clean and dry; keep food covered; destroy crumbs; control sources of infestation; inspect all incoming foodstuffs; eliminate damp areas, dripping drains, overflowing sinks, pipe leaks; close all openings in ceilings, floors, walls; keep storage area clean; do not leave dirty dishes or food scraps out at night; use chemical controls; use the proper chemicals; do not store chemicals around food!
Ants	Live in communities where they store food and raise their young; some like sweets, others like meats	Transport wastes and filth on their feet and bodies to food	Be careful to dispose of waste; do not leave food open; keep garbage cans clean; find the hill in which they live and use chemical controls
Rodents	A half-inch crack will admit a young rat or an adult mouse; they are resourceful, dislike open places, move along walls, leave a dark, greasy trail; they gnaw at edges of doors and on wood panels; rodents will eat any kind of food regardless of freshness or decay; they prefer comfortable living quarters close to humans; they live 2–3 years and produce 5 liters of 6–9 rats a year; they are good swimmers, travel in sewers, build nests in rubbish heaps, under lumber piles, in boxes, in cellars, under floors, between floors and walls; rats can leap 2–3 feet in air	They may carry fleas on their bodies that transmit typhus fever and bubonic plague; urine and feces infect food; rat tissues may contain trichinosis parasites that infect hogs and are transmitted to humans; hogs sometimes eat rats, and humans eat hogs	Eliminate nesting places by building them out of the structure; seal holes in walls, around pipelines, doors, windows, and ventilation grilles; deprive of food; keep garbage tightly covered; protect food; practice good housekeeping; use rodenticides under supervision of an exterminator service
Mosquitoes	Breed in water, drains, rain pools, and barrels; life cycle is 10 days; they multiply rapidly	They carry disease on and in their bodies and transmit to humans by biting (directly into human blood)	Inspect breeding places frequently; put screens on doors and windows; use chemical control as appropriate
Lice	Eggs, called nits, hatch in 2–3 weeks	Cling to hair of host; carrier of typhus and relapsing fever; increasing problem in schools	Chemical controls
Dirty food handler	Inability to adhere to highest standards of personal cleanliness; cannot be trained or will not follow rules and regulations	Unclean clothes and body	Enforce all sanitation rules; do not hire; if hired, fire at once
Birds Droppings	Can contaminate food	Can pass diseases such as Avian flu	Keep loading dock clean Check windows for openings Check storerooms for nest

eliminated from storage and foodservice areas. Carelessness will result in the spread of disease and costly spoilage. The best method of control is a clean environment and a pest-control contract with a pest company that sprays and follows up with visits on a monthly basis. It is unwise for foodservice professionals to use sprays, chemicals, or insecticides around food. A number of chemicals can cause problems. Never use a chemical that is not approved for use in foodservice operations. Check local and state regulations relating to the "safe use" of traps, gel tapes and other items used to control pest.

Pests may enter the facility despite good housekeeping and control. They come in on customers or in baggage and packages, as well as in supplies from warehouses. This is especially the case with roaches, ants, and flies.

Foodservice managers need to check for infestations. Areas where pests are most often found are garbage, floor drains, dark and damp areas, dumpsters, racks and shelves, bottle and can return area, doors, windows, and other openings. Pest infestation is often found outside the facility in pallets, containers, lumber, and construction materials. The garbage area where garbage is stored until removed is a haven for roaches, ants, and mice and in some area raccoons, squirrels, and opossums. The area should be kept clean at all times.

A system called **intergraded pest management (IMP)** uses a variety of techniques and focuses on prevention. The following should be implemented:

- Seal pipes, conduits, and duct penetration in exterior walls.
- Screen all windows, vents, louvers, and exhausts with mesh screens.
- Install a steel plate across the entire width of the bottom of the outside door to reduce clearance to less than one-quarter inch.
- Inspect ventilating and heating exhausts on roofs for signs of bird activity.
- Place filters on exhaust hoods.
- Put fasteners on floor drains.

- Repair any broken water lines, leaks, and small plumbing channels in floors for refrigeration lines.
- Inspect all incoming deliveries for pest infestation.
- Check and repair wall cracks, door frames, and switch boxes.
- Check produce area for roach infestation.
- Monitor all dry products in storage area.
- Check compressor areas.
- Keep area clean and sanitized.
- Hire a licensed **pest control employee/operator**, a person trained and licensed in pest management and control.

The service manager needs to work closely with the engineering and housekeeping staffs to ensure that inspections are made of the outside area. Joint department policies and procedures need to be in place for maintaining the equipment and outside areas. Work orders for extra-needed maintenance should also be in place. A pest control activity record should be kept that records the pest incidence, control action taken, and the dates, times, and initials of the person or persons who took the actions.

SUMMARY

Foodservice directors must adhere to prescribed guidelines that guard against food-borne illness due to food contamination. The model suggested for the design, development, and implementation of an effective sanitation program, HACCP, is a self-evaluation system for the control of food-borne illness and time–temperature abuse. The seven principles of HACCP were thoroughly discussed.

The proper use of cleaning compounds; germicides and sanitizers; and agents for cleaning and sanitizing equipment, utensils, and service ware. Methods for proper handling and storage of clean equipment and utensils and an operation's self-evaluation of its sanitation program were given. Because pest infestation is a foodservice problem, pests were identified with methods for control.

KEY TERMS

Acidic cleaners
Air gap
Alkaline cleaners
Backflow
Chlorine disinfection
Cleaning
Cleaning schedule
Critical control points
Critical limits
Cross-connection
Detergent
Documentation for verification

Flowchart
Germicides
Hazard Analysis Critical Control Point (HACCP)
Iodine
Neutral cleaners
Pest control
Potable water
Quaternary ammonia compounds
Sanitizers
Sanitizing
Seven principles
Surfactants

1. What are the methods that will need to be taken to implement an HACCP process?

2. How do you implement a program in regard to maintaining healthy employees?

3. Construct a master cleaning schedule while seeking input from employees.

4. What is the role of the foodservice director when participating in a self-evaluation of the department; a local, state health inspection; and a TJC, OBRA, CMS, OSHA, or HACCP inspection; and taking corrective action for deficiencies?

5. Distinguish between the various cleaning agents and their use.

6. How do you work with an outside pest control profession to eliminate any pests?

7. Explain how to contact maintenance for corrective action for securing department/building against pests.

CHAPTER 15

SAFETY, SECURITY, AND EMERGENCY PREPAREDNESS

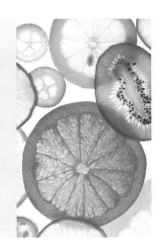

LEARNING OBJECTIVES

- Define safety and security issues in the physical facility to include ergonomic conditions and universal precautions.
- Interpret MSDS sheets for employees before they are used in the facility.
- Develop an in-service for all employees in the Hazard Communication Standards.
- Describe appropriate storage of chemicals used in a foodservice.
- Discuss the responsibility of the organization as it relates to workplace violence.
- Develop a disaster and emergency preparedness plan for the establishment's geographical area.
- Arrange for a specialist to provide education on fire safety.

A PRIMARY RESPONSIBILITY of health care foodservice professionals is to help ensure the maintenance of safe working conditions, equipment, and practices that promote a safety mind-set among employees, staff, and vendors. The most effective way this is accomplished is through a department safety plan that complements and reinforces the larger facility's safety efforts while ensuring compliance with all federal, state, and municipal codes and standards for occupational safety and health.

A critical part of safety is the security measures that help protect food, supplies, equipment, employees, and customers. This occurs on two levels—internally and externally. Internal security in foodservice has to do with instituting policies, procedures, and controls that ensure against jeopardizing employees, customers, food, equip-

ment, and inventory, whereas external security has to do with guarding against threats from outside the department. These include theft by visiting relatives, nondepartmental personnel, and even delivery and catering personnel.

No safety program would be complete without provisions for *disaster and emergency planning*. Floods, earthquakes, hurricanes, tornadoes, power outages or reductions, massive accidents (plane crashes, for example), workplace violence, and bioterrorist acts using nuclear, biological, or chemical agents can pose a threat to foodservice operations.

This chapter addresses these three areas—safety, security, and disaster or emergency preparedness—as they relate specifically to foodservice operations. The chapter examines safe working conditions including ergonomics, Occupational Safety and Health Administration (OSHA) requirements, Hazard Communication standards formerly called "the right to know," self-inspection of safety training programs, fire safety, and first aid.

Techniques for internal and external security are presented, along with a summary of key areas of security concerns for a foodservice operation. The chapter includes a disaster assessment form and information for designing and implementing a disaster-planning program. Because some events are beyond a facility's control, the chapter discusses limited measures to be taken in the event of flood, earthquake, power outage or reduction, and massive casualties (for example, from plane crashes, damaging weather, or civil unrest). Throughout all such contingencies, the foodservice director's role and responsibilities are clearly delineated.

SAFETY

Safety is every employer's and employee's responsibility and not a chore left to the safety committee. The attitudes and examples set by

FIGURE 15.1 Foodservice Safety Checklist

Check your department for the following unsafe procedures and unsafe conditions. How does the department rate?

Unsafe procedures

	Yes	No
1. Failure to look where you are going	___	___
2. Failure to observe your surroundings (such as standing too close to a steamer)	___	___
3. Improper handling of knives	___	___
4. Reaching for falling objects, especially knives	___	___
5. Not paying close attention to the use of sharp tools (such as knives, choppers)	___	___
6. Failure to use leg and thigh muscles when lifting heavy objects	___	___
7. Failure to use safety guards on slicers, grinders, choppers	___	___
8. Failure to use handles when opening or closing doors	___	___
9. Failure to get first aid for accident victims	___	___
10. Failure to keep everything in its proper place	___	___
11. Engaging in horseplay	___	___
12. Entering doors without looking to see if someone is on the other side	___	___

Unsafe conditions

	Yes	No
1. Spillage	___	___
2. Wet, dirty, greasy, slippery floors, glass or food on floor	___	___
3. Pot handles protruding from stovetops	___	___
4. Cluttered storage of mops, buckets, and supplies	___	___
5. Overheated or cold work areas	___	___
6. Unsafe ventilation	___	___
7. Inadequate lighting	___	___
8. Electrical machines left plugged in/running	___	___
9. Walk-ins do not have inside door releases (all employees should be taught how to get out of a walk-in if they are shut in one)	___	___
10. Dull knives	___	___
11. Frayed electrical cords or use of extension cord	___	___
12. Sharp knives left in a sink of soapy water	___	___
13. Poorly maintained equipment	___	___
14. Poorly trained employees	___	___
15. Safety guards missing	___	___

managers influence employees' safety practices. The manager should always think "Safety first."

The foodservice operation can be an unsafe working area if employees have not been trained in safety, safe handling of equipment, safety procedures, and safe environmental conditions. The foodservice operation engages in many complex activities that can lead to accidents.

Figure 15.1 presents a safety checklist to evaluate unsafe procedures and unsafe conditions. If any of these procedures or conditions are checked "no," corrective action needs to be taken at once by the person responsible for providing a safe working environment. The employees are responsible for following established policies and procedures. Policies and procedures need to be posted, and employees need to be trained in safety procedures and retrained as often as appropriate. The foodservice director needs to observe employees' safety habits and make corrections on the spot.

Figure 15.2 lists basic safety tips for the kitchen area. These tips need to be posted in the production area.

Accidents and Injuries

An *injury* is the result of an accident such as a fall, cut, or burn. An *accident* is an event that is unexpected or unforeseen, resulting in injury, loss, or damage. It is an unplanned event that interrupts an activity or function. An occupational illness may result from exposure over time to a hazard. Regardless of the accident, an employee should submit an accident report that documents the nature of the injury or illness; when, where, and how the accident occurred; and any circumstances that surround the accident. It is the responsibility of the foodservice director, the foodservice safety officer, and the facility safety officer to investigate the accident and determine what actions need to be taken to prevent a reoccurrence. Staff may need additional training, equipment repaired, or hazards in the workplace corrected.

Accidents may be numerous in foodservice operations, but many accidents can be prevented. If accidents are constantly occurring in the department a study needs to be conducted to

FIGURE 15.2 Basic Safety Tips for the Kitchen

1. Safety is everyone's business. Report any unsafe conditions you see to your supervisor.
2. When you see anything on the floor that does not belong there—anything from a spill to an object—either mop or pick it up immediately.
3. Report all defective equipment. Obey safety rules when you are working with any equipment, electrical or not.
4. Walk, do not run, in kitchen or cafeteria area.
5. Avoid horseplay and practical jokes. Harmless fun can result in harmful injury.
6. Store clean equipment in proper place.
7. Never leave electrical equipment running and unattended.
8. Never jerk electrical cords from the socket by the cord. Remove the cord by pulling the plug.
9. Do not attempt to operate equipment until you have been thoroughly trained in its use.
10. Never try to repair frayed cords yourself. Report them to your supervisor.
11. Do not use extension cords on electrical equipment. If cord on equipment is too short, report it to your supervisor.
12. Never mix chemical cleaning products; always use products as instructed by supervisor and manufacturers' directions.
13. Always wear personal protective equipment when using cleaning products.
14. Never leave mops, dust mops, or mop buckets in hallways or in front of doors.
15. Know where all firefighting equipment is located; know how and when to use each fire extinguisher.
16. Know fire and disaster procedures.
17. Report all injuries, no matter how small, to your supervisor.
18. Always complete an accident form and give to the supervisor for filing.
19. Think safety; you may pay for carelessness forever.
20. Use "Wet Floor" signs when mopping.
21. Require staff to wear skid-proof shoes.
22. Keep crates, garbage cans, and boxes out of hallways.
23. Replace broken tiles and torn carpet immediately.
24. Keep doors and drawers closed.

---

determine why. Could it be that the wrong employee was hired or that the employee had not been properly trained to do the job; or most/all accidents occurred in the same work area? If one or two employees are the ongoing reason for accidents the foodservice director will need to do a one-on-one retraining program. If these employees continue to be involved in accidents corrective action needs to be taken, including transfers, or termination. Safety is every manager's and employee's responsibility. Accidents do not just happen; something causes them, and most of them can be controlled.

A foodservice operation should have an accident prevention program that evaluates all accidents and, as a result, develops policies, procedures, and monitoring techniques to eliminate the accidents. Accidents are expensive because of lost time and productivity, possibly disabling or life-threatening results including death, increased insurance premiums, increased overtime, employee compensation claims, litigation, reduced employee morale, and investigation by OSHA. Most accidents are the result of human error. Many of these accidents involve the use of knives, high-powered machinery, spills of hot food, burns, trying to catch a falling objects, lifting heavy products, and slipping/falling on wet or greasy floors. Posted next to food choppers, cutters, slicers, and steam equipment are guidelines on how to use and clean the equipment.

Liberty Mutual Insurance Company has listed the 10 leading causes of injuries and illness that account for 86 percent of the

$38.6 billion in wages and medical payment employers paid in 1998 (latest information available), however the estimate may be as high as $125 billion to $155 billion when all other indirect charges are included.

Cuts, burns, and falls account for most of the accidents that occur in foodservice, according to the Liberty Mutual. In 2002 causes and cost (in billions of dollars) to employers of workplace injuries are as follows:

Causes	Percent of Workers	Nationwide Direct Compensation Cost
Overextension—injuries caused by excessive lifting, pushing, pulling holding, carrying or throwing an object	25.57%	$9.8 billion
Falls and body reactions:	11.46%	$4.4 billion
Bodily action—injuries resulting from bending, climbing, loss of balance and slipping without falling	9.35%	$3.6 billion
Being struck by an object	8.94%	$3.4 billion
Repetitive motion	6.10%	$2.3 billion

Source: Liberty Mutual Group, "Workplace Injury Causes and Costs: Liberty Mutual Releases Study on Top 10 Workplace Injuries," *Water & Wastes Digest*, www.wwdmag.com/workplace-injury-causes-and-costs

Employees should be well trained in safety procedures. The organization must have policies and procedures that are followed and monitored. The policies need to clearly define drinking and drug abuse, fighting among employees and other inappropriate conduct while an employee is on duty. Management should provide personal protective equipment (PPE) for use, as in some cases the use of PPE can prevent accident or injuries.

All equipment should be maintained in safe working order at all times. As applicable, contracts with outside manufacturers may be appropriate. Employees should never be allowed to "repair" equipment without specific training.

Risk Management

Risk management is a management tool concerned with minimizing the liability of an organization in such areas as work-related illness, accidents, and injuries to employees that occur in the workplace as a result of the organization's negligence.

When employees or customers are injured and the organization is adjudicated to be at fault, the organization must pay. If OSHA imposes a fine, this will be an additional cost. These increased costs have an overall effect on the organization because fewer funds are available to operate the organization.

In addition to safe working conditions, an effective safety program depends on several factors: established work-safety procedures, thorough training and continual self-evaluation, good fire-prevention practices, and adequate first-aid training. OSHA places legal responsibility on all employers for providing a safe working environment. In practice, primary responsibility for enforcing safety rules and employee compliance in following them is the responsibility of department-level managers. The Joint Commission (TJC) manual describes basic safety procedures for health care institutions, including the food and nutrition service department. In many organizations, a safety committee composed of employees is appointed or elected. The committee works with each department director to implement a meaningful safety program.

The scope of responsibilities for the foodservice safety committee varies, depending on size and complexity of the department. Some committee functions include:

- Conducting a safety self-inspection to identify hazardous conditions that could result in injury to employees and customers
- Investigating all accidents or events for a previous month (or other time period determined appropriate for the operation) and recommending steps to prevent accident or event recurrence and to analyze trends
- Documenting all accident prevention recommendations and forwarding the reports to the safety officer and as appropriate to upper management
- Monitoring all safety-training records, noting discrepancies, and recommending actions to correct discrepancies
- Following up on previous safety self-inspections to verify that corrective actions have been implemented and to identify any other problems

- Maintaining a safety committee notebook with minutes of meetings, correspondence regarding committee recommendations, and safety inspection reports
- Recommending content of safety-training programs
- Conducting an audit of the safety program and identifying any areas that need modifying
- Providing in-service training, follow-up and as appropriate use corrective action if unsafe acts by the same employee continue to occur

Even though the committee may assume a leadership role in planning and implementing a safety program, success of the program depends on the cooperation of all employees and support of department management.

Working Conditions

Before safe working policies and procedures can be developed and enforced, the basic physical safety of the foodservice department's facilities and equipment must be ensured. Fundamental requirements include:

- Adequate working space
- Safe clearance for aisles, doors, loading stations, and traffic areas
- Adequate lighting and ventilation
- Sufficient number of well-marked exits
- Guarded stairways and platforms
- Clean, dry floor surfaces free of hazards
- Suitable storage facilities for food and other supplies
- Electrical and gas equipment constructed and installed in accordance with applicable standards and codes (the National Sanitation Foundation codes, Underwriters' Laboratory codes, and National Electrical codes, as well as any state and local regulations)
- Properly grounded and insulated electrical equipment
- Guards and enclosures for potentially dangerous equipment
- Noise levels within those set by OSHA regulations
- Complete, posted operating instructions on or near every piece of equipment
- Locks that open from the inside on walk-in refrigerators and freezers
- Proper insulation or protection from heat-producing equipment, water heaters, condensing units, compressors, and water pipes
- Sharp knives that are properly stored

The regulations of federal, state, and local governments also dictate standards for safe working conditions, and government authorities are empowered to conduct inspections of health care institutions. In addition, TJC and CMS base their accreditation of individual facilities on their compliance with its published standards, as verified by periodic on-site surveys.

Occupational Safety and Health Administration

The William Steiger Occupational Safety and Health Act of 1970, enacted by Congress in April 1971, mandated safe and healthful working conditions, that the workplace environments be free of recognized hazards likely to cause serious physical harm or even death. The act established *OSHA* as the federal agency that administers legislation within the U.S. Department of Labor. The goal of the act is "to assure, so far as possible, safe and healthful working conditions, and to preserve human resources for every working man and woman." Even with this goal every year more than 6,000 Americans die from workplace injuries, an estimated 50,000 people die from illnesses caused by workplace chemical exposures, and 6 million people suffer nonfatal workplace injuries. Injuries alone cost the economy more than $110 billion a year. OSHA has been criticized due to the number of rules, overzealous enforcement, and burdensome rules. There have been complaints that the "one-size-fits-all" regulatory approach has treated conscientious employers no differently from those who put workers at needlessly risk. These two realities mean that OSHA, in the next 25 years, must do two things: *increase* the protection of worker health and safety, while *decreasing* red tape and paperwork.

The act covers every employee of a private commercial business with one or more employees. (Different federal laws and government agencies regulate other workplaces, and so their employees are not covered by OSHA regulations.) Health care institutions of all kinds fall under the jurisdiction of OSHA, although state and local governments are exempt from these standards. Individual states also have the power to establish occupational safety programs for their employees.

OSHA Record Keeping

An OSHA regulation (29 CFR 1904.2–8) requires that employers gather and record all available information about work-related accidents and illnesses that occur in the workplace. Federal regulations require employers with eleven or more employees at any time during the preceding calendar year to complete OSHA Forms 100, 101, and 102, to be maintained for five years (excluding the current year). Forms 100 and 101 must be kept current to within six days. Form 102 must summarize all occupational injuries and illnesses for each calendar year and be posted in the workplace no later than February 1 each year and remain posted until March 1. The forms must be posted even if there were no injuries or illnesses during the calendar year, with zero entered on the total lines. Employers must keep records of all work-related accidents and illnesses, including those that result in any of the following:

- A fatality
- A loss of consciousness
- A lost workday or workdays
- A need for medical treatment
- An employee's transfer or termination
- A death or the hospitalization of five or more employees
- A need for employees to be advised of excessive exposure to hazardous substances

In addition, employers are required to post one full-size (10-inch-by-16-inch) OSHA poster (OSHA 2203), or a state-approved poster where required, in the workplace. The purpose of the poster is to inform employees of their rights under OSHA regulations.

OSHA also encourages states to develop and operate their own OSHA-approved workplace safety and health programs, which the federal agency monitors to determine its level of commitment and effectiveness. OSHA uses quarterly reports and semiannual evaluations as tools to oversee state plans, and each quarter states having their own programs submit a summary of their enforcement and standards activities. After analyzing each state's progress toward meeting its standards and enforcement goals, OSHA conducts investigations of the performance of individual states and summarizes its findings in a comprehensive report that is submitted to the state every six months. The state is then given an opportunity to respond to the report and the recommendations.

OSHA Inspections

To determine whether a workplace is safe and healthful, OSHA officials are allowed to enter a place of business at any time for purposes of inspection. They may do so either in response to complaints filed against an employer or as part of a random inspection. On-site inspections also are conducted when OSHA has reason to suspect imminent employee endangerment and when a fatal accident or other catastrophe has occurred at the work site.

Certain circumstances usually surround an OSHA inspection of a foodservice facility, for which advance notice of the visit may or may not have been given. On announcing himself or herself and showing adequate identification, the compliance inspector performs the following activities:

- Reviews all accident report forms on file.
- Inspects records of workplace illnesses and injuries.
- Requests the name and address of the company physician or staff members trained in administering medical aid.
- Checks the supplies in the first-aid kit.
- Asks questions concerning the number of people working on each shift, the number of supervisors and workers on staff, and the classification of staff members by job and gender.
- Reviews the department's safety-training programs.
- Requests that a ranking supervisor and a shop steward (if the institution is unionized) accompany him or her on the tour of the department.
- Talks with employees about safety topics.
- Points out hazards or unsafe conditions such as oil, debris, and trash in traffic and work areas.
- Checks all machines, electrical equipment (including plugs) for proper grounding, ladders, tools, and storage areas.
- Notes the location, application, and last testing date of each fire extinguisher.
- Reports to the supervisor (and to the shop steward in unionized institutions) any unsafe actions observed among workers.

- Makes written comments on all violations cited.
- Talks with individual employees previously cited for violations to determine the best way to correct the safety problems.

After the inspection, citations and penalties (if any) are issued if the organization was found to be in violation of OSHA standards. The seriousness of the violation determines whether a fine is levied or legal action is taken.

OSHA Hazard Communication Standards (29CFR1919.1200)

The *Hazard Communication Standard* is the centerpiece of the workplace rights movement. This movement went into effect in 1985 and has now expanded to cover almost all workplaces under OSHA. To assure compliance with 29CFR1910.1200, Hazard Communication OSHA requires employers to establish *hazard communication* programs to transmit information on the potential hazards of *chemicals* to their employees by means of labels on containers, MSDS, training programs, and a written hazard communication program. The employer is also required to maintain a list of hazardous chemicals in the workplace. Implementation of these hazard communications will ensure all employees have the "right-to-know" the hazards and identities of chemicals they work with, and will reduce the incidence of chemically related occupational illnesses and injuries.

Chemical manufacturers and importers who produce, manufacture, or import hazardous chemicals are required to prepare technical hazard information to be used on labels and MSDS to accompany the hazardous materials. The exceptions to this rule include:

- **The MSDS must indicate that trade secret information is being withheld.**
- **The MSDS must disclose information concerning the properties and effects of the hazardous chemical, even if actual chemical identity is withheld.**
- **The trade secret information must be disclosed to a doctor or nurse in a medical emergency.**
- **In nonemergency cases health professionals can obtain a trade secret chemical identity if they can show they need it for purposes of health protection and if they sign a confidentiality agreement.**

OSHA and other U.S. agencies have been involved in a long-term project to negotiate a globally harmonized approach to informing workers about chemical hazards. OSHA is revising its HazCom Standards to make it consistent with Global Harmonization Standards (GHS). The new standards will include more consistent information and definitions for hazardous chemicals and a standard approach to conveying information on MSDS. At the present time hearings have been scheduled on this proposal.

Material Safety Data Sheets

Chemical manufacturers and importers must supply an MSDS for every hazardous chemical they produce or import. MSDS must be ordered at the same time all chemical products are ordered. Employees who receive chemical products **must** verify that the MSDS is either already on file or a new MSDS accompanies the product at the time of receipt. If there is no MSDS the person receiving the product may: refuse the product from the supplier or receive the product, order an MSDS directly from the manufacturer, and hold the product for final distribution until the MSDS arrives. When chemicals are stored off-site the chemicals will be transferred in original containers to the user site with an accompanying MSDS.

The supervisor in the area where the chemical is to be used must maintain an MSDS. The information must be written in plain English, be readily available to designated employee representatives and OSHA officials, and must include both the scientific and common names of the chemical (for example, sodium hydroxide or caustic soda).

The OSHA HazCom specifies the required elements that must be on an MSDS plus other important data. MSDS Form 174(OMB#1218–0072) is the MSDS form from the U.S. Department of Labor's Occupational Safety and Health Administration. This form can be downloaded. The MSDS usually contains more information than required by OSHA, but not less. The form cannot be changed without federal regulation changes.

All MSDSs must contain at least the information listed in Exhibit 15.1, with no spaces left blank.

EXHIBIT 15.1   Material Safety Data Sheet

Material Safety Data Sheet May be used to comply with OSHA's Hazard Communication Standard, 29 CFR 1910.1200. Standard must be consulted for specific requirements.	U.S. Department of Labor Occupational Safety and Health Administration (Non-Mandatory Form) Form Approved OMB No. 1218–0072
IDENTITY (As Used on Label and List)	Note: Blank spaces are not permitted. If any item is not applicable, or no information is available, the space must be marked to indicate that.

Section I

Manufacturer's Name	Emergency Telephone Number
Address (Number, Street, City, State, and ZIP Code)	Telephone Number for Information
	Date Prepared
	Signature of Preparer (optional)

Section II—Hazard Ingredients/Identity Information

Hazardous Components (Specific Chemical Identity; Common Name[s])	OSHA PEL	ACGIH TLV	Other Limits Recommended	% (optional)

Section III—Physical/Chemical Characteristics

Boiling Point		Specific Gravity (H2O = 1)	
Vapor Pressure (mm Hg.)		Melting Point	
Vapor Density (AIR = 1)		Evaporation Rate (Butyl Acetate = 1)	

Solubility in Water

Appearance and Odor

Section IV—Fire and Explosion Hazard Data

Flash Point (Method Used)	Flammable Limits	LEL	UEL

Extinguishing Media

Special Fire Fighting Procedures

EXHIBIT 15.1 *(Continued)*

Unusual Fire and Explosion Hazards

(Reproduce locally)   OSHA 174, Sept. 1985

Section V—Reactivity Data

Stability	Unstable		Conditions to Avoid
	Stable		

Incompatibility (Materials to Avoid)

Hazardous Decomposition or Byproducts

Hazardous

Polymerization	May Occur		Conditions to Avoid
	Will Not Occur		

Section VI—Health Hazard Data

Route(s) of Entry:	Inhalation?	Skin?	Ingestion?

Health Hazards (Acute and Chronic)

Carcinogenicity:	NTP?	IARC Monographs?	OSHA Regulated?

Signs and Symptoms of Exposure

Medical Conditions
Generally Aggravated by Exposure

Emergency and First Aid Procedures

Section VII—Precautions for Safe Handling and Use

Steps to Be Taken in Case Material Is Released or Spilled

Waste Disposal Method

Precautions to Be Taken in Handling and Storing

EXHIBIT 15.1 (*Continued*)

Other Precautions

Section VIII—Control Measures

Respiratory Protection (Specify Type)

Ventilation	Local Exhaust	Special
	Mechanical (General)	Other

Protective Gloves	Eye Protection

Other Protective Clothing or Equipment

Work/Hygienic Practices

*U.S.G.P.O.: 1986—491—529/45775

Hazard Training Programs As mandated by OSHA's revised standard, employers must implement a hazard training and communication program for all employees. Training should cover:

- Location and availability of the written hazard program (described in the next subsection)
- Identity of hazardous chemicals being used in the workplace
- Specific physical and health hazards of individual chemicals
- Protective measures to take when hazardous chemicals are in use
- How to read and interpret information on chemical labels and MSDSs
- Where and how to get additional information
- How to use personal protective equipment or clothing to avoid exposure to hazardous chemicals
- Symptoms of exposure, including the effects of contact, inhalation, or overexposure
- First-aid measures to take in the event of contact or symptoms of overexposure
- Demonstration of first-aid procedures and identification of who can administer treatment

- What should be done in the event of a spill or other accident

The following individuals should be included in the in-service session, especially if a new chemical is involved: the user(s), the supervisor(s), and an individual with firsthand knowledge about the chemical (for example, the distributor's sales representative or a manufacturer's representative). The chemical and its MSDS should be used as visual aids during the session. All in-service sessions should be documented. Employees should be retrained at least once a year on the safe use of hazardous chemicals in their work area.

Written Hazard Communication Programs

To comply with OSHA's requirement for a written program, the health care organization's foodservice department must address in writing specific issues related to hazardous chemicals in the workplace. This mandate encompasses labeling and other written forms of conveying information. A written communication program, then, should include at least four components: labeling, MSDSs, a written prospectus of the employee training program, and employees' "right to know."

EXHIBIT 15.2 Employee Chemical Information Request Form

This form is provided to assist employees in requesting information concerning the health and safety hazards of toxic substances found in the workplace.

Please print:

1. Name _____   4. Department _____

2. Job Title _____   5. Ext. _____

3. Supervisor _____

Describe briefly the toxic substance you are exposed to:

1. Trade name _____

2. Chemical name or ingredient (if known) _____

3. Manufacturer (name and address if known) _____

4. Does substance have a label?   Yes ·   No ·

If yes, copy information on label.

5. Physical form of substance: Gas ·   Liquid ·

                                   Dust ·   Solid ·

                                   Other ·

6. Any other information that will identify the substance (the circumstances of exposure, other characteristics of the substance, etc.): _____

_____

_____

7. If you have specific questions, write them below. _____

_____

_____

_____   _____

Employee Signature   Personnel Signature

_____   _____

Date   Date & Time

Source: Developed by Ruby P. Puckett©.

Labels and other forms of written or graphic warning (for example, symbols) must be supported by a description of the labeling system used. Labeling includes the written information on in-house containers, written designation of responsible person(s) for monitoring labeling procedures and receipt of labels from manufacturers, and procedures for updating label information.

The *material safety data sheet (MSDS)* component includes identification of person(s) responsible for obtaining and maintaining MSDSs. It also includes a description of how employees can obtain access to MSDSs and the procedures for updating or requesting them.

A *written description* of the prospectus of an employee hazard communication program should be accessible. It can be kept on file in a supervisor's office or posted prominently throughout the department.

OSHA's Hazard Communication Standards, described earlier, must be delineated in plain English (and predominant second language, if applicable) and be current, available, and accessible to employees in their work area. This component of the mandate includes the following disclosures:

- Employees are to have access to the hazardous chemicals list for their work area (see the sample request form in Exhibit 15.2).
- Employees are to be informed of the hazards associated with chemicals contained in unlabeled pipes and where hazards are present in their work area.
- The written hazard communication program is to be accessible to all employees.
- All MSDSs are to be readily available during working hours.
- Employees must be informed of OSHA's Hazard Communication Standards.

Open and honest communication is essential when it comes to complying with the hazard communication standard. Exhibits 15.3 and 15.4 are examples of forms that can be used in a written hazard communication program. In addition to OSHA standards, TJC and CMS have certain requirements for managing a safe environment for all employees.

EXHIBIT 15.3   Change in Product or Material Safety Data Sheet

Answer all the questions that apply to this change and date, sign, and route to safety officer. Maintain copy for departmental files. For new product, attach material safety data sheet (MSDS) to form.

Department name: _____

New product name: _____

Old product name: _____

Potential hazardous chemicals: _____

Reason for change: _____

Cost: Yes _____ No _____ Change in contract: Yes _____ No _____

Change in distributor: Yes_____ No_____ No longer available: Yes_____ No_____

New MSDS information: Yes_____ No_____

Improved product (less hazardous): Yes_____ No_____

Other (explain): _____

Action: _____

Secured copy of MSDS for new product: Yes_____ No_____.

Secured copy of MSDS for improved product: Yes_____ No_____

*MSDS deleted for product no longer available, but copy filed with safety officer: Yes_____ No_____

New MSDS sheet filed in department and with safety officer: Yes_____ No_____

Other users notified about change: Yes_____ No_____

Materials removed from inventory: Yes_____ No_____

Disposed in an environmentally safe manner: Yes_____ No_____

Employers provided training on change: Yes_____ No_____

Additional comments _____

_____

_____

_____   _____   _____
Director   Department   Date

Note: Must be kept on file for 30 years.
Source: Form developed by Ruby P. Puckett©.

EXHIBIT 15.4   Hazard Communication Monitoring Checklist

Using this checklist, review the area and put a checkmark under Yes or No for each question. For all No answers, review existing policies and procedures and take action as appropriate.

		Yes	No
A.	Chemicals		
	Is chemical storage cabinet or space locked?		
	Is list of approved chemicals posted?		
	Are there unauthorized chemicals in area?		
	Is there a warning about mixing chemicals?		
	Is formula posted for ppm (parts per million) for disinfection or sanitation mixtures?		
B.	Labels on Containers		
	Are there labels on all containers, including any squeezable bottles, cans, and the like?		
	Is the original container labeled or tagged with the identity of the chemical?		
	Does label have warning signal or word?		
	Does label have hazard statement?		
C.	MSDS Sheets		
	Are up-to-date material safety data sheets (MSDSs) available for all approved chemicals?		
	Are MSDSs readily available to all employees?		
	Is there a method for updating information?		
	Date of last update: _____		
	Do employees know how to interpret data?		
D.	Policies and Procedures		
	Are there written policies and procedures for:		
	Request for addition or deletion of specific chemicals?		
	Storage of chemicals?		
	Personal protective equipment?		
	Use of specific chemicals?		
	Mixing of chemicals?		
	First aid?		
	Emergencies and emergency telephone numbers?		
	Others as applicable?		
	Are policies and procedures available to all employees?		
	Are employees and management aware of their responsibilities?		
E.	Orientation, Training		
	Have all new employees been oriented concerning Hazard Communication?		
	Has training been scheduled for all employees for all shifts?		
	Have all management and employees completed the required annual training?		
	Is training documented?		
	Filed in personnel file?		
	Have complaints, questions, or concerns of employees been addressed?		
	Have safety officer check and dispose following required rules, regulations, and laws.		

Source: Form developed by Ruby P. Puckett©.

OSHA Blood-Borne Pathogens OSHA recognized the need for a regulation to protect health care workers against the health hazard of exposure of blood and other potentially infectious materials (including blood-borne pathogens) and to reduce their risk of exposure. OSHA's regulations on blood-borne pathogens were published in 1991, in the *Federal Register* under 20CFR1920.1030 and became effective in March 1992.

Most foodservice facilities and departments are not considered at-risk units; however, the exposure education and training are required. Each occupationally exposed employee must be given free information and training; training must be provided during work hours. New employees must receive training at the time of their initial assignments and orientation (Exhibit 15.5). All employees must receive annual training within one year of previous training and additional training when existing tasks are modified or new tasks are assigned that involve occupational exposure to blood-borne pathogens.

The training must be comprehensive and include the following items:

- Information on blood-borne pathogens
- OSHA regulations
- Employer exposure control plan and how to obtain a copy of the plan
- Information on the epidemiology and symptoms of blood-borne diseases
- Ways in which blood-borne pathogens are transmitted
- Information on how to recognize tasks that might result in occupational exposure
- Personal protective equipment
- Information on types, selection, proper uses, location, removal, handling, decontamination, and disposal of personal protective equipment
- Information on hepatitis B vaccination
- Who to contact in case of an emergency
- How to report exposure incident, post exposure evaluation, and follow-up
- Warning labels and color coding

Training must be comprehensive. The person conducting the training must be knowledgeable in the subject matter. The information provided must be written and appropriate in content and vocabulary to the educational level, literacy, and language of the audience.

EXHIBIT 15.5 New Employee Orientation Checklist for Hazard Communication (OSHA)

Employee name: _____ Date of training: _____

Job title: _____

Supervisor: _____

Facility-wide orientation (conducted by safety officer):

_____ Facility's safety and health policies and procedures

_____ OSHA Right-to-Know—Hazard Communication

_____ Material safety data sheet (MSDS)—What are they? function?

_____ Other as appropriate

A check (✓) indicates new employee attended the facility-wide orientation conducted by:

_____   _____

Safety Officer   Date

First-day orientation, area-specific orientation:

_____ Review of job duties that require the use of chemicals and types of hazards.

_____ Tour chemicals storage area.

_____ Explain and demonstrate how to read container label.

_____ Location of personal protective equipment (PPE) and how to use.

_____ MSDS review, location of sheets, and chemicals used in work area.

_____ Review of approved chemicals to be used in work area.

_____ Caution about mixing chemicals with other chemicals.

_____ Procedure for chemicals to be mixed with water.

_____ Emergency procedures, telephone numbers, and locations of telephones.

_____ Required attendance at annual training.

_____ Employee's right to request additional information.

_____ Questions.

A check (✓) indicates that the new employee has been provided information concerning Hazard Communication.

Completed by _____   Date _____

Employee signature _____   Date _____

Return completed checklist to employee's department file, with copy to safety officer.

Source: Developed by Ruby P. Puckett©.

Universal Precautions

The single most important measure to control the transmission of hepatitis B virus and human immunodeficiency virus (HIV) is to treat all human blood and other potentially infectious materials as if they were infectious for HIV. Other contagious diseases also need to be treated as dangerous; they include chicken pox or scabies, various flus, multidrug-resistant Staphyloccus aureus (MRSA), as well as major pandemic outbreaks. Application to this approach is referred to as *universal precautions* (Figure 15.3). Blood and other infectious materials should be considered as potentially infectious materials. These fluids cause contamination.

Methods of Control

Engineering and work practice controls are the primary methods used to control the transmission of hepatitis B virus and HIV. Personal protective clothing and equipment also are necessary when occupational exposure to blood-borne pathogens remains even after instituting these controls.

Engineering controls reduce employee exposure in the workplace by either removing or isolating the hazard or isolating the worker from exposure. Suction apparatus, self-sheathing needles, and special containers for contaminated sharp instruments are examples of engineering controls.

FIGURE 15.3 Universal Precautions

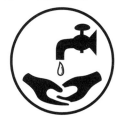

Hands
Must be washed before
and after patient care

Gown
Indicated if soiling
is likely

Gloves
Indicated for touching
blood and body fluids

Mask/Eye Wear
Indicated if splashing in
face, eyes, mouth is likely

Sharps
Dispose properly;
no recapping

Engineering controls must be examined and maintained, or replaced, on a scheduled basis. Applicable engineering controls that apply to long-term health care workers include, but are not limited to, the following:

• Use puncture-resistant, leak-proof containers to collect, handle, process, store, transport, or ship blood specimens and potentially infectious materials. Label these specimens if shipped outside the facility. Labeling is not required when all specimens are handled using universal precautions and when specimens are kept within the facility.

• Use puncture-resistant, leak-proof containers, color coded red or labeled according to the standard, to discard contaminated items such as sharps, broken glass, scalpels, or other items that could cause a cut or puncture wound.

• Use puncture-resistant, leak-proof containers, color coded red or labeled, to store contaminated reusable sharps until they are properly reprocessed.

Engineering controls are to be used in combination with work practice controls.

Proper work practice controls reduce the likelihood of exposure by altering the manner in which a task is performed. All procedures involving blood or other potentially infectious materials must be performed in a manner that will minimize spattering, splashing, and spraying and the generation of droplets. Safe work practices include, but are not limited to, the following:

▪ Do not eat, drink, apply cosmetics or lip balm, or handle contact lenses in areas of occupational exposure.

▪ Do not mouth pipette or suction blood or other potentially infectious materials.

FIGURE 15.4 Biohazard Symbol

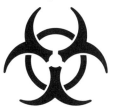

Biohazard Symbol

Note: Label requires a fluorescent orange or orange-red label with the biological hazard symbol, along with the word "BIOHAZARD" in contrasting color, affixed to the bag or container.

▪ Do not store food or drink in refrigerators or other locations where blood or potentially infectious materials are kept.

▪ Wash hands when gloves are removed and as soon as possible after skin contact with blood or other potentially infectious materials.

▪ Never recap, bend, or remove needles by hand unless the employer can demonstrate that no alternative is feasible or that such action is required by a specific medical procedure. When recapping, bending, or removing contaminated needles is required by a medical procedure, this must be done by mechanical means, such as the use of forceps, or a one-handed technique.

▪ Never shear or break contaminated needles.

▪ Discard contaminated needles and sharp instruments in containers that are closable, puncture-resistant, leak proof, and color coded red or labeled with the biohazard symbol (see Figure 15.4); ensure that containers are accessible, maintained upright, and not allowed to overfill.

The foodservice director or designee should be knowledgeable about the entire plan and the possible risks to the staff.

Work Safety Policies and Procedures

To ensure a safe workplace, before developing policies and procedures the foodservice director, the chairman of the department safety committee, and the engineer need to do a "walk-through" of the department to identify any hazards and ensure that any problems are immediately corrected and addressed in the policies. Once a safe working environment has been established, policies and procedures that support safe working habits must be developed by the foodservice director or designee, approved by the institution's administration or safety committee, and implemented by both management and the employees. Basic safety rules for foodservice workers are:

- Always wear safe clothing and shoes. (Most departments require employees to wear standard uniforms and hard-toed, low-heeled, rubber-soled shoes. Heavy coats and gloves should be worn in walk-in refrigerators and freezers. Bracelets and dangling earrings should not be worn.)
- Use ladders to reach supplies and equipment stored on high shelves.
- Use the protective guards and safety devices supplied for potentially dangerous machines and equipment, such as meat slicers.
- Use appropriate tools for opening cartons and other containers.
- Follow safe procedures for lifting heavy objects (see Figure 15.5).
- Use dry potholders or cloths to handle hot utensils.
- Maintain good housekeeping conditions in all work areas by keeping equipment clean and by properly storing equipment and supplies not in use.
- Carefully follow the established operating instructions for all tools, equipment, and machines.
- Use other personal protective equipment as appropriate. Personal protective equipment may include gloves, gowns, aprons, goggles, face shields, or ventilation devices. Gloves may be disposable nonlatex gloves or heavy-duty utility gloves.

The foodservice director and supervisory personnel are responsible for establishing and maintaining a safe working environment for all foodservice employees. There are a number of ways in which this can be accomplished:

- Perform regular and thorough department inspections. The sample checklist in Exhibit 15.6 can be used as an inspection model.
- Appoint a department safety committee.
- Analyze every work-related accident and then correct any problems identified.
- Take immediate action when employees behave inappropriately (for example, engage in horseplay or in fighting), show evidence of substance abuse, or express poor attitudes toward their work.
- Train employees to be safety conscious.
- Maintain records of training.
- Know what to do after an on-the-job accident.
- Be sensitive to employees' work-related problems and avoid placing undue pressure on them in the workplace.
- Teach employees proper motion economy
- Review the work design/layout and make any simple changes. If more expensive work is needed, place an emergency work order requesting the work be accomplished. Justify the need and the cost as appropriate.

Safety Training and Self-Inspection of Safety-Training Programs

The foodservice director and all foodservice managers are key people in developing a safety-minded workforce. Safety training begins with a new employee's first day on the job and is reinforced by leadership style and regularly scheduled training sessions. (Posters and safety reminders are one way to help keep employees alert to safety procedures. Check www.business.com/guides/workplace-health-and-safety-posters-3100/ for workplace safety posters and signs.)

It must be *vital* that employees report any safety hazards immediately to get the problem corrected quickly. The entire department should be periodically inspected for safety compliance in addition to scheduled inspections of equipment by manufacturers' representatives or by the institution's maintenance supervisor. Local fire departments can assist in fire-prevention training. Regular safety-training programs should include at least:

- Procedures for safely lifting heavy objects
- Procedures for handling hazardous materials
- Procedures for ensuring fire safety
- Procedures for reporting on-the-job accidents
- Procedures for disaster and emergency preparedness (TJC, CMS and other surveying agencies rules, regulations and standards)

A system for self-inspection of department safety programs should be conducted at regular intervals. Exhibit 15.6 can be used as a safety evaluation checklist and as a basis for developing a self-inspection program. Employees should participate in developing and enforcing the department's safety program.

Fire Safety and Prevention

The danger of fire in the foodservice department is always present. All employees should know and practice the department's fire-prevention and fire-response procedures, revised and reviewed annually, as well as those developed for the institution as a whole. The department should post its procedures and provide in-service training on how to react to different types of fires.

FIGURE 15.5 Safe Lifting Procedure

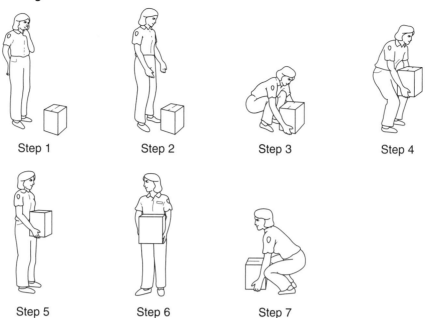

Step 1	Step 2	Step 3	Step 4

Step 5	Step 6	Step 7

Step 1. Approach the load and size it up (weight, size, and shape). Consider your physical ability to handle the load.

Step 2. Place your feet close to the object to be lifted, 8 to 12 inches apart for good balance.

Step 3. Bend your knees to the degree that is comfortable and get a good handhold. Then, using both leg and back muscles,

Step 4. Lift the load straight up, smoothly and evenly, pushing with your legs and knees. Keep the load close to your body.

Step 5. Lift the object into carrying position, making no turning or twisting movements until the lift is completed.

Step 6. Turn your body with changes of foot position after looking over your path of travel to make sure it is clear.

Step 7. Remember that setting the load down is just as important as picking it up. Using leg and back muscles, comfortably lower the load by bending your knees. When the load is securely positioned, release your grip.

Source: R. P. Puckett, Dietary Managers Training Program, Division of Continuing Education, University of Florida, 2009.

EXHIBIT 15.6   Example of a Safety Checklist

SAFETY CHECKLIST

Checked by: _____   Date: _____

Standard	Deficiency		Comments	Date Corrected
	No	Yes		

Personnel

1. Signs prohibiting unauthorized people from entering the foodservice department are posted.
2. All personnel have participated in a safety program.
3. Personnel are lifting heavy objects properly.
4. Authorized protection is used to prevent burns when handling hot pots and pans.
5. Chopping, cutting, and slicing are done on cutting boards.
6. Knives and other sharp objects are stored in a manner to prevent accidental cuts.
7. Plastic gloves and aprons are not worn in the hot food preparation areas.
8. Long hair is properly covered.
9. Wearing dangling jewelry is prohibited in work areas.
10. Only shoes with enclosed toes and low heels are worn.
11. Step stools or stepladders are used to reach items that are stored on high shelves.
12. Wet floor signs are used to warn personnel and customers.

Fire

1. All personnel have participated in fire prevention and emergency training.
2. All prevention instructions are posted.
3. Department policies and procedures for fire safety are reviewed annually.
4. Fire extinguishers are strategically placed.
5. Fire extinguishers are clearly labeled for class of fire.
6. Fire extinguishers are periodically checked for adequacy of pressure and chemicals.

Electricity

1. Routine inspections are made of electrical equipment and outlets by the maintenance department.
2. Foodservice personnel have been trained in safe use of electric powered equipment.
3. Electric cords and plugs are in good repair.
4. Personnel immediately report any damaged or malfunctioning electrical connections or equipment to their supervisor.
5. All electrical equipment is properly grounded.
6. Power to meat slicers and mixers is disconnected when the equipment is being cleaned.
7. Equipment guards (on meat slicers and similar equipment) are in place at all times.

Facilities and Equipment

1. Walls do not protrude that would obstruct traffic areas.
2. Storage drawers are kept closed.
3. Placing pots and pans on the floor in traffic areas is prohibited.
4. Floors in food production and refrigerated and dry storage areas are regularly cleaned, to prevent slips and falls.

EXHIBIT 15.6 (*Continued*)

Standard	Deficiency		Comments	Date Corrected
	No	Yes		
5. Storage areas are provided with proper shelving.				
6. Heavy items are stored on lower shelves.				
7. Cleaning supplies and other chemicals are in an area separate from food storage.				
8. Adequate lighting is provided in storage areas.				
9. Light fixtures are in good working order.				
10. Adequate lighting is provided in customer service area.				
11. Adequate lighting is provided in food production areas.				
12. Carts are provided for transport of supplies.				
13. Step stools and ladders are kept in good repair.				
14. Refrigerators and freezers are equipped with inside door release devices.				
Plumbing				
1. Plumbing, steam, temperature gauges are regularly checked by maintenance department.				
2. Personnel have been trained in proper use of steam-heated equipment.				
3. Personnel have been trained in proper use of steam-cleaning equipment.				
4. Personnel immediately report any plumbing or steam malfunctions to their supervisors.				
5. All drains are flowing freely.				
6. All exposed water and steam pipes are protected with insulated covering.				
Cleaning and Disposal				
1. Personnel are trained in proper use of all cleaning supplies and chemicals.				
2. Personnel are trained in proper use of dish-washing equipment.				
3. Wood or metal textured platforms are used in the dish-washing and pot-and-pan-cleaning areas to prevent slips and falls.				
4. Water temperatures are constantly monitored and as necessary recorded.				
5. There are no obstructions in the traffic lane of the dish-washing and pot-and-pan-cleaning areas.				
6. Adequate scraping space is provided.				
7. Adequate drying space is provided.				
8. Adequate dry dish storage space is provided.				
9. Provision is made for safe disposal of chipped, cracked, or broken dishes and cutlery.				
10. Pot-and-pan-washing areas are provided.				
11. Adequate pot and pan storage space is provided.				
12. Garbage disposals are maintained in safe, clean, operating condition.				
13. Trash is disposed in tied plastic bags.				
14. There is a designated, temperature-controlled, trash and garbage storage area.				
15. Garbage and trash disposal areas are free of spills.				

Source: Developed by Ruby P. Puckett©.

FIGURE 15.6 Know Your Fire Extinguishers

To Operate
Read Instructions; some vary

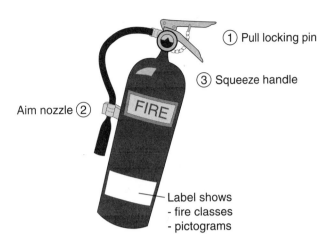

① Pull locking pin

③ Squeeze handle

Aim nozzle ②

Label shows
- fire classes
- pictograms

FIGURE 15.7 Types of Fire Extinguishers

Water (cools, soaks)

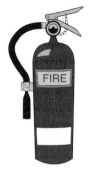

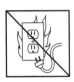 For ordinary combustible fires

NOT flammable liquids or electrical fires

Dry Chemical (smothers)

 Regular type

For flammable liquids and electrical fires,
NOT ordinary combustibles

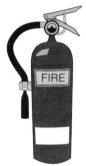

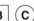 Multipurpose type

For ordinary combustibles, flammable
liquids, and electrical fires

Electrical fires and grease fires are the two leading types of fire in foodservice departments. One is due to misuse or negligence with regard to electrical equipment; the other arises from grease buildup on stoves and hoods, grills, and other appliances. The Underwriters Laboratories 300 Standard, which took effect on November 21, 1994, set new and more stringent standards for the design and installation of fixed fire suppression systems in restaurants. This standard addresses kitchen exhaust hoods, dry chemicals, and liquid agent fire suppression. If changes are made to the facility, the existing system must comply with the new standards.

Employees must be trained in evacuation procedures and receive annual training on the use of portable fire extinguishers. Annual maintenance must also be performed, and monthly inspections may also be required. Employees must know how to use fire extinguishers and select the appropriate extinguisher for each of the five classes of fire. A fire *extinguisher* is a special container for an agent like water or chemicals (Figure 15.6). It is designed to put out small fires, not big ones. The five classes of fire are described as follows:

1. *Class A fires* involve ordinary combustible items such as wood, paper, and cloth. Extinguishers for use on Class A fires are marked with a triangle and a capital letter A.
2. *Class B fires* involve flammable liquids such as fuel oil, gasoline, paint, grease, and solvents. Extinguishers for use in Class B fires are marked with a square and a capital letter B (see Figure 15.7).
3. *Class C fires* involve electrical equipment such as overheated fuse boxes, conductors, wiring, and motors. Extinguishers for Class C fires are marked with a circle and a capital letter C.
4. *Class D fires* involve metals such as magnesium and sodium and require a special dry powder extinguisher; Extinguishers for Class D fires are marked with a star and the letter D. Class D extinguishers are rarely, if ever, found in a foodservice department.

5. *Class K* was recently assigned to fires involving cooking media (grease, fat, and oils) in commercial cooking appliances. Because oils have a wide range of auto-ignition temperatures, these fires are unlike almost all other fires. Auto-ignition occurs when the oils reach high temperatures, typically above 400°F. When this occurs, the entire mass of oil must be cooled below its auto-ignition temperature to be extinguished.

- Class K extinguishers must be installed adjacent to all commercial cooking locations. Class K extinguishers contain BC Purple K dry chemicals, which get their name from the odor and the purple crystals used in the extinguisher.

To use a fire extinguisher, remember the acronym *PASS*:

Pull the pin
Aim the nozzle at the base of the fire
Squeeze the handle
Sweep from side to side at the base of the fire

Fire extinguishers, which should carry the certification of a nationally recognized laboratory such as Underwriters' Laboratory (**UL**), must be checked periodically by the fire department to determine whether they are fully charged and whether the fire retardant contained in the cylinder is less than 12 months old. In 2003 the National Fire Protection Association updated its standard, which requires that service collars be used on extinguishers. At specific service intervals and when most extinguishers undergo recharging, it is required that the valve be removed and the extinguisher be examined internally. This new standard requires the use of an external "verification of service" collar, which is installed between the cylinder and the valve of the extinguisher. This collar provides proof that the unit was taken apart and subjected to maintenance. This collar bears the name of the serving company, date of service and the initials of the service person. Extinguishers should be recharged. They should be mounted higher than 5 feet if they weigh 40 pounds or less or at least three and a half feet off the floor if they weigh more.

In addition to an adequate supply of correctly located fire extinguishers, at least one automatic sprinkler with adequate pressure, capacity, and reliability, should be in place. Water-flow alarms should be provided on all sprinklers. The system should be periodically inspected and maintained. Shutoff valves in all air ducts located over cooking equipment and heat sources should be provided and inspected at least once a year.

Dry chemical or carbon dioxide firefighting systems should be inspected and tested at least once a year by the fire department and reports of the inspections kept on file. All dry chemical and carbon dioxide systems should benefit from regular maintenance.

Fire Drills

Employees on all shifts must participate in departmental and facility fire drills at least annually. They should know where the exits and emergency routes are (all exit signs should always be lighted and free of obstructions). Employees should know the location of all fire alarms and how to contact the facility operator, administration, or safety officer to report a fire. As part of the in-service training, all employees should be taught how to use a fire extinguisher correctly and the location of the extinguishers. Evacuation routes should be clearly marked. When a fire occurs, employees must act immediately. The first three minutes are the most critical. All employees need to know the acronym RACE:

> **R**escue patients
> **A**ctivate an alarm or call operator to announce fire code
> **C**onfine the blaze
> **E**xtinguish, if it is a small fire; otherwise, evacuate

If your or an employee's clothing is on fire: *STOP, DROP, and ROLL*

First Aid

Most health care institutions have specific policies and procedures for the treatment of injured employees. In many organizations, employee health departments handle minor injuries. However, serious injuries and illnesses are always referred to emergency departments. Emergency telephone numbers (poison control, trauma units) should be posted near each telephone. If deemed appropriate, first aid should be provided immediately.

OSHA's regulations (29 CFR 1910–151) state that provisions for first aid must be made in the workplace if there is no infirmary, clinic, or hospital near the workplace that can be used for the treatment of injured or sick employees. Health care institutions may offer immediate first aid on the premises; however, OSHA requirements for employee first-aid treatment programs may provide helpful guidelines for foodservice directors responsible for managing first-aid programs in their departments:

- At least one employee on each shift should be qualified to give first aid, including cardiopulmonary resuscitation and the Heimlich maneuver. The employee providing first-aid treatment should follow designated procedures to protect himself or herself from communicable diseases.
- First-aid supplies should be readily available and accessible in the work area.

Foodservice directors can contact their state public health departments for regulations that govern first-aid programs in the workplace. For example, some states have passed laws that require employees in public eating establishments to be trained in performing the Heimlich maneuver. When feasible, foodservice directors should encourage workers certified in this technique to train other employees. Posters are available from the National Restaurant Association.

Workplace Violence

Workplace violence is violence or the threat of violence against workers. It occurs at or outside of the workplace and can range from threats and verbal abuse to physical assaults and homicide, one of the leading causes of job-related deaths. Workplace violence is a growing concern for employers and employees nationwide.

Each year more than 2 million American workers are victims of workplace violence, Workplace violence can strike anyone, anywhere and at any time, no one is immune. Some jobs propose a greater threat: persons who handle money; delivery persons, mail carriers, food deliverers (pizza deliverers especially); service workers (especially those who work in high crime areas); and health care providers—home health nurses, physical therapists, social workers; probation officers, police, and taxi drivers.

Employers have a responsibility to protect their employees. TJC suggests that all employees be required to attend a workplace violence program as part of orientation. Policies and procedures, employees handbooks, and other organization manuals should contain information on what to do to protect themselves and what to do following an incident of workplace violence.

The Department of Labor, OSHA has developed a *Fact Sheet on Workplace Violence* that will be helpful in developing information for yourself and the employees. Contact OSHA at www.osha.gov or send a fax request to 202-693-2498.

SECURITY

Theft is a major problem not only by foodservice employers but also for employers generally. Employee theft amounts to a loss of more than $25 million annually. It has been estimated that 85 percent of all employees have stolen from their employers. In addition, persons not employed by the operation can take money and property unlawfully. Foodservice theft can encompass money, food, beverages, supplies, and equipment, so department security should involve implementation of internal and external controls to protect all cash, merchandise, equipment, and supplies.

Perhaps the greatest theft is that of "stealing time and use of electronic equipment and telephones for personal use." Employees who surf the Internet for nonorganization business, pay bills, or check bank accounts online while on duty are stealing from their employer, reducing productivity, and not fulfilling their job tasks. Due to the increased misuse employers have devised systems to monitor the employee use of telephones and electronic equipment. Employees have been terminated when misuse is discovered. Employees who surf the net for pornography while on duty have been terminated immediately. Employees who use the Internet to send harassing messages or explicit sexual messages to employees have also been fired and in a number of cases legal action has been brought against the sender. Detailed policies and procedures must be in place and become a part of the orientation. The policies must include how, when, who, and what the telephone and electronic equipment may be used for. The consequences of failure to follow the policies and procedures must also be spelled out.

The most vulnerable areas for foodservice are purchasing, receiving, storage, inventory control, production, cafeteria, vending, and catering services. Each of these areas poses a unique opportunity for theft and requires specific control procedures.

Both internal and external security primarily is the responsibility of the foodservice director, although this responsibility cannot be accomplished without the assistance of departmental staff and the larger facility's security department. Forming a partnership between organizational and departmental security teams is imperative. Employee cooperation in preventing and reporting theft is essential to internal and external security efforts.

Internal Security

Internal security primarily deals with the department's employees. This does not mean, however, that foodservice directors should overlook the fact that nondepartmental employees (or persons outside the institution) may commit theft. Some causes of employee theft include:

- *Poor employee morale:* Anger and resentment may make certain employees feel that the employer "owes them something," or they want to strike back.
- *Leadership deficiency:* Apathetic or poor supervision, management complacency and carelessness, or poor examples set by supervisory and management staff (for example, wastefulness or failure to enforce disciplinary policy) can give the wrong message to employees.

- *Uncompetitive wage structure:* Inadequate wages compromise employees' ability to manage their incomes or meet their expenses and thus may invite temptation to theft.
- *Temptation:* Some people are completely honest, others are incorrigibly dishonest, and still others are only as honest as circumstances permit. Employee access to cash, food, supplies, and equipment should be restricted and closely (but diplomatically) monitored.
- *Rationalization:* People may distance themselves from their actions by viewing their theft not as stealing from a unique entity (their employer) but, rather, as taking from an anonymous large corporation that can "afford the loss."
- *Kleptomania:* Certain persons have a persistent neurotic impulse to steal that is not driven by economic motive.
- *Thrill factor:* Stealing presents a challenge—a titillating taboo—to some people.
- *Personal problems:* Substance abuse, stress, family crisis (divorce, for example), and escalating bills may drive an otherwise responsible worker to desperate acts.

To discourage *pilferage* in the foodservice department, managers need to deal with the problem immediately, persistently, and consistently. Firm corrective action, enforcement of well-defined policies and procedures that are applied fairly, continuous job-enhancement training, and effective supervisory techniques that boost morale are some deterrents to this problem. Also important are written and well-publicized internal and external security policies and procedures (within the limits of what reasonably should be disclosed). For example:

Security begins with the employment process. Check references and, if possible, talk directly to an applicant's previous employer(s). During the screening phase, watch for gaps in job history, references that appear professionally unrelated, questionable addresses or telephone numbers of references, or a Social Security prefix that does not match an applicant's reported birth state. Another cautionary signal is a space left blank on that portion of an application form that asks whether an applicant has been convicted of a felony or misdemeanor.

- Provide new employees with complete and thorough training and orientation to departmental policy and procedures.
- Occasionally check content of packages taken by employees from the department, **only** if allowed by facility policies or laws of city or state.
- Routinely check content of trash carts and garbage containers.
- To the extent possible, maintain only one employee entrance and exit that are visible to supervisory staff.
- Lock-and-key procedures should be clear-cut, with key-assignment logs maintained and a sign-out procedure for keys kept in a central lockbox. Duplication of keys should be prohibited. Those locks and combinations to which former employees had access should be changed—especially if the reason for release from employment was security related or if an employee's exit was less than amicable.

As noted earlier, unique security problems can occur in purchasing, receiving, storage, inventory control, production, and services (including cafeteria, vending, and catering). Two security problems in the purchasing area that require careful monitoring are potential collusion between purchasing personnel and distributors and the ordering of excess items that can increase inventory and, with it, the possibility of theft.

Security problems in receiving, storage, and inventory control will affect the quality and quantity of available supplies and, therefore, the cost of food and supplies. Receiving is vulnerable because it is possible for either delivery or receiving personnel (or both jointly) to short items or substitute lower-quality items and then sell the original items for personal profit. Unless merchandise is immediately accounted for and stored on receipt, the potential for theft is heightened. In a foodservice operation, expensive and high-demand items such as alcoholic and carbonated beverages, knives and other small utensils, or candy may have to be placed in locked storage areas.

A variety of measures can be implemented to prevent pilferage in the production area. Close (but nonthreatening) supervision of activities will reduce employee consumption or removal of leftovers or their unauthorized preparation of food items for personal consumption. Meat and cheese are the two most frequent targets of theft from the production storage area. Therefore, cases of meat placed in refrigerated or frozen storage should be opened and inventoried one by one. Again, controlled access to production storage areas is recommended.

Unique security problems in the service areas—the cafeteria, vending, and catering operations—are pilferage of food and supplies and control of cash. Commonly, theft in this area ranges from a cashier's charging friends less for meals to not charging for one or more individual items, to "no-sale" transactions or "over-rings" from which the cashier pockets the customer's money. Sometimes a cashier may leave a register unlocked for another employee to take money. Vending machine operations represent another territory susceptible to pilferage, especially if department employees are responsible for filling machines and counting money. The following examples have been observed by managers:

- Products are given away to other employees while machines are being filled.
- Change is removed from the change return while the door is open (an area often not secured by vending machine equipment design).
- Money is removed directly from the deposit area if the moneybox is left unlocked. Machines with currency changers are especially vulnerable.

Security measures that can help control service-area pilferage and cash loss are summarized below.

- Monitor portion control and storage of leftovers carefully.
- Purchase cash registers designed with as many safeguards as possible.
- Review all voided transactions, overcharges or over-rings, shortages, and "no sales" daily.

- Designate a supervisor to complete or verify cash register currency, coin counts, and reports.
- Monitor cashier's techniques (such as placing extra money into or taking money from the register) to evaluate his or her accuracy and honesty.
- Insist that cash register drawers remain locked at all times when they are not in use.
- Insist that cashiers give a cash register receipt to every customer to prevent possibility of receipt over-rings and to permit customers to compare change with the charge.
- Purchase vending machines equipped with electronic counters that reconcile money.
- Promote installation of locks on all vending machine money boxes to eliminate employee access to currency.
- Delegate the duties of filling machines and removing money to different employees to allow for double-checks.
- Make provisions for a security escort during removal of money from cash registers and vending machines.
- Provide a security escort during deposits from vending and other cash operations.

External Security

External security involves preventing the loss of items once they have left the immediate area. This means securing items from other hospital departments or from customers and protecting the department's property and employees from outsiders.

Food theft may be committed by taking items from patients' or residents' trays or sometimes consuming entire meals. Service ware is another favored area for theft, one attributed mostly to other staff, and represents up to 75 percent of the supply costs for a hospital foodservice department. Food, trays, bowls, and so on are frequently lost following catered events, when employees may pilfer food or property. The same policy that prohibits foodservice employees from taking leftover food also should apply to all other employees, including administrative staff.

By no means is theft the province of employees only. Patients, residents, and family members are not exempt from temptation. For example, they may take service ware as souvenirs, for use at home, or because they feel an item is paid for in the cost of their stay. One hospital implemented a unique approach to this problem: the addition of a service ware check-off section on the menu, labeled "for foodservice use only," whereby service personnel listed any service ware not returned with a patient tray. The operation reduced losses of flatware and service ware by 55 percent and 50 percent, respectively.

Systems must be in place to prevent unauthorized outsiders from entering the department and to monitor authorized entrants. This should be done for security and sanitation purposes. Again, maintaining one entrance and exit for employees and authorized personnel is a good measure. All outside doors should be kept locked except for deliveries. Distributors' representatives should have specific times and days allowed for visits and should not be allowed to enter the department from the dock area. Employees' visitors should be limited to the authorized break area and should never be allowed to enter restricted areas (such as production and storage areas).

A formal external security program should be designed in cooperation with the facility's larger security unit. Many of the techniques used in internal security apply to external security measures. (Chapter 22 also discusses some design features that enhance security efforts.) Specific external security strategies may include:

- Supervisors and security personnel routinely check doors to ensure that they are locked.
- Electronically monitor the dock to ensure that shipments are taken to their intended destinations in the foodservice department. Assigning a supervisor in the receiving area when large deliveries are received is recommended.
- Security should be provided the date, approximate time, and name of deliveries and refuse pick-up
- All sales representatives need to be informed to check in with security to receive a visitor's pass before going to the foodservice department.
- Monitor exits at shift changes to scrutinize employees' packages.
- Boxes on the premises should be broken down before the employee can remove them from the department.
- Rotate supervisors on all shifts to other shifts occasionally.

Securing and protecting the foodservice department rely on partnerships between the management staff and the security unit and between employees and management. To prevent loss, all functions of the department must be considered and appropriate policies and procedures established and consistently implemented.

DISASTER AND EMERGENCY PREPAREDNESS PLANNING

For purposes of this discussion, disasters can be classified as either external or internal. External disasters take place outside the institution but affect its operation. Examples of external disasters include natural calamities such as damaging snowstorms, hurricanes, earthquakes, and accidents (such as plane crashes, explosions, fires, and mass food poisonings) resulting in large numbers of casualties. External disasters also include national emergencies such as riots, wars, and terrorist attacks. External disasters can overburden an institution owing to the volume of casualties the institution may have to handle. They also can affect the institution's ability to provide services—for example, when a flood or a hurricane damages or incapacitates the institution's facilities.

Internal disasters occur within the institution and damage its facilities or threaten the well-being of its patients or residents and employees. Examples of internal disasters include fires, bomb threats, power outages, and radiation accidents. The health care institution's overall disaster plan should include policies and procedures for handling external and internal disasters that occur in their geographic area.

Design of the Disaster Plan

TJC has recently revised its standards for Emergency Management (EM) as a new and complete section of standards rather than have standards in several other sections (see "Evaluation of the Joint Commission Emergency Management Standards," www.nvha.net/bio/posting.jcstandards.pdf). These standards include required emergency management drills and exercises for all departments, all employees, on all shifts. All departments need to identify their strengths and weaknesses for preparedness. These drills need to be based on realistic events that could occur in their local area, be of sufficient length and complexity that challenges the organization's capacity and capability. Administration and the emergency preparedness director are responsible for the organization's plan. In conjunction with the emergency preparedness director, each department develops plans for their department that become a part of the total plan. The foodservice plan is important as it is responsible for food and water. Figure 15.8 is a general form that can be used to determine the department's readiness and assist in developing a plan for the department.

TJC revised standards include six critical functions. Each of these critical areas supports an "all hazard" approach rather than each individual hazard. The six critical functions are:

1. Communicating during emergency conditions
2. Managing resources and assets during emergency conditions
3. Managing safety and security during emergency conditions
4. Defining and managing staff roles and responsibilities during an emergency
5. Managing utilities during emergency conditions
6. Managing clinical activities during emergency conditions

OBRA and long-term surveys standards use "F Tags" as guidance for surveyors. These regulations are F517 and F518. Other tag numbers include F454 fire safety and F 455 emergency power. TJC standards are E.C. 4; 7.20; 7.40; I.M. 2.30 and I.C. 6.10. Regularly check all regulatory agencies for changes/updates.

The institution should appoint a disaster committee, with representatives from various departments within the facility. Their responsibilities include developing and maintaining the disaster plan and coordinating disaster drills throughout the institution.

The committee also should coordinate with local and state government agencies, the local chapter of the Red Cross, local law enforcement officials, local civil defense authorities, and local fire and rescue departments.

Because disasters can happen at any time or any place, in many forms and with a varying degree of severity, a comprehensive disaster plan should delineate written procedures designed to ensure quick and efficient response to an external or internal disaster. The plan also should include provisions for responding to specific kinds of disasters (such as power outages, plane crashes). Among factors to be covered in specific disaster plans are:

- Allocation of supplies and labor (who is responsible) especially food and water.

FIGURE 15.8 Disaster Assessment Checklist

This form is to be used to assist in the foodservice department to review the department disaster plan and readiness in case of a disaster. To be filled out by the foodservice director and used as a primary guide in developing/updating the disaster plan.

- Is the disaster plan up to date, signed, and posted?   Y_____ N_____
- Is the call list updated to all new hires?   Y_____ N_____
- Is a step-by-step plan for fire and natural disasters posted?   Y_____ N_____
- Do employees know how to handle a bomb threat, workplace violence?   Y_____ N_____
- Who is responsible for activating the foodservice plan?   _____
- Disaster planning discussed in orientation?   Y_____ N_____
- Documented in employee files?   Y_____ N_____
- Have all employees received in-service training to include:
  1. Layout of department and facility to include exit and evacuation routes? Y_____ N_____
  2. Location of electrical panel, fuse boxes, emergency lights, flashlights? Y_____ N_____
  3. Location of main shutoff valves for water, gas?   Y_____ N_____
  4. Location of fire extinguishers, sprinkler system?   Y_____ N_____
  5. What to do in a natural disaster, a terrorist attack?   Y_____ N_____
  6. Has all technological information been copied, stored off site?   Y_____ N_____
  7. Records maintained for attendance at inservice?   Y_____ N_____
- Have employees participated in a drill within the last year?   Y_____ N_____
- Deficiencies found, were they corrected?   Y_____ N_____
- List equipment that is on emergency power.
- Date of last emergency power tested: _____
- A source of potable water available?   Y_____ N_____
  1. Someone trained in methods of purification?   Y_____ N_____
  2. Materials available to use to purify water?   Y_____ N_____
- The required amount of food/water on hand?   Y_____ N_____
- Is there a plan for the provision of food to patients/residents, employees, families, media, volunteers,   Y_____ N_____
  emergency preparedness team, clergy, and an influx of persons seeking aid?
- Have disaster menus been planned, food for menus on hand?   Y_____ N_____
- A Memorandum of Understanding between the department and vendors to provide food, water, and   Y_____ N_____
  supplies during a disaster?
- Are security systems in place?   Y_____ N_____
- A disaster call or alert system been explained to employees?   Y_____ N_____
- Policies and procedures implemented for:
  1. Utilization of volunteers?
  2. Training volunteers in safe food handling?
  3. Priority of persons to be fed?
  4. Who maintains the communication post?
  5. Callback procedure
  6. Location and use of food and water for disaster
  7. Safety of delivery of food
  8. Safe food handling during a disaster
  9. Sanitation of area, waste management
  10. Personal hygiene and hand-washing procedures
  11. Use of chemicals—use of PPE
  12. Role of foodservice in organization procedures
  13. Monitoring of food and supplies
  14. Unauthorized people in any area of foodservice
  15. Methods for feeding patients/residents in case of no electricity, no operable elevators, and shortage of personnel
  16. Responsibilities of all foodservice personnel during a disaster
  17. Plans for disasters that are most likely to occur in your locality
  18. Telephone numbers of outside agencies, health care facilities, restaurants, dry ice and ice houses, and others as appropriate

Use this checklist to help develop the department plan. Serve on the facility disaster committee; work with the facility disaster preparedness director for input and assistance, as needed, to develop your plan; coordinate your plan with other departments; and provide cooperation where needed.

developed by Ruby P. Puckett copyrighted

- Responsibilities of specific departments and guidelines for interdepartmental cooperation.
- Provisions for caring for existing patients or residents and for incoming disaster casualties.
- Provisions for dealing with victims' families, clergy, and media representatives.
- Evacuation plans.
- Security of the personnel and the buildings.
- A plan to handle stress of employees/families.

A system for notifying the institution's employees of an impending disaster is vital to effective disaster planning. Every employee should be able to recognize the public address code or light signal used to announce disaster status in the institution, and evacuation routes should be posted. In addition, the addresses and telephone numbers of all staff and employees should be kept up to date so that in the event of an emergency, off-duty personnel could be called in. The list should be arranged by department, with the name of the department head at the top. It also might help to arrange employees' names according to their geographical locations throughout the city so that personnel who reside closest to the disaster area are to be called first. Supervisors should maintain copies of the call list at home as well as in the office.

The plan should include a list of vendors and other suppliers with telephone numbers, a list of emergency supplies and location of where stored, preplanned menus, water purification supplies, computer backup information, layout of area where the data is stored off-site, security measures, ingress and egress doors, and how to report suspicious activity or persons. Primary vendors and the foodservice department need to have a signed memorandum of understanding (MOU). This memorandum is an agreement that the vendor will do all the company can to meet the needs of the facility/department in case of an emergency.

Health care institutions should conduct regular disaster drills and disaster training programs for all staff members and employees on all shifts. These programs should describe types of potential disasters for the specific geographic area and procedures to be followed during each. The roles and responsibilities of individual employee positions should be explained, and the following questions addressed:

- What identification should the employee wear during a disaster?
- Where should the employee report for work?
- To which department or supervisor should the employee report?
- What duties and responsibilities should the employee perform?
- What should the employee's work priorities be?
- Where will the employee be able to find needed supplies?
- What will be the official communication system?
- What should the employee do once the disaster is over?

Foodservice Department Disaster Plan

The foodservice department plan is to ensure continuous operation and safety while remaining consistent with the plans of the larger health care facility. To ensure this objective, the director (or designee) should confer with the institution's disaster-planning team in developing and updating the department plan.

Developing the Foodservice Department Disaster Plan

As indicated earlier, the foodservice department's written disaster plan should support the institution's overall disaster plan and be specific to that institution and geographic location. In maintaining and developing the department plan, the director or designee will need to:

- Learn the institution's overall plan for handling internal and external disasters.
- Train the foodservice staff to perform their roles in handling potential disasters.
- Know the amount of nonperishable food that must be kept on hand for emergencies according to state law.
- Perform regular checks of stores of emergency food and supplies and rotate, use, or replace them as necessary.
- Reassess the effectiveness of the disaster plan at regular intervals by participating in disaster drills.
- Upgrade the department's emergency call list whenever there is staff turnover or there are changes in personnel addresses or telephone numbers.

The director may decide to appoint a department disaster-planning committee to develop and update the department's plan. Whether the foodservice director handles disaster planning or delegates to a committee, the plan should include provisions for the following items:

- A *signed memorandum of understanding (MOU)* between the foodservice department and other health care facilities, restaurants, hotels, grocery stores, and regular suppliers saying they can or will provide assistance in case the facility foodservice operation is damaged.
- *Methods of alert of impending dangers*: The plan should include the alarm system, coded intercom messages, evacuation routes, emergency telephone numbers, and addresses of person in charge with backup person. Internal procedures should include a call list of employees, vendors, and other suppliers; a list of emergency supplies and where stored; preplanned menus; water purification procedures; backup data on employees' records and inventory; security measures such as identification badges, ingress and egress doors, and how to report suspicious activity or persons.
- *Water*: Procedures need to ensure that some potable water is always on hand and an agreement made with suppliers to provide needed potable water.
- *Menus*: Menus should be planned to use foods that will spoil first, especially when there is no electrical power. Menus should be simple so that as few items as possible need to be served. If there has been a refrigeration problem, the freshness of all milk and milk products must be carefully evaluated before being served. Within the first 24 hours of a disaster, meals probably will continue to be served. They should be as simple and nutritious as possible under

the circumstances. The type of menu and service depends on the number of people to be fed and what equipment and personnel are available. When possible, consideration should be given to local food preference. Preparation and service procedures for the first 24, 48, and 72 hours after a disaster should be covered in the foodservice department's disaster plan.

• *Supplies*: The plan should include provisions for maintaining supplies adequate for at least 72 hours at all times. These supplies should include disposable dishes and flatware, cleaning and disinfecting compounds, garbage bags, and sterile and potable water supplies.

• *Sanitation*: The plan should outline procedures for maintaining sanitation at all times during a disaster. Careful attention should be given to checking for spoiled food, sanitizing pots and pans, and cleaning the food production work area. Food safety for temperatures, cross-contamination, and employee hygiene should be outlined.

• *Communications*: Communications should be developed to expedite information and provide for efficiency of continuous operations.

• *Security*: Security measures should cover food, supply, and employee safety. Provisions against intruders (looting) should be made. Especially during this period, employees should wear or carry identification cards at all times.

• *Use of volunteers/employees from outside of the foodservice department*: The disaster plan should describe the circumstances under which it would be appropriate to use workers from outside the department to perform foodservice tasks. When staff shortages make it necessary to use unskilled workers, for example, the tasks and roles they are to perform should be clearly delineated and their work carefully supervised.

• *Service priorities*: Priorities should be established for providing foodservice during emergencies. The needs of existing patients or residents and disaster victims should be met first, and then staff and employee needs should be served. Of lower priority would be service to members of the press, law enforcement officers, families of victims, and so on.

• *Coordination*: The external plan will need to be coordinated and incorporated into the organization's overall policies and procedures and coordinated with law enforcement agencies, civil defense, local and state fire departments, and rescue and ambulance teams. When applicable, the Red Cross and the military should be included.

• *Participation*: Employees on all shifts should participate in a preparedness drill, know their responsibilities, and act accordingly. Employees should be reminded to always carry identification, money in small bills, have a full tank of gas in automobile, and always let someone know where they are.

• *Clean-up*: Once the disaster is over there will be a need for clean-up. The foodservice director or designee will need to tour the area with engineering and, as applicable, the local FEMA or Red Cross to assess the damage and determine how to begin to clean up. Everyone should be aware of ants, cats, dogs; large animals such as cows, horses; and wild animals such as squirrels, snakes, raccoons, and other animals because they are frightened and may attack. Do not pick them up. Check the entire department for downed electrical wires, broken water lines, and gas leaks. If there is an odor of gas report it immediately and leave the area; do not light a match. When cleaning up and discarding boxes, equipment, and food follow the local codes and FEMA recommendation. Do **not** allow employees to enter the department until the area has been approved for employees to enter.

Planning for Various Disasters

Like the institution's disaster plan, the foodservice department plan should include specific provisions for a variety of natural disasters common to the facility's geographical area. For example, earthquake planning is especially important in California, Alaska, Washington, and Oregon. Disastrous snow and ice storms should be planned for in the Midwestern, Northeastern, and Mountain states. Floods occur in all areas of the United States, but institutions located in floodplains along waterways should be especially careful to plan for these relatively common disasters. Power shortages and failures often accompany natural disasters, and even summer thunderstorms, winter blizzards, and short-term localized power blackouts can put health care institutions on a disaster footing without warning.

Power Failures The electrical power supplied to health care facilities by local utilities can be cut off or decreased as a result of equipment failures, blackouts, brownouts, and natural disasters such as storms, floods, and earthquakes. The problem can last a few minutes or several days. When it is clear that the power may be off for more than a few minutes, the institution's procedures for handling power failures should be followed. The following steps may also be helpful:

- Immediately seal the door frames of all freezers with insulating tape and block the thresholds of walk-in freezers and refrigerators with blankets or other nonporous materials to keep warm air from entering.
- If possible, keep perishable food cold with dry ice. Keep a list of vendors, telephone numbers, and addresses and an MOU with companies.
- Use food stored in refrigerators first because it is the most perishable.
- Seek the help of local vendors or other health care institutions who may not have been affected, for help in storing some of the frozen food.
- Supply consumers with disposable service ware to make up for limited hot water supplies and unworkable dishwashers.
- Clean pots, pans, utensils, work surfaces, and other preparation equipment with sanitizing agents.
- Keep all refuse in heavy-duty bags and if possible maintain scheduled pick-up.

Floods and Hurricanes The National Weather Service issues watches and warnings to alert the public of impending danger. When these watches or warnings are received, the foodservice director in correlation with the organization's disaster teams should immediately activate the procedures for "before the storm." Once the storm hits, the action plan should be implemented, and once the storm is over, follow the procedures for after the storm.

Facilities located in flood-prone areas should formulate disaster plans that provide for enough food, equipment, and service ware to serve patients and personnel for five to seven days. Where floods are likely to occur due to seasonal river flooding or hurricanes, the foodservice department's production and storage areas are best located above ground level to prevent contamination from floodwaters, which contain dirt, sewage, dead animals, snakes, and fuel oil. However, most foodservice storage areas are located at or below ground level, so the storage area for disaster supplies should be well above ground level.

Winter Storms   The National Weather Service issues winter watches and storms. It is vital that the foodservice director act immediately. Be aware that employees may not be able to report to work due to road conditions and that there may be power outages. The plan for winter storms must cover a number of scenarios. In many parts of the United States, travel can become difficult or impossible during heavy snow and ice storms, limiting access to health care facilities. When this happens, employees may be forced to remain at the institution until surface transportation is restored. Therefore, contingency arrangements should be made for the delivery of food and supplies by air or mobile snow vehicles.

Heat Exhaustion   The National Weather Service issues temperature, heat indexes, and other weather each day. Data may also be found on the web for cities/states and broadcasts on radio and television and other electronic devices.

Heat-related problems should be carefully handled and information concerning heat-related problems posted throughout the department. Excessive heat causes death. When heat reaches 85° inside and stays there for four hours the medical examiner or county health department should be called for help.

There are three types of heat problems that must be addressed in the emergency plan. They include *heat cramps, heat exhaustion*, and *heat stroke*. When an employee exhibits the signs or symptoms of a heat stroke immediate action must be taken. **Delay can be fatal**.

Other natural disasters include, tornadoes, earthquakes, thunder and lightning, mudslides, uncontrolled fires, tsunamis, and volcanic eruptions. Plans should be in place for each of these types of disasters if there is a possibility that they may occur in your geographic area.

Bioterrorism   *Bioterrorism* is a threat to health care organizations and to the population as a whole. Bioterrorism includes nuclear, biological, and chemical agents (NBC). The use of these agents would have an effect in many areas, including the food supply. The biological agents may be delivered by means of infected animals or contaminated animal products, aerosols, contaminated food and water, ticks, rodents and their fleas, deer flies, mosquitoes, algae, crabs, octopus, yellow rain, and secondary person-to-person contact.

Nuclear agents include dirty bombs, which are a source of radiation. Radioactive fallout over a limited area is the result of an explosion. Many symptoms of radiation sickness will usually appear between one and six hours after exposure. Symptoms include headaches, nausea, vomiting, and diarrhea. If a nuclear attack should occur, leave the contaminated area immediately and get inside the nearest building. Remove clothing and shower as soon as possible. The plan for nuclear activity should include how to handle contaminated food from direct contamination, indirect contamination, and induced radiation.

Food may be contaminated by fallout miles away from the blast site. Nuclear contamination of food is detected by using a Geiger counter to determine the degree of radioactivity. Food that has nuclear contamination does not appear or change in any noticeable way without the use of testing with a Geiger counter.

The federal governmental and the military have developed methods for detecting nuclear, biological, and chemical contamination. They have also developed methods to be used to decontaminate the food or else throw it away (destroy it).

The preferred method of disbursement of biological and chemical agents is spraying. Be aware of unusual spraying and discarded spray devices.

Chemical agents are chemical substances that are intended for use in military operations to kill, seriously injure, or incapacitate people. Excluded from this definition are riot control agents, herbicides, and smoke and flames.

Chemical bioterrorism of food is usually accomplished by *chemicals* that enter the processing plant with raw materials or ingredients, chemicals used in the plant to support manufacturing processes, and chemicals used for sanitation purposes.

The following are the most common chemical agents:

- Nerve agents such as sarin, soman, VX, GF, and tabun, with variable symptoms depending on the agent, but major symptoms include runny nose, constricted pupils, tightness in the chest, blurred vision, nausea, vomiting, convulsions, loss of control of bodily functions, and respiratory tract paralysis. These agents have an odor of fruit or fish. Antidotes are available.
- Blistering agents such as nitrogen mustard and lewisite agents cause symptoms of eye and airway irritation, tearing, chemical skin burns and blisters, pulmonary edema, respiratory tract failure, and gastrointestinal and hematopoietic effects. They have an odor of garlic, onion, horseradish, or mustard; there is no antidote.
- Blood agents such as hydrogen cyanide, cyanide chloride, and hydrogen sulfates cause symptoms of confusion, dizziness, increased breathing and heart rate, convulsions, and asphyxia. They have a faint odor of bitter almonds; the antidote must be given immediately.
- Choking agents such as phosgene gas cause symptoms of eye and airway irritation, pulmonary edema, and choking. They have an odor of fresh-cut hay, grass, or corn, and there is no antidote.

Biological threats are probably the easiest to bring into the country (facility or department), but many agents are difficult to grow and break down quickly when exposed to the sun. Biological agents are infectious bacteria, viruses, or toxins that are used to produce illness or death in animals, plants, and humans. The Centers for Disease Control and Prevention (CDC) has listed the following agents to be of high priority:.

- Anthrax is a bacterium, exposure to which leads to flulike symptoms, difficulty breathing, shock, and if not treated, death. It is not contagious and can be treated with antibiotics.
- Smallpox is a virus that causes symptoms of fever, vomiting, headache, backache, and rash on face, hands, and forearms. It is transmitted by close contact with an infected person, and it can be treated with a vaccine.
- Plague (caused by the bacterium *Yersinia pestis*) has a rapid onset of feeling ill, muscle pain, cough with bloody sputum, skin and fingernails turning blue, and throat swelling that can lead to respiratory tract failure. It can be treated with antibiotics.
- Botulism, caused by the neurotoxin *Clostridium botulinum*, can destroy the nervous system and cause blurred vision, dry mouth, general weakness, poor reflexes, difficulty in swallowing, and death. It can be treated with antitoxins.
- Tularemia is caused by bites from ticks or biting flies and is characterized by fever, pneumonia-like illness, deep chest pain, swollen lymph nodes, respiratory tract failure, shock, and death without treatment. It can be treated with antibiotics and antimicrobial drugs.
- Hemorrhagic fever is a group of viral illnesses that can be mild to life threatening. Symptoms are fever, fatigue, dizziness, muscle aches, and exhaustion; in severe cases, there is bleeding under the skin, in internal organs, and from the mouth, eyes, and ears. There is no treatment, cure, or vaccine. It is spread by rats, mice, mosquitoes, ticks, or infected people.

Other biological agents of concern can affect the food supply. They include the following list of organisms:

- *Listeria monocytogenes*
- *Salmonella* species, as used by the Bhagwan Shree Rajneesh group in restaurants and grocery stores in Oregon; 750 cases were reported but no deaths; egg recall of a billion eggs, many people were hospitalized
- *Echerichia coli* 0157:H7 usually found in ground meat—there have been numerous recalls in the past years affecting hundreds of people
- *Shigella* species, used by a laboratory technician in Dallas; all those infected survived
- The epsilon toxin of *Clostridium perfringens*

Salmonella, Shigella species and *E. coli* are considered bacterial diarrheal problems; *Shigella* species and *E. coli* are considered to represent the greatest risk. There are no vaccines available for this group of food-borne illnesses, but treatment is available.

Bovine spongiform encephalopathy (mad cow disease) comes from eating brains or spinal matter from an infected cow. Persons develop a related brain-wasting illness, a variant of Creutzfeldt-Jakob disease. A mixture of meat from a "mad cow" could be shipped all over the world and some of it eaten before it could be recalled.

Centralization of food processing, production, destruction, or misrouted foods, especially raw foods, and the possibility of infection of domestic animals make food a tool of bioterrorism. The food we eat may travel more than a thousand miles from field to table, making it vulnerable to attack.

Water The CDC has identified two major biological threats for contaminating water: *Vibrio cholerae* and *Cryptosporidum parvum. C. parvum* was responsible for an outbreak in the water supply in Milwaukee. Chemicals that may present a problem are cyanide and mercury. The concern for water safety is low due to the treatment methods used in water treatment plants.

The plan for nuclear, biological, and chemical disasters should be similar to the plan for all disasters. It should address the following actions:

- Reduce fear, anxiety, and panic, remain calm, be more proactive.
- Develop a plan for each contingency; be aware of the "real risk."
- Develop a communication plan.
- Know the location of emergency suppliers.
- Develop food safety and sanitation procedures.
- Develop security measures for food, suppliers, and personnel; check all incoming food and note discrepancies, including time of delivery or different driver and truck.
- Develop guidelines for interacting with the media.
- Have a procedure for products that may be contaminated by germs, bacteria, fire, contaminated water, and radioactivity.
- Have alternative water supply and water purification kit.
- Know how to secure all entry and exit doors, loading docks, dumpsters, and trash removal areas by keeping doors locked as appropriate.
- Institute a procedure for backup and storage of computer records (financial and personnel).
- Store off-site blueprints of department.
- Know how and when to report suspicious activity, unusual odors, or loitering of unauthorized people.
- Train all personnel, beginning with the orientation process.
- Conduct drills, evaluate procedures, and make any necessary changes.
- Treat everything unusual as a threat and alert the organization's security officer.
- As applicable, install alarms and video surveillance on doors and loading docks.
- Be informed and keep employees informed.

To help employees to remain calm and assist them in preparing for any disaster, employees should be given information on how to protect themselves and their families. They will need to:

- Store up on food, formula, or other nutritional feeding supplements as appropriate; water; disinfectants; battery-operated clock; radio; extra batteries; cellular telephone; extra medication; blankets; extra clothing; water purification kit or other methods to purify water; plastic trash bags; waterproof matches; first-aid kit; candles; and disposable flatware and dishes. These supplies need to be stored off the floor in a temperature-regulated area, free from pests, and rotated as needed.

- Have money on hand in change and small bills.
- Always let family know where you are; decide on a meeting place for family if away from home.
- Use fireproof containers to store important documents. Store such items as wills; birth certificates; and ownership of homes, cars, and the like.
- Keep auto filled with gas at all times.
- Be aware of the status of alerts. Follow the directions of the response team. Try not to panic.

Check with the Association of Food and Nutrition Professional for articles and other materials on disaster planning. Many utilities and large grocery stores also have additional information, as does the Red Cross.

ERGONOMICS

Work-related *musculoskeletal disorders (MSD)*—such as tendinitis, carpal tunnel syndrome, and low back pain—are leading causes of suffering and disability in the workplace. The average cost to business is $29,000 per MSD. The number of MSD has constantly been increasing and now accounts for 6 out of 10 new occupational illnesses reported to the Bureau of Labor Statistics and most included disorders were overexertion and repeated trauma.

Ergonomics is the science of creating a good fit between workers and working environment. It was first used in 1970 by the automotive industry to design car interiors that were more functional and easier to use.

Ergonomics is part of the program standards of OSHA. The purpose of the standard is to reduce the number and severity of musculoskeletal disorders (MSDs) caused by exposure to risk factors in the workplace. (This standard does not address injuries caused by slips, trips, falls, vehicle accidents, or similar accidents.) Managers, supervisors, and employees should be trained in their roles, the recognition of MSD signs and symptoms, the importance of early reporting, the identification of MSD hazards in jobs in the workplace and the methods taken to control them and should review the program for effectiveness and correction of problems. All current and new hires must be provided basic information on MSD during orientation and as needed to correct a practice. Employees who have not been trained in MSD should never be allowed to perform a job for which they are not qualified. The director must control MSD hazards, and records must be maintained.

The revised OSHA standards concerning MSD have been relaxed and OSHA is working with business and labor on ergonomics initiatives, including training and education, technical assistance and regulatory support. OSHA's efforts will reward high-performance employers, support employers requesting assistance, and address employers who fail to keep workplaces free of recognized and serious ergonomically related hazards.

MSDs are subtle injuries, which over time affect the musculoskeletal region of the body such as muscles, tendons, and nerves at body joints, especially the hands, wrists, elbows, shoulders, neck, back, and knees. It is the buildup of trauma that causes the disorder. Serious risk factors for MSDs involve *repetitions* such as repeating the same motion every few seconds or repeating a cycle of motions or using an input device in a steady manner for more than four hours total in a workday.

Force factors are those such as lifting a specific amount of weight a specific number of times per day, pushing and pulling, pinching an unsupported object weighing two or more pounds per hand, gripping an unsupported object, and repeatedly raising and working with the hands above the head or elbows above the shoulders for more than two hours per day.

Awkward positions are those using the back, hands, fingers, or neck. Contact stress and vibration involve the use of tools.

A number of these factors may be found in foodservice operations such as the repetitive motions of data entry and cash register use. Force factors of lifting are found in workers in receiving and storage areas and those working in awkward positions that may include loading and unloading food carts.

The foodservice director has the responsibility to prevent or reduce MSDs through observation, training, following guidelines as established by OSHA and other professional organization such as physical and occupational therapy. Ergonomics has to do with safety of personnel, both short and long term. Whenever ergonomic equipment space is designed so workers do not overexert themselves, money can be saved from worker's compensation, overtime, and improved morale.

With the assistance of an occupational and physical therapist, the director should minimize the risk by developing ways to reduce repetitive motion and force factors and implement a program that will eliminate awkward postures. If necessary, tools should be purchased that will help employees to work in a more natural position. It may also be necessary for employees to see a physician who may find it necessary, for a definitive diagnosis, to do a physical examination, lab work, nerve test, X-rays, CAT scan, MRI, bone scans, joint aspiration, and arthroscopy procedure. When an employee complains of ergonomic pain the foodservice director should immediately seek help for the employee.

Employees need appropriate tools and equipment to do their job; they also need to have a workstation designed for the specific task to be performed. Tables and desks should not be too low or too high. They should be at a height where the task can be done within two inches above or below the elbow. The work area could be arranged where tools are within 16 inches of the body. Stepladders or stools should be used to reach materials in high places. For employees who transport goods, a handcart with vertical handles should be used. Employees such as stock clerks who lift objects should follow correct lifting procedures.

In March 2003, OSHA announced the first of four in a series of industry-specific guidelines for the prevention of MSDs in the workplace. The guidelines are recommendations for employees to reduce the number and severity of workplace injuries. OSHA emphasizes that specific guideline implementation may differ from site to site. The agency recommends that all facilities minimize the manual lifting of residents in all cases and eliminate such lifting when possible. The four-pronged approaches include guidelines, enforcement, research, and assistance.

For computer and cash register users, the information technology department and occupational therapist should customize the work area. Progress should be monitored when changes are made to ensure that the changes have not created more MSD hazards.

SUMMARY

The foodservice director has a responsibility to provide a work environment that protects employees from injury and complies with OSHA and other health and safety regulations. The department should have an established safety program that includes designated safety procedures, continuous self-inspection, comprehensive training, and an effective fire-prevention plan. This chapter describes working conditions, OSHA regulations, safety policies and procedures, components of safety training, fire-safety measures, and first-aid guidelines.

Protecting the foodservice department against theft requires implementing internal and external security controls. Theft-prevention techniques are presented for various functional areas. However, no security technique can succeed without a strong partnership between the foodservice security team and the larger facility's security unit or between management and employees.

A foodservice department must be prepared to respond to any kind of disaster—earthquake, flood, damaging snowstorms, power outages or reductions, and the like. To do this, the department should establish a disaster plan that complements the institution's plan and meets TJC and other regulatory agencies standards. Disaster training should be an ongoing effort, as should participative disaster drills. Employees must also be protected against injury on the job by being provided training before using tools, including the appropriate tool for the task, and proper ergonomic techniques for the required task.

KEY TERMS

Accidents
Bioterrorism
Blood-borne pathogens
Chemicals
Class A fire
Class B fire
Class C fire
Class D fire
Class K fire
Disaster and emergency planning
Electronic security
Ergonomics

Extinguisher
Hazard communication
MOU
Musculoskeletal disorder (MSD)
OSHA
PASS
Pilferage
Risk management
Safety
STOP, DROP, ROLL
Universal precautions
Workplace violence

DISCUSSION QUESTIONS

1. What are some methods that can be used to reduce injuries and accidents to employees?
2. Interpret MSDS sheets and explain why some chemicals may not appear on a MSDS.
3. Why is the Occupational Safety and Health Act important? Give reasons that changes need to be made to the original law. Include ergonomics.
4. Explain the importance of record keeping and what records must be kept.
5. What responsibilities does a foodservice director have in safety, safety inspections, and the safety committee?

6. Name the methods to provide fire safety education.
7. What is the effect of theft on the department budget and productivity, and what policies and procedures need to be developed? Include those that relate to the use of telephone and electronic equipment and include the consequence of not following the procedures.
8. What do you do in case of workplace violence?
9. Explain the importance of having an emergency preparedness plan for the geographic location of the facility. How would you help the department proceed in case of a major disaster?

CHAPTER 16

MENU PLANNING

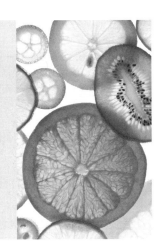

LEARNING OBJECTIVES

- Use the 2010 U.S. Dietary Guideline and My Plate and develop a "life-style change" for persons who are 15 percent overweight.
- Plan menus that are age-appropriate and meet the medical and nutritional needs of the customer while maintaining fiscal responsibility.
- Evaluate menus for aesthetic factors.
- Construct a customer satisfaction survey form.
- Explain at least three different types of menu systems, providing advantages and disadvantages for each.
- Utilize the master menu; plan the most used medical nutrition therapy diets.

THE MENU IS one of the most important plans a health care foodservice director and the team develop because the menu serves as a primary control for the operation. A menu is a list of food items offered to a customer from which to make a choice and affects almost every aspect of the foodservice operation. It can be viewed as the hub around which all other functions revolve. The menu determines what foods are to be purchased, produced, and served; affects the number and type of personnel hired; and has implications for kitchen design and equipment selection. The menu provides the basis for further departmental planning (for example, service expansion) and serves as a major determinant of purchase scheduling and, ultimately, the financial status of the operation.

In the system model, the menu is the primary control of the foodservice system. The input leads to transformation, which leads to output, with constant feedback. The menu controls all other sub-

systems, such as procurement, production, sanitation, maintenance, distribution, and service. The subsystems within the system may vary depending on the foodservice organization.

Aside from listing the food items offered to target markets, the menu serves other internal and external purposes. Internally, it provides crucial information to foodservice employees by specifying what items are provided. This enables employees to select which food and supplies to purchase, menu items to prepare, and service arrangements to provide.

The menu also functions externally to communicate the operation's offerings to potential customers. Because the menu facilitates communication between the foodservice operation and its customers, it also serves as an important marketing tool. In addition, a food operation's menus may even influence customer perceptions about the facility's overall quality of care. Therefore, the menu should be based on information about customers' wants and needs as identified by the facility's marketing information system. The menu should be compatible with the rest of the operation in the level and diversity of services offered and marketing mix, for example. It should also be useful in implementing the operation's marketing plan. The menu-planning process must produce a menu designed to satisfy customers and the marketing objectives specific to a particular operation.

In this chapter, critical elements of effective menu planning are discussed. Some of these are food preferences based on specific sources of information and changing trends, nutrition requirements among different customer markets, budgeted resources, availability, and skill levels of the foodservice labor force, and a number of other factors covered at length.

Menu specifications are covered. Considerations such as target markets, meal plans, meal patterns, and types of menus used throughout an operation drive these.

The menu-planning process is described in detail so that a menu planner will have a clear picture of what goes into the research, design, implementation, and follow-up evaluation of a good menu. Different types of menus—normal diets, modified diets, and special-service diets (such as gourmet selections)—also are addressed.

The chapter also includes brief summaries of four areas and several related methods and techniques of particular importance to foodservice managers and menu planners. These are (1) menu format, which addresses the design of the menu as an effective communication and marketing tool; (2) pricing strategies, which describe several approaches to arriving at what to charge for menu items; (3) menu evaluation, which gives suggestions for review of menu performance before and after implementation; and (4) menu-planning computer applications, which point out some advantages and limitations of computer-assisted menu-planning programs.

PLANNING CONSIDERATIONS

Because of its impact on the success of a health care foodservice operation, the menu must be developed with great care. The following factors should be considered:

- Food preferences of customers, especially sociocultural factors and linguistically worded food items, ethnic favorites, culture
- Nutrition requirements of group(s) being served, activity level
- Budget allocations within the department
- Availability and skills of foodservice workers
- Type of equipment, avoiding the overuse of one piece for preparing the menu items
- Amount of time required to prepare and serve the food
- Current marketplace conditions and availability of specific food supplies
- Legal responsibilities to follow federal, state, and facility guidelines
- Type of production and service system in use
- Amount of space and type of storage, preparation, and service equipment available
- Truth in describing the product you plan to prepare and serve
- Aesthetic of the menu—color, texture, form/shape, consistency, preparation and temperature (hot and cold), variety and balance
- Awareness of cultural, religious, and regional food preferences, economic background of the customers
- Environmental issues—local farmers, convenience food
- Mission, values, and philosophy of the organization and department
- As part of the continuous quality improvement program

In modification of the menu, consider:

- Physical limitations—eyesight, hearing, chewing, and swallowing
- Diseases (renal, diabetes, etc.)

- Allergies
- Need to increase or decrease calories, nutritional deficiency
- Recovery from illness, surgery, or trauma
- Dementia or other psychological conditions
- Food lore, fads, or aversion to certain foods

Food Preferences

Food preferences are defined by customer wants and are based on personal, cultural, and regional factors. A health care foodservice operation's marketing information system should provide information about specific food preferences of the operation's target markets. Informal and formal methods can be used to collect data about how patients, employees, staff, visitors, and guests will react to various foods and food combinations.

Sources of Information

Informal observations made in the dining room, the cafeteria, and patients' rooms, for example, can provide valuable insight on preferences. Formal methods—questionnaires, for example—provide information about preferences for menu items already served or new items under consideration. Specifically, patient satisfaction questionnaires may measure reactions to menu items served during a patient's stay. Observations of plate waste for specific entrées, either by visual assessment or by weight, can reveal much for purposes of menu planning. To predict preference or acceptance of specific items, rating forms designed for respondent ranking can be used. This measure generally uses a Likert-type scale. With a Likert scale, customers indicate their attitudes by checking how strongly they agree or disagree with a statement, ranging from "very positive" (extremely high preference) to "very negative" (extremely low preference). The number of alternatives ranges from three to nine. Preferences for food combinations (for example, cranberry sauce or cranberry relish with turkey, raisin sauce or mustard sauce with ham, dumplings or biscuits with beef stew) also can be determined using this technique.

Food preference and acceptance surveys are particularly important when a limited menu or a nonselective menu is used. Most consumers enjoy frequently being served favorite foods; thus, less-preferred foods should not be repeated too often. Nutrition assessment procedures may also provide essential information about eating behaviors that can be used in planning menus for patients on regular or modified diets.

Trends

In a facility where the population changes frequently, it is important to survey food preferences frequently to keep menus current. Even with this information in hand, the task of menu planning is far from easy. Menu planners must keep pace with changing trends to develop new and creative ideas.

Changing Tastes Most major foodservice trade journals track and report the popularity of specific menu items. It is critical that the menu planner keep up with these reports so that the operation's menus can be modified accordingly. For example, the move to organic foods and the whole push to sustainability have a major impact on menu planning. For example, fried chicken, a staple in the 1970s and 1980s, is rarely found on menus today.

Trade journals also report that consumers prefer more flavors in their foods, primarily due to the growing popularity of spicier ethnic and regional foods. Of particular popularity are Japanese, Latin American, and European cuisines, followed by Chinese, Mexican, and Italian menu items. In today's society, with the major concern of obesity in the population, most foodservice operations are offering many of the more popular diet food items on their menus. Current trends also indicate the growing popularity of specialty soups and sandwiches, along with increased interest in vegetarian entrées. The menu planner must assess these trends in relation to the preferences indicated by the operation's target markets.

Changing Demographics and Sociocultural Influences The changing demographics described in Chapter 1 have implications for the menu-planning process. Most important among these is the aging of the population. The older adult will represent a larger percentage of the general population but will also present an increase in the need for health care services. Some of the baby boomers and older adults are leaving their homes and moving into residential facilities. The menu planner needs to pay close attention to this market segment when developing patient menus and when planning community ventures such as home-delivered or congregate meals.

Another important segment identified in Chapter 1 is the baby-boom generation, a segment currently at or approaching middle age to older adults. Most baby-boom households had children, whose menu preferences become important when the children become customers. Many of these children are accustomed to eating meals away from home and have developed strong preferences. When it comes to satisfying this segment, a number of them may still seek fast foods but many of them are changing their lifestyles to more healthy eating—organic, locally grown. The menu planner should carefully review trade journals to identify changing trends and creative ways to provide foodservice to the customers. Children will present a challenge to the menu planner, especially given the increase in obesity of children.

Cultural diversity of the general population continues to increase. The most rapid growth has been, and will continue to be, in the Hispanic and Asian populations. As nonwhite minorities make up an increasingly larger percentage of the patient and employee segments, menu planners must assess and modify menus to appeal to these markets. Other points to consider include religion, regional food habits, food preferences, and comfort foods.

Changing Habits In addition to monitoring the tastes and demographic makeup of their customers, menu planners must analyze their customers' food attitudes and behaviors. An increased commitment to and concern for health and nutrition have important implications for menu planners. The move to more fresh foods that have been grown and produced without pesticides and fertilizer, and the concern with healthful eating, continues to grow and has resulted in changes in the consumption of specific foods and menu items. Today's literature contains many references to the changing habits of the population that include a decrease in fat consumption, especially saturated fats and cholesterol, and for some a reduction of white flour and refined sugar products.

Attitudes will change as each new dietary regiment becomes popular and promises to reduce weight. The number of "fad" diets that are advised, by all forms of media, can be staggering. Many of these type of dieters "yo-yo"; others are committed and seek the assistance of registered dietitians to help plan a lifestyle change. Unfortunately, many people still believe in the magic "pill" or "diet" to reduce weight; they may stay on the diet until they lose weight but then gain it or more back because they did not make the necessary changes in their lifestyle. To meet the wants of committed weight-loss customers, the menu planner should incorporate creative, flavorful menu items that conform to dietary guidelines for good health. However, the United States is facing a crisis of obesity, due in part to the "supersizing" of meals in fast-food outlets, the extra-large servings offered at some restaurants, and the lack of exercise and control of food intake. There are still other reasons for the obesity crisis, and they include the trend of working longer hours, watching television, and becoming sedentary, while constantly "snacking" on high-calorie carbohydrate foods. Most obese people do not regularly exercise, resulting in their intake being greater than their output. Menu planners have an increasingly difficult problem in trying to meet the needs of a diverse population.

Customers continue to eat more meals away from home and at less-regular hours, a lifestyle change that provides both an opportunity and a challenge for health care foodservice operators. Other considerations when planning menus include age, sex, occupation, health status, marital status, disposable income, religious preferences, level of education, and nationality. This is particularly the case with breakfast, which has increased in importance as a meal eaten away from home. Because breakfast preferences vary widely among individuals, breakfast menus should offer a range of choices but without wasting food. To enhance breakfast sales, menu planners have incorporated more diverse menus, convenient hours of service, and, in some cases, spirited marketing strategies. To provide menu items that meet customer wants, the menu planner should continue to monitor changing trends in the market and customer demands.

Nutrition Requirements

Although it is important to focus on customers' wants, the specific nutritional needs or requirements of individual customers and groups of customers also should be considered. The nutritional needs of the general customer segment, which is composed of employees, staff, visitors, and guests, are discussed first, followed by a brief discussion of the patient market.

Dietary Guidelines for Americans 2010

Increased awareness of the importance of nutrition to health has prompted menu planners to consider the nutritional quality of their menu items offered to general customer markets. The major concern is obesity and a sedentary lifestyle. This lifestyle increases the likelihood of developing major health problems (diabetes, cardiovascular disease, etc.). Although numerous plans have been developed for the general population, one specific guide is particularly valuable when considering menu planning for this segment: *Nutrition and Your Health: Dietary Guidelines for Americans* (revised in 2010). The U.S. Department of Agriculture (USDA) and the U.S. Department of Health and Human Services developed these guidelines. Key recommendations are:

- Balance calories to manage weight
  Reduce calorie intake to manage body weight, eat fewer calories
  Reduce intake of saturated fats, added sugar, and alcohol
  Be physically active each day—30 to 60 minutes of moderate exercise each day and reduce time spent in sedentary activities
  Maintain appropriate caloric balance through each stage of life
- Reduce food and food components
  Reduce daily sodium to less than 2,300 mg and after age 51 reduce to 1,500 mg/day (other ethnic groups or disease entities may need to further reduce sodium intake)
  Consume less than 10 percent of calories from saturated fatty acids, replace with monounsaturated and polyunsaturated fatty acids
  Consume less than 300 mg/day of cholesterol
  Limit foods that contain synthetic sources of trans fats, such as partially hydrogenated oils and other solid fats
  Reduce the intake of calories from solid fats and added sugar
  Limit foods that contain refined grains plus solid fats and sugar
  Limit alcohol—up to one drink per day for women and two drinks per day for men and only for adults of legal drinking age
- Foods and nutrients to increase
  Guide your food choices while staying within energy needs
  Increase vegetable and fruit intake
  Eat a variety of vegetables, especially dark green, red, and orange vegetables and beans and peas
  Increase whole grain consumption, consuming at least one-half of all grains as whole grains
  Choose carbohydrates wisely for good health, increase fiber intake to 14 grams per 1,000 calories
  Reduce added sugar, especially in sugar-sweet beverages
  Increase intake of nonfat or low-fat milk and milk products such as yogurt, cheese, or fortified soy beverages
  Choose a variety of protein foods
  Increase the amount and variety of seafood by replacing some meat and poultry
  Choose foods that provide more potassium, calcium, and vitamins A, C, D, and E
  Choose foods high in antioxidants
  Keep food safe to eat

There are also guidelines for women becoming pregnant, women who are pregnant, and individuals 50 years and older

- Choose sensibly
  Choose a diet that is low in saturated fat, trans fat and cholesterol, and total fat between 20 and 35 percent of total of energy (caloric intake)
  Weekly consumption of two servings of fish, particularly fish rich in EPA and DHA
  Choose beverages and foods to moderate your intake of sugars
  Choose and prepare foods with less salt, keep salt intake to 2,300 mg per day, and increase the intake of potassium
  If you drink alcoholic beverages, do so in moderation—one drink per day for women and two drinks per day for men. One drink is defined as 12 ounces of regular beer, 5 ounces of wine (12 percent alcohol), or 1.5 ounces of 80-proof distilled spirits.

A significant new element is the "keep food safe" guideline, which finds the USDA advising consumers on the need to keep and prepare foods safely in the home and recommending that they keep preparation areas and utensils clean; separate raw, cooked, and ready-to-eat foods; cook food to safe temperatures; and chill perishable food promptly (see Chapters 13 and 14).

The *My Plate* (www.ChooseMyPlate.gov; see Figure 16.1) has replaced the Pyramid Steps to Healthier You. My Plate was developed to make it easier for people to understand food groups and serving sizes. Basic suggestions are to:

- Balance calories (reduce portions)
- Increase certain foods (vegetables, fruits, and whole grains)
- Reduce other foods (sodium and sugary drinks)

FIGURE 16.1   Choose My Plate

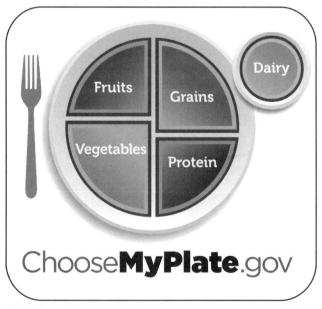

Source: ChooseMyPlate.gov.

The plate is brightly colored, which helps people understand what they need to eat. The plate is divided into four colored sections representing vegetables, fruits, grains, and protein, with dairy on the side. The chart makes it easier for customers to choose nutritious foods. It is suggested that customers try to make half the plate fruits and vegetables, eat more whole grains, and do not oversize the portions. It is also suggested that rather than using a 12-inch plate, an 8-inch plate would be more appropriate.

The My Plate website also includes the concept of "equivalents" in ounces to help understand portion sizes. It also makes daily recommendations based on age, gender, and an assumption of 30 minutes per day of moderate exercise.

Menus will need to be planned to meet these new guidelines—for example, offer more vegetables, smaller portions of lean meat or protein food, fruits (rather than high-sugar desserts), and whole grain bread and cereals. Dairy could be reduced fat milk or other dairy products (use ice cream sparingly).

Carefully choose fats to try to avoid trans fats; keep saturated fats and cholesterol as low as possible. Check labels of all fats and other products before purchasing or offering to the customer.

Foodservice has a great opportunity to develop new menus, to train personnel, and to post the plate poster in the department as well as the cafeteria. Another suggestion is to develop fliers for patient trays explaining My Plate and the reason behind the menu change. Use your creativity!

Patient Market

In foodservice operations that provide three meals a day, as is the case with most health care establishments with inpatient service, menus should follow the *Dietary Reference Intake* (DRI). The DRI includes four types of reference values: Estimated Average Requirements (EAR), Recommended Daily Allowance (RDA), Adequate Intake (AI), and the Tolerable Upper Intake Level (UL). The primary goal of these dietary reference values is to prevent nutrient deficiencies and reduce the risk of chronic diseases such as osteoporosis, cancer, and cardiovascular diseases. Menu planners should evaluate regular patient menus to determine that they indeed satisfy the DRI. In cases where a patient's medical condition requires modifications to the regular menu, the menu planner should refer to the health care operation's dietary manual.

Budget Allocations

The menu is the major factor in establishing and controlling food costs. With some effort and imagination, a skilled menu planner can design a menu that offers variety, interest, and appeal and still remains within most budgets while being planned around up-to-date, tested recipes. Keeping a running total of the cost of items on the menu as it is being planned allows the planner to balance high-cost items with low-cost items so that total daily costs can be kept within the limits of the budget. However, the same cost level should be maintained from day to day rather than balancing overbudget days with days on which the cost is considerably less than the budgeted daily average.

This approach works well for controlling costs with nonselective menus, provided the cost information is current and projected market conditions are considered when menus are planned far in advance. When a selective menu is offered, a forecast of the demand for each item must be determined before total cost per meal or patient day is computed.

When menus are planned for employees and guests, cost and selling price must be considered. The selling price should cover ingredients, labor, specified overhead, and profit. (Specific pricing techniques are discussed later in this chapter.) Accurately forecasting demand is difficult because the selling price itself affects the demand for individual items on the menu. Keeping careful records of the popularity of various food items can sharpen the forecast when the same combination of food items is offered again.

Availability and Skills of Foodservice Workers

The availability and skills of production personnel must be considered in menu planning, but they need not limit menu variety and quality. Menu items that require considerable skill and time to prepare can be purchased from commercial manufacturers that supply all or most of the labor involved in preparation. Therefore, menu items that cannot be produced on the premises with available personnel and equipment can still be part of the menu in most operations when the cost of prepared foods fits into the budget.

Employee expectations and satisfaction also should be considered. Plans should be made for the average level of skill and energy, but whenever possible, challenges should be offered to employees who seek to enhance their job skills.

Preparation and Scheduling Requirements

Overloading production schedules by poor menu planning can lead to tired, frustrated employees. Menus that balance the production workload from day to day and leave time for other essential tasks help foster positive employee attitudes.

In the past, managers relied primarily on their intuition and experience in making estimates of the labor involved in preparing individual menu items. Today, however, researchers use industrial engineering methods to determine foodservice production times. Reliable estimates of the total preparation time for each menu item will help managers plan the menu mix, schedule personnel, forecast labor costs, and develop effective menu-pricing systems. Basically, the food for properly planned menus can be produced within the allotted time by employees working at a steady but unhurried pace. Most employees can adjust to occasional miscalculations in the amount of preparation time needed, but they become frustrated and angry when crises become routine. Also, low productivity results when the employees' productivity and skills are underutilized as a result of poorly planned menus or when labor time is not adjusted downward to accommodate the use of more prepared foods.

Physical facilities such as the layout, design, age, and condition of equipment also influence the preparation and scheduling requirements.

Marketplace Conditions

Several factors affect the supply and price of foods in the marketplace. Three of these are weather conditions, supply cycles, and geographical location.

Weather conditions may dictate sharp short-term fluctuations in supply and price of fresh produce. Favorable weather conditions can result in an unexpected abundance of produce at lower prices, but adverse conditions can bring higher prices and shortages. Fruits and vegetables grown for processing are also affected, with resulting supply problems that may extend over several months.

As for *supply cycles*, improvements in food processing, distribution, and storage technology have increased the availability of many foods throughout the year. However, seasonal fluctuations still occur for some fresh fruits and vegetables that are marketed in unprocessed form.

Geographical location may determine the type and quality of food products available. In today's (and projected) economy, location cost will probably be passed on to the buyer as gas prices continue to fluctuate. Improvements in transportation have eliminated this problem for many products, especially with the refrigerated and frozen carriers. However, other products still may not be available in the ready-to-serve state to hospitals or nursing homes in rural areas. It is suggested that foodservice establishments purchase locally, provided the sellers meet all applicable codes.

Technological advances in growing and processing foods may become a factor in menu planning. It may become necessary to identify food items that contain genetically modified foods, foods that have been irradiated, and what percentage of a food is organic.

Production and Service Systems

For production systems in which foods are prepared, held hot or cold, and served on the same day, menus may be limited by the amount of time available for food preparation between meals. The menu planner should try to spread the workload as evenly as possible among employees over the workday and still avoid holding conditions that may damage food quality.

In production systems that incorporate a thermal break, time limits may not be as severe. Once food is produced, it is held in a chilled or frozen state until served. Service deadlines do not limit the production schedules in these two systems, although not all food items are suitable for these holding methods without extensive ingredient or process modification. Menu planners must be completely familiar with the problems associated with certain menu items and revise production procedures accordingly.

The critical relationship between menu items offered and service system selected must be considered. The method of service and the distance that trays or bulk food must be transported can limit the types of menu items that can be served successfully. For example, fried eggs, pancakes, omelets, and ice cream can deteriorate in quality if too much time passes between preparation and service. Or the number of sauces and casserole dishes may have to be limited in bulk-food distribution because of space limitations in food carts for the extra containers and because of the extra handling required at the point of service. Room service in all health care facilities and the cafeteria, buffet, and wait service in long-term care facilities can eliminate some of these problems.

Space and Equipment

Successful menu planning cannot take place without factoring in the amount and type of available storage space for holding foods before, during, and after preparation. Purchasing policies need to consider storage facilities so that deliveries are scheduled in a way that ensures adequate food supplies.

Equipment capability also must be considered during menu planning because a menu item cannot be produced unless the necessary equipment is available when needed. Unfortunately, many small foodservice operations do not have labor- and time-saving equipment such as mechanical slicers, shredders, choppers, and peelers that allow production of more complicated products. Although this equipment is expensive, it can increase productivity and enhance menu variety. In menu planning, demands on equipment must be balanced to avoid overloading ovens, steam equipment, and other production facilities.

Aesthetic

Aesthetic literally means art, beauty, and good taste. Aesthetic can be accomplished when the planner thinks what causes a menu to be in "good taste, artful, and beautiful." Customers want the food to have a balance of flavor, color, texture, form/shape, consistency, variety, temperature (hot and cold), and preparation methods. When planning menus the planner needs to be able to visualize how the food will look on the serving plate, how it will taste, and whether there will be variety in preparation. More information on aesthetic is described later in the chapter under menu features.

When planning menus for a health care facility, plan the house diet and then modify for medical nutrition therapy diets. Use as many foods from the house diet as possible on the modified diets. Liberalizing diets is the best method to use in menu planning.

Other Considerations

Recent census reports (see Chapter 1) indicate that we are a mobile society made up of cultural, ethnic, and economic backgrounds. When planning menus the planner needs to have marketing information of the customers it serves (see Chapter 3). In a number of cities and states ethnic population is the majority. Ethnics and cultural preferences must be considered. Religious customs that avoid certain foods and the food preferences of geographic region of the nation need to be noted. It is prudent to know religious customs and whether some foods must be eliminated for these groups or if certain foods need to be eliminated for a specific time period. Language differences from English may be a problem. It may become necessary to seek the assistance of translators.

With global travel and influx of people from other nations many "new" items are now appearing on menus. Know your customers, and offer what is best for your geographic location. Education, economic backgrounds, and the move for a sustainable environment and level of activity influence menus. For example, in most university communities all four of these influence the menu—in relation to the type of food and preparation, the need for calories to meet the needs of students. A number of colleges and universities have moved to being more sustainable—supporting local farmers, organic foods, green buildings, and leaving no carbon footprint; this shift in customer preference is having a major impact on the entire foodservice operation.

Pitfalls

There are a number of pitfalls in the menu planning process. One is the overuse of items that are favorites of the menu writer to the exclusion of other items. Second is using the same item over and over. An example would be mashed potatoes rather than using a variety of preparation methods for potatoes. The meal at which this most often happens is breakfast. Discuss with your vendor new food items that may be available and how they will still meet the budget if added to the menu. Continue to review trade magazines for the newest trends in food items and preparation skills. Use your imagination.

A major pitfall is in not following the "truth in menu" law (sometimes referred to as "accuracy in menu").

Truth in menus involves honesty in pricing and precisely stating the price. When placing and describing an item on a menu the planner must be accurate in describing the preparation style, ingredients, origin, portion size, and health benefits. You must not misrepresent your menu item. For example, if you describe an item as 6 ounces wild salmon from Alaska, grilled served with a lemon sauce, you **must** serve this item as described; to do otherwise you are being fraudulent in your claim and not in compliance with the law. (This is a federal law that is more than 1,000 pages long and is overseen by dozens of agencies and administrative entities. To avoid fines and other legal charges be honest in what is printed on a menu and what is served.)

The federal government mandates that menus be followed, planned in advance, and **posted**. Deviation from the posted menu is allowed only if a patient refuses the food. Any other change made to the posted menu must be noted in writing, with the reason why (unavailable, price increase, etc.) and kept on file for the duration of the posted menu. If there are local or state regulations concerning posted menus they must also be followed. Laws change—know and follow the laws.

Menu Revision

In health care facilities menus have a tendency to become boring with the possible loss of customers, especially in employee cafeterias. Menus need to be occasionally revised for the following reasons:

Holidays and theme days. Menus for holidays should be changed to offer the "traditional" foods served during this celebrated time. This is especially true for patients and employees working on the holiday because they are not home with family. Theme-day menus offer a change in the routine and can be fun especially in long-term care facilities.

Seasonal change. Menus can reflect foods that are available during a certain season. During the warm/hot months the menu should be lighter and offer as many fresh and raw foods as possible. During the cold weather the menu should offer thicker soups and perhaps heavier meals.

Customer survey results. The input from customer surveys must be taken seriously if a number of customers have the same negative comment. When customers note that the suggestions were taken seriously they are more inclined to be "better" customers.

Plate waste and sales volumes studies. All foodservice directors need to periodically do a plate-waste study and a sales analysis to determine what menu item is most often left uneaten or is a low purchase. The foodservice director should then investigate the causes and if appropriate immediately remove the food item from the menu.

Change in service. When changing from one type of menu service to another, menus must be changed to meet the needs of the new system, for example, from a selective menu to room service.

Availability and cost. There are times due to weather conditions that food on a preplanned menu may not be available. In these instances, the item will need to be removed and another item replace it. Availability and cost go hand-in-hand. When cost goes above a set price allocation for the item it must be removed from the menu. For example, if lettuce goes from $10 per case to $20 a case, a substitute for lettuce must be found as this increase in cost would cause a variance in the budget that must be justified. In examples like this it is a good idea to let customers know why the change was necessary.

MENU SPECIFICATIONS

The foodservice director must establish basic menu specifications before planning any menus. To begin, the foodservice director needs to appoint a menu committee composed of the chef/head cook, patient hostess, dietitian, purchasing manager, catering manager, nonpatient manager, head cashier, tray line supervisor, and several regular customers. This committee will review all survey results and tabulate positive and negative comments concerning food and service, complete a week of food plate waste studies, and interview patients and nonpatients using a standardized form for questions. The chef/head cook needs to be prepared to discuss equipment use; the storeroom manager will let everyone know the storage capacity for dry, refrigerated, and freezer storage and what foods are on hand. The registered dietitian (RD) will provide input concerning the nutrition of the menu. Once all data is collected the committee meets to discuss existing problems and possible problems with a new menu system.

The foodservice director will explain the number of target markets or customer groups for which menus will be developed, along with any special services offered by the department that needs to be discussed. The number of menus that must be developed to meet the needs of different customer groups must be specified. Next, a meal plan and menu pattern appropriate for each customer group must be determined. Finally, such issues as the degree of selection and repetition to offer customers should be specified.

Target Markets

As described in Chapter 3, market segmentation can be one of the foodservice director's most powerful marketing tools for help in determining the markets or customer groups, along with those specified by health care administration, for which menus will be developed. The most significant distinction is the categorization of potential customers as either patients or nonpatients. Consumer wants and needs with regard to food differ between the two groups, thus influencing the planned menus. The patient customer group can be further segmented based on medical condition, age, and gender, whereas the nonpatient group typically is composed of employees, staff, visitors, and guests. Special services offered by the hospital or the foodservice department (or both) may provide the opportunity to serve other markets or groups as well. Examples of special services include child-care centers, home-delivered meals for senior citizens, or catering services for off-premises customers. Once the target markets have been selected, the director must determine how many menus to develop. Only then can the menu-planning process proceed to the next step: determining the appropriate meal plans for each customer group.

Meal Plan

The number of meals offered during each 24-hour period varies according to the *meal plan* and type of facility, for example, a cancer or pediatric unit. Choosing the patient meal plan appropriate for the facility is an administrative decision that requires input from other patient care departments and the medical staff, if appropriate. For example, the nursing, radiology, and physical therapy departments must schedule patient treatment around mealtimes. Therefore, because meal plans and schedules affect these other departments, their needs should be considered.

The *three-meal plan* follows the traditional breakfast–lunch–dinner or breakfast–dinner–supper pattern. However, because of changes in American food habits and problems associated with labor scheduling and availability, four- and five-meal plans are being adopted by some health care institutions, with many using room service. With any meal plan, no more than 14 hours should pass between the last meal of one day and the first meal of the next (see CMS and local regulations).

The director and the nonpatient manager must determine appropriate meal plans for nonpatients. Again, the customers' wants and needs regarding the number and scheduling of meals must be balanced with the resources required to support these plans. Based on this type of analysis, weekend brunches have met with success among health care foodservice operations. As mentioned earlier, customers' food habits reflect a move away from the traditional three-meal plan to more frequent dining at less-regular hours. This, along with the realization that potential customers are available 24 hours a day, should be considered when establishing the meal plan for other customer groups. Viewing this situation as an opportunity, the foodservice director should collect information

from these potential customers to develop cost-effective meal plans. Special attention should be given to meal plans that address the needs of the evening and night-shift employees of the health care operation.

Menu Pattern

Translating the daily food needs of customers into attractive and appealing meals requires good organization. For inpatients or residents, the normal diet—also known as the *regular, general,* or *house* diet—is the starting point for planning because it is the basis for all diet modifications. Planning and producing modified diets is easier when the normal diet menu includes several foods that can also be served on modified diets. However, variety in the general menu should not be restricted by this consideration; only slight changes in certain menu items will make them suitable for modified diets.

The menu planner uses the normal diet and the minimum daily requirements to develop the patient *menu pattern*, which simply lists the food components to be offered at each meal. For example, the traditional menu pattern for a three-meal plan includes:

- Breakfast
  Fruit or juice
  Hot or cold cereal
  Meat or meat alternative
  Bread and butter or margarine
  Beverage
- Lunch
  Meat or meat alternative or soup and sandwich
  Vegetable, salad, or both
  Bread and butter or margarine
  Dessert or fruit
  Beverage
- Dinner
  Appetizer or soup or juice
  Meat or meat alternative
  Potato, rice, or pasta
  Vegetable
  Fruit or vegetable salad
  Bread and butter or margarine
  Dessert
  Beverage

The traditional menu pattern may offer more food than is necessary because most healthy adults do not consume this many courses at their meals when at home. This pattern should be analyzed to see if the number of courses can be reduced and still meet customers' nutritional requirements.

The number of items offered at each meal on each day should be about the same to ensure that the recommended number of servings from My Plate are served, to maintain an even level of food intake from day to day, and for cost accounting. Menus also need to meet the *Dietary Reference Intake* for Vitamins A, C, and E and selenium, as foods high in these vitamins and minerals are high in antioxidants.

Menu patterns for nonpatient customer groups also must be established. The menu patterns established for these groups should balance customers' wants and needs; applicable regulations or requirements, such as with menus for child-care facilities; those resources required to support the menu patterns; and the effect of the menu patterns on profitability of nonpatient foodservice operations. It is helpful to use a form specifically designed for menu planning so that meals for customer groups conform to the standard set for the facility.

Printed Menus

The method used to present a menu to a customer has a significant effect on the foodservice operation and on sales in the nonpatient area. The menu design and format should appeal to customers to stimulate sales and influence them to select food they want to eat. The foodservice director and production staff with, as appropriate, a consultant choose the menu cover, color, print size, and message that will go on the outside of the menu.

The cover of the menu should be designed to complement the overall theme of the operation. The name of the facility should go on the cover. The menu size will depend on the number of items being offered, amount of copy to describe each item, and the print size. The weight, quality, and color of the paper add to the overall impression.

The sequence of the placement of menus may follow the progression of the meal or a focal point on the menu (when a daily special "meal" is listed). Most health care organizations use a three-hole perforated design for selective menus. The layout may be breakfast, lunch, and dinner or lunch, dinner, and breakfast. The layout will depend on the food production system and distribution of the meal trays. Room service menu may contain a large variety of items, but may remain the same for weeks.

The typeface must be large enough and legible enough to allow customers (patients) to read the description. The most common typeface used is Times New Roman. It may be set in uppercase, lowercase, or italics. There should be a space between each line. Black print is the easiest to read and the most acceptable regardless of the color of the paper. The inside of the menu should use descriptive words to identify a food item. The wording should be accurate to enable customers to visualize the food item. Avoid terms or phrases that do not tell customers what the food is unless a description is provided. Misleading names given to the menu item are illegal (see discussion under pitfalls).

The menu is an important marketing tool for all customers. In nonpatient areas, menu boards and signage should be posted that describe the food and beverages that are available for purchase. Menu boards should be designed to attract attention, provide information with print size larger enough to be read before selecting food items, and be tailored to each operation. Menu boards come in a variety of sizes and shapes and may be illuminated and custom designed.

Types of Menus

Once the meal plan and menu pattern for each customer group have been developed, additional menu specifications must be established. These focus primarily on the degree of menu selection and repetition offered to customers.

Selection

Menus are basically three types: single use, static, and cycle. The single-use menu is designed for one use and not used again. These menus are used for special events and fine dining where the chef changes the menu daily. The *static menu* remains the same from day to day, such as a restaurant-style menu and in some instances the room service menu. This menu is often found in fast-food outlets and specialty eating places such as a barbecue house or delicatessen. The *cycle menu* is different every day and is used for a specific time frame such as eight days or three weeks and then repeated. Cycle menus need to be changed often to meet the demands of customers. Menus may also offer no choice, limited choices, or a wide variety of choices. Airline foodservices are a good example of those offering no choice, and meal programs for the elderly offer limited choices.

Menus may also be classified by the method of pricing. In an *à la carte menu*, food items are priced individually. Using this type of menu, customers select only the foods they want. The *table d'hôte menu* offers a complete meal for a fixed price. A *du jour menu* offers the menu of the day with no substitutions. It must be planned and written daily.

Menus can be nonselective, selective, or a combination (for example, a choice of entrées could be offered, but other menu items would be fixed). A nonselective menu gives patients no choice in what is served. Although many foodservice directors believe that such a menu saves time, money, and waste, patient dissatisfaction can outweigh such perceived advantages. Even when nonselective menus are carefully planned, some patients may be dissatisfied because they are obliged to eat unwanted foods or leave them as plate waste. However, in many extended-care facilities, nonselective menus are used frequently because residents are incapable of making their own choices. In some long-term care and residential facilities that have dining room service, meals are served buffet style. Although there may be no choice of entrée, starch, and vegetable, a variety of salads, breads, desserts, and beverages may be offered.

A *selective menu* offers three obvious advantages: patients can choose what they want, the amount of plate waste can be lowered, and food costs can be reduced. These advantages are especially attractive when an expensive entrée is paired with an inexpensive one, thus allowing the lower-cost item to offset the more expensive one. When patients choose their own food, they are more likely to eat everything served. They may even choose fewer items than would have been served on a nonselective menu. For example, when bread and a starchy vegetable are offered, a patient may select only one of the items.

A selective menu requires that the foodservice department prepare several different menu items for each meal but in smaller quantities than would be needed for a nonselective menu. Therefore, even a facility with limited equipment and personnel can offer a diverse and interesting menu. Careful item pairing will balance workload, equipment use, and costs. Carefully planned selective menus also include options that can be used on modified diets. To help ensure that patients select a nutritionally adequate diet, menu items often are grouped in categories from which a specified number of selections can be made, or specific starches and vegetables may accompany each entrée. Using selective menus for patients on modified diets also can be an effective aid in teaching patients to manage their own diets. To realize the benefits of this type of menu, selective menus should be reviewed for unnecessary selections and variety.

The major disadvantage to a selective menu is patient disappointment as the food selected for today is usually served the next day. Patients selected the items today so they make the assumption that the food will be served today and when the trays arrive and their selection is not served they think they have received the wrong tray. Patient education is important when using selective menus. If a patient nutrition associate is not available to assist the patient in their selection it is suggested that a **bold** message be on the menu explaining that today's selection will be served tomorrow.

Cycle, Static, and Single-Use Menus

Menu planning in many institutions is streamlined by using a cycle menu, in which a set of carefully planned and tested menus is rotated for a specified number of days, weeks, or months. During a given cycle, no menu is repeated. Depending on the average length of stay, the cycle in an acute-care hospital may be 5, 7, 8, or 14 days. Longer cycles are followed in long-term care facilities and for employee cafeterias.

Cycle menus require careful planning and can be either selective or nonselective. When the system is first instituted, the first cycle can be regarded as a test period, after which adjustments are made to increase the attractiveness of meals, to avoid preparation or service difficulties, or to reduce costs. Cycle menus should also be adjusted with the changing seasons, marketplace conditions, and particularly with a change in customer base. As a rule, menus should be reviewed periodically and changed whenever suppliers introduce new and appealing food items or food formats. The cycles should be flexible enough to feature holiday foods or to adjust to other social activities, particularly in extended-care facilities. A balanced level of item popularity should be maintained throughout the cycle. In addition, the beginning and the end of the cycle should be different from one another so that the foods offered show variety. Repeating food items on the same day of every week should be avoided.

Once established, a cycle menu saves time and labor in menu planning, food procurement, and food production. Purchase orders should be filed with the menus to simplify future purchasing and production forecasts. When menus are used over a period of time the employees become more efficient and effective because they are accustomed to the menu. Some patients may enjoy the cycle menu because they know what to expect and may look forward to their favorite meal. The actual rates of selection for each item should be recorded so that accurate demand forecasts can be made each time the cycle is repeated. The cycle menu is also useful as a training device because it enables employees to become familiar with the production of each item and enhances organizational and time management skills.

Some health care foodservice operations offer a *static menu* (or set menu) to their customer groups. This menu resembles a restaurant menu in its variety and number of selections and remains the same from day to day, with the possible exception of one or more daily specials. A static menu can simplify purchasing, production, service, and management of the foodservice operation. However, the characteristics of each customer group, such as patient length of stay, should be analyzed closely to determine if this type of menu is appropriate for any of the operation's customer groups.

The third type of menu based on repetition is the *single-use menu*, which is planned for a specific meal on a specific day, possibly not to be used again in the identical form. The most likely use of this type of menu in a health care operation would be for catered events or as a monotony breaker in the employee cafeteria.

MENU-PLANNING PROCESS

A primary purpose of planning menus is to prepare and serve nutritious foods that meet the budget allocation as well as the needs of the target market. (See earlier for appointing a menu planning committee.) Many decisions must be made before the process can begin, including:

- Layout and design of menu
- Number of choices to be offered
- How many meals
- Type of menu
- Length of menu
- Flexibility for special occasions
- Frequency of revision

Menus need to be planned in advance to have them printed, purchase needed food and supplies, standardize new recipes, and determine if the skills needed are available. In health care, a nutritional analysis of each menu should be made in advance. If brand names are used, the available product must be the one that is advertised on the menu; that is, if one brand name for a beverage is given, another brand should not be used. How the food is prepared—such as baked, broiled, fried, and so forth—should be described where appropriate.

The menu planner should organize the procedure and schedule adequate time and resources for this activity. The committee should gather all reference materials needed for the task, including previous menus, inventory lists, standardized recipes, market reports, results of food preferences and acceptability studies, trade publications, other manuals, and the like. Usually these are available from professional foodservice and health care associations. A standard menu-planning form (which lists meal patterns, meals served, and days of the week in the period being planned) should be used.

New items on the menu will need to be evaluated for ability of staff and equipment, cash value, and customer satisfaction. Cash value and customer acceptance may include determining whether it is more feasible to purchase a ready-to-serve product even though it may be more costly, or use raw ingredients, which is more labor-intensive and the resulting labor expense reduces the advantage of the lower food cost.

Patient Menus

In a health care operation, the primary customer groups are patients/clients. When planning patient menus, the menu planner must weigh the planning considerations described earlier in this chapter, particularly the challenge of balancing patient needs (nutritional requirements) with patient desires (food preferences). To help meet this challenge, a systematic planning process that starts with normal diets should be followed.

Menu-Planning Steps

When planning a menu, first select the *meat* or *meat alternative entrées* for the main meals over the entire menu cycle. If the lunch or noon meal is the heavy meal fill in the entrée for the entire menu period and then choose the entrée for the dinner meal. Entrée choices are made first so that other foods served for each meal can complement and enhance the entrée. Given that entrée items are the costliest and because most of the food dollars go for main dishes, the frequency of their use must be controlled. It is helpful to make a list of possible meat and meat-alternative entrées to use in menu planning.

Once the entrées have been selected for both the noon and dinner meal, consider the entrée for the main meal first and then the entrées for the other meals; choose the accompanying *vegetables* and *potatoes, rice,* or *pasta* on the basis of their color, form, texture, and flavor. A colorful vegetable in whole, sliced, diced, or mashed form makes the meal more attractive. Crisp vegetables complement a soft or creamy main dish.

Next, select *salads* that contrast with the rest of the meal in color, flavor, and texture. For example, chilled salads complement hot entrées. Main-dish salads, chef salads, and cold plates that include salads also are popular entrées. Soup and sandwich or soup and salad may be planned as a total meal. The soup should be hearty cream-style soup and the sandwich or salad should be large and include some protein food item.

Vary the type of *bread* served from meal to meal. Include yeast breads, quick breads, sweet breads, specialty breads, popovers, biscuits, cornbread, bagels, and English muffins.

Select *desserts* that complete and balance the meal in flavor and texture and sometimes in caloric content. Fresh, canned, and frozen fruits are offered as alternatives to desserts in many health care institutions. Limit empty-calorie desserts. An edible garnish should be planned for each meal and incorporated into the master menu.

Offer the most popular *beverages*. Most institutions provide coffee, tea, and other hot beverages and milk in various forms. Many people prefer low-fat or skim milk to whole milk; chocolate milk may appeal to some patients.

When an *appetizer* is offered make sure it blends with the rest of the menu; for example, tomato juice and tomato soup on the same menu is poor planning. Appetizers may vary in amount, taste, and variety.

Plan the *garnish* for those items that would be enhanced by one, such as on desserts, main meal plates, and so on.

Plan breakfast menus last. Although breakfast menus are simple, they should provide interesting food variations from day to day. Plan a good source of vitamin C. Some menus offer grits and oatmeal each morning plus an assortment of cold cereal. Nontraditional items such as breakfast sandwiches, wraps, bagels, and biscuit

sandwiches are popular and add variety to the breakfast menu. There are many new and innovative breakfast items that need to be tested for acceptance. Always offer a good source of vitamin C in either juice or fruit. Trade journals can suggest creative ideas for breakfast menus that are simple yet nutritious, appetizing, and attractive.

The last menu that needs to be planned is called an *alternate menu* or *menu substitute*. There are times when a patient does not like or want what is on the main menu or has an allergy to a specific food.

A menu substitution list should be available to the floor hostess, who may suggest a substitute. A copy should be posted in the diet office to help nursing and foodservice meet the needs of a patient. However, some substitutions should be available at all times. When a substitute is made it must follow CMS standards that state "the substitute must equal in value in calories, protein and so forth as the meal/food that is being replaced."

A diet *spreadsheet* is helpful in menu planning. A spreadsheet displays the menu offerings and portion sizes for each diet, for each meal, and for each day of the cycle. The spreadsheet lists the regular diet and then each modified diet for three meals. The menus should be as simple as possible with no more restrictions than is medically required. When at all possible liberalize the diet, especially in long-term care operations. Make the menus "healthy" by following the Daily Guidelines for Americans 2010 discussed earlier in this chapter.

Some patients on regular diets may have needs that differ from the general patient population such as a disability or hearing or sight problems. This is particularly the case with children and older adults. For children hospitalized and separated from the familiarity of parents and homes, food takes on added significance. Meals should not only satisfy the nutritional requirements and appetites of hospitalized children but also be fun to eat. The use of special bags and containers for meals helps eliminate some of the fear of being in a hospital. In facilities where there is a large playroom, ambulatory children should be allowed to eat as a group in a relaxing, nonthreatening atmosphere. Familiar foods such as peanut butter and jelly sandwiches, grilled cheese sandwiches, and hot dogs should be offered. The idea is to have the children *eat*. Each family should be consulted about its child's food preferences and eating habits. Menu items should suit the child's age and developmental stage. Menus will need to be modified, which includes modifying (grinding or pureeing) the physical form of food if necessary. Raw fruits and vegetables that can be eaten as finger foods usually are much more popular than traditional salads. Finger food may also be necessary because the child or adult may lack the strength in their upper extremities or may lack coordination. Other ideas for finger foods include using strips of meat rather than whole pieces, cookies rather than cake, drinking cups for soup. Some children may need the assistance of an adult when using dips for dipping the finger foods. In the cases of swallowing problems a speech therapist should be consulted for recommendations for tube feeding or other methods of feeding to keep the nutrition level appropriate during therapy or recovery. Children age 2 to 5 years prefer simple foods over mixed dishes; gravies and cream sauces should be avoided in favor of colorful, attractive, and easy-to-handle foods. Midmorning and midafternoon snacks also are options and may be needed to meet the nutritional needs of the children.

Menus should be planned for various age groups, such as 2 to 5 years, 6 to 12 years, and 13 to 18 years. Many pediatric hospitals and institutions use specially designed menu forms with attractive colors and artwork. Nutrition education, particularly for children who may be on modified diets, can be incorporated in an appealing way. For example, menus can be designed to teach children about vegetables and fruits by using pictures and personifying each one with a name. Explanations of the body's nutritional needs could be included on the cover of the menu. Coloring books that teach the principles of good nutrition could be distributed at the time each child is admitted to the facility.

Menus for school-age children (including adolescents) need to be adjusted for their nutritional needs and their activity level. Food preferences of this age group, still distinctly different from those of adults, should be carefully considered. A sample pediatric menu for normal diets is shown in Figure 16.2.

The second group that may require special attention from the menu planner is older adults whose nutritional needs differ from those of younger adults only in the number of calories required. Older adults, because of their decreased physical activity levels and the slowing of their body processes, need fewer calories. Frequently, older persons need better nutrition from their meals than they have been receiving, particularly if they live alone or have a physical ailment that limits their food intake or digestion. Lack of motivation to prepare or consume meals on a regular basis may lead to overweight or underweight in this population.

Planning menus for older adults presents many challenges, particularly in long-term care facilities. For one thing, when older persons enter a long-term care facility, the change from a familiar to an unknown environment often produces marked psychological reactions, such as feelings of rejection, insecurity, and despondency. Often new residents express these feelings by complaining about the food, refusing to eat, or insisting on eating only common and familiar foods. For this reason, obtaining a complete profile of the patient's eating habits soon after admission is important. The resident's family and friends can provide additional information along these lines.

The procedures for planning meals for older adults are the same as those followed for planning menus for younger adults on a normal diet, but the quantity and form of foods can be varied to suit the special needs of this group. Note, however, that although the loss of teeth or poorly fitting dentures may make chewing more difficult for some, it should not be assumed that all older adults in this category need soft or finely ground foods. Offering a variety of food textures and colors in each appetizing meal stimulates interest and appetite. Never puree if ground is okay, and never grind if whole works well. When a selective menu format is feasible, individual preferences can be taken into consideration.

The following is important information that needs to be discussed with administration, nursing, and other health care providers. **Food Code 2009 3–201.11 Compliance with Food law (B). Food prepared in a private home may not be used or offered for human consumption in a food establishment.**

Menu Planning for Modified Diets

It has been recommended by the Academy of Nutrition and Dietetics in a position paper that a more liberal approach to diet modification has many advantages including patient's satisfaction and in most cases improves food intake and decreases the possibility of weight loss and malnutrition. A liberalized diet reduces the number of modified diets that need to be planned. Diets may be combined, especially where sodium and sugar are restricted.

After the regular diet menu has been planned, soft and liquid diets and other modified diets can be planned, with substitutions made only as necessary to conform to the prescribed diet as stated in the organization's dietary manual. One advantage of this approach is that it keeps the number of modified-diet foods at a minimum, thus eliminating the need to prepare many small batches of such foods and reducing labor costs.

An alternative to this type of menu for long-term pediatric patients, who may be mobile, would be to set up the playroom for meal service. In advance, provide the patients with a select menu that would offer high-quality food but akin to fast food. Serve the food in an attractive sack or box. Include crayons, small books, or other educational toys. This gives patients and families an opportunity to interact and reduces the stress of hospitalization.

Because variety is an important element of a satisfying and appealing foodservice, the menu planner should double-check at the end of the planning process to make sure that repetition has been kept to a minimum. Offering a variety of flavored seltzer waters, herbal teas, frozen yogurts, frozen-flavored ice sherbets, and ice cream can enhance even liquid diets. The menu repeat form in Figure 16.3 is a useful tool that helps control repetition. The form can identify individual items that appear on the menu too frequently. When this is disclosed, a similar food can be substituted to add variety to the planned menu. For example, mashed potatoes might be replaced with diced or au gratin potatoes. Or pudding, canned fruit, or ice cream might be offered in place of gelatin on certain menus.

Menu Planning for Special Services

Offering options in foodservice is one way to increase patient satisfaction and improve how the surrounding community views the hospital. Some patients are even willing to pay extra for special services. To satisfy these demands, many health care institutions have implemented gourmet meal programs and guest trays for family members.

A health care gourmet menu is much like a hotel room service menu in that menus are made available in patients' rooms, and patients or their visitors may call the foodservice department directly to request service. The order is taken and the price of service is verified over the telephone. After the department checks the patient's diet prescription to verify that the selection is allowable, the order is given to the appropriate production employee for preparation. A foodservice employee who collects cash or credit card payment for the service then delivers the food to the patient's room.

Gourmet meal programs may include wine with meals, an on-demand meal schedule, and tasty meals presented with flair.

FIGURE 16.2 Pediatric Menu for Normal Diets

BREAKFAST
Please circle your selections

Eye Openers
Orange juice, Apple juice, Cranberry juice, Tomato juice, Prune juice, Banana, Fresh fruit in season

Cereals
Buttered grits, Hot oatmeal, Cornflakes, Rice Krispies, Puffed Rice, Raisin Bran, All Bran, Frosted Flakes, Apple Jacks, Puffed Wheat

Breakfast Entrées
Scrambled egg, Poached egg (Or), Cheese omelet, French toast w/syrup, Whole wheat waffles/syrup, Pancakes w/syrup and fresh fruit, Country sausage patty, Crisp bacon, Grilled ham patty

Breads 'n' Spreads
Croissant roll, Breakfast roll, Hot biscuit, Fruit muffin, Bran muffin, Bagel w/cream cheese, Donut, Toasted English muffin, Margarine, Jelly, Honey

Beverages
Milk, Low-fat milk, Buttermilk, Chocolate milk, Hot chocolate

LUNCH
Please circle your selections

Savory Beginnings
Vegetable juice, Apple juice, Tossed green salad, Potato salad, Cranberry juice, Fruit cup, Tangy coleslaw, Strawberry-gelatin salad, Fruit flavored or plain yogurt, *Soup of the day*, Cottage cheese, Lettuce/tomato slice

Dressings:
French, Blue cheese, Thousand Island, Italian, Creamy, Ranch

Main Course Selections (choose one):

Hearty Hot Entrées
*Specialty of the house, Roast beef w/gravy, Fish sticks w/ketchup, Hamburger on bun, Vegetarian manicotti

Deli Delights
Ham on white bread, Breast of turkey sandwich platter, Peanut butter and jelly sandwich, Grilled cheese sandwich

Meal of a Salad
Chef's salad bowl, Tuna salad platter

*Comes with starch and vegetable. Choose salad and dessert.

Hot Vegetables of the Day
Whipped potatoes, Steamed rice, French-fried potatoes, Green beans, Whole baby carrots, Broccoli, Whole kernel corn

Breads 'n' Spreads
Hot roll, Cornbread (Mon.–Fri.), Margarine, Whole wheat bread, White bread, Jelly

Sweet Endings
Fruit pie, Lemon pie, Applesauce, Sliced peaches, Cherry gelatin w/whipped cream, Orange sherbet, Fresh fruit in season, Vanilla ice cream, Chocolate pudding, Oatmeal cookie, Baked custard (available Mon.–Fri.), Vanilla wafers

Beverages
Milk, Low-fat milk, Buttermilk, Chocolate milk, Hot chocolate, Iced tea, Lemonade

SUPPER
Please circle your selections

Savory Beginnings
Vegetable juice, Apple juice, Tossed green salad, Potato salad Lettuce/tomato slice, Cranberry juice, Fruit cup, Tangy coleslaw, Soup of the day, Cottage cheese, Fruit-flavored yogurt

Dressings:
French, Thousand Island, Blue cheese, Italian

Main Course Selections (choose one):

Hearty Hot Entrées
*Specialty of the house, Pizza, Baked ham, Spaghetti w/meat sauce, Hot dog on a bun w/trimmings, Peanut butter and jelly sandwich

*Comes with starch and vegetable. Choose salad and dessert.

Deli Delights
Ham on white bread, Pimento cheese on whole wheat, Chicken salad on whole wheat

Hot Vegetables of the Day
Whipped potatoes, Steamed rice, Macaroni and cheese, Green beans, Whole baby carrots, Broccoli, Whole kernel corn

Breads 'n' Spreads
Hot roll, Cornbread (Mon.–Fri.), Margarine, Whole wheat bread, White bread, Jelly

Sweet Endings
Fruit pie, Lemon pie, Brownie, Fresh fruit in season, Baked custard (available Mon.–Fri.), Sliced peaches, Orange gelatin w/whipping topping, Lime sherbet, Vanilla pudding, Small sugar cookies, Applesauce, Crackers, Potato chips, Honey, Strawberry ice cream, Vanilla ice cream, Oatmeal cookie, Chocolate chip cookie

Beverages
Milk, Low-fat milk, Buttermilk, Chocolate milk, Hot chocolate, Iced tea, Lemonade

Gourmet meal tickets usually are sold in the gift shop and are purchased by friends or family members for patients who are well enough to enjoy the meals. A typical gourmet menu is shown in Figure 16.4.

Because gourmet meal service can be costly to start up and maintain, before it is offered, the foodservice director and the institution's administrators must weigh realistically the investment expenses against potential benefits for the institution. Start-up and operating expenses may include the following features:

- Special linens and serving tables
- Fresh flowers for the table setting
- Wine service (possibly a wine steward) [may need approval of physician and administration—check concerning a liquor license]
- Design and printing of special menus
- Special food items (such as expensive meat cuts and fresh or out-of-season produce)
- Additional labor for food preparation and individualized service
- A special marketing program for the service

A word of caution: Despite the tight constraints of today's health care environment, some institutions have initiated gourmet meal service programs only to discover, unfortunately, that they are expensive and used little by their patient population, especially with the shortened lengths of stay and the greater acuity of patients. Preliminary market surveys that look closely at patient demographics (especially lifestyle and income levels) will indicate the level of interest in, and affordability of, gourmet meal service. In addition, an informal survey of other health care operations that offer the service would be informative.

Once gourmet meal service has been instituted, it must be adequately marketed to potential customers. Information about the program should be included in the patients' information directory or notices placed in patients' rooms and in the gift shop. When possible, advertisements in local newspapers and other media are helpful.

Other Types of Service Menus

There is a growing tendency to provide on-demand meals and room service. *Room service* in a health care institution is similar to hotel room service. Menus are available in the patients' rooms, and patient and visitor may call the foodservice department or go online to order a meal. The order is taken and the order is verified over the phone or online. A patient's diet order must be verified to determine if the selection is allowable; the order is then given to the appropriate production employee for preparation. The food is then delivered to the patient's room

Room service appears to be successful in meeting the new demands and new needs of patients. Because foodservice must be available 24 hours a day, seven days a week, this service results in providing patients what they want and when they want it.

There are many steps involved before implementing a room service program/menu. It takes time to do the research, surveying facilities that have implemented the service, writing a justification and discussion and approval from administration before the service can be implemented. Room service is an excellent idea; however, it may not be applicable for all facilities. The following questions will

FIGURE 16.3   Menu Repeat Form

Item Served	Monday			Tuesday			Wednesday		
	B	L	D	B	L	D	B	L	D
Scrambled eggs	X		X					X	
Mashed potatoes		X			X			X	
Gelatin			X		X			X	X

FIGURE 16.4   Sample Gourmet Dinner Menu

Please circle your selection.
Dinner

Relish tray seasonal vegetables	Chilled cranberry, V-8, and/or grape juice	
Dressing		
Soup du jour	or	Lightly creamed mushroom soup
Lamb chops with mint jelly	or	Grilled salmon, blueberry compote
Caesar salad	or	Sliced tomatoes, Mozzarella cheese, vinaigrette
Potatoes in butter sauce	or	Rice pilaf
Asparagus spears with hollandaise sauce	or	Steamed broccoli
Fresh-baked WW rolls with butter	or	Fresh-baked WW rolls and margarine
Tray assorted pastries	or	Tray of fruit with assorted cheeses
Coffee or Herbal tea	or	Seltzer water or iced or hot tea or coffee

Condiments: Horseradish, cream, sugar, lemon, salt/pepper, Mrs. Dash
Complimentary Beaujolais
A gourmet vegetarian meal may be requested

need to be explored and answered in the request and justification for the change in service. The foodservice director will need to evaluate and justify the effect of such a service on at least the following by asking:

- Will the cost of implementing the service for labor, menu style, and supplies increase?
- Will it reduce the cost per meal?
- Will it increase hours of service?
- Will the capital budget cover capital expenses for equipment or renovation?
- Will staff accept the change? What additional training is needed?
- Will physicians and nurses support the change?
- Will patient satisfaction increase from the current level?
- Will this change meet the needs or demands of patients?
- Will there be a reduction in error or duplicate trays?
- Will the service increase revenue?

(See Bibliography for more information on cost, procedures needed to be followed, and labor requirements; see entries by Norton and others concerning room service.)

Spoken Menu

In most health care facilities, less than 47 percent of selective menus are filled out by the patient or patient's family. In searching for improved service and reduced cost, many health care facilities have implemented the spoken menu. A spoken menu is similar to restaurants that tell customers what is on the menu. The menu or order is filled out for each patient by a food and nutrition service representative who verbally describes the menu to patients by 9 A.M. for lunch and 2 P.M. for dinner and the next day's breakfast.

The items from appetizer to dessert are recited, and the patient accepts the entire menu or is offered an alternative for foods they dislike. The food and nutrition representative would say to the patient, "Ms. Brown, for lunch today we have Choice 1 or Choice 2 available or a choice from each available menus." The foodservice representative then describes the menus, answering the patient's questions. Once completed, the representative should ask: What selections would you like? Patients can ask questions about the selection if they are unfamiliar with the selection described. The representative also describes the side dishes and the dessert of the day. The patient does not select the side dishes or desserts because they are part of the meal. The patient also chooses the beverage. If a patient hears a choice he or she does not like, the patient tells the representative, who offers a substitute for the entrée. The foodservice representative always carries the list of substitutes that are available for that day and the substitutions that are always available.

During lunch service, the process is repeated for dinner and next day's breakfast. The representative records the patient's selection by a number on a menu card, which the tray line personnel use when they assemble trays and the tray passers use to identify the patient to whom the tray should be delivered.

The use of a spoken menu provides both advantages and disadvantages. The following are the advantages for a department:

- The diet office can be deleted.
- The diet office duties can be reassigned to patient representatives.
- The organization is flattened.
- Patients receive immediate answers to questions about items on the menu.
- Printed menu cost is nearly eliminated.
- Tray line service has less difficulty in deciphering the menu.
- Fewer mistakes are made when preparing and serving patient trays.
- Foodservice personnel have more interaction with patients.
- Patient education can begin on the first visit as the patient representative explains the menu items and, as appropriate, their modification for medical nutrition therapy.
- Production requirements are reduced.
- Food cost is decreased.
- Quality is improved due to production start time.
- Patients are more satisfied.

The following are disadvantages of the spoken menu:

- The staff is unable to forecast the number of servings because production for most items does not begin until three to five hours before service.
- A well-developed training program must be in place and ongoing.
- Patient representatives must be motivated and knowledgeable concerning the products on the menu; if they are not, patient satisfaction may become a problem.

Preselected Menus

Because patient stays are getting shorter, the need for a multiweek selective menu cycle has become less important. Foodservice departments can now offer patients' favorites and prepare them better.

For a variety of reasons, more hospitals are using a preselected menu system. One of the major reasons for the change is financial. A preselected menu is given to a patient on admission to the hospital or is in the patient's room. One entrée is offered daily for a predetermined menu cycle period with a number of standard, well-accepted food items. A foodservice representative visits a patient after admission to elicit food dislikes and allergies and records the information in a computer. Using the computer, an individualized menu can be printed for each patient from the master menu preplanned by the menu committee. Lunch is ordered at breakfast time.

The use of the preselected menu has the following advantages:

- Eliminates menu printing, distribution, and collection.
- Reduces food cost by 10 to 20 percent over a selective menu—because of fewer leftovers.
- Reduces staff needed for production and tray line service (labor cost).
- Places focus on quality by doing a few things well.
- Screens for patients' special needs.
- Ensures that a patient receives a balanced diet.

Bedside Menus

The bedside menu-entry system is one where patients input requests into a handheld computer that the foodservice representative uses to input data or by use of the bedside phone. The computer contains the same-day menu for lunch and dinner, chef specials, and other items. The *bedside menu* eliminates the need for paper menus, which means savings to the department. However, each computer may cost as much as $1,000 and will contain more than 100 orders. This type of system is connected to the patient information system and is updated, allowing the department to know of any diet order changes within several hours. When using the bedside phone, the patients press a predetermined code on their phone to access menu ordering. A customized voice confirms name, room number, and diet order. After confirmation, the system provides meal options to the caller. The patient uses the digits on the keyboard to select menu items. This information is then forwarded to the foodservice department, where a meal ticket is printed. The menu data are given to the staff for production and service. The cost of the system for software and hardware programming and special application is expensive.

Foreign Language Menus

As part of The Joint Commission, health care providers have the responsibility to meet the needs of patients with cultural or religious differences and those with physical or mental disabilities. The foodservice department needs to have information available on a variety of food restrictions due to cultural or religious beliefs. There should also be information on where to acquire kosher foods and a list of persons who are multilingual and who could provide assistance to patients and staff. In areas where a large percentage of the population are non-English speaking or reading, menus should be provided in the prevalent non-English language. Personnel should be available to assist patients who are blind, deaf, handicapped, or illiterate.

Long-term facilities are offering new ways to provide foodservice to its residents. This includes buffets where residents may select the foods they want. Menus are liberalized, therefore there is no problem with modified diets unless a resident is on a modified diet. Restaurant service is also offered, where a waiter takes the resident's food order from a menu.

In health care facilities some patients will be unable to eat at the time meals are served. There are a number of reasons for this such as missed meals due to surgery, tests and/or other procedures, late admissions, and a "radical diet change" such as from clear liquid to regular. These residents are served a *late tray*.

Late tray service can be expensive and in some instances produce complaints. It is wise to have set menus for late trays as food left on a hot steam table for more than 30 minutes to an hour after the tray line has been completed has deteriorated in quality and may be unsafe to serve. The late tray menu will need to be attractive and the food well prepared. In most instances a cold meal would be the best choice.

When room service is implemented in a health care foodservice, "hold" and late trays become less of a problem and can lead to improved patient satisfaction.

Nonpatient Menus

In addition to patients, or the primary target market, most health care foodservice operations provide services to employees, staff, and visitors. As described earlier, the wants and needs of these groups, as identified by the marketing information system, should be considered during menu planning.

Employees, Staff, and Visitors

The menu planning committee should pay special attention to the facility's cafeteria menus that serve employees, staff, and visitors. A well-managed cafeteria can be a showcase for the high-quality food served as well as a profitable operation. When most of the cafeteria items come from the general patient menu, it is recommended that additional items be provided, especially if the menu offered to patients is nonselective. Even when selective menus are the basis of the general patient menu, a cafeteria menu that includes more variety can attract additional customers.

Cafeteria menus should keep customers coming back by offering a variety of foods. Theme or special-event days have been successful in attracting customers, but they usually can be scheduled for only one day each month. To help make customers happy, special health-promoting menus can be offered that include calorie and nutrition information and recipes for favorite items. Other techniques for increasing cafeteria revenues include offering special foods during slow periods, providing take-out services, and selling holiday desserts. Menus that offer a variety of cold and hot deli sandwiches, salads, main-dish salads, and salad plates also are popular and other fast-food options have been well accepted. Variety is needed to keep the operation's employees interested, particularly if the menu is on a relatively short cycle. One or more daily specials can be offered, and some of the items on the general patient menu can be combined for a single-price meal. Consideration should be given to the price mix of cafeteria menu items to ensure affordable alternatives to customers as well as a range of appeal.

Cycle menus can be used in cafeterias as well as for patient service. However, the cycle should be several weeks long when employees use the cafeteria for meals. The many advantages of cycle menus prevail, with the added advantage of balancing appeal and selling price considerations for the cafeteria.

In acute care hospitals and other short-term care facilities that have a relatively large number of visitors and outpatients, it may be advantageous to make food available in the cafeteria, in the coffee shop, and from vending machines for most of the day. When there is no coffee shop in the facility, several cold items (sandwiches, rolls, doughnuts, juices, ice-cream products, desserts, and beverages) easily can be provided in a designated area of the cafeteria. Providing microwave ovens that can be operated by customers or employees allows customers to reheat prepared foods during hours of limited cafeteria service.

Community Residents

Some health care foodservice operations have implemented services for outside customer groups such as community residents. Depending on the location of the operation and its foodservice facilities, workers from nearby medical clinics and businesses may be attracted by the facilities' realistic prices and quick service. Serving Sunday brunches, providing delivery service for office parties, and giving weekend and evening discounts to senior citizens are other ways to market the department's services.

Some directors are increasing department revenues by adding off-premises catering services to their business mix. However, this may require nonprofit hospitals to establish a for-profit catering venture. Because of the implications for the hospital's tax status and the effect on the operation's public image, hospital administration must decide whether to compete with the commercial foodservice sector by providing non-hospital-related catering services. If off-premises catering is implemented, the foodservice director may want to expand in-house menus to appeal to a wider variety of catering customers and to develop a reputation for full service.

MENU FORMAT

Because the menu is an important marketing tool, its format must be designed to ensure effective communication. Therefore, the menu planner writes the final menus out in two different formats, one for purchasing, production, and service personnel and the other for patients and other customer groups. The menu used in the kitchen usually provides the names and numbers of the recipes to be followed and the production forecast. Information on portion sizes, special comments about the recipes, and advance preparation requirements can be added. The name of each menu item should be specific. For example, the kind of fruit juice, the flavor of gelatin, the type of bread item, and so forth should be stated if not already specified in the recipe. This information ensures that the intended balance of flavors, colors, and textures will be produced.

Patient Menus

Selective menus distributed to patients should be informative, accurate, attractive, and easy to understand. Terms used should be clear, simple, and comprehensible to readers who may be seriously ill or sedated or who may not be fluent in English. Nutrition education information, which can also be included with patient menus, might include general dietary guidelines distributed with all regular menus. Informative notes on modified-diet menus could include explanations of the special dietary needs of patients with diabetes and those with high cholesterol levels. Menus also could contain entertainment features such as crossword puzzles, nutrition trivia questions, or coloring pages for children. Specially designed forms can be used to make menus more appealing. Forms should be consistent in format and give clear directions for marking choices. An example of a restaurant-style menu used in a hospital is reproduced in Figure 16.5.

Nonpatient Menus

If foodservice is provided to nonpatient customers, appropriate menu formats must be developed to provide adequate communica-

tion between the operation and these customers. An appropriate format for the cafeteria would be a menu board. Lettering used on a menu board should be legible and large enough for ease of viewing by customers with differing visual acuity. The board also should be designed to allow changes to be made easily.

In more upscale operations where table service is provided, a printed menu should be developed. Design features include the menu cover, visual format and layout, copy (text), and graphics (pictures). Menu production features deal with typeface style, paper, ink color, and color of graphics. Menu design should reflect current cultural trends, which may mean that customers favor designs that are simple and light (not too crowded or "busy"). In-house desktop publishing can produce menus appropriate for many occasions. However, because of its importance as a marketing tool and the cost of producing this type of menu, the foodservice director might consider contracting for the services of a menu design consultant.

PRICING STRATEGIES

Pricing the services provided by a foodservice operation is an extremely important task. The process starts with the cost of producing individual menu items and eventually affects whether the operation achieves its profitability objectives while maintaining quality and cost-effectiveness of service.

Pricing Considerations

To determine what to charge for specific menu items, a number of factors must be considered. Key among these are:

- Customer mix, as described by the marketing information system
- Product mix, including the type of menu item, the style of service, and the meal occasion or time of dining
- Psychological effects of pricing such as perceived value, price spread between items, and "odd-cents" pricing
- Past prices that customers may have paid for the same menu items
- Competitors and their prices for similar products
- Profit objective as specified in the department marketing plan

Pricing Methods

Approaches to menu pricing vary, and no one method predominates. Accurate records are needed, such as items' sales records, standardized recipes, standardized portions, and cost history. There are seven quantitative methods, six of which follow:

1. The factor system, also called mark-up system
2. The prime cost factor
3. The actual pricing method, or all costs plus profit
4. The overhead-contribution system
5. The gross profit system
6. The base price method

FIGURE 16.5 Restaurant-Style Health Care Menu for Normal Diets

BREAKFAST
Please circle your selections

Eye Openers

Orange juice	Tomato juice	V-8 juice
Apple juice	Prune juice	
Cranberry juice	Banana	
	Fresh fruit in season	

Cereals

Buttered grits	Shredded Wheat
Hot oatmeal	Puffed Rice
Cornflakes	Raisin Bran
Rice Krispies	All Bran

Breakfast Entrées

Scrambled egg	French toast w/syrup	Egg/bacon tomato wrap
Poached egg (Or)	Pancakes w/syrup	Whole wheat waffles
Cheese omelets		
Country sausage patty		
Crisp bacon		
Grilled ham patty		

Breads 'n Spreads

Croissant roll	Fruit muffin	
Breakfast roll	Bran muffin	
Hot biscuit	Bagel w/cream cheese	
Donut	Toasted English muffin	
Margarine	Honey	Fruit toppings
Jelly		
	Syrup	

LUNCH
Please circle your selections

Savory Beginnings

Vegetable juice	Cranberry juice	Soup of the day
Apple juice	Fruit cup	Cottage cheese
Tossed green salad	Tangy coleslaw	
Fruit-flavored yogurt		
Potato salad	Lime gelatin with cottage, pecan and pear salad	
	Lettuce/tomato/onion slice	

Dressings:

French	Blue cheese	Thousand Island
		Italian
		Vinegar/olive oil

Main Course Selections (choose one):

Hearty Hot Entrées

*Specialty of the house	Mushroom burger w/Swiss cheese
Roast beef w/gravy	Vegetarian manicotti
Baked fish w/lemon	

*Comes with starch and vegetable. Choose salad and dessert.

Deli Delights

Ham on rye sandwich	Meal of a salad
Breast of turkey sandwich platter	Chef's salad bowl
Grilled cheese sandwich	Tuna salad platter
	Cottage cheese and fresh fruit

Hot Vegetables of the Day

Whipped potatoes	Green beans	Broccoli
Steamed rice	Whole baby carrots	Whole kernel corn

SUPPER
Please circle your selections

Savory Beginnings

Vegetable juice	Cranberry juice	Soup of the day
Apple juice	Fruit cup	Cottage cheese
Tossed green salad	Tangy coleslaw	Fruit-flavored yogurt
Potato salad	Strawberry gelatin with pineapple and strawberries salad	

Dressings:

French	Blue cheese	Thousand Island
		Italian
Vinegar/olive oil		

Main Course Selections (choose one):

Hearty Hot Entrées

*Specialty of the house	Spaghetti w/meat sauce
Roast beef w/gravy	Hot dog on a bun w/trimmings
Baked ham	

*Comes with starch and vegetable. Choose salad and dessert.

Deli Delights

Ham on rye sandwich
Pimento cheese on whole wheat
Chicken salad sandwich on whole wheat

Hot Vegetables of the Day

Whipped potatoes	Green beans	Broccoli
Steamed rice	Whole baby carrots	Whole kernel corn
Macaroni and cheese		

FIGURE 16.5 (Continued)

Beverages

Coffee	Milk
Caffeine-free coffee	Low-fat milk
Hot tea	Buttermilk
Herb tea	Chocolate milk
Hot chocolate	
Lemon	
Nondairy creamer	
Artificial sweetener	

Breads 'n' Spreads

Hot roll	Whole wheat bread	Melba toast	
Cornbread (Mon.–Fri.)	White bread	Crackers	
Margarine	Jelly	Potato chips	Honey

Sweet Endings

Cherry pie	Sliced peaches	Vanilla ice cream
Lemon pie	Strawberry gelatin w/whipped topping	Chocolate ice cream
Cheesecake		Orange sherbet
Brownie	Coconut cake with lemon filling	
Chocolate pudding		
Fresh fruit in season	Baked custard (Mon.–Fri.)	

Beverages

Coffee	Milk	Lemonade	
Caffeine-free coffee	Low-fat milk	Nondairy creamer	
Hot tea	Buttermilk	Artificial sweetener	Sliced lemons
Herb tea	Chocolate milk		
Iced tea	Hot chocolate		

Breads 'n' Spreads

Hot roll	Whole wheat bread	Melba toast	
Cornbread (Mon.–Fri.)	White bread	Crackers	
Margarine	Jelly	Potato chips	Honey

Sweet Endings

Fruit pie	Sliced peaches	Vanilla ice cream / Fresh fruit in season
Lemon pie	Black cherries, pecans, and Bing cherries in gelatin w/whipped topping	Chocolate ice cream
Cheesecake		Sherbet
Chocolate cake double dark chocolate frosting	Vanilla pudding	
Fresh fruit in season		
Oatmeal raisin cookie	Baked custard (Mon.–Fri.)	

Beverages

Coffee	Milk	Lemonade
Caffeine-free coffee	Low-fat milk	Nondairy creamer
Hot tea	Buttermilk	Artificial sweetener
Herb tea	Chocolate milk	
Iced tea	Hot chocolate	

Each method has its advantages and disadvantages. Generally, methods that account for more variables, such as different categories of costs, also require more precise information.

The remaining or seventh method focuses on the costs to produce specific menu items. Many operations mark up a product by a standard percentage over food cost such as 30 to 65 percent with 40 percent being the standard. In the *factor method*, the targeted food cost percentage of the operation is divided into 100 to determine a factor; thus, for a food cost percentage of 35 percent, the factor would be 2.86 (rounded). The menu price is then determined by multiplying the raw food cost by the factor

$$\text{Raw food cost} \times \text{Factor} = \text{Menu price}$$

In this example, if the raw food cost for a menu item is $1.03, the menu price would be calculated based on the following formula:

$$\$1.03 \times 2.86 = \$2.95$$

The remaining cost-based methods work in a similar manner but take into consideration other areas of costs such as labor, variable costs, fixed costs, and profit. Although this is an advantage over the factor method, extensive cost records must be maintained, and computer-generated data may be necessary to support these systems.

The *prime cost factor* considers raw food and direct labor costs. The direct labor cost is the only cost that involves production; it does not include other costs, profits, or any other perceived valued. The *actual pricing method* includes all costs plus a required profit to determine selling price. Included are raw food cost, labor cost, variable cost, fixed cost, and profit. The *overhead-contribution* system is a modification of the actual pricing method. The menu price would be the actual cost of food, actual labor cost, other variable costs, and fixed cost and profit. The advantage of this method is that it contains all costs and the direct profit in the selling price of the menu item. The *gross profit method* is designed to determine a specific amount of money that should be made from each customer—that is, every customer should pay a specific amount to cover nonfood costs and profit. For example, taking the menu price of an item, the item cost is subtracted, and the difference is the gross profit. With the *base pricing method*, menu items are priced at a certain level to satisfy the market and then worked backward to determine the amount to spend on raw ingredients. Computers are now being used to determine this cost. This pricing method is rarely used in health care institutions.

Other Pricing Considerations

Other pricing considerations need to be evaluated. An item sold for $1 sounds more expensive than one sold for 99¢. Therefore, *odd-cents pricing* appears to be a bargain. Odd pricing includes prices that end in odd numbers, usually 5s and 9s; prices that end in a number other than a zero; and prices below a zero. In expensive, fine-dining restaurants, pricing is usually stated in whole numbers, such as $22.

In many cafeterias, delicatessens, and salad-and-sandwich operations, food items may be priced by the ounce. The price must cover raw food, labor, and profit. By the ounce is frequently self-service, and the customers decide what and how much to place in a container. The customer proceeds to the cashier, who weighs the product and tells the customer the cost (cash registers are programmed to determine price). Or in a deli, a sandwich may have 2, 3, 4, or more ounces of meat or cheese and is priced to the ounces requested.

Another method is "what the traffic will bear." This means that you need to know what the competition in your local area is selling the same type of items for. For example, a coffee house may sell a "plain" cup of coffee for $1.50 and you are selling the same coffee for a $1.25, you would be okay. However, if a deli is selling sub sandwiches for $4.49 and you are selling them for $5.75, you may want to make a change.

Pricing must be set on the profit projection goals of the department and the approval of administration. Some organizations offer a reduced price for food as a fringe benefit and not as a profit.

MENU EVALUATION

Because of its effect on the foodservice operation's success, an effective menu evaluation system must be established to provide mechanisms to measure menu performance before implementation, with a focus on specific menu features. After implementation, menu performance must be evaluated for customer acceptability and contribution to the financial status of the department. These processes are described next.

Menu Features

Once the menu-planning process is finished, the proposed menus should be evaluated by dietitians to see whether all nutritional objectives have been attained, by foodservice department managers to determine whether the department's resources have been used effectively, by the production supervisor to determine equipment use and skills of personnel, and by customer focus groups to disclose whether the menus will be appealing to customers. The following list, which describes the characteristics of a good menu, can easily be used as an evaluation checklist:

- *Menu pattern:* Each meal is consistent with the established menu pattern (that is, room service, spoken menu, and so forth) and includes all food components and portion sizes specified as necessary to meet the customers' nutrition requirements and, at the same time, minimize plate waste.
- *Color and eye appeal:* The color combinations in each meal are pleasant and blend well, and a variety of colors are used in each meal. Attractive garnishes are included when appropriate.
- *Texture and consistency:* A mix of soft, creamy, crisp, chewy, and firm foods is included in each meal.
- *Flavor combinations:* Food flavors are compatible yet varied. Having two or more strong-flavored foods (such as broccoli, onions, turnips, cabbage, and cauliflower) in the same meal has been avoided. Combinations of foods with similar flavors (such as tomato juice with macaroni–tomato casserole and macaroni and cheese with pineapple–cheese salad) also are avoided.

- *Sizes and shapes:* Meals include a pleasing variety of food sizes and shapes. Having several chopped or mixed items in the same meal (such as cubed meat, diced potatoes, mixed vegetables, and fruit cocktail) has been avoided.
- *Food temperatures:* A balance between hot and cold items is offered for each meal. The climate or season of the year (or both) also is a consideration in selecting food temperatures. For example, cold vegetable soups are appropriate in summer, whereas hot bean soups are more suited to cold weather.
- *Preparation methods:* Offering more than one food prepared in a particular manner in a meal has been avoided. A balanced distribution of creamed, boiled, fried, baked, and braised foods is offered each day.
- *Popularity:* Popular and less-popular foods are part of the same meal when a selection is offered. Serving all popular foods at one meal and all less-popular foods at another has been avoided.
- *Day-to-day distribution:* The types of food offered for consecutive meals and on consecutive days are varied in ingredients and in preparation method. For example, the menus avoid offering meat loaf at lunch and another ground beef entrée for dinner or supper. Variations in the foods offered the same day each week are planned. Serving hot dogs every Monday and chicken every Sunday, for example, has been avoided.
- *Customer preferences:* The menus are appropriate for the cultural, ethnic, and personal food preferences of the operation's customers. The menu planner's own food prejudices are not taken into consideration.
- *Availability and cost of food:* Seasonal foods are used frequently. High- and low-cost foods are balanced within each day's menus and throughout the menu cycle so that budget constraints and customer pricing demands are met.
- *Facilities and equipment:* The equipment available is adequate to produce high-quality menu items. Equipment use is balanced throughout the day and the menu cycle. Menu items are compatible with the capacities of transport and service equipment. Enough serving dishes of appropriate sizes and types are available for the attractive presentation of menu items.
- *Personnel and time:* The department's staff—that is, the number of workers and their skill levels—is adequate for the preparation and service of items on the menu. The department's workload is balanced from day to day and week to week. Adequate time is available for producing and serving the foods on the menu.
- *Menu form and presentation:* Descriptions of the menu items are specific, appealing, and accurate. The menu follows a consistent and accepted sequence of consumption. (This information is a type of continuous quality improvement. It needs to be recorded and kept on file; see Chapter 4.)

After correcting any problems noted during the pre-implementation evaluation, the menu planner should recheck the menus one final time. This procedure should be followed every time menus are planned, but less time is required when cycle menus are used. Whenever a menu is actually produced, any problems encountered should be noted on the master menu form and the appropriate changes made before repeating the menu in another cycle. Records should be maintained concerning the problem and how it was solved. These records then are used when the next cycle of menus is planned.

Menu Performance

Regardless of how perfect a menu may appear to be, all menu planners must face the periodic elimination and replacement of menu items. Therefore, methods to evaluate menu effectiveness must be employed, ranging from simply counting the number of items selected or sold to computerized monitoring of consumption practices. Both customer acceptability and menu engineering (using popularity and profitability of menu items as bases for making changes) are key evaluation measures.

Acceptability by Customers

Surveys help determine customer acceptance of various menu items. The form in Exhibit 16.1 asks for customer comments on specific new menu items. Exhibit 16.2 shows a multipurpose survey that asks for suggestions and comments from cafeteria customers on various services and food items. Keeping precise sales histories on menu items helps in forecasting demand and in eliminating unpopular items from the menu. Observing plate waste is another good way to assess the customer acceptance of various menu items. The management of the foodservice department must establish minimum standards of acceptability based on customer input. If the acceptability of a menu item falls below the standard, a change must be considered (another continuous quality improvement method).

Menu Engineering

Menu engineering is a method used to evaluate the effectiveness of an operation's current menu while providing the basis for future menu-planning decisions. Various theories of menu engineering have been proposed. One method categorizes menu items based on both profitability and popularity. One of the more popular methods uses three categories based on the contribution and volume of each menu item. The category in which a menu item is placed determines whether the item will be retained (on the current and future menus), repositioned (perhaps as a side dish), or eliminated (from all present and future menus). These techniques can be time-consuming without the assistance of a computer software program.

EXHIBIT 16.1   Customer Survey Form for a New Menu Item (A continuous quality improvement form)

We need your assistance in helping us to meet our goal of serving you high-quality food that tastes good. Please share your comments with us about this new menu item by filling out this questionnaire and dropping it in the suggestion box located in the cafeteria.

1.   Menu item (Name) _____

2.   Menu item served at proper temperature?   Yes   No

3.   Menu item cooked properly?   Yes   No

4.   Did the item have eye appeal?   Yes   No

5.   Did you like the taste of new menu item?

    Enjoyed _____

    Acceptable _____

    Disliked _____

6.   Did size and shape enhance product?   Yes   No

7.   Is there anything you can recommend to improve this menu item? _____

Source: Developed by Ruby P. Puckett©.

COMPUTER APPLICATIONS

Computer-assisted procedures are used for menu planning in some facilities. To take advantage of the computer's speed, accuracy, and capacity, menu-planning information must be expressed in quantitative terms. Programs can be designed to plan menus that consider labor and raw food costs, nutrient content, color, consistency, frequency, and other factors. However, two variables—nutrient content and raw food cost—are the most widely used in current computer-assisted menu-planning programs.

The greatest obstacle to computer-assisted menu planning has been the absence of sufficient data about each variable. Unless the foodservice department uses standardized recipes for every item produced, there is little point in planning menus that accurately fulfill nutrient requirements and meet cost limitations. The ingredients used in each recipe must be issued through a controlled procedure, and production workers must follow recipes exactly.

Food composition data must be available for each food item. However, values for some items on the market either are not available or differ from those stated in government handbooks. Nutrient data for many products must be obtained from their manufacturers. In some cases, the foodservice director must develop the data.

The menu planner must specify such variables as the frequency with which menu items may be served and the food combinations allowed on one menu. This process involves coding for ingredients, color, flavor, shape, and other factors in such a way that the computer can identify these considerations and deal with them. Menu cost is a combination of raw food cost and labor cost. Yet, because accurate production time data are not available for most food items and are difficult to obtain, precise planning for labor costs may be impossible. Flexibility in adjusting to the special needs of customers or incorporating new items is severely limited as well. These are a few of the problems involved in computer-assisted menu planning that have led many operations to continue using manual procedures. Applications in which the computer is used to support the menu-planning process, such as with menu engineering, have been more successful.

EXHIBIT 16.2 Survey of Suggestions and Comments from Customers (another continuous quality improvement form)

Several changes are occurring within the Department of Food and Nutrition Services to better meet the needs of our customers. We have changed our menu, and we are providing additional services such as Healthful Food for Life. These changes are for you! Therefore, we want your ideas and opinions on how the new menu and additional services can best meet your needs. Please share your comments and suggestions with us so that we can meet our primary goal—pleasing you!

1. Age _____   Sex _____

    Years employed at hospital _____

2. Have you read any of the "Good News" handouts?

    Yes _____   No _____

    If so, did you find them interesting and informative?

    Yes _____   No _____

    Would you like us to provide them on a regular basis?

    Yes _____   No _____

3. Have you tried the Healthful Foods for Life menu?

    Yes _____   No _____

4. Did you find the Healthful Foods for Life menu worthwhile?

    Yes _____   No _____

5. Which one of the following types of foods do you prefer?

    Mexican _____   Seafood _____

    Italian _____   Vegetarian _____

    Southern _____   Other _____

6. Do you find that the new menu meets your food preferences?

    Yes _____   No _____

7. Please share any additional comments or recommendations.

    _____

    _____

    _____

8. If you would like to be interviewed, please leave your name and phone number during the day. We will contact you to arrange an appointment.

    Name _____   Telephone _____

Note: It is difficult to determine a percentage of answers (such as Excellent, Good, and so forth) with this survey. The Likert Scale of analysis would not work with it.
Source: Developed by Ruby P. Puckett©.

SUMMARY

In many respects, the successful operation of a foodservice department depends on the effectiveness and appropriateness of the department's menus, which can affect perceptions of the facility's overall quality of care. In today's competitive environment, the revenue brought in by various foodservice department ventures can make a valuable contribution to the hospital's profits—or losses. Menu planning involves designing meals that meet the nutritional needs of a variety of customer groups, both patient and nonpatient. At the same time, menus must fulfill the customers' appetite for good-tasting and attractive food.

À la carte menu

Actual pricing method

Base pricing method

Bedside menu

Demographics

Dietary Reference Intake

Du jour menu

Factor method

Gourmet meal

Gross profit method

Meal plan

Menu pattern

My Plate

Odd-cents pricing

Pricing strategies

Room service

Sociocultural influences

Static menu

Table d'hôte menu

DISCUSSION QUESTIONS

1. What are the various types of menus and when is the most appropriate time to use them?

2. How can you incorporate My Plate in planning menus for all ages?

3. How would you plan a "liberalized" regular selective menu and modify it for the most difficult medical nutrition therapy requirements?

4. What questions would you ask on a customer satisfaction survey?

5. Using an existing health care menu, evaluate it for the aesthetic factors outlined in this chapter.

6. What method would you use for pricing menu items for an employee cafeteria? Why did you choose this method?

CHAPTER 17

PRODUCT SELECTION

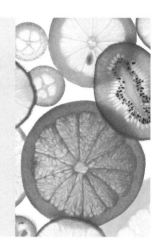

LEARNING OBJECTIVES

- Describe the systems model and how it applies to food selection.
- Identify various grades of veal, pork, eggs, seafood, fruits, vegetables, and dairy products.
- Inspect foods to ensure they meet quality and wholesome food.
- Write accurate measurable specifications for all food, small equipment, and utensils.
- Discuss the advantages and disadvantages of genetically modified, irradiated, cloned, and organically grown food.
- Define: various classifications of vegetables, botanical types of fruits, teas, dairy products, pastas.
- Describe the intended use of food products.
- Use cost-effectiveness in selection of food and small equipment.
- Investigate methods to become a sustainable foodservice operation.
- Follow all rules, regulations, and laws that relate to food selection.

PRODUCT SELECTION (food, preparation equipment, and service ware) is a critical factor in meeting customer expectations, adhering to nutrition guidelines, and containing expenses for a health care foodservice operation. The purchasing agent for the department must be knowledgeable about food and ingredients, menu patterns, production and service systems and the move to a more sustainable system before he or she can select food supplies with any degree of accuracy and cost-effectiveness.

In this chapter, basic information is presented on all the food groups—meats and seafood, eggs and egg products, milk and other dairy products, fruits and vegetables, grains and cereals, and beverages. Specifically, topics on meat inspection, meat grades, meat specifications, and processed meats are presented. The same is done for most of the other food groups so that a purchaser can make informed and economical choices that will complement rather than hamper operation controls. The latest technology for protecting the food supply is also described. Sustainability is briefly mentioned here as well in previous chapters and in future chapters.

Food substitutes and equivalents are addressed, as are national and local regulations regarding interstate and intrastate purchasing decisions. Food nutrients, federal standards of quality, and methods of food processing also are described. For example, the fat content of dairy products, moisture content of dehydrated foods, and hydrogenation features of various oils are examined. This is a long chapter. You are not expected to know and keep all this information in your head. The most important information will be designated by this symbol:$^{\Delta}$.

In the system model, the first process in the transformation system is procurement (Figure 17.1). There must be constant feedback at all steps of the system and subsystems. *Procurement*, the first subsystem, is defined as securing needed food, supplies, and equipment for the production subsystem, the second subsystem in the transformation system. Procurement also includes following all laws, regulations, and ethical considerations; maintaining the established budget; keeping records; and securing products to assist in meeting the customers' needs and wants (outputs).$^{\Delta}$ The procurement subsystem has numerous activities or processes that must be carried out, as shown in Figure 17.2. Each of these activities has laws, regulations, contracts, policies, and procedures that must be followed. Constant feedback needs to be made to the foodservice

FIGURE 17.1 Procurement System Flowchart

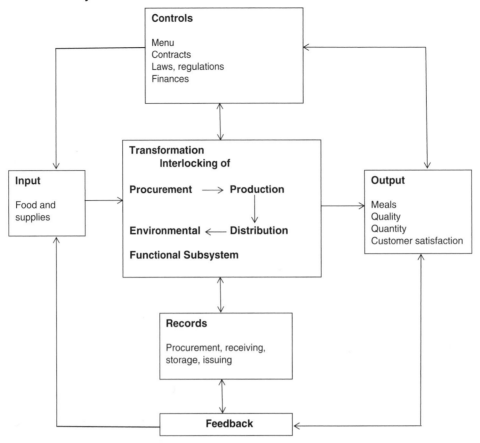

Source: Ruby P. Puckett© revised 2010.

FIGURE 17.2 Procurement Subsystem Flowchart System

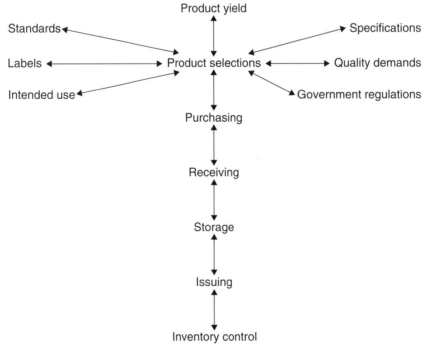

Source: Ruby P. Puckett© revised 2010.

director to ensure that needed supplies have been acquired ethically and are accounted for by an audit trail.

As noted in Figure 17.2 the system has many interlocking processes. The transformation subsystem cannot be completed without procurement (securing food), production (changing food into edible process, Figure 17.1). Once these two transformations are completed the finished product is distributed to the customer.

To produce food the environment must be kept clean; employees must follow the hygiene process, equipment is cleaned, and waste is appropriately handled.

PRODUCT STANDARDS

Once the menu has been planned, the product is selected for the specific cycle of the menu. Quality food and supplies need to be specified for the intended use of the product. Food standards are then developed that describe characteristics for a specific product and provide a quality reference such as the grade of the product. The U.S. Department of Agriculture (USDA) sets quality standards for meat, poultry, eggs, dairy products, fruits, vegetables, and nuts. The U.S. Department of Commerce (USDC) sets quality standards for fish and seafood.

The U.S. Food and Drug Administration (FDA) determines and enforces standards of identity, quality, and fill. *Standards of identity* define what a food product must contain to be called a certain name—for example, the grade of meat. *Standards of quality* describe the ingredients that go into a product and apply mainly to fruits and vegetables. The standards limit defines the number and kinds of defects permitted. The standards establish minimum quality requirements. A good example is fruit cocktail. *Standards of fill* regulate the quantity of food in a container. They tell a packer how the container must be filled to avoid deceiving consumers. All these standards are mandatory for foods in interstate commerce and may be voluntary for others.

The FDA is responsible for enforcing federal labeling requirements. A food is considered misbranded if the label does not include adequate or mandatory information or provides misleading information. The Fair Packaging and Labeling Act ensures that the consumer can obtain accurate information on quantity and content from a food label. Nutritional information is mandatory on labels only for foods for which a nutritional claim is made or that have added vitamins, minerals, or protein.

The Farm Security and Rural Investment Act of 2002 requires that all beef, lamb, pork, fish, fruits, and vegetables include a country of origin on each package and places the task of creating the regulations for those stickers on the USDA.

The country-of-origin labeling has the power of choice as a benefit. The information given to the consumer must be accurate, and food retailers and wholesalers are responsible for every mislabeled item, even if the supplier is at fault[△] (all of the above).

Legislation

Legislation related to the foodservice industry makes it the most controlled industry in the United States. The USDA, the FDA, the Public Health Service, and the USDC are government agencies that establish laws that must be followed. Each agency has its own responsibility for ensuring the safety of the food supply. In addition to the federal government controls, there are state and local regulation, plus survey standards from various organizations that must be met.

Technological events have led the FDA to establish standards for *food irradiation* and *genetically engineered* (modified) foods. Irradiation of foods has been approved since 1960 but has gained new acceptance in recent years. According to the CDC, food irradiation is a "new" technology that can eliminate disease-causing germs, does not cause food to become radioactive, does not cause dangerous substances to appear in the foods, and does not change the nutritional value of the food. The CDC has stated that food irradiation holds great potential for preventing many food-borne diseases that are transferred through meat, poultry, fresh produce, and other foods. Irradiation is considered a food additive and is regulated by the FDA. Irradiation is the exposure of a substance to gamma rays. The amount of radiation absorbed by a food is measured in units called **kilorays**. Irradiation is used to inhibit the sprouting of tubers in potatoes; delay the ripening of some fruits and vegetables; control insects in fruits and stored grains; and reduce parasites in foods of animal origin as well as fresh and frozen red meats, including beef, lamb, and pork, to control disease-causing microorganisms.[△]

All foods that have been irradiated must be labeled with the international symbol (Figure 17.3) and contain the words "treated by irradiation."

Genetically Modified Foods

The FDA regulates *genetically modified foods* (GM) for safety. Genetically modified foods are crop plants used for food by humans and animals that have been modified by a molecular biological process known as recombinant DNA technology. Recombinant DNA technology produces a new combination of genes by splicing in new genes or suppressing or eliminating existing genes. Through this process, the genetic makeup of a food can be modified. These plants have been modified in the laboratory to enhance desired traits such as increased resistance to herbicides, improved nutritional content, reduced spoilage, and improved flavor.

There are two types of GM foods that are that modified and will not be discussed here. A *genetically engineered* (GE) organism is one that is modified using techniques that permit the direct transfer or removal of genes in that organism.[△]

It is estimated that 60 to 70 percent of food products in retail stores already contain genetically modified ingredients. More than 40 genetically modified products have been approved from fields to store. Some of these products are tomatoes, soybeans, corn, potatoes, cotton, rice, papaya, squash, sugar beet, cantaloupe, canola (rapeseed oil), and flax. Soybeans and corn are the largest crops that have been genetically modified. Recently the FDA approved the GM of salmon, the first fish product to be GM.

The health concern is the potential for GM foods to cause allergies. Specific proteins in milk, eggs, wheat fish, tree nuts, peanuts, soybeans, and shellfish cause 90 percent of all food allergies. If a protein from one of these food types were to be incorporated into a food that normally would not have this protein, people who are

FIGURE 17.3 International Irradiation Logo

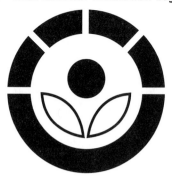

allergic to these proteins could unknowingly consume such a food and suffer an allergic reaction. The FDA has put measures into place to prevent this from happening by requiring producers of a GM food product present an evidence base that they have not incorporated any allergenic substances into their product. When this evidence cannot be produced, the FDA requires a label to be put on the product to alert consumers.

Cloned food is the exact genetic copy of another. There are a number of types of cloning. The sheep Dolly, the first mammal to be cloned, was created by reproduction cloning. There are strict rules/guidelines on cloning, especially of humans. Cloning is used in hundreds of species, including goats, sheep, cows, mice, pigs, cats, dogs, and rabbits. In 2010 the FDA approved the cloning of salmon.

Currently the FDA has policy guidelines about food product labeling. These guidelines apply to food and food ingredients, including products developed through biotechnology. New foods that contain a new substance or an allergen that is new to that food or that exhibit a different level of certain dietary nutrients or increased toxins are required to be tested before being marketed. If a product is one of the categories approved by the FDA, that food would be labeled with information about the food's content and characteristics. However, if a peach is a peach—whether produced through conventional breeding techniques or through biotechnology—no special label is required. At present, the FDA does not require genetically modified foods to be labeled; however, it has developed a guiding document for companies that wish to declare genetically enhanced ingredients in their food. A number of alternative proposals are being considered concerning the labeling of foods obtained through biotechnology.[△]

Organic Standards

The USDA has also developed nutritional "organic standards" for agricultural products. The labeling must be consistent from coast to coast. The USDA has adopted the National Organic Program (NOP), which certifies organic foods based on the standards developed by the NOP. Supermarkets must also display organic foods separately from nonorganic products.[△]

The USDA organic seal appears on foods labeled as:

- *100 percent organic:* Products made entirely from organic ingredients

- *Organic:* Products containing 95 percent organic ingredients
- *Made with some organic ingredients:* Products containing 70 percent organic ingredients
- *Some organic ingredients:* Products containing less than 70 percent organic ingredients (Dimitri and Greene, 2002)[△]

Organically grown foods must not contain synthetic herbicides, insecticides, or fertilizer, and must be produced without exposure to human waste. Milk must come from cows raised on pastureland free of all chemical compounds. To be considered organically produced, animals and poultry must not have been given growth hormones or antibodies, no genetic modification.

When purchasing "locally grown organic foods" it is important that the foodservice director and purchasing agent determine if the grower is a certified organic grower; that the company and grower fully comply with all safety requirements and comply with all local rules and regulations. This is especially important when local meat, milk, eggs, seafood, and produce come from smaller farms. Be sure to ask (and verify) the state of sanitation of "food sheds and employees who are processing the food," pest controls of farms and processing sheds, and if potable water is used for cleaning the products. All growers, regardless of the operation's size, should follow Good Agriculture Practices (GAP) and manufacturers should follow Good Manufacturing Practice (GMP). The USDA has an audit verification program for compliance with GAP and GMP for fruits and vegetables. When purchasing locally the "buyer needs to be aware."

Adulterated food is food that has had substances added that could cause health problems. The food is usually prepared in filthy, unsanitary conditions and may have nails, bones, hair, decomposed animals, or diseased animals in the food. The FDA inspects meat, fish, dairy products and fresh and processed fruits and vegetables for unsafe residue levels. The FDA publishes a list of what is commonly known as *Generally Recognized as Safe* (GRAS). This list has been verified by evidence-based science (see Chapter 13).[△]

Labeling

Food product sellers provide nutrition labeling. Such labeling contains information on the nutritive content of the food. Food nutritional labeling is used only if a food is fortified, a nutritional claim is made, or the food serves a special dietary purpose. Figure 17.4 shows the standardized information required by law.

Considerations pertinent to purchasing equipment—utensils, service ware, dinnerware, and hollowware, for example—are discussed. Upon completing this chapter, foodservice directors and purchasing agents will be able to communicate freely and collaborate on purchasing decisions that facilitate departmental and organizational goals, profitability, and service delivery.

MEAT AND MEAT PRODUCTS

Meat is the most costly component of the daily menu, but it also is one of the most important sources of protein in the diet and must be selected carefully for use in the foodservice department. Both wholesomeness and quality of meat products must be considered,

FIGURE 17.4 Standard Label Information

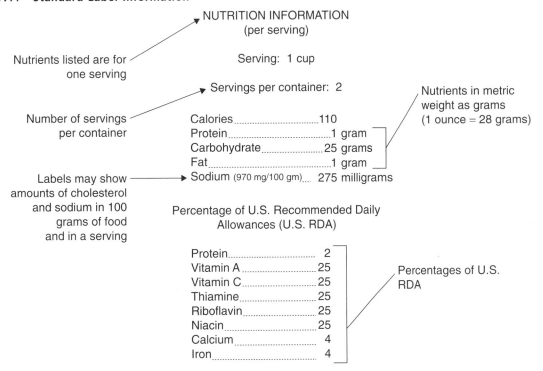

NUTRITION INFORMATION
(per serving)

Nutrients listed are for
one serving

Serving: 1 cup

Servings per container: 2

Number of servings
per container

Calories 110
Protein ....1 gram
Carbohydrate ....25 grams
Fat ....1 gram
Sodium (970 mg/100 gm) ... 275 milligrams

Nutrients in metric
weight as grams
(1 ounce = 28 grams)

Labels may show
amounts of cholesterol
and sodium in 100
grams of food
and in a serving

Percentage of U.S. Recommended Daily
Allowances (U.S. RDA)

Protein 2
Vitamin A 25
Vitamin C 25
Thiamine 25
Riboflavin 25
Niacin 25
Calcium 4
Iron 4

Percentages of U.S.
RDA

keeping in mind that various cuts are marketed in different-quality grades. The cut and grade of meat selection should be based on the meat's intended use. Purchasers must be familiar with meat inspection variables, grades of meat, market forms of meat, meat specifications, and processed meats.

Meat Inspection

Meat products sold in interstate commerce must be inspected for wholesomeness and stamped for approval. Figure 17.5 illustrates the federal stamps that are affixed to carcasses of meat, on the label of processed meat, or on a meat product if the product has met specific standards. Each label designates that the product has been examined for disease and that any unwholesome part has been removed and destroyed, that the meat has been handled and prepared in a sanitary manner in a processing plant that meets federal sanitation standards, and that no harmful substances have been added to the meat. The combined letter and numeric designation in certain inspection stamps identifies the plant at which the meat was processed and inspected.[Δ]

Products purchased from processing plants within a certain state must meet minimum state sanitation criteria. The criteria and inspection program vary significantly from state to state and may not always be reliable. With the increased concern regarding the safety of meat, purchasing agents should carefully consider the risk and liability implications of purchasing meat that has not met federal standards. For purchases made locally, it is advisable to tour the plant and obtain a copy of the standards.

The stamp or seal *kosher* ("fit to eat") refers to the ritualistic manner in which meat was slaughtered and butchered by a *shochet*

(a religious slaughterer) according to Orthodox Jewish dietary law. The symbol does not guarantee the wholesomeness or quality of the meat but indicates approval by the Union of Orthodox Jewish Congregations that the meat has met the standards of kosher and *kashrut* ("Jewish dietary laws"). There is confusion concerning the certifying agencies such as VHM, Chaf K, Kehilloh, Star K, and others. Many rabbis use their own symbol or just a plain **K** to designate a product's kosher status. The most common kosher agencies in the world include O/U, O/K, Star K, and KOF-K.

Meat Grades

The USDA has an established voluntary system for grading the quality of products. There are two types of grade: *yield grade* and *quality grade*.[Δ] All operations use quality grade when selecting meat because it is a measure of the palatability—that is, the eating quality—of the product. Operations that purchase wholesale or primal cuts need to know the desired quality and yield grades. *Quality grades* are based on the following criteria:

- Shape or conformation of the carcass
- Class (kind) of animal
- Sex of animal
- Amount of exterior fat (finish)
- Amount of inter-muscular fat (marbling)
- Firmness of lean and fat

Yield grades are based on the amount of external fat, internal fat, size of the rib-eye area, and carcass weight. These are used only at the wholesale level. Quality grade refers to palatability or the overall

FIGURE 17.5 Grade Stamps and Inspection Marks Used for Meat, Poultry, Eggs, and Seafood

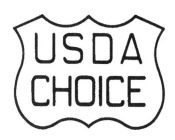

Federal grade stamp for meat

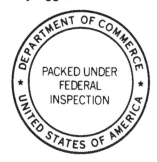

Federal inspection stamp for seafood

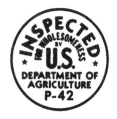

USDA poultry inspection mark

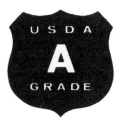

USDA poultry grade mark

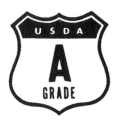

USDA shell egg grade mark

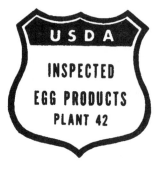

USDA egg products inspection mark

taste appeal, tenderness, juiciness, and flavor of cooked meat. It is based on two factors, the amount of marble in the meat and the age of the animal.△

Each general type of meat (described in the following subsections), poultry, and eggs is graded according to a specific set of requirements. After the grading process, the external surface of the meat carcass is marked with a shield indicating the federal grade (Figure 17.5). Because grading is not required by law, the food buyer must specify on the purchase order the USDA grade of meat desired when graded meat is to be purchased.

Beef

Beef is graded for quality according to eight USDA *beef grades*: "prime," "choice," "select," "standard," "commercial," "utility," "cutter," and "canner." Beef also is graded according to a system of yield grades, which are guides to the amount or cutability of usable meat in a carcass.△ Carcasses with high cutability combine a minimum of fat covering with thick muscling and yield a high proportion of lean meat. The USDA yield grades are numbered 1 through 8. The yield grades reflect differences in yields of boneless, closely trimmed, retail cuts. The yield grades also reflect overall fatness of carcasses and cuts. Yield 1 represents the highest yield of retail cuts and the least amount of trim, and Yield 8 indicates the lowest yield of retail cuts and the highest fat trim. Assigning yield grades for beef is a nationwide uniform method of determining "cutability" differences among carcasses. *Cutability* is the amount of salable meat obtained from a carcass as boneless, semiboneless trimmed, and retail cut from the round, loin, rib, and chuck sections.

Prime grade is the most tender, juicy, and flavorful beef available on the market because of its abundant marbling and thick external fat cover; it comes from young cattle. However, the external fat cover and marbling give prime beef a high fat content, which is unacceptable in many health care institutions. In addition, the price per pound for all USDA prime cuts usually is too high for most health care institutions to use except for special occasions, and the supply of this high-quality beef is limited.

Choice grade is of high quality but has less fat than prime grade. More choice-grade beef is produced than any other grade, and most consumers and institutions prefer it because of its tenderness and flavor. Rib and loin cuts are tender and can be cooked by dry-heat methods. Other cuts such as round or chuck also are tender and have a well-developed flavor when prepared by moist-heat methods.

Cuts of *select grade* have less marbling within the muscle and a thinner fat cover. The meat is relatively tender, but it lacks much of the juiciness and flavor associated with higher grades of beef. Rib and loin roasts and steaks prepared by dry-heat methods can yield fairly satisfactory products, but other cuts are best prepared by moist-heat methods.

Standard grade comes from young cattle and has traces of marbling. Commercial grade is produced from mature animals and lacks the tenderness of the higher grades. Institutions find it economical to use this grade for ground beef and stew meat, which becomes tender and full-flavored when cooked slowly with moist heat.

The three other USDA grades for beef—*utility, cutter,* and *canner*—usually are not sold as fresh beef. Instead, they are used in processed meat products.

Lamb

The five USDA grades for lamb are "prime," "choice," "select," "commercial," "utility" and "cull."[△] The standards for these grades are similar to those for beef. Choice or good is the grade selection usually specified for institutional use. *Utility* and *cull grade* lamb is used primarily in processed meat products. Maturity is the most important characteristic in quality grading. There are three maturity classes: A grade refers to lamb Class 1; B, yearly mutton class; and C, mutton Class 3. Mutton begins with USDA choice, as the top grade and is followed by good, utility and cull The yield designation range from 1 to 5, the rating being determined by the amount of fat covering the outside of the carcass and the fat deposited inside.

Veal

Veal is meat from calves up to 4 months of age that are milk or formula fed. The six USDA grades for veal are "prime," "choice,"

"select," "standard," "commercial," "utility," and "cull."[△] A veal carcass of *prime grade* is superior in quality and has thick muscling and firm, fine-textured flesh. The cut surface of the flesh looks and feels velvety and is light pink to a darker pink. The bones are small in relation to the size and weight of the carcass.

The carcass of *choice grade* is moderately blocky and compact, with fairly thick fleshing. The flesh is firm and finely textured and may look and feel moist; it may be dark grayish pink to red. The bones are moderately small in proportion to the size and weight of the carcass.

A carcass of *good grade* is blocky and compact, with thin fleshing and no evidence of plumpness. The flesh is moderately soft and on a cut surface looks and feels moist. The bones are large in proportion to the size of the carcass.

A carcass of *standard grade* is not thickly fleshed and has a higher proportion of bone to meat. Moist-heat methods of cooking are needed to produce juicy meat with a well-developed flavor. The two other grades of veal, utility and cull, are rarely used in institutional foodservice operations.

Pork

Pork is produced from young animals and is less variable in quality than beef. The USDA rates pork according to two quality levels: acceptable and unacceptable.[△] The USDA grades for pork are numbered from 1 to 4 for animals of acceptable quality. Grade differences are related to the ratio of lean to fat and the yield of the loin, the ham, the picnic, and the Boston butt. Pork that is not acceptable for use as fresh meat and pork that is watery and soft are graded *utility.* The yield grades for pork are similar to those for beef, but the grades for pork reflect the differences in carcass yield for the four major cuts rather than the differences in eating quality. Most pork marketed today is Grade 1 or 2. If a foodservice operation purchases carcass or packer-style (split-carcass) hogs, the following guidelines should be used to assess quality:

- *Cuts:* Muscles should not have more than a moderate amount of interior fat.
- *Bones:* Bones should be porous with cartilage present. Avoid brittle or flinty bones.
- *Lean:* Color should range from light pink to bright red and be smooth and finely textured, similar to veal.
- *Fat:* Fat should be firm, creamy white, and evenly distributed.
- *Skin:* The skin should be smooth, thin, and pliable.

Market Forms of Meats

Meat can be purchased in several market styles: by the half- or quarter-carcass, in wholesale or primal cuts, or in oven-ready or portion-control cuts.[△] Carcasses and primal cuts seldom are used in most foodservice departments today because of the amount of chilled storage space, cutting equipment, and skilled labor needed to prepare them for use. In addition, disposing of bones and other waste is a problem. Also, it is difficult to use all the different meat cuts effectively within a menu cycle. Carcasses and primal cuts are

TABLE 17.1 Primal Cuts of Beef, Veal, Pork, and Lamb△

Beef	Veal	Pork	Lamb
Chuck	Shoulder Jowl	Shoulder	
Rib	Rib	Boston shoulder	Rib (rack)
Short loin	Loin	Loin	Loin
Sirloin	Sirloin	Leg	Sirloin
Round	Round Spare ribs	Leg	
Tip	Breast	Picnic shoulder	Breast
Flank	Shank	Foot	Shank
Short Plate			
Brisket			
Foreshank			

Source: National Life Stock and Meat Board; National Cattlemen's Beef Association.

not even available from many institutional meat purveyors because suppliers purchase only the wholesale cuts they use most frequently and break them down into the oven-ready and portion-control cuts used by their foodservice customers.

The advantages of using oven-ready and portion-controlled meats are many. Roasts can be purchased in uniform sizes, weights, and trims. This gives the foodservice director greater control over portion yields and cost per serving. Specification of serving size for individual portion cuts offers maximum control of production quantity and quality, with little or no waste. Greater customer satisfaction can be achieved because each person receives the same-size portion.

Chuck, rib, loin, round cuts of beef come from the upper half of the animal. Brisket, flank, short plate and foreshank come from the lower back of the animal. Retail cuts come from primal cuts.

Meat Specifications

The United States Department of Agriculture (USDA) through its Agricultural Marketing Service (AMS) develops and maintains the *Institutional Meat Purchase Specifications (IMPS)* for meat and meat products. There are 10 documents that make up the IMPS series and include:

General Requirements
Quality Assurance Provisions
    Fresh Beef . . . . Series 100
    Fresh Lamb and Mutton . . . . Series 200
    Fresh Veal and Calf . . . . Series 300
    Fresh Pork . . . . Series 400
    Cured, Cured, and Stored, and Fully
        Cooked Pork Products . . . . Series 500
    Cured, Dried, and Smoked Beef Products . . . . . . Series 600
    Edible By-Products . . . . Series 700
    Sausage Products . . . . Series 800

These specifications are recommended for use by any meat product procuring activity. For assurance that procured items comply with these detailed requirements, the USDA, through its Meat Grading and Certification Board (MGCB), provides a voluntary Meat Certification Service. For labeling purposes, only products Certified by the MGCB may contain the letters "IMPS" on the product label.

All meat products should be purchased according to specifications that are based on a sound knowledge of the factors that influence preparation needs. A *specification* is a clear and concise but complete description of the exact item desired so that all vendors have a common basis for price quotations and bids. As such, it is an essential communication tool between buyer and seller. Specifications should be realistic and should not include details that cannot be verified or tested or that would make the product too costly. Without up-to-date product information, specifications are useless. The specific information varies with each type of food, but all specifications should include at least the following information:△

- Clear, simple description using common or trade or brand name of product; when possible, use a name or standard of identity formulated by the government such as IMPS
- Amount to be purchased in the most commonly used terms (case, package, or unit)
- Name and size of basic container (10/10# packages)
- Count and size of the item or units within the basic container (50 pork chops, 4 ounces each)
- Range in weight, thickness, or size
- Minimum and maximum trims, or fat content percentage (ground meat, 90 percent lean and 10 percent fat, referred to as 90/10)
- Degree of maturity or stage of ripening
- Type of processing required (such as individually quick-frozen [IQF])
- Type of packaging desired
- Unit on which price will be based
- Weight tolerance limit (range of acceptable weights, usually in meat, seafood, and poultry)

Foodservice departments that purchase relatively small quantities of meat may not find it practical to follow the lengthy specifications found in the IMPS or to use the Meat Acceptance Service. When these standards are not utilized the foodservice director, chef, and purchasing agent should work closely with the meat provider. When possible they should visit the meat facility to determine if sanitary techniques are being used, if the plant is clean, well maintained in all areas of the operation; if the employees seems well versed in their job task and safety and sanitation. They also need to know if the facility is government inspected and the meat meets the IMPS standards.

For best quality, meat items that will be used within three to five days after delivery (within one day for ground meat) should be purchased frozen.△ The blast freezing process used by meat purveyors provide the best conditions for quality retention. The common practice of foodservice departments freezing fresh meat usually results in quality deterioration because most foodservice freezers have the capability of holding frozen meats in a frozen state but not of freezing meat rapidly. The exception would be if there is a blast freezer within the department.

Regardless of how much meat is purchased at any one time, the written specifications to be given the vendor should include the following information:[Δ]

- Government inspected (when buying locally be aware of this requirement) (mandatory)
- Name of the cut
- Requirements for boning, rolling, and tying (if applicable)
- USDA grade or other quality designation
- Weight/thickness of cut or individual portion (state tolerance allowed)
- Fat tolerance
- IMPS or MBG number (if applicable)
- Chilled or frozen delivery
- Packaging or number of units per shipping container

Following are some examples of specifications that adhere to these rules:

- Beef, inside round roast, USDA Choice, 8 to 10 pounds, chilled, 32- to 40-pound polylined boxes preferred
- Beef, ground (special) bulk, USDA standard or commercial, 10 to 15 percent maximum fat content, blast frozen, 10-pound bag. Must specify the amount of fat.
- Bacon, sliced, layout pack, skinless, cured and smoked, Select No. 1, 8- to 12-pound bellies, 18 to 22 slices per pound, chilled, 10- to 15-pound polylined boxes preferred

Processed Meat

Processed meat is a term used to identify meat that has been changed by cooking, curing, canning, drying, or freezing or by a combination of these processes. Meats commonly described as processed include sausages, cold cuts, ham, bacon, and frankfurters. Some are fully cooked and can be served as purchased, whereas others require heating. Table 17.2 lists the characteristics of common processed meats.

Ready-to-serve are meats that have been precooked and may be either refrigerated or frozen and only require reheating. In health care foodservice they may be used as the main protein item or as a back-up item. These types of items work well when room service is used for patient meal service. Beef and pork are the two most used items. Beef and pork may be cooked as roasts and hams, as well as a variety of other forms. Heat-and-serve items are also being used more often to reduce labor cost. Heat-and-serve items include pre-formed sausage patties, ham, pork chops, and spare ribs. It is a good idea to determine how these convenient items would fit your food and labor budget.

Game Meats

Game meat is the flesh of animals such as bear, ostrich, and game animals. Meat that comes from wild animals and birds that are hunted is considered game meat. Most game meat found on menus is raised, slaughtered, and processed under voluntary inspection programs administered by the USDA and for the purpose of commercial foodservice operations. Federal, state, and local laws protect many wild animals, plants, and birds that are endangered and threatened. The flesh of these animals cannot be sold for any purpose. Game meats raised on farms are provided a diet different from their wild ancestors. Wild game meat includes:

- Birds: wood pigeon, duck, pheasant, quail, rock and ring dove, squab, woodcock, pigeon and ostrich
- Animals: antelope, wild bear, boar, wild buffalo, deer, kangaroo, alligator,* frog* (in frog legs), whale,* turtle,* musk ox, and rabbit (in some locations, squirrels and other small wild animals are used as sources of protein for home use)

The North Dakota Department of Health (NDDH) and the Minnesota Department of Natural Resources (MN DNR) have recently released independent studies that provide recommendations for minimizing lead exposure to hunters and other individuals who consume game meat harvested with lead-based bullets. The recommendations from both studies are: (1) children under the age of six and pregnant women should not consume game harvested with lead bullets; (2) encourage liberal trimming of wound channels; (3) grinding of venison is the most likely to contain lead, therefore (4) grinding surface of meat processing equipment be routinely cleaned, even between individual cuts of meat.

It is recommended that that game meat be cooked thoroughly, including bones and scraps fed to dogs. It is also suggested that turning bear meat into jerky is not safe because smoking preserves the meat from rotting but does not kill worms found in the meat.

SEAFOOD

More than 200 kinds of seafood are on the market today, including freshwater and saltwater fish and various kinds of shellfish. All fish are broken down into two broad categories—fish and shellfish.

Fish have gills, backbones, and fins while shellfish have shells of varying forms. Fish can also be classified as *saltwater* or *freshwater fish*.

Seafood is the general term applied to all edible aquatic organisms that come from rivers, lakes, seas, and oceans. The kinds and prices of fresh fish and shellfish products available vary with the

---

*Location of facility will determine the use of these animals. These items are often found on "specialty restaurant menus" or menus for special occasions. Note that whale is not available in countries that have signed the international treaty against whaling.

TABLE 17.2 Common Processed Meats

Meat	Description
Bacon	The cured and smoked belly of the hog. Available sliced shingle style or on parchment paper ready to grill or precooked.
Beef, dried	Also known as chipped beef. A slow-cured product made from beef round; cured, smoked, dehydrated, and thinly sliced. Available in cans, jars, and vacuum packages.
Bologna	Made of cured beef and pork; finely ground with seasonings similar to those in frankfurters. Available in rings, rolls, or slices of various diameters; fully cooked and ready to serve. • Beef bologna: Made exclusively of beef and has a definite garlic flavor. • Meat bologna: A mixture of beef and pork. • Poultry bologna: Made of chicken or turkey or a combination of chicken and turkey.
Bratwurst	Pork or a pork and veal mixture, highly seasoned, made in links slightly larger than frankfurters. Available both fresh and fully cooked.
Braunschweiger	Liver sausage that has been smoked after cooking or includes smoked meats as ingredients.
Chorizos	Dry pork sausage of Spanish origin; meat coarsely cut, smoked, highly spiced and hot to the palate; size similar to large frankfurters or bulk style.
Ham	Cured pork leg available with bone in or boneless; sold in a variety of forms, dry cured or with water added for economy, tenderness, and a juicy flavor. Generally supplied fully cooked and ready to heat and serve.
Knockwurst (or knackwurst)	Similar in ingredients to frankfurters and bologna, with garlic added for stronger flavor; made in wide natural casings or in skinless style; fully cooked but usually served hot; also known as Knoblauch or garlic sausage.
Liverwurst, liver sausage	Finely ground selected pork and livers; seasoned with onions and spices; may also be smoked after cooking or may include smoked meat such as bacon.
Luncheon meat	Chopped pork, ham, and/or beef, seasoned and ready to serve. Available in loaves, in cans, and in vacuum packages, sliced.
Mettwurst	Cured beef and pork ground and lightly seasoned with allspice, ginger, mustard, and coriander; smooth, spreadable consistency; cooked before serving.
Pastrami	Flat pieces of lean beef, dry cured, rubbed with a paste of spices, and smoked.
Polish sausage	Coarsely ground lean pork with beef added, highly seasoned with garlic; frequently referred to as kielbasa, once a Polish word for all sausage.
Pork sausage, fresh	Made only from selected fresh pork; seasoned with black pepper, nutmeg, and rubbed sage; sold in links, packaged patties, or bulk; thorough cooking required.
Pork sausage, fresh country style	Made of selected fresh pork; ground more coarsely than other fresh pork sausage; generally sold in casings, but also in bulk and links; thorough cooking required.
Pork sausage, smoked country style	Fresh pork sausage, mildly cured and smoked; thorough cooking required.
Salami	General classification for highly seasoned dry sausage with characteristic fermented flavor; usually made of beef and pork; seasoned with garlic, salt, pepper, and sugar; most air dried and not smoked or cooked.
Salami, cooked	Made from fresh meats; cured, stuffed, then cooked in a smokehouse at high temperatures; may be air dried for a short time; softer texture than dry and semidry sausages (cooked salamis are not dry sausage); refrigeration required.
Salami, Cotto	Cooked salami; contains whole peppercorns; may be smoked as well as cooked.
Salami, Genoa	A dry sausage of Italian origin; usually made from all pork but may contain a small amount of beef; moistened with wine or grape juice; seasoned with garlic; cord wrapped lengthwise and around the sausage at regular intervals.
Salami, Italian	Includes many varieties named for towns and localities (for example, Genoa, Milano, Sicilian); principally cured lean pork, coarsely chopped and some finely chopped lean beef added; frequently moistened with red wine or grape juice; usually highly seasoned with garlic and various spices; air dried; chewy texture.
Salami, kosher	All beef; meat and processing under rabbinical supervision; mustard, coriander, and nutmeg added to regular seasonings.
Smoky links	Coarsely ground beef and pork; seasoned with black pepper; stuffed and linked like frankfurters.
Sausage, Thüringen style	Made principally of ground pork; may also include veal and beef; seasoning similar to that in pork sausage, except no sage is used; may be smoked or unsmoked.

geographical location of the facility and the season of the year. Because frozen fish and shellfish products are widely available and easy to use, most foodservice departments use frozen rather than fresh seafood. Most kinds of frozen seafood are available throughout the year.

Nutritional concerns for omega-3 fatty acids and high-quality protein, which are essential for cardiovascular function, joint health, brain function, and blood sugar metabolism plus other health concerns, has increased fish usage, therefore taxing the supply and resulting in increased prices for many of the most popular species. To meet the demands, *aquaculture* (fish farming) is now being used to control production of such fish as trout, catfish, tilapia, and salmon, which are the most common fish grown on a fish farm. Large quantities of chemicals are used in aquaculture including antibiotics, pesticides hormones, anesthetics, vitamins, minerals, and anti-parasitical substances often dumped directly into ocean water. As the demand for fish continues to increase, more fish will be grown on "fish farms." About one-third of the world's seafood is produced on a fish farm. Consequently, many less-familiar fish are being marketed in fresh and frozen forms. Because many of these fish are satisfactory and economical, they deserve consideration.

Fish may be sold by different names in different parts of the country. For example, bass has many names: the Pacific bass may be called rockfish, sea bass, or striped bass; the Atlantic variety may be called striped bass, sea white bass, or common bass. Seafood may also be known as saltwater fish (cod, flounder, tuna, salmon, sole), freshwater fish (trout and catfish), mollusks (mussels, clams, oysters, scallops), or crustaceans (crabs, lobsters, shrimp).[△]

Fish may also be sold by approximate fat content, especially for health care facilities.

The most used oily fish include:

Fish	Fat	Saturated	Unsaturated
Mackerel, fried	12 g	2.2 g	9.2 g
Salmon, steamed	11.0 g	2 g	9.5 g
Trout, steamed	2.6 g	0.7 g	1.8 g
Tuna in brine	0.5 g	0.3 g	0.2 g

Some fish may be common to a particular area but are frozen and shipped to other areas of the country for consumption. Some of these include:

- Redfish: Common to the South Atlantic and the Gulf of Mexico
- Halibut: Common to both the Pacific and the Atlantic
- Mullet: Common to the South Atlantic and the Gulf of Mexico
- Northern pike: Common to Canadian lakes
- Pompano: Common to the South Atlantic and the Gulf of Mexico
- Salmon: Common to the North Pacific
- Scrod: Common to the North Atlantic
- Whitefish: Common to the Great Lakes

Inspection for sanitary conditions and wholesomeness—which is required for meat, poultry, and egg products—is not as widely applied to seafood. The FDA and U.S. Public Health Service Food Code states that "fish that are received for sale or service shall be commercially and legally caught or harvested and approved for sale or service." The Seafood Quality and Inspection Division of the National Marine Fisheries Service, USDC, conducts a voluntary seafood inspection program on a fee-for-service basis for processors and other interested parties. Contract plant inspection means that the processing plant, equipment, and food handlers have met all required sanitation standards. In addition, a federal inspector has examined samples of the product and found it to be safe, wholesome, and properly labeled. Most seafood plants have implemented the hazard analysis critical control point system to ensure the safety of seafood.[△]

Seafood packed under federal inspection bears a statement of inspection on the label or the *"Packed Under Federal Inspection"* (PUFI) mark (see Figure 17.5). Product grading, which is voluntary, is an additional guarantee to consumers that the product meets a certain level of quality. Graded products may bear the appropriate grade mark: USDC grade A, B, or C. The grade stamp signifies that the product meets the following criteria:[△]

- The product, by type, is clean, safe, and wholesome.
- The specified quality standard as indicated by grade designation has been achieved.
- The condition of the establishment in which the fish was processed was acceptable as required by food control authorities.
- The product was processed under supervision of federal food inspectors and was packed under sanitary conditions.
- The common or usual name is accurately reflected on the label.
- Market form—whole, *eviscerated*; seafood, alive, whole shucked, and so on.[△]

The grading service is used primarily by large processors and only rarely by small ones. However, fresh and frozen products of excellent quality can be obtained from uninspected sources when the vendors are reputable and are known to follow adequate sanitary standards.

Fresh Fish

High-quality fresh fish has firm, elastic flesh with a smooth, slippery slime and shiny surface. The eyes should be bulging and clear, the gills should be pink to bright red, and there should be no strong "fishy" odor. As fish deteriorates, the slime becomes more viscous (sticky) and grainy, the odor changes from smelling like seaweed to smelling like ammonia, and the flesh softens.[△] Because fresh fish deteriorates rapidly, great care must be taken in handling it during harvesting and processing. This task becomes more difficult when markets are far from the source. For this reason, a large percentage of fish on the market is sold frozen.

Frozen Fish

Frozen fish, if properly processed, packaged, and stored, shows no sign of freezer burn. Packages are free from dripping and ice. Individually quick frozen fillets and steaks are best to purchase (except for breaded fish products). The fish should have little or no odor. If handled properly, frozen fish will remain in good condition for relatively long periods. If the fish is purchased as a ready-to-cook breaded product, the ratio of fish to breading should be checked to ensure that the department is getting its money's worth of fish.[Δ]

Shellfish

Shellfish (crab, lobster, clams and oysters) is marketed live and should be alive when purchased or cooked whole in the shell, headless (usually shrimp with the head and thorax removed), or shucked (shellfish such as oysters removed from the shell). The meat can be purchased fresh or frozen, cooked or raw, plain or breaded, and canned. Shellfish purchased live in the shell must be kept alive until cooked. Buyers of fresh shellfish should be well acquainted with their source of supply and should check to make sure that the products have been harvested from uncontaminated waters.[Δ] A high proportion of shellfish is imported, frozen, and the quality characteristics of frozen shellfish are the same as those described for other frozen fish.

Market Forms of Fish and Shellfish

Fresh and frozen fish are available in several forms, some of which are as follows:

- *Whole or round:* Just as it comes from water; sometimes scales are removed.
- *Whole and dressed:* Scales, entrails, and usually the head, tail, and fins are removed.
- *Dressed:* Scales, head, tails, fins, and entrails removed.
- *Steaks:* Cross-sectional slices are cut from large dressed fish with the skin off, usually five-eighths- to three-quarter-inch thick; must specify portion size.
- *Fillets:* The sides of fish are cut lengthwise, away from the bone; fillets are practically boneless and come with or without skin.
- *Drawn:* Eviscerated through a small opening but not split; gills and scales may be removed, but head and tail still on.
- *Butterfly fillet:* Both sides of the fillet connect at the top.
- *Portions and sticks:* Large, solid, frozen blocks of boneless fish are machine cut. Pieces are dipped in batter or breading and may or may not be partially cooked. The designation precooked means that only the batter or breading is cooked and that the fish is raw. Fillets are available in many shapes and sizes and are ready to cook as purchased.

Currently, many other seafood products are processed and sold in convenience form, either frozen or in a freeze-dried state.

Frozen fish fillets or portions may be filled with stuffing, sauce, or nuts. Shrimp and crab are available freeze-dried, which helps reduce the amount of labor involved in preparation. Both products can be stored for long periods because they are cooked and cleaned before being frozen, freeze-dried, or canned. Reconstitution in water takes little time, the flavor and color are good, and the cost may be less than that of the fresh product at certain times of the year.

Specification for Fish and Shellfish

When developing specifications for fresh or frozen fish and shellfish, the following information should be included:[Δ]

- Species (kind) of fish or shellfish—must be specific
- Origin—freshwater, saltwater, or farm raised
- The PUFI seal or grading stamp, if applicable (USDC grade and inspection stamp)
- Market form or portion shape and size
- Raw or precooked, plain or breaded
- Chilled or frozen
- Quantity per package
- Additives such as sulfites or tripolyphosphates; if no additives permitted, state in specification
- Seafood comes from an HACCP-certified plant, inspected by USD of Commerce, Seafood Inspection Service
- Only varieties that are controlled by the Fishery Laws of the United States will be accepted
- Style and size
- Substitutions must be approved by the foodservice before delivery
- Certificate must be given for each order of seafood and product must be traceable

Some sample specifications include:

- Cod, breaded, 6 ounces for deep-fat frying, frozen, 10°F on delivery in refrigerated truck, USDC Grade A or equivalent; 10 6-pound boxes per case, price per case
- Salmon, Alaska Coho, 8-ounce steaks for grilling, fresh, may be farm raised, but no GM salmon, 35°F on delivery in refrigerated truck, USDC Grade A, packed, 20-pound carton, PUFI seal, price by pound
- Pollock, from North Atlantic Ocean, boneless skinless fish sticks, lightly breaded, IQF, to be oven baked, 10°F on delivery in refrigerated truck, Mrs. Paul's™ breaded fish sticks, each stick to weigh 1.2 ounces, with 70 percent solid fish, 30 percent breading, packed in 10-pound carton, price by carton
- Shrimp, United States from the South Atlantic or Gulf of Mexico, no imports, pink shrimp, fresh, never frozen, shelled, deveined, 20 per pound, delivered at 35°F in a refrigerated truck, USDC Grade A, packed bulk, 10-pound cases, price by case

Canned Fish

Many kinds of canned fish products are available, including salmon, tuna, mackerel, crab, shrimp, sardines, clams, oysters, herring, anchovies, and caviar. Of these, only salmon and tuna are available in several species and styles. Some canned fish is canned in spring water, others in oil. All may have added herbs or sauces.

On the Pacific Coast, salmon usually is sold by species name because of the differences in color, texture, and flavor among species. *Chinook* (or king) salmon, for example, which ranges in color from white to deep salmon, is the highest-quality salmon and therefore the highest priced. Little of this salmon is canned because most is sold fresh or smoked. *Sockeye* is the reddest of all varieties, is of high quality, and also is high in price. Silver, medium-red, or *Coho* salmon, usually a rich orange color slightly touched with red, is widely used for canning. Pink or *humpback* salmon is lighter in color but has excellent flavor and is good for use in many combination recipes. *Chum* or *keta* salmon is light colored and bland in flavor.△

Tuna canned in the United States is produced from four species of the mackerel family: *albacore, yellowfin, bluefin,* and *shipjack.* Albacore has the lightest meat and is the only tuna that may be labeled *white meat.* The other species are labeled *light meat.*

Canned salmon and tuna are available packed in oil, water, and brine. Four styles of pack are available: fancy or solid pack, which must contain 82 percent solid pieces; chunk style, in which 50 percent of the weight must be pieces ½ inch or larger in diameter; flakes, in which 50 percent or more of the pieces are less than ½ inch in diameter; and grated. Specifications for canned fish should state the species and variety, packing medium, style of pack, size of can, and number of cans per case. Some sample specifications include:△

- Tuna, solid pack, fancy white meat (albacore), water pack, six 64-ounce cans per case
- Tuna, solid pack, fancy light meat, water pack, 24 6½-ounce cans per case
- Salmon, pink, PUFI, six 64-ounce cans per case

The FDA recommends that all women who are pregnant, may become pregnant, nursing mothers, and young children abstain completely from shark, swordfish, king mackerel, and tilefish because of the high levels of *mercury* contamination that may be particularly harmful to unborn babies and the developing nervous system of young children. The FDA also recommends eating no more than 12 ounces of fish and shellfish lower in mercury, including shrimp, canned *light* tuna, salmon, pollock, and catfish. It further advises keeping up to date on local fish safety warnings and, if there is no advisory available, not to eat more than 6 ounces of local-caught fish weekly.

Some religions have rites and rituals concerning the use of certain fish.

POULTRY

Poultry products or domesticated birds are used extensively in foodservice menus because of their great versatility in both general and modified diets. Poultry, also called *fowl*, includes chicken, turkey, duck, Rock Cornish game hen, and geese. Poultry is classified by kind and age of the bird. Kind includes chicken, turkey, duck, and goose; class indicates the age of the bird and the tenderness of the meat. Class also indicates cooking method. Most young birds are of either sex, the exception being the capon chicken, which is a surgically desexed male chicken. The availability of poultry is rarely a problem because the production and processing techniques used today provide a consistent supply of the desired kind, quality, and quantity of poultry in almost any season. Prices fluctuate according to market conditions and the prices of red meats, but in general most poultry products are less expensive than other meat items.

Market Forms of Poultry

Many of the different market forms of poultry are popular because they save time in preparation and eliminate waste. Turkey roasts of boneless white, dark, or mixed light and dark meat are available in a range of weights. They are marketed raw, usually seasoned, and ready to cook from the frozen state. Frozen, cooked, and diced white or dark meat of chicken or turkey, separate or mixed, is an ideal product for use in many foodservice recipes. Cooked fried chicken products, breaded or battered, are available in a wide range of portion sizes and styles.

All poultry products should be handled carefully after delivery, and they should be refrigerated or frozen under the conditions appropriate and recommended for specific items. Microorganisms grow readily, particularly on the surface of the body cavity. If chicken is delivered in ice when received, remove from ice and store for 1 to 2 days (NO MORE) and refrigerate at 35°F to 38°F. All precooked or uncooked frozen products should be thawed under refrigeration or reheated without thawing. Frozen raw poultry is best thawed in a refrigerator for the specified hours (chicken) or days (turkey). Frozen poultry may also be thawed under running water (not a good choice due to shortage of water and increased cost) or wrapped in watertight bags or heavy paper and in a cold-water bath of approximately 70°F (21°C). Water must be *changed frequently.* Chicken and turkey may be thawed in a microwave oven as part of the cooking process. **Never thaw chickens or turkey on a counter nor overnight on a counter**. To hasten the thawing process, remove the neck and giblets from the internal neck cavity of whole fowl.△

Poultry Specifications

The USDA grades for poultry are U.S. Grade A, U.S. Grade B, and U.S. Grade C. U.S. Grade A is the grade commonly found in the market. Poultry may be purchased whole, halves, quarters, or pieces of the whole fowl, or by selected items such as breast or thighs and skin on or off, boneless. Cut-up pieces frequently cost more due to labor cost, developed specifications for whole poultry carcasses and parts.△ Specifications should be based on the following eight standards:

1. *Kind* refers to the species, such as chicken, turkey, duck, capon, goose and quail.

2. *Class* refers to physical characteristics related to age and sex, as follows:
   - Broiler-fryer chicken: A young chicken of either sex, 9 to 12 weeks old, weighing 1½ to 4 pounds, ready to cook
   - Roaster chicken: Young chicken of either sex, 3 to 5 months old, weighing 4 to 6 pounds or more, ready to cook
   - Hen or stewing chicken: Female chicken, older than 10 months, weighing more than 4 pounds, ready to cook
   - Rock Cornish game hen: Female chicken, 5 to 7 weeks old, weighing less than 2 pounds, ready to cook
   - Fryer-roaster turkey: Less than 16 weeks old, weighing 3 to 7 pounds, ready to cook
   - Young hen or tom turkey (or young turkey): 16 to 24 weeks old, weighing 8 to 16 pounds (hens) or 16 pounds or more (toms), ready to cook
   - Yearling or mature turkeys: Older than 12 months and of heavy weight
3. *Grade* refers to the quality of the product and is determined by factors such as conformity, fleshing, fat covering, and freedom from various types of defects such as cuts, tears, broken bones, and discoloration. The USDA grades for ready-to-cook poultry are A, B, and C. Almost all chicken or turkey marketed fresh-chilled or frozen is Grade A; Grades B and C are used for processed forms. All poultry must be inspected for wholesomeness. Inspection and grade marks for poultry are shown in Figure 16.5. Birds that have a wing, tail, or drumstick missing because of damage during processing but whose eating quality has not been affected are labeled "Parts missing."
4. *Style* indicates whether the bird is to be cut up or left whole. When ready-to-cook poultry is purchased, the buyer's preference for parts, quarters, eight-piece cut, nine-piece cut, breasts, legs, thighs, boneless, and so forth should be indicated.
5. *State of delivery* indicates whether the poultry should be delivered fresh-chilled, frozen, or cooked and frozen and in a refrigerated truck with temperature monitored during delivery from 32°F to 35°F on delivery if fresh.
6. *Weight or size* indicates weight range allowable for individual birds, or ounces per portion for convenience forms, or both.
7. *Delivery unit* refers to weight or number per delivery box or package refrigeration, packed in ice, and so on.
8. *Mandatory inspection.*

   Some sample specifications for poultry are:
   - Chicken, U.S. Grade A, 2½- to 3-pound broiler, quartered, fresh, chilled, or frozen as specified, temperature monitored during transport and available to foodservice department
   - Chicken, boned, cooked, ready to use, minimum of 91 percent meat, maximum of 6 percent broth and 3 percent fat, natural proportion of light and dark meat, seasoned with salt only, six 30-ounce rolls per case, prepared under continuous USDA inspection

- Chicken, diced, ½-inch cubes, mixed meat, cooked, frozen, three 10-pound polybags per case
- Chicken, fryer, cooked in batter, frozen, nine-piece cut, quartered or individual parts, 9 pounds per case
- Turkey, young hen, U.S. Grade A, whole, fresh or frozen, 12 to 14 pounds
- Turkey, young tom, U.S. Grade A, whole, fresh or frozen, 20 to 26 pounds
- Turkey breast, U.S. Grade A, boneless, frozen, uncooked, natural skin cover, four 8- to 10-pound polybags per case
- Turkey, diced, ½-inch cubes, white, dark, or mixed meat, cooked, frozen, three 10-pound polybags per case
- Turkey ham, cooked, frozen, two 7- to 8-pound polybags per case
- Turkey franks, chilled, 10 per pound, 10 pounds per case

EGGS AND EGG PRODUCTS

Egg production is a highly automated business that yields superior fresh eggs for the foodservice and retail markets. Modern technology and the federal regulations covering shell eggs, as stated in the Egg Products Inspection Act of 1972, prevent the distribution or use of eggs that have not been graded.

Grades of Shell Eggs

The USDA provides a voluntary grading service for producers of shell eggs. Eggs that have been graded under this program can be identified by the official USDA shell egg grade symbol on the package (see Figure 17.5). The symbol indicates that the eggs have been graded for quality under both federal and state supervision.

Grades refer to the interior quality and condition of the egg and the appearance of the shell. Official consumer grades are U.S. Grade AA, U.S. Grade A, and U.S. Grade A Medium. The higher-quality eggs—Grades AA and A—have a firm and thick white, a well-rounded high yolk, and a delicate flavor. They are ideal for any purpose but are particularly good for frying and poaching when appearance is important. Grade A eggs are less expensive than Grade AA and are entirely satisfactory for the same purposes as the higher grade. Grade B eggs have thinner whites and somewhat flatter yolks that may break easily. They are less expensive and are suitable for general cooking and baking.[Δ]

Weight and Size of Shell Eggs

Shell eggs also are classified according to size, although size has no relation to quality. Large eggs can be of any quality, just as eggs of any quality can be of any size. Official size categories are based on the minimum weight per dozen. Eggs for institutional use are sold in cases of 30 dozen and half cases of 15 dozen. The official size categories and weights per dozen and the minimum weights per case, excluding the weight of the container, are listed in Table 17.3. The most common sizes are extra large, large, and medium.

The weight of cases of eggs received from various suppliers should be checked periodically. An empty carton that contains the filler flats should be weighed to get an approximate weight of

TABLE 17.3 Official USDA Size Categories for Shell Eggs[△]

U.S. Weights or Classes, Size	Minimum Weight per Dozen, Ounces	Minimum Weight* per 30-Dozen Case, Pounds
Jumbo	30	56 lbs.
Extra large	27	50½ lbs.
Large	24	45 lbs.
Medium	21	39½ lbs.
Small	18	34 lbs.
Peewee	15	28 lbs.

*Weight may include corrugated fiber case and filler between layers of eggs.
Verified by Egg Board 1981 and 2010.

the carton. Then a full case should be weighed and the results, minus the weight of the carton, checked against the weights given in Table 17.3.

Price Consideration in Purchasing Eggs

The size and grade of eggs purchased should depend on the price per ounce and the intended use of the eggs. In some areas, shell color can affect the egg's price even though color does **not** affect its grade, nutritional value, flavor, or cooking performance. Egg prices vary by size for the same grade, but the degree of price variation depends on the supply of the various sizes. To determine which size is the most economical, the price per ounce of various sizes should be compared by dividing the price per dozen by the weight in ounces for a dozen eggs of a particular size. For example, if large eggs are 80 cents per dozen, with a minimum weight of 24 ounces for a dozen eggs of that size, the price per ounce would be 3.3 cents. Medium eggs at 70 cents per dozen, weighing 21 ounces per dozen, also would cost 3.3 cents per ounce. In this case, either size would be an equally good buy. However, medium eggs at any price per dozen over 70 cents would cost more per ounce than large eggs at 80 cents per dozen and would not be a good buy.[△]

Egg Products

Egg products are a convenience item for foodservice operations and commercial food manufacturers. Whole eggs, yolks, whites, and various blends can be obtained in liquid, frozen, and dried forms.

The Egg Products Inspection Act of 1970 requires that liquid, frozen, and dried egg products be inspected under the USDA's continuous mandatory inspection program. This requirement applies to products shipped between states, within a state, and in foreign commerce. The official USDA egg products inspection mark (see Figure 18.5) means that the products were processed under continuous supervision of a USDA-licensed inspector, that the products were processed in an approved plant that had adequate facilities, and that the products were pasteurized in accordance with USDA requirements and were truthfully and informatively labeled.

Institutional packs of liquid, frozen, and powdered eggs are available in various sizes. Containers for frozen packs range in size from 3 to 45 pounds. Many foodservice operations find the smaller containers, which resemble half-gallon milk cartons, to be the most convenient to use within a short time after thawing. The containers should be stored at 0°F (−18°C) or below and thawed under refrigeration. Dried egg products also are available in many pack sizes, and the 5-pound container is the easiest to use. Because dried egg products can be contaminated easily and deteriorate in quality rapidly, they should be stored in the refrigerator in a tightly covered container.

The foodservice buyer should become familiar with the product variety provided by local vendors and develop specifications in accordance with need and market availability. Table 17.4 summarizes the manufacturing and inspection specifications for several egg products.

Specification for Eggs and Egg Products

Specifications for fresh eggs should include the form, quality designation, size, and unit of purchase. Shell eggs should be received clean and sound and not exceed the restricted egg tolerance for U.S. Grade B. Raw shell eggs must be received in refrigerated equipment that maintains an ambient air temperature of 45°F (7°C) or less. Once received, they should be refrigerated at 45°F (7°C) until used. No quality designation (such as grade) is used for egg products because they are not graded; the words "USDA inspected" are used in place of a grade. Some sample specifications for eggs and egg products follow:

- Eggs, fresh, Grade AA, large, 45-pound net per 30 dozen cases, 45°F when delivered on refrigerated truck, price by crate
- Eggs, frozen, whole, pasteurized, homogenized, USDA inspected, six 4-pound pouches per case, delivered at −10°F in a refrigerated truck
- Eggs, pasteurized, dried whole, six 3-pound cans per case

Salmonella infection is a concern in eggs. Salmonella (Chapter 13) may be found in the intestines of chickens. These bacteria may be passed from the intestine tract to the hands of the cooks and then to the food. Hand washing is vital when handling eggs. Eating raw eggs in drinks (eggnog) can be dangerous and is discouraged.

Eggs should be delivered in refrigerated trucks and immediately refrigerated, in the delivery case and used by date stamped on the carton. Do not store eggs at room temperature. If eggs are not delivered in a refrigerated truck and are warm when they arrive at the loading dock it is wise to refuse them.[△]

MILK AND OTHER DAIRY PRODUCTS

Effective sanitation in production, transport, and processing is the key to high-quality milk and other dairy products. Milk is one of the most perishable of all foods because of its nutrient composition and fluid form. Milk is an ideal medium for bacterial growth. It must

TABLE 17.4 Manufacturing and Inspection Specifications for Selected Egg Products

| Specification | Liquid or Frozen | | | Solids | | | | | | |
| | | | | Whites | | Whole | | Yolk | | |
	White	Yolk[a]	Whole	Spray Dried	Pan Dried	Plain	Free Flowing[b]	Plain	Free Flowing[b]	Scrambled Egg
Moisture, %	—	—	—	8.0	14.0	5.0	3.0	5.0	3.0	2.5
Total solids, %	11.0	43.0	24.7	—	—	—	—	—	—	—
Crude protein, %	10.0	14.0	12.0	80.0	74.0	45.0	45.0	30.0	30.0	34.3
Total lipids, %	Nil	28.0	10.5	±0.02	Nil	40.0	40.0	56.0	56.0	36.5
pH	8.9 ± 0.3	6.2 ± 0.1	7.3 ± 0.3	7.0 ± 0.5	5.5 ± 0.5	8.3 ± 0.3	8.3 ± 0.3	6.4 ± 0.3	6.4 ± 0.3	
Carbohydrates[c], (%)	—	—	—	Glucose free	Glucose free	SOP	SOP	SOP	SOP	17
Total microbial count, grams	<5,000	<5,000	<5,000	<10,000	<10,000	<10,000	<10,000	<10,000	<10,000	<10,000
Yeast, grams	10 max.	10 max.	10 max.	10 max.	10 max.	10 max.	10 max.	10 max.	10 max.	—
Mold, grams	10 max.	10 max.	10 max.	10 max.	10 max.	10 max.	10 max.	10 max.	10 max.	—
Coliform, grams	10 max.	10 max.	10 max.	10 max.	10 max.	10 max.	10 max.	10 max.	10 max.	—
Salmonellae, grams	Negative[d]	Negative	Negative	Negative	Negative	Negative	Negative	Negative	Negative	Negative
Granulation	—	—	—	100%[e]	SOP	100%	100%	100%	100%	—
				USBS 60		USBS 16	USBS 16	USBS 16	USBS 16	
Others[f]	—	—	—	—	—	—	—	—	—	—

[a]Egg yolk contains 17 percent egg white; natural egg yolk contains about 52 percent solids.
[b]Free-flowing products contain less than 2 percent sodium silicoaluminate.
[c]Most egg white solids are desugared. Whole egg and yolk products are desugared if specified on purchase (SOP).
[d]Negative by approved testing procedures.
[e]U.S. Bureau of Standards (USBS) Screen No. 80.
[f]Additives and performance specifications may be specified on purchase.
Source: American Egg Board.

be protected against contamination and delivered and stored above 40°F. For this reason, the regulations concerning sanitary production of dairy products are strict. The U.S. Public Health Service's Milk Ordinance and Code is the basis for state and local milk regulations. The Grade A classification for milk and milk products is a designation based on compliance with sanitation requirements of applicable laws. Only Grade A pasteurized milk can be shipped interstate, and in most states it is the only grade available for purchase and use as a fluid product. A foodservice buyer should be familiar with all state and local regulatory standards that apply to the *suppliers* with whom he or she deals.

Grades of Milk

Grades$^\triangle$ are related to the conditions under which milk is produced and handled and the bacterial count in the final product. *Pasteurization* destroys pathogenic (disease-causing) organisms and most other bacteria commonly found in milk. Most fluid milk is *homogenized*, a process that divides the fat globules into tiny particles that remain in permanent suspension in the milk. FDA standards for the composition of milk specify the minimum amount of milk solids and milk fat contained in milk or cream products.

Forms of Milk and Dairy Products

Milk and dairy products are available in a wide variety of forms. The most familiar are whole milk, skim milk, low-fat milk, cultured buttermilk, cream, evaporated milk, sweetened condensed milk, and a number of other forms as described in the following subsections.$^\triangle$

Whole Milk

According to FDA standards, whole milk must contain at least 3.25 percent fat and 8.25 percent milk solids (may have added vitamins A and D, approximately 150 calories per 8 ounces, and approximately 300 milligrams of calcium). This applies to plain or flavored milk.

Skim or Nonfat Milk

To meet FDA standards, skim milk, plain or flavored, contains less than 0.5 percent fat and at least 8.25 percent milk solids. Total solids can range from 8.0 to 9.25 percent and, depending on state standards, may have vitamins A and D added; it contains 80 calories and 300 milligrams of calcium per 8 ounces.

1 Percent Low-Fat Milk

Low-fat milk must be fortified with vitamin A at levels specified by FDA regulations. Fortification with vitamin D is optional. Standards for milk products in certain states may vary from federal standards, which require that low-fat milk in plain or flavored form contain at least 0.5 to 2 percent fat and 8.2 percent milk solids, with 100 calories and 300 milligrams of calcium per 8 ounces.

2 Percent Low-Fat Milk

Low-fat milk must be fortified with vitamin A. Fortification with vitamin D is optional. The fat content is at least 2.0 percent and the solids without fat are 8.2 percent. Low-fat milk contains 120 calories and 300 milligrams of calcium per 8 ounces.

Cultured Buttermilk

Cultured buttermilk, which has a characteristic flavor that is produced by bacterial fermentation, is processed from pasteurized skim milk or whole milk to which lactic acid and bacteria have been added. Partial fermentation produces some coagulation of the milk protein. Small butter granules may be added. Buttermilk is a by-product of butter production. No federal standards have been established for buttermilk.

Flavored Milk

Flavored milk may be whole, low fat, or fat-free. Chocolate, strawberry, and other flavors may be added to the milk. This causes a variation in the calories and carbohydrates but not the protein content.

Lactose-Free Milk

Lactose-free milk$^\triangle$ contains lactose that has been broken down to make it easier to digest. Lactose, an enzyme, has been added to assist people with lactose-intolerance problems in digesting and absorbing the lactose in milk.

Organic, Fiber-Added, and Acidophilus Cultured Milk

Organic milk$^\triangle$ comes from cows that are raised on a pastureland free of all chemical compounds.

Fiber$^\triangle$, such as cellulose gel, is added to low-fat milk to enrich the texture. The milk has a thicker consistency and a whiter color due to the addition of natural coloring agents. The milk has fewer calories than fat-free milk and more calcium due to enrichment.

Acidophilus-cultured milk$^\triangle$ is low-fat or fat-free milk that is cultured with Lactobacillus acidophilus to digest the lactose. Lactose-intolerant people can often tolerate this form of milk.

Eggnog

Eggnog contains milk products, cooked egg yolks, egg whites ingredients, and sweeteners. It also contains salt, flavoring, stabilizers, and color additives. Eggnog must not contain less than 6 percent milk fat and 8.25 percent milk solids without fat. Eggnog must be pasteurized.

Goat's Milk

Goat's milk$^\triangle$ is easily digested, but it quickly deteriorates and becomes odoriferous. The main difference between goat's milk and cow's milk is in the fat and protein structure. Goat's milk contains only traces of the major protein of cow's milk. It is usually sold in an evaporated form packed in a can or dried.

Cream

Several forms of cream are commonly available. Half-and-half, by federal standards contains 10.5 to 18 percent fat, and light cream contains 18 to 30 percent fat. Light whipping cream contains 30 to 36 percent fat and heavy whipping cream contains 36 percent or more. "Coffee creams" are available as "no-fat half-and-half" and in a wide variety of flavored creamers.

Evaporated Milk

Evaporated milk is prepared by removing about 65 percent of the water from fresh whole milk. The milk-fat content is no less than 7.5 percent, and the milk-solid content is no less than 25.5 percent. Evaporated milk must contain 25 international units of vitamin D per ounce; the addition of vitamin A is optional. Evaporated low-fat and skim milks are also available, which are useful in reducing the amount of fat in the diet.

Sweetened Condensed Milk

Another type of milk used occasionally is sweetened condensed milk. This product is made from whole milk by removing about half the water and adding 40 percent sugar in the form of sucrose, dextrose, or corn syrup before evaporation takes place. The product contains not less than 7.5 percent milk fat and 25.5 percent total milk solids.

Yogurt

Yogurt△ is a cultured product that can be made from whole milk, low-fat milk with added milk solids, and skim milk with added milk solids. It is available plain or in flavors and with various levels of fat content. Because of the variation in yogurt composition, buyers should check local sources for product information and nutrient composition.

Sour Cream and Sour Half-and-Half

Sour cream and sour half-and-half are cultured milk products that can be used in foodservice operations. Cultured sour creams contain not less than 18 percent milk fat and cultured half-and-half about 12 percent milk fat. Sour half-and-half can be substituted for the richer product in most recipes and is less expensive.

Nonfat Dry Milk

Nonfat dry milk is economical for institutional use in cooked and baked products. Standards in the United States for grades of nonfat dry milk are U.S. Extra Grade and U.S. Standard Grade. Nonfat dry milk contains no more than 5 percent moisture and no more than 1.5 percent milk fat, unless otherwise specified. Instant nonfat dry milk, made by a special process that gives it improved solubility, is the most popular form. However, noninstant nonfat dry milk also is available and can be used satisfactorily in baked products when mixed with the dry ingredients. Fortification of nonfat dry milk with vitamins A and D is optional and, if desired, should be stated in the specification.

Dry Buttermilk

Dry buttermilk is another useful product for baking purposes. The grades for this product are the same as for nonfat dry milk. All dry milk products are made from pasteurized milk. Dry buttermilk is more stable than fresh buttermilk.

Other Types of Milk

Other types of milk△ are available in some markets. Most of these milks come from mammals native to a specific geographic location and include milk from camels, water buffalo, llamas, yak, and reindeer. These milks vary in tastes and nutrients and in some the fat content is higher than in cow's milk. Milk is also available from soy and almonds. Shelf-life milk is a good product to include for emergency supplies both as individual and larger servings.

Ice Cream

Federal standards for ice cream specify a minimum content of 10 percent milk fat and 20 percent milk solids. The quality of ice cream is related to its composition, the quality of its ingredients, the weight per gallon, and the quality and quantity of flavoring materials. Differences in these components influence the price of the various products and brands. Ice cream is available in a wide variety of forms suited to foodservice use, including such time-savers as individually wrapped slices and individual cups. Novelty items add variety to a menu.

Ice Milk and Sherbet

Ice milk, hardened or soft, is available in a wide variety of flavors. Ice milk contains at least 2 percent milk fat and 11 percent milk solids. Fruit sherbets contain a minimum of 1 percent milk fat and 2 percent milk solids. Because compositional requirements vary from state to state, food buyers must be familiar with state regulations.

Specifications for Milk and Milk Products

Written specifications for milk and other dairy products△ are just as important as specifications for other foods. Additions or deletions from the following sample specifications may be needed to suit particular situations:

- Milk, whole, homogenized, pasteurized, fortified with vitamins A and D, minimum 3.25 percent milk fat, half-pint cartons

- 2 percent reduced-fat milk, homogenized, pasteurized, minimum 2 percent milk fat, fortified with vitamins A and D, half-gallon cartons, priced by half gallon
- Buttermilk, cultured, homogenized, pasteurized, minimum 8.25 percent milk solids, quart cartons, added vitamins A and D, priced by carton
- Cream, half-and-half, pasteurized, 10.5 to 18 percent milk fat, pint cartons, priced by carton
- Milk, nonfat, dry, instant, U.S. Extra Grade, 5-pound bag, priced by bag
- Yogurt, nonfat, minimum 8.5 percent nonfat solids, 0.5 percent milk fat, plain-flavored, 8-ounce cartons, priced by case

NONDAIRY SUBSTITUTES FOR MILK AND CREAM

Cream substitutes, dessert toppings, and imitation milk are among a group of products developed as substitutes for dairy products. There are no compositional standards for these products, so food buyers must check the ingredient lists provided by the manufacturer. Some nondairy products, including many coffee whiteners, contain no milk or other dairy products and are available fresh or frozen in liquid or powdered form. Dessert toppings are marketed in pressurized containers and in powdered or frozen form. The stability of nondairy toppings and their low cost compared with dairy products have made them extremely popular for foodservice use.

Imitation milk, available in some states, can have utilitarian value for some modified diets. These products combine fats or oils other than milk fat with food solids but exclude milk solids. Sodium caseinate is frequently used as the protein source.

Cultured nondairy sour cream is another imitation dairy product. Lauric acid oils—including coconut oil, hydrogenated coconut oil, and palm kernel oil—are frequently used in this product. The manufacturer should be consulted for specific content information.

NATURAL, PROCESSED, AND IMITATION CHEESES

More than 2,000 varieties of cheeses are available that have tremendous potential for use in interesting menus and are a challenge to the food buyer. Making good cheese purchases requires a knowledge of the quality and flavor characteristics of each cheese and of the ways it can be used.

Natural cheeses are made from whole, partially defatted, or skim milk, depending on the variety of cheese. Federal standards of identity specifying the processing methods and setting minimum fat and maximum moisture contents have been established for the primary cheese varieties. *Cheese* is classified by origin, consistency, texture, color, shape, coating, flavor, basic ingredient, and normal ripening period.[△]

Varieties of Natural Cheese

Natural cheeses are classified into several groups by degree of hardness: soft, such as cottage cheese, ricotta, and cream cheese; semisoft, such as brick, Muenster, and mozzarella; hard, such as cheddar and Swiss; and very hard, such as Parmesan and Romano. Further distinctions are made on the basis of the organism (bacteria or mold) involved in the ripening process and the length of ripening or aging.

Cheddar Cheese

Cheddar is a whole-milk cheese that is perhaps the most popular of all the natural cheeses in the United States. Also known as American cheddar, it can be identified by its shape or style and classified as longhorn or daisy. In addition, it is often identified by the locale where it was produced, such as Wisconsin, Vermont, or New York. Standards for cheddar cheese specify a minimum of 50 percent milk-fat content and a maximum of 39 percent moisture by weight. The USDA grades for cheddar cheese—AA, A, B, and C—are based on the cheese's flavor, body, texture, color, and appearance. Some states also have their own grades.

Flavor terminology also is used to specify age of the cheese. As cheddar cheese ages, its flavor becomes sharper. The market flavors available are fresh or current; medium, mild, or mellow; aged or sharp; and very sharp. Aged cheddar melts faster and produces a smoother product than cheese less than three months old.

When purchasing cheddar cheese, the desired form and size should be specified: 20-, 40-, or 60-pound blocks; 12-pound cylindrical longhorns; 20-pound cylindrical daisies; 5- to 20-pound loaves; or any other size or form available from vendors. Sliced forms also are available. In addition, the desired degree of aging and USDA or state grade should be specified.

Swiss Cheese

Swiss cheese, produced from pasteurized whole and skim milk, has a lower fat content than cheddar cheese. Standards require a minimum of 43 percent milk fat and no more than 41 percent moisture. The characteristic holes, or "eyes," are formed when bacteria produce gas bubbles during the aging process. The activity of bacteria also creates the sweet, nutty flavor characteristic of Swiss cheese. USDA-graded Swiss cheese is available. Aging for three to nine months is typical, although the desired aging should be specified.

Cottage Cheese

Cottage cheese is the soft, uncured curd from pasteurized skim milk. Cream is added to the dry cheese curd to make creamed cottage cheese. The milk-fat content and moisture should not be less than 4 percent and 80 percent by weight, respectively, in the finished product. Creamed or dry cottage cheese comes in small curds, with particles about one-eighth to one-quarter inch in diameter, and in large curds, with particles up to three-eighths inch. Specifications for this product should state the curd size to be ordered. Cottage cheese is available in many container sizes, from 1 to 30 pounds. Because cottage cheese, particularly large-curd cottage cheese, has a limited shelf life once the container has been opened, the quantities served and how long a container lasts should be considered when purchasing the product.

Other Natural Cheeses

Because the variety of natural cheeses is so extensive, other specific types are not described here in detail; Table 17.5 gives examples of cheese classifications and describes the characteristics of commonly used cheeses. Except for mozzarella, federal grades and standards have not been established for most of the varieties listed. However, familiarity with the quality standards of various manufacturers and careful product evaluation will help food buyers select high-quality cheeses.

Processed Cheese

Pasteurized processed cheese is a blend of two or more varieties of the same cheese or two or more varieties of different cheeses, fresh

TABLE 17.5 Common Cheeses

Cheese	Description
American (pasteurized process)	Semisoft to soft; light yellow to orange; mild. Made of cow's milk (whole), cheddar, and/or Colby cheese.
Blue	Semisoft; white with blue-green mold; flavor similar to Roquefort. Made of cow's milk (whole).
Brick	Semisoft; smooth; light yellow to orange; flavor mild but pungent and sweet. Made of cow's milk (whole).
Brie	Soft; edible white crust; flavor resembles Camembert. Made of cow's milk (whole, low-fat, or skim).
Camembert	Soft; almost fluid; mild to pungent flavor. Made of cow's milk (whole).
Cheddar	Hard; smooth; light yellow to orange; mild to sharp. Made of cow's milk (whole).
Colby	Soft and more open in texture than cheddar; white to light yellow, orange mild. Made from cow's milk (whole).
Cottage	Soft; moist, delicate, large or small curd. Mildly acid flavor. Unripened; usually made of cow's milk (skim). Cream dressing may be added to cottage dry curd.
Cream	Soft; smooth; buttery; mild, slightly acid flavor. Unripened; made of cream and cow's milk (whole).
Edam	Semisoft to hard; rubbery; mild, sometimes salty flavor; cannonball shape. Made of cow's milk (low-fat).
Feta	Soft, flaky, white. Made from cow, sheep, or goat milk.
Gorgonzola	Semisoft, less moist than blue; marbled with blue-green mold; spicy flavor. Made of cow's milk (whole) or goat's milk or mixture of these.
Gouda	Hard; flavor like Edam. Made of cow's milk (low-fat).
Gruyère	Hard with tiny gas holes; mild sweet flavor. Made of cow's milk (whole).
Monterey Jack	Semisoft (whole milk), hard (low-fat or skim milk); smooth; mild to mellow. Made of cow's milk (whole, low-fat, or skim).
Limburger	Soft; strong, robust flavor, highly aromatic. Made of cow's milk (whole or low-fat).
Muenster	Semisoft; flavor between brick and Limburger. Made of cow's milk (whole).
Mozzarella	Semi soft, creamy white; may be molded into various shapes, Made of cow's milk whole or low fat.
Neufchâtel	Soft; creamy; white; mild flavor. Unripened or ripened 3 to 4 weeks. Made of cow's milk (whole or skim) or a mixture of milk and cream.
Parmesan	Very hard (grating) granular texture. Made of cow's milk (low fat).
Provolone	Hard, stringy texture; bland acid to sharp, usually smoked flavor; pear, sausage, or salami shaped. Made of cow's milk (whole).
Ricotta	Soft, moist, and grainy, dry. White, bland, but semisweet. Made from whey and whole or skim milk, or whole and low fat milk.
Romano	Very hard, brittle rind, granular interior, comes in various sizes, sharp, when aged piquant. Made from low fat cow's milk, goat milk, or a mixture of cow and goat milk.
Roquefort	Semisoft; white with blue-green mold; sharp, piquant flavor. Made of sheep's milk.
Stilton	Semisoft; white with blue-green mold; spicy but milder than Roquefort flavor. Made of cow's milk (whole with added cream).
Swiss	Hard with gas holes; mild, nutlike, sweet flavor. Made of cow's milk (low-fat).

and aged, which are heated to stop further ripening. The varieties are noted on the product's label. Emulsifying agents are added to yield a smooth texture and prevent separation. Because of the heating process, the texture and flavor of the cheese remain constant after processing.

Pasteurized processed cheese is similar to natural cheese, except that the former has a lower fat content, a higher moisture content, and added whey or milk solids. Other ingredients, such as sausage, vegetables, and nuts, are sometimes added. Processed cheese usually has a less-pronounced cheese flavor than natural cheese but melts more readily during cooking.

Pasteurized processed cheese spread has less fat and more moisture than the other products already described. It is soft and can be spread with a knife. A stabilizer is usually added to prevent separation of the ingredients. None of the processed cheese products are federally graded.

Imitation Cheese

The Filled Cheese Act of June 6, 1896, imposed a tax on cheese and licensed its manufacture and sale under special labeling and packaging procedures. Various states also imposed other restrictions that inhibited or discouraged the development of filled-cheese products. The Filled Cheese Act was repealed in October 1974. As a result, filled-cheese foods are now subject solely to the provisions of the Federal Food, Drug, and Cosmetic Act and the Fair Packaging and Labeling Act. Today, they move freely in interstate commerce as nonstandardized foods, but their sale is prohibited in some states.

At present, two types of imitation cheese are available to consumers, those made with skim milk plus vegetable fat and those made with calcium caseinate or sodium caseinate plus vegetable fat. Most of these products have the body, texture, and appearance of regular cheese, although some consumers find the flavor to be different. Cheese substitutes also are functionally equivalent to their natural cheese counterparts. Various convenient package sizes are available for foodservice use.

Cheese Specifications

Sample specifications[△] for cheese include:

- Cheese, American, processed, medium blend, pasteurized, six 5-pound blocks
- Cheese, cheddar, natural, U.S. Grade A, medium aged, six 5-pound blocks
- Cheese, mozzarella, part skim, low moisture, six 5-pound blocks
- Cheese, cottage, creamed, minimum of 2 percent milk fat by weight, maximum of 80 percent moisture, small curd, 5-pound container

Soy Protein

Soy protein isolate is the most refined form of soy protein, and is mainly used in meat products to improve texture and eating quality. Soy isolates contain about 90 percent protein. *Soy protein concrete*

is soybeans without water-soluble carbohydrates. It contains about 70 percent protein. *Textured soy protein* (TSP) is made of soy protein concentrate, giving it some texture. TSP is available in a variety of forms and contains about 70 percent protein.[△]

Soybeans belong to the legume family, containing no cholesterol, low in saturated fat, and the only vegetable protein that contains all eight essential amino acids. Soybeans are also a good source of fiber, iron, calcium, zinc, and B vitamins. Soy protein is used to replace animal proteins in individual diets.

Recent studies have shown an increased use in soy protein especially for individuals who are obese, have cardiac problems, cancer, and infants with lactase deficiency. Infant formulas must be coordinated with the pediatric physicians and the "house" formula. TSP products need to be kept on hand for persons on vegetarian diets and for others who desire this type of food. The best method to determine type, cost, and intended use of soy products is to discuss the products with a vendor, as well as reviewing trade magazines and evidence-based information. There are also a number of "soy only" companies that can offer assistance.

FRUITS AND VEGETABLES

A significant amount of information is needed to purchase fresh or processed fruits and vegetables. As with other food products, it is important to select the form (fresh, canned, or frozen), style, and quality best suited to the planned use. The *Blue Goose Purchasing Guide to Fresh Fruits and Vegetables* and *Produce 101* are excellent references for use in purchasing fresh produce. *Fruit* is defined as the edible portion of mature and flowering products of a tree or plant that contains ripened seeds and edible flesh, such as peaches. Many fruits are usually eaten raw but may also be cooked using a variety of preparation methods.[△]

Grades of Fruits and Vegetables

The USDA's Agricultural Marketing Service has developed quality grade standards for fruit and vegetable products. The grading of fresh, frozen, and canned fruits and vegetables is voluntary. Any grower, processor, or buyer who wants the product graded requests and pays for the grading service.

For wholesale purposes grading is important for pricing of fruit. The Agricultural Marketing Service of the USDA is responsible for the grading standards. These grades are:[△]

U.S. Fancy Premium produce
U.S. No. 1 Chief trading grade
U.S. No. 2 Intermediate quality grade
U.S. No. 3 Lowest commercially useful grade

The container containing federal grade will be marked with an official USDA grade shield or label stating, "Packed under continuous Inspection of the U.S. Department of Agriculture."

After a USDA inspector has graded the products, they can be labeled with the U.S. grade name. When a product is labeled with one of the official grade names, such as Fancy, but without the prefix "U.S.," that product still must meet the USDA's standard for the grade, whether or not it has actually been inspected.

Although most fresh fruits and vegetables are sold wholesale on the basis of U.S. grades, not many are marked with the grade when they are resold. The typical range of grades for fresh fruits and vegetables includes U.S. Fancy, U.S. No. 1, and U.S. No. 2. For some products, there are grades above and below this range.

Grades for canned and frozen fruits and vegetables packed under continuous USDA inspection bear the U.S. grade: U.S. Grade A (Fancy), U.S. Grade B (Choice for fruits and Extra Standard for vegetables), and U.S. Grade C (Standard). Grade A fruits and vegetables are the most tender, succulent, and uniform in size, shape, and color. Grade B is good quality, but Grade B fruits and vegetables may be slightly less uniform in size and color, and the products may have a few blemishes. Grade B fruits usually are packed in heavy syrup. Grade C products are of good quality, just as wholesome and nutritious as the higher grades, and they may be the best buy for use in combination recipes when appearance is not important. Grade C fruits are mature and usually are packed in light syrup. Grade C fruits also are used in most water-packed and low-calorie fruit products.

Most processors and distributors have their own quality control programs and quality designations, whether they use USDA's grading service, and most pack more than one grade of product. Food buyers should be aware of the various quality designations used by the processors and distributors in their areas.

Net Weights of Canned Fruits and Vegetables

Various federal and state laws require that a statement of net quantity appear on the label of canned fruits and vegetables. However, none of these laws specifies what the labeled weight or volume should be for these products. The fill, which affects the net weight or volume, varies with each product, but cans must be as full as practical, usually about 90 percent.

Classification of Vegetables

The classification of vegetables is by a specific part of the plant, as follows:△

Classification	Example
Roots	Carrots, radishes, beets
Bulbs	Onion, garlic
Tubers	Sweet and white potatoes
Leafy	Lettuce, spinach, and most greens
Stems	Celery
Flowers	Broccoli
Fruit	Squash, cucumbers
Seeds	Peas, beans

Exotic Vegetables

Exotic vegetables are being added to menus due to the cultural diversity of the population, worldwide business, and worldwide travel. Some of these vegetables and some origins are listed here.

- Bamboo shoots
- Watercress
- Artichokes
- Bean sprouts
- Escarole
- Chicory
- Bok choy
- Swiss chard
- Sorrel leaves
- Daikon (Japanese radish)
- Fava beans
- Kohlrabi
- Soybeans
- Rutabagas
- Chiles (hot peppers)
- Water chestnuts (used in Asian cooking)
- Taro root (China and Hawaii; used in poi)
- Apio
- Nopales (cactus pads)
- Malanga (yautia; tubular tropical plant)
- Jicama (similar to potato)
- Squash (Cocozelle, Turk's turban, spaghetti, banana)
- Tomatillo ("little tomato"; Mexico)
- Chinese snow peas
- Cassava (also called yucca; native of South America)
- Noni (Indian Mulberry; Polynesian; used for medicinal purposes; called a "gift from God")

Consideration in Buying Fruits and Vegetables

The intended use of fruits and vegetables and the size of the container to select should be considered before fruits and vegetables are ordered for use in the foodservice department. These two considerations are discussed next.

Intended Use

The customer makeup of the area served and the intended use△ of a product determines which product style to buy, and the product style affects the cost of fruits and vegetables. Canned whole fruits and vegetables usually cost more than cut styles but should be used when appearance is important. Short cuts, dices, and vegetable pieces are the least expensive and are good for use in soups and stews. Less-perfect fruits can be chosen for cooked desserts and mixed salads when appearance is not important.

When fresh fruits and vegetables are purchased, the quality, variety, and size of the produce needed should be considered. For some fresh items, the labor and waste involved in trimming and preparation should be considered. For example, fresh broccoli requires some preparation time, and some net loss occurs from trimming stems and cutting bunches into uniform serving sizes. Apples purchased for eating raw are different in variety and size from those purchased for cooking.

Container Size

The container size△ selected can affect cost, quality of food, and ease of handling. Using large containers can involve a lower cost per serving if the quantity of food they contain can be used while the food is at peak quality. If purchased in too large a unit, some food may have to be discarded due to staleness or spoilage, thus increasing food costs.

The No. 10 can, packed six per case, is the most common packing container for canned fruits and vegetables. It weighs 6 pounds and 9 ounces or 3 quarts or 12 cups. A 46-ounce can, sometime referred as a *3CYl*, holds approximately 1 quart 14 fluid ounces or 5¾ cups and used for juices. For items used in smaller quantities, such as some modified foods, No. 303 cans, packed 24 per case, may be a better purchase size. A 303 can weighs approximately 1 pound, or 15 fluid ounces and holds 2 cups. There are other container sizes that may be used, such as a No. 2½, weight of 1 pound 13 ounces or one pint, 10 fluid ounces or approximately 3½ cups.

Frozen vegetables are most commonly found in 2- or 2½-pound packages and are packed 12 per case. However, some are available in 20-, 30-, and 50-pound packages.

As stated earlier, the acronym IQF used in relation to frozen fruits and vegetables means individually quick-frozen. Pieces of the product are frozen separately and then packed loosely so that the right amount of product can be measured without having to thaw the whole package. Generally, IQF fruits and vegetables are available in 2½-pound packages and in 20-pound polybags; sometimes they are available in larger quantities.

Fresh fruits and vegetables are usually purchased by weight, but in some cases the count per shipping container also should be specified. Many different sizes of cartons, boxes, and other shipping containers are used for fresh produce, depending on the type of product and where it is produced. A list of common container sizes for fresh fruits and vegetables is available from the United Fresh Fruit and Vegetable Association in Washington, DC.△

To retain their color and flavor, many fruits are packed in sugar syrup. Because fruit-to-sugar ratios vary, suppliers should be consulted for specific information.

All fruits including bananas, citrus, and especially all melons should be thoroughly washed before being served.△ Browning of the cut surface of some raw fruits such as apples, peaches, and bananas, is due to oxidation.

Various Types of Vegetables

Vegetables are the edible portion of plants. They may serve as a main dish; salad when mixed with other vegetables, meat, cheese, or fruits; snacks; or accompanying an entrée. Vegetables are seasonal but are usually available year-round through imports. Vegetables are a good source of carbohydrates, fiber, and vitamins and add color to menus. The My Plate suggests that the daily intake of vegetables should be three to five servings per day. Vegetables should always be cleaned before eating or cooking. They should never be overcooked.△ A limited list of vegetables follows.

Beans

Beans are available in many varieties. Green, snap, and wax beans are slender and snap easily. Overly mature pods contain large beans. Beans may be purchased frozen, fresh, canned, whole, cut, and julienne (French cut).

Broccoli

Broccoli is the number-one choice of vegetables. Broccoli should be firm, dark green, and have compact bud clusters. Stalks, branches, and buds are eaten. It is a healthy food. It may be purchased frozen, fresh, chopped, whole, or florets or mixed with other vegetables such as cauliflower.

Cabbage

Many varieties of cabbages are available—green, crinkle leaf, red, Chinese—but a common factor of quality includes solid, heavy heads (just how solid depends on the variety). The color should be typical for the variety, without yellow or wilted leaves (which indicate age). Heavy outside leaves should be trimmed back. The stem end should be dry. Broken or burst heads and excessive softness indicate poor quality. Cabbage may be cooked or served raw. Cooked cabbage does not freeze well, but it can be frozen raw. Cabbage is purchased by the pound. The weight of a head varies with the variety; 2 to 5 pounds is the best institutional size, with 3 pounds being ideal in some varieties. Sauerkraut is processed cabbage. Cabbage may be purchased in airtight bags—shredded (for coleslaw), chopped. Bag should be stamped with a "use by date."

Carrots

Carrots are available year-round. For institutional use, carrots should be bought with the tops cut back to less than 1 inch. Carrots should be at least 3 inches long and have blunt ends (tapering carrots have high peeling loss). Diameters should not be less than three-quarter inch or more than 2 inches. Miniature carrots often called *Belgium carrots* and are an excellent item. They can be purchased raw—ready to eat—or canned. Raw carrots may also be shredded, chopped, and sealed in an airtight bag stamped with "use by date." Carrots may also be used in cakes and salads.

Celery

Celery, mainly the Pascal variety, is available all year. Clean, brittle stalks and bright green leaves indicate good quality. Celery should be about 16 inches long and have straight, well-bunched stalks. A bunch of celery is made up of all the stalks. The best size for institutions is 1- to 1¾-pound bunches. U.S. No. 1 is the grade for institutional use and is the equivalent of U.S. Grade A for the consumer market. It may be served cooked or raw. Celery is especially good when mixed with other dishes.

Corn

Corn may be yellow or white; most commercial varieties are yellow. Fresh corn should have rounded, bright plump kernels and a fresh greenish husk. Corn may be fresh, frozen, or canned. Fresh corn, with a small amount of husk to cover the kernels, is excellent when cooked in a microwave oven. Hominy is another form of corn.

Cucumbers

Good-quality cucumbers are crisp, have a good even shape, and are of medium size (2½ inches in diameter and 5 or 6 inches long). A bushel weighs about 48 pounds. Cucumbers are usually served raw in salads and sandwiches.

Greens

Many varieties of greens are available: spinach, turnip, collards, Swiss chard, mustard, kale, beet tops, endive, and dandelion. Greens should be tender, young, crisp, green, and free of blemishes. They may be served raw or cooked. They may be fresh, frozen, or canned. When purchasing fresh they must be cleaned. Many raw greens are available already cleaned and ready for used. Varieties may be mixed to cook.

Legumes

Legumes include black-eyed peas, kidney beans, lentils, limas, navy beans, Northern beans, garbanzo beans, red beans, soybeans, and split peas. They contain a high level of incomplete protein and are used heavily by vegetarians. Legumes are available dry, fresh, frozen, and canned.

Lettuce

Lettuce is available in several varieties: iceberg, or crisp head; Boston, or butter head; Bibb; cos, or romaine; leaf, or bunching; and stem. Lettuce is in good supply throughout the year in most places. Lettuce leaves should be bright, fresh, and clean. The head should be large and well packed for variety. "Well-trimmed" means that no more than three wrapper leaves remain, none of which is large or coarse.

Lettuce can also be purchased chopped or shredded in various sizes and packaged in airtight bags with a "use by" date on the bag.

Onions

Onion varieties include yellow (Spanish), white, green, and red. They have a strong flavor. Newer varieties called sweet, Texas, and Vidalia are milder than Spanish onions. Onions may be purchased raw—chopped, shredded, sealed in a bag with a date stamped with a "use by date." Onions may be served raw, cooked, or in combination. They are available dry, frozen, and fresh.

Potatoes

Potatoes are the most commonly eaten vegetable in the United States. They are available in white, red, yellow, and russet varieties.

They should be smooth, well shaped, and firm. They may be purchased canned, fresh, frozen, or dehydrated. Raw potatoes may be purchased as whole, shredded, diced, and so forth. Examine bags for discoloring and blemishes. There should be a "Use by date" stamped on the bag. Potatoes may be fried, boiled, baked, mashed, and so forth.

Sweet Potatoes or Yams

Yams are moister and sweeter than sweet potatoes and are orange to copper color. Sweet potatoes are light yellow and dry and mealy inside. Both are available fresh, canned, frozen, and dehydrated. They may be baked, boiled, fried, or candied. They can be used in pies, custards, cakes, cookies, or as a starch for a menu item.

Real yams are starchy, tuberous roots of several tropical, climbing plants of the yam family (genus Dioscorea) and are widely grown in the tropics for food. A moist, orange variety of sweet potato is frequently called a *yam* in the United States.

Tomatoes

Tomatoes are highly perishable. Vine-ripened tomatoes, for example, are generally available only in the locality where they are grown, unless the new "hard" tomato is available (developed at the University of Florida). Thus, tomatoes for shipping to distant markets are picked before they are fully ripe and then are ripened under artificial conditions (in much the same way as bananas). The best-quality tomatoes are fully ripened on the vine before harvesting. The sizes of tomatoes are small (less than 3 ounces), medium (3 to 6 ounces), large (6 to 10 ounces), and very large (more than 10 ounces). Tomatoes are mostly marketed in lugs that contain 30 to 32 pounds.

Other Frequently Used Vegetables

Bell peppers are green, yellow, or red. They are available year-round and are an excellent source of vitamin C. They can be purchased raw and frozen—the frozen variety is best used in cooked foods.

Asparagus may be green or white, green grown commercially and must be kept cold after harvesting or it will deteriorate rapidly. Asparagus is expensive and be canned, fresh, or frozen.

Botanical Types of Fruits

Fruits are classified by botanical type and include:

Type	Example
Dupes	Smooth skin, simple seed surrounded by edible flesh (peaches apricots, plums, nectarines, and cherries)
Pomes	Smooth skin covering an enlarged fleshy area, which surrounds a central core containing seeds (apples, pears, and quinces)
Berries	Succulent and pulpy, embedded with tiny seeds (strawberries, raspberries, blackberries, cranberries, loganberries, huckleberries, gooseberries, and grapes)

Type	Example
Citrus	Enclosed in skin of various thickness and relatively smooth surfaces (oranges, lemons, limes, tangerines, kumquat, citron, mandarin oranges, and grapefruit)
Melons	Rough or smooth outer skin, fleshy, contains seeds (watermelons, casaba, cantaloupe, honeydew, Crenshaw, Persian)
Tropical fruit	Grown in the tropics (bananas, plantain, pineapple, avocado, fig, dates, mango, papaya, pomegranate, kiwifruit)

Types of Fruits

Fruits are a seasonal item, but because of imports they are usually available fresh year-round. Fruits are grown on bushes and trees, with the exception of grapes and melons that grow on vines. Fruit may be purchased fresh, frozen, dried, and canned. Fresh fruits are usually purchased "in season." Fruits add carbohydrates, fiber, and color to menus. My Plate food guide recommends that four servings of fruits should be eaten each day. Fruits may be used to accompany an entrée, as a dessert, snack, or when mixed with other ingredients, as a salad.△ Bananas are the most commonly eaten fruit in the United States. The following is a list of the more poplar fruits and is not all-inclusive for each fruit.

Apples

Most apples are picked and stored so that fresh apples are available year-round. Apples that are in season and harvested in the fall and winter have the best keeping qualities.

There are more than 28 varieties of apples. Different varieties are suitable for different uses (Table 17.6). Apples to be eaten raw should be crisp, juicy, and have moderate to low acidity and high sweetness. When baked, a good baking apple is soft, moist, firmly textured, with a skin that will hold the apple's shape. Some apple

TABLE 17.6   Apple Varieties

Variety	Season	Raw	Cooking
Baldwin	Oct. to Mar.	Fair	Good for all
Cortland	Oct. to Feb.	Good	Good for all
Delicious, red	Sept. to Apr.	Excellent	Poor for all
Delicious, golden	Sept. to Mar.	Excellent	Poor for all
Jonathan	Oct. to Feb.	Excellent	Good for all (not baked)
McIntosh	Oct. to Apr.	Excellent	Good for all
Rome Beauty	Nov. to Mar.	Good	Excellent, especially baked
Stayman	Dec. to Apr.	Good	Good for all
Winesap	Dec. to May	Excellent	Excellent for pies
York Imperial	Oct. to Mar.	Excellent	Poor for all

varieties are more suitable for applesauce or for pies than others, although canned apples are now being used for these purposes in many foodservices.

Size is another factor that affects raw apples. It may be stated as count (the lower the count, the larger the apple and the fewer there are in a box or case). Size is also stated by diameter, which ranges from 1¼ to 3¾ inches. The best all-round size is 2½ inches (113 count, or medium-size). Peeling loss is about 25 percent.

Color is a factor in grading and depends on the variety.

Apples may be fresh, canned, dried, or frozen. They may be used as a dessert, in pies cakes, cookies salads, juice, and in combination with other fruits, vegetables, or meats. Many apples are being imported from New Zealand, Chile, and other countries. Many apples are produced in Washington and North Carolina. The wax coating on apples and other fruits is a protective coating to reduce moisture loss to protect against shriveling and against decay. The coating extends the quality of the fruit. Wash apples before using.

Bananas

Bananas must be picked and shipped green to develop proper flavor. Ripening is accomplished in special rooms with controlled temperature and humidity. Fast ripening takes place in 3 to 4 days, medium in 5 to 7 days, and slow in 8 to 10 days. "Hand ripe" means the skin is a bright yellow color with no trace of brown. The fruit is firmly textured and slightly astringent in flavor. Bananas need approximately three days at room temperature to ripen. "Turning ripe" means the skin is pale, the tips are green, and it has little, but sharply astringent, flavor. These need five to six days to ripen at room temperature. About three medium-size bananas make up a pound. Peeling loss averages about 33 percent. Bananas may be eaten raw at any meal, as well as baked in pies, cakes, and breads. They should be washed before using.

Berries

Berries are the most delicate of fruits. They may be served raw, as juices, or in cakes, pies, jams, and jellies. Berries include strawberries, blueberries, raspberries, blackberries, and huckleberries. Seasons vary, but due to imports berries are usually available all year. They can be fresh, frozen, or canned. Grapes may be dried to raisins. Grapes may be purchased by the bunch in a lug. Wash before using.

Melons

Slightly larger than an average cantaloupe, honeydew melons weigh 6 to 6½ pounds. Signs of maturity are referred to as full-slip, with softening at the blossom end, and a typical odor. (A sour odor indicates overripeness and spoilage.) There are three stages of full-slip, depending on the degree of ripeness (and the color of the skin). If the stem is still partially attached, it is called half-slip. If the stem does not come free from the fruit, the melon was green when it was picked. The flesh is a delicate greenish white. It is excellent with lime juice sprayed over cut surfaces. Honeydew melon may be served at breakfast, as a dessert, or in combination. It may be frozen. It should be washed before slicing.

The peak season for cantaloupes is from July to October. Cantaloupes picked at the "full-slip" stage of maturity show a clean tear at the stem end. Cantaloupes average 12 ounces to 4 pounds in weight. Those 5 inches in diameter weigh 20 to 24 ounces each.

Other melons are muskmelon, Crenshaw, casaba, and Persian. Casaba has soft, yellowish white flesh. The Crenshaw melon is a cross between the casaba and Persian melons; it is salmon-color inside and has a rich flavor. Wash all melons before cutting.

Oranges and Other Citrus

Most citrus fruits are picked before they are ripe. Orange coloring may be added to the rind; citrus may be purchased fresh, canned, or frozen. It is best when packed in its own juice. The two most common types of oranges in the United States are Valencias and navels. Valencias are most often used as juice; the navels are ready-to-eat. Navels are orange in color; the bottom is the "beginning of an orange within an orange." It is seedless, easily peeled, and sectioned. Citrus fruit is high in vitamin C. It includes oranges, grapefruit, tangerines/tangelos, lemons, limes, and mandarin oranges. Oranges and grapefruit are often served as juice. Recent studies have shown that using grapefruit products interferes with certain medications. Some health care facilities have eliminated grapefruit products from menus and will only serve them if it can be verified that the customer is not taking one of the medicines. Peak season is from late October until March. Lemons are available all year and usually come from Arizona and California. They are used in drinks, pies, cakes, and teas, and may be added to some cut fruit to prevent browning. Limes are similar to lemons and are used in the same manner. Limes are green and lemons are yellow. Limes are not as shelf-stable as lemons. All citrus should be washed before using for food preparation or serving.

Peaches

Peaches are highly perishable and cannot be shipped fully ripe. They are picked before maturity and should be selected on the basis of plumpness, color, and firmness of flesh. Well-known varieties are Elberta, Golden Jubilee, and Hall. Some peaches have white flesh. As with all fruit, they should be washed before using.

Pears

Pears are picked when slightly immature. The color of the skin and the softness of the flesh indicate full ripeness. They can be stored for long periods at 30°F to 32°F. They will ripen in three to five days at 60°F to 65°F. Pears are sized in counts; the best size for institutional use is 110 to 135 per case. Some varieties of pears mature during summer, others during winter (Anjou, Comice, and Winter Nellis). They should be washed before using.

Pineapples

Pineapples are mild-flavored sweet tropical fruits that are available year-round. They may be canned or fresh. Canned pineapple is available sliced, crushed, cubed, as spears, or as juice. The fruit is best when it is packed in its own natural juice. The interior fruit is yellow. It may be used in salads, cakes, pies, sauces, and in combination dishes.

Watermelon

U.S.-grown watermelons are on the market from June to September, their fresh attractive appearance and symmetrical shape identifying mature watermelons. The color should be typical for the variety, but the lower side should be yellowish. There should be a bloom over the cut surface, giving it a velvety look. A hard white streak through the length of the red-to-pink interior flesh is known as *white heart*. This indicates poor quality, but it cannot be detected until cutting. The best weight for institutional use is about 28 pounds. It can be used for dessert or in combination. It does not freeze well. Wash before cutting.

Other Important Fruit

Even though some people think of **avocado** as a vegetable, it is a fruit. (The best way to determine a fruit or vegetable is that if the product continues to ripen after it is picked it is a fruit.) Avocados are highly perishable. There are two kinds—the California variety (Hass)—with a thick, pebbled skin that changes from green to purplish-black as it ripens. It may weigh a half-pound. The other variety is from Florida and contains less fat and is larger than the Hass avocado.

Cherries Cherries may be sweet or sour; they may be black (Bing), red, or light white sweet cherries (Rainer cherries, which are the most expensive; with a light skin, any sign of bruising is noticeable). The black Bing cherries are round with an extra-sweet taste. The inside flesh is reddish-purple and is usually black when completely ripe. Most Bing cherries come from Washington and are available from May to August. Some black cherries may be available in the fall and winter but these are imported. Wash before eating. The maraschino cherry is made from Royal Ann cherries. Coloring is added and the seed removed before packaging.

Plums Most plums come from California. There are more than 100 varieties of plums; the most popular are black, red, green, or Japanese or European variety. The Japanese types are red or black with a juicy yellow or reddish flesh and are eaten raw. The European types are blue or purple with a golden flesh and are either cooked or dried, the dried being called prunes. Wash before eating the fruit raw or preparing to cook.

Kiwi Fruit Kiwi fruit comes from New Zealand. It is fuzzy brown on the outside and green with black seeds inside. It is excellent eaten raw and a great addition to fruit salads.

Mangoes Mangoes are a popular fruit that comes Mexico, Florida, Haiti, South and Central America. They have an orange flesh that may be eaten raw or dried. Gently wash before eating. Dried ones are excellent snacks.

Dried Fruits

Dried fruits are firm and bright in color. Drying reduces the fruit's moisture. Adding sulfur dioxide during drying prevents discoloration. Commonly dried fruits are raisins or dried grapes (they may be dark or light, seedless or seeded), prunes or dried plums, apricots, dates, apples, peaches, pears, and pineapples. Raisins, dates, and prunes are the most commonly used dried fruits. Dried fruits are usually soaked in water and then simmered in water for cooking; sugar and spices may be added. They may be used in salads (raisins, dates), breads, cakes, compotes, pies, muffins, and puddings, or eaten as is.

Exotic Fruits

As mentioned earlier for "Exotic Vegetables," many *exotic fruits* are available for health care menus. Such fruit as kiwi fruit, carambola (star fruit), guava, plantain, lychee, and UGLI[R] fruit add color and taste to fruit salads or as a garnish. These fruits are tropical, with guava coming from Mexico and South America and UGLI[R] from Jamaica. In addition to these more commonly used exotic fruits, the following are gaining a foothold in the United States. Most of these seven fruits are considered tropical.

1. **Rambutan**: Native of Malay, Southeast Asia—resembles Lychees—popular garden fruit—fruit is sweet and juicy and used in jams.
2. **Jackfruit**: Native to southwestern India, Bangladesh, Philippines, and Sri Lanka—one of the largest tree-borne fruits in the world—juice around the seeds taste similar to pineapple, but are milder and may be canned or made into chips.
3. **Passion fruit**: Native of South America, grown in India, New Zealand—soft juicy interior full of seeds—used in other juices to enhance flavor. There are two types: one gold and one purple.
4. **Kumquat**: Native of China—related to the citrus family—eaten raw.
5. **Dragon fruit**: Native to Mexico, Central and South America-fruit from several cactus species—sweet delicate taste and creamy pulp—can be made into wine or juice, flowers are eaten or used for tea.
6. **Guava**—Native to Mexico and Central America—contains as many as 535 seeds.
7. **Rose apple**: South Asia—smells and tastes a lot like roses. They spoil very quickly after being picked and therefore are rarely found in markets around the world. Rose apples can be eaten raw or boiled in water to make rose water. All fruits should be washed before eating or preparing for cooking.

Grading Fruit

Fruits are graded as follows:[Δ]

- Canned fruits:
  U.S. Grade A or U.S. Fancy
  U.S. Grade B or U.S. Choice
  U.S. Grade C or U.S. Standard
- Frozen fruits:
  Grade A or Fancy
- Fresh fruits:
  U.S. Fancy
  U.S. No. 1
  U.S. Extra No. 1
  U.S. No. 2
  U.S. combination

Fruit and Vegetable Specifications

Specifications for fresh, frozen, and canned fruits and vegetables should include the following information:[Δ]

- Name of product
- Style or type of product (whole, cut, trimmed, and so forth)
- USDA grade, brand, or other quality designation
- Size of container or shipping container
- Quantity or weight per shipping unit
- Other pertinent factors, depending on the product (packing medium, syrup density, variety, stage of maturity, drained weight, and so forth)

Specifications for fruit and vegetable products should be based on the quality and type of product needed in a particular operation. Some sample specifications for fruit and vegetable products follow:

- Bananas, fresh, No. 1, green tip, six 8-inch, 40-pound carton
- Fruit cocktail, canned, U.S. Grade A (Fancy), heavy syrup, minimum drained weight 72 ounces, six No. 10 cans per case
- Blueberries, frozen, whole, U.S. Grade A, IQF, 20-pound box
- Cabbage, fresh, green, U.S. No. 1, 11/2- to 2-pound heads, 50-pound mesh sack
- Corn, canned, yellow, whole kernel, U.S. Grade A (Fancy), vacuum packed, minimum drained weight of 70 ounces, six No. 10 cans per case
- Broccoli, frozen whole spears, U.S. Grade A, 12 2-pound packages per case

Dehydrated Fruits and Vegetables

Sun-dried dehydrated fruits and vegetables have been available to U.S. consumers for many years. Today, freeze-drying, dehydration, and vacuum drying are used. Sulfur oxide fumes are used in drying some fruits, especially orange colored, to preserve the color. Dried fruit should be firm but pliable. More and more dehydrated products, particularly potatoes, are used in foodservice operations. Two basic types of dehydrated products are available: regular moisture and low moisture. Regular-moisture products contain 18 to 20 percent of the food's original moisture. Apples, apricots, raisins, dates, cranberries, guava, peaches, and prunes are available in this form. Low-moisture dehydrated products contain only 2.5 to 5 percent moisture; these foods are less perishable. Onions, parsley, green peppers, potatoes, garlic, and many other vegetables are sold in this form.

Two processing methods for drying foods are used. In warm, dry areas of the country, fruits are dried in the sun. In colder climates, foods are dried by vacuum dehydration, a process that involves vacuum chambers and exposure to dry, warm inert gas.

Federal standards of quality exist for nearly all dried and low-moisture fruits. These standards are U.S. grades A, B, and C. No standards are available for low-moisture vegetables except for dried legumes (beans, peas, and lentils). Nearly all peas and lentils and about a third of all beans are officially inspected before or after processing, even though retail packages seldom carry the federal or state grade stamp.

The USDA grades for dried legumes are generally based on the food's shape, size, and color and on the presence or absence of foreign material. State grades are based on quality factors similar to those for federal grades. The low grades usually contain more foreign material and more kernels of uneven size and nonstandard color. The high grades are U.S. No. 1 for dry, whole, or split peas, lentils, and black-eyed peas. USDA No. 1 Choice Handpicked or simply handpicked are the high grades for Great Northern, pinto, and pea beans. U.S. Extra No. 1 is the high grade for lima beans, large and small.

The specifications for dehydrated fruits and vegetables should call for a clean product that has been prepared and packed under sanitary conditions. The product should have a bright color and good aroma.

Specifications for dehydrated potatoes should include the style required: flaked, granulated, sliced, or diced or many additional products that have been added such as garlic, parsley, and cheese. In addition, it should be specified when instant mashed-potato products are to include dry milk, vitamin C, or both. Other important considerations are the quality and yield of instant dehydrated potatoes. The actual number of pounds the product yields in the reconstituted state should be checked against the yield given on the label. Cooking a sample of dehydrated potato products is the best way to check their quality.

Some sample specifications for dehydrated foods follow:

- Potatoes, red bliss, sliced with some skin in place (cross-sliced one-eighth-inch thick), dehydrated, maximum of 7 percent moisture, four 5-pound bags per case
- Potatoes, instant, granules, without milk, Fancy, six 10-pound bags per case
- Beans, dry, navy, U.S. Grade No. 1, 25-pound bag
- Peas, dry, split, green, U.S. Grade No. 1, 25-pound bag
- Raisins, processed, Thompson seedless, natural, U.S. Grade A, small, 30-pound box

FATS AND OILS

Foodservice operations use several kinds of shortening and oil products. Manufacturers offer specific products for baking, frying, and general cooking purposes.

Animal Fat—Lard

Lard$^\triangle$ is fat rendered from hogs. Its quality varies according to its color, texture, and flavor. The shortening ability and texture of lard are well suited for use in pastry. However, ordinary *leaf lard* is not satisfactory for frying because its smoking point is lower than that of vegetable oils. Hydrogenated lard is of higher quality and has a higher smoking point than leaf lard. Blends of lard and tallow (rendered from cattle and sheep) are marketed, as well as blends of meat fat and vegetable shortenings. These products are suitable for most general cooking purposes. Also available are hydrogenated meat-fat shortenings that are designed for stability in deep-fat frying. Lard is rarely used in health care foodservice operations. Lard can become rancid and have a strong odor. Lard should be stored in the refrigerator.

Animal Fat—Butter

Butter is made by churning milk and cream until the cream breaks into fat particles. For commercial use pasteurized milk and sweet or sour cream are used. It can be sour creamed or lactic acid bacteria may be added to the sweet cream. Color can be added to give the product a yellow color. Once the butter has been removed the left-over product is buttermilk. The butter is removed, washed, salted, and is worked to remove excess buttermilk. Some butter does not have added salt and is referred as *sweet butter*. **Butter by law must contain no less than 80 percent milk.**

Butter grades have been established the USDA. There are four grades for butter based on quality scores: with taste and smell accounting for the majority of the score, the rest of the score includes body, color, and salt.

The grades, based on a numerical point system, are Grade AA 93 score, Grade A 92 score, Grade B 90 score, and Grade C 82 score.

For food production butter is usually purchased in 5-pound cartons. Butter is also sold by quarter pound, pound, and patties. Patties are sold 72 to 90 per pound in 5-pound cartons. Each patty is individually wrapped in foil, or in small cups with covers. Butter may also be sold whipped form. The quality desired, style, number of chips per pound, and total weight of the container should be included in a specification for butter.$^\triangle$

Trans Fats and Hydrogenated Shortenings

Trans fat is made when manufacturers add hydrogen to vegetable oil through a process called *hydrogenation*.$^\triangle$ Hydrogenation increases the shelf life and flavor stability of foods containing these fats. Trans fat is found in vegetable shortening, some margarines, crackers, cookies, snack foods, and other foods made with or fried in partially hydrogenated oils. Unlike other fats, most trans fat is formed when manufacturers turn liquid oils into solid fats like shortening and hard margarine. A small amount of trans fat is found naturally, primarily in dairy products, some meats, and other animal-based foods. Trans fats must be listed on the label of contents.

Hydrogenated vegetable shortenings can be used for many food production purposes. The process of hydrogenation changes vegetable oils from liquid form to a solid form that is creamy and plastic at room temperature. Fully hydrogenated vegetable shortening is used in baking—especially crackers and cookies—grilling, and other cooking operations. Commercial shortenings, for the most part, are mixtures of unsaturated (monounsaturated and polyunsaturated) and saturated fatty acids combined with glycerol. Unsaturated fats are beneficial when consumed in moderation, but saturated and trans fats are not.

Vegetable Oils

Vegetable oils△ for general and specialized uses include those from a single source and blends of several different vegetable oils. Monounsaturated fats include olive and canola oil. The most widely used vegetable oils are those from corn, cottonseed, soybeans, olives, and peanuts. Corn, sunflower, and safflower oils are polyunsaturated, are more unsaturated than the other common oils, and therefore are being incorporated into many new products. Most vegetable oils are deodorized, bleached, and clarified for use in foods, but any of these processes may be omitted in the making of specialized oils. The quality of vegetable oils can deteriorate from exposure to air, light, and moisture. Oils also can become cloudy under cold conditions if they have not been winterized, a process that keeps them clear at refrigerator temperatures. Cooking oils not processed in this way become solids at low temperatures.

Olive Oil

Olive oil△ is made from only the green olive fruit. Olive oil may be made by the pressure applied by hand to produce oil; this method produces a small amount of oil from olive paste. This method is called *cold pressing*. Due to demand and to extract more oil hot water was applied to the olive paste to improve the flow of oil. This is method is called *first pressing*.

There are a number of types of olive oil. The color, consistency, and flavor vary. This is usually due to geographic area where the olive was raised, difference in varieties, and weather conditions. The types include:

- *Extra virgin oil:* Made through the cold pressing method, has less than 1 percent acidity
- *Virgin olive oil:* Made from olives riper than those used in extra-virgin oil, produced in the cold pressing method, and has a higher acidity level of 1½ percent acidity
- *Refined olive oil:* Made by refining the virgin olive oil, tasteless, off-flavor, unpleasant odor, and an acidity level of 3.3 percent
- *Pure olive oil:* Comes from either the second cold pressing or chemical extraction of the olive mash left over from the first cold pressing, lighter in color, bland taste, an all-purpose oil with no nonolive oil mixed in.

Oils and Shortening for Deep-Fat Frying

Shortenings and oils that were specifically designed for good performance in deep-fat frying are best for foodservice use. Oils with high smoking points are needed to help prevent fat break-down. A minimum smoke point of not less than 426°F should be specified.

Fat and Oil Specifications

Before products for deep-fat frying, baking, and general-purpose cooking are purchased, detailed information about their ingredients and performance should be obtained from their manufacturers. Specifications for these products may be similar to the following:△

- Oil, mixed (cottonseed, soybean, and corn), 5-gallon container
- Shortening, all vegetable, high ratio, no trans fat, must not be partially hydrogenated or fractionated, 50-pound container
- Shortening, all vegetable, all purpose (smoking point 435°F [223°C]), no trans or saturated fats, 50-pound container
- Shortening, liquid, all vegetable with stabilizer, contains no trans fat (smoking point 440°F [227°C]), three 10-quart, six 5-quart, or six 1-gallon containers per case

Margarine

Margarine is manufactured under federal standards of identity and must contain 80 percent fat, 1 percent milk products, 9,000 international units of vitamin A, and not more than 15 percent moisture and 4 percent salt. The kinds of fat used in the manufacture of margarine must be listed on the label. Soybean and cottonseed oils are the primary ingredients. Margarine may be made from partially hydrogenated vegetable oils as well as saturated fats. Margarine should be purchased without trans fats and saturated fats. Choose soft margarines (liquid, tub, or spray) because they contain less saturated and trans fat and are lower in trans fats than solid, hard margarine and animal fats, including butter. If animal fat is used, the margarine must be manufactured under government inspection. Margarine for cooking can be purchased in one-pound packages. For table use, chips and patties are available in different sizes and with and without trans fats. Many states have laws requiring foodservice operators to inform customers when margarine is used as a table spread. The information needed in written specifications is similar to that needed for butter.

GRAINS AND CEREALS

Grains are seeds of the grass family. Cereal is named after the Roman goddess of grain, Ceres. Cereals and grains are excellent sources of fiber, B vitamins, and iron. They are complex carbohydrates; fiber is the indigestible part of plant foods. Most grains are similar, being made up of *endosperm*, the outer layer, a source of soluble fiber, B vitamins, carbohydrates, and protein; *bran*, the largest part of the grain but not by weight, a source of B vitamins, trace minerals, and insoluble fiber; and *germ*, the sprouting section of the seed.△

Foodservice operations, especially those that prepare bakery products from scratch, may select several kinds of flours. Pasta and rice products are basic elements of the menu in health care institutions, as are breakfast cereals.

Types of Flour

Several types of flour made from different kinds of wheat are available for specific uses. Flours are classified by their density (hard, semi-hard, or soft), color, protein strength, and use. Hard or bread flours have a higher protein content than other types of flour. These proteins help form gluten, the strong, elastic structure needed in yeast-leavened dough. Flour may be enriched. The FDA inspects and approves the use of flour treatments and additives that are used to improve appearance, storage, and batter performance.

All-Purpose Flours

All-purpose flours can be blends of hard wheat flours, soft wheat flours, or both hard and soft wheat flours. Although all-purpose flours are suitable for many purposes, they are not as satisfactory as bread flour for baking high-rising breads. However, all-purpose flour can be used for almost any other baked product with excellent results. All-purpose flour is available bleached or unbleached. Self-rising, all-purpose flour also is available; this flour contains baking powder, baking soda, and salt.

Pastry and Cake Flours

Pastry and cake flours usually are milled from soft wheats and are used mainly in pies, cakes, and other desserts. These flours have a lower protein content and a higher starch content than other flours. When purchasing white flour products, the buyer should specify that the flour be enriched with thiamin, riboflavin, niacin, and iron. Fifty- and 100-pound bags are the most convenient sizes for food-service use.

Whole Wheat or Graham Flour

Whole wheat or graham flour is made from the entire wheat kernel with only the outer bran layer removed. Because the wheat germ, which is high in fat, is left in whole wheat flour, it becomes stale or rancid when not stored properly.

Rye Flour

Rye flour, made from rye grain, contains the proteins needed for gluten formation in bread baking but not in the same proportion as in wheat flour. For this reason, some wheat flour is used in rye bread recipes. Rye flour may be mixed with wheat, or it may be whole rye flour with unground rye or berries.

Soy Flour

Soy flour, with varying amounts of fat removed, is high in protein. Incorporation of some soy flour into bakery products improves their protein content, moistness, and tenderness.

Organic Flour

Organic flour is from wheat and other grains that are grown without chemicals; the designation "organic" for flour is not standardized because it varies from state to state. Organic flour is grown and stored without the use of synthetic herbicides or insecticides. No toxic fumigants may be used to kill pests in the grain, and no preservatives may be added to the flour, packaging, or food product. To be 100 percent organic, all of the above must be observed.

Other Flours

Bread flour is white flour that is a blend of hard, high-protein wheat with a greater gluten strength.

Self-rising flour is when one-half teaspoon of salt and 1½ teaspoon leavening is added to one cup of all-purpose flour. This is not to be used for yeast bread making.

Semolina is a hard spring wheat with a high gluten content, granular, and resembles sugar; used to make couscous and pasta products. It is enriched.

Whole wheat flour comes from spring wheat, high-protein content, and low starch. It's made by grinding the whole wheat kernel or recombining the white flour, germ, and bran that was separated at milling. There is little difference in method except coarseness and fiber content.

Flour Specifications

Specifications for flours$^\triangle$ commonly include the percentage of protein required and the ash content. The following examples illustrate suggested specifications for some wheat flours. Specifications also contain origin, type of wheat, purpose, composition, package, and price.

- Flour, U.S. and Canada grown, wheat, white, all-purpose enriched, 0.46 percent maximum ash, 9 percent minimum protein on 14 percent moisture basis, 50-pound bag, priced per pound.
- Flour, a blend of hard U.S.-grown wheat, bread, enriched, 0.46 percent maximum ash, 9 percent minimum protein on 14 percent moisture basis, 50-pound bag, priced per pound.
- Flour, whole wheat or graham, 1.9 percent maximum ash, 11 percent minimum protein on 14 percent moisture basis, 25-pound bag.

Other Grains

Barley is not eaten as a food; instead, it is converted into malt for beer production or to feed for animals. Pearl barley is a form that is used in foodservice operations especially for soups mixed with meats.

Buckwheat is the seed of a plant related to rhubarb; it is a plant source of complete protein. It is available as buckwheat flour; kasha; buckwheat groats; whole, medium, or fine grind; or cream of buckwheat.

Couscous is the milled endosperm of hard durum wheat known as semolina. It comes in bulk or instant form.

Oats

For centuries oats$^\Delta$ were used as animal food. When evidence-based science researched oats and found that they help reduce cholesterol in humans and that they contained complex carbohydrates, protein, minerals, vitamins, and soluble and insoluble fiber, their use became popular. Today oats may be served hot as instant or long-cooking oatmeal with a variety sugars, syrups, nuts, and fruit added. They are also served as ready-to-eat cereal such as oat flakes, clusters, or mixed with other grains.

Types of Pasta

Enriched macaroni products are made from wheat. High-quality macaroni products are made from hard amber durum wheat, which yields glutinous flour. The wheat is milled into a golden-toned, coarse product called semolina, into granules that contain more flour, or into flour itself. Water is added to a mixture of durum meal or flour, semolina, and farina to make dough that is forced through dies to make tubular macaroni products and cord-like spaghetti. Because enrichment of these products with thiamin, riboflavin, niacin, and iron is not mandatory, the buyer must specify that the product be enriched. Macaroni products can be made with other kinds of wheat flours, so durum wheat pasta products should be specified for high quality.$^\Delta$

Noodle products are similar in composition to macaroni except that they contain liquid eggs, frozen eggs, dried eggs, egg yolks, dried yolks, or any combination of these at a minimum level of 5.5 percent.

Vegetables and spices added to pasta provide color; for example, pasta can be purchased in various colors, flavors, and shapes. Green pasta contains spinach, red pasta contains tomato, orange pasta contains saffron, and deep red pasta contains hot pepper. Some packages of pasta may contain one or more of these.

Pasta Specifications

Examples of pasta specifications include:

- Macaroni, shell, 100 percent durum, enriched, small, 10-pound box, price by box
- Egg noodles, durum, enriched, broad, 10-pound box, price by box
- Spaghetti, 100 percent durum, enriched, angel hair, 10-pound box, price by box

Corn and Cornmeal

Corn may be white, yellow, mixed white and yellow, blue and red. White or yellow corn is used to make *hominy* using a lye treatment to remove the bran and germ leaving the endosperm of the corn. Grits are coarsely chopped hominy and can be made from yellow or white corn. White grits are preferred in the South. White, blue, and red corns are processed into "corn chips."

Cornmeal, made from white or yellow corn, is available in either coarse or fine grinds. Enrichment with B vitamins and iron is common but not mandatory; calcium is another optional enrichment ingredient. Regular cornmeal, which contains most of the corn kernel, contains more than 3.5 percent fat. Degermed cornmeal has a fat content of less than 2.25 percent. Self-rising cornmeal, with added baking soda, baking powder, and salt, also can be purchased. Common purchase units are 5- and 25-pound bags. The size that best suits an institution's needs should be selected. If only small amounts are used at any one time, smaller bags are easier to handle. A sample specification for cornmeal would include the following information: white, enriched, self-rising, 25-pound bag.

Types of Rice

Rice can be classified as short, medium, or long grain. China produces about 90 percent of the world's supply of rice. Each type has different cooking characteristics. For example, short-grain rice tends to be stickier after cooking and is suitable for use in recipes in which it is used as an extender and binder. Both medium- and long-grain rice remains separate and more distinct in form after cooking. Varieties of rice include pearl (American and California), short grain (Calora, Magnolia, Zenith), and medium grain (Blue Rose, Early Prolific). Rice is available in several forms: regular milled white, parboiled or converted white, precooked white, and brown or husked.$^\Delta$

Regular White Rice

Regular milled white rice has the outer hull removed and is polished. Because this processing removes significant amounts of B vitamins and some minerals, enrichment is desirable and should be specified in the purchase order. A sample specification for white rice would include the following information: milled, long grain, enriched, U.S. Grade 1, 25-pound heavy bag.

Converted Rice

Parboiled or converted rice is regular white rice treated to retain its B vitamins by either parboiling or subjecting the rice to steam pressure before hulling. After cooking, the grains tend to be more separate and plump and have better holding qualities than regular white rice.

Precooked Rice

Precooked rice is milled, cooked, and dehydrated. It usually is enriched.

Brown Rice

Brown rice has only the rough outer husk removed and thus has a higher calorie, protein, and mineral content than enriched white rice. The firmer texture and characteristic nutty flavor have helped increase the popularity of brown rice. It is well suited to many kinds of recipes and is a staple of vegetarian fare. The specification information needed is similar to that for other kinds of rice.

Wild Rice

Wild rice is not rice but the seed of a grass-like plant. Because it is more expensive, it usually is purchased as part of a mixture that includes white or brown rice and that often is preseasoned. Relatively small quantities of wild rice produce large cooked yields because wild rice continues to absorb water throughout the cooking process.

Breakfast Cereals

Many kinds of hot cooked cereals can be found on menus in health care facilities. These include oatmeal (rolled oats), farina, grits, cream of wheat, cream of rice, and rolled wheat. Regular, quick-cooking, and instant forms are available for many of these products. Except for the whole wheat products, enrichment should be specified.

Ready-to-eat breakfast cereals add great variety to breakfast selections. Individual boxes and ready-to-serve individual bowl packs are available for the most popular varieties. If patients are unable to handle individual boxes, bulk retail packages should be considered. These are less expensive but require more labor to serve. Sweetened cereals cost more per ounce than unsweetened cereals.

Ready-to-eat cereal may contain a mixture of wheat, rice, or corn (or all of these). Dry cereals may contain a sweetening agent, salt, flavorings, coloring agents, antioxidants, preservatives, and additional fiber. Most cereals are fortified with vitamins and minerals; some meet 100 percent of the minimum daily requirement. Dry cereal may be shredded, flaked, puffed, or granular. Dry cereal may also have nuts, fruits, marshmallows, or other foods added.

A specification could read as follows: Individual boxes, fortified low-fat bran flakes with added sweet raisins, with 100 percent daily value of 11 various vitamins and minerals.$^\Delta$

Following are sample specifications for two types of cooked breakfast cereal:

- Farina, enriched, regular, six 5-pound packages per case, priced per case
- Cereal, whole wheat meal, malted, six 5-pound packages per case, priced per case

OTHER STAPLES

Many other food items are staples in foodservice operations, but purchasing decisions for these are easier to make than for the products covered thus far. For example, many kinds of prepared bread and bakery products are available. Developing specifications requires knowledge of local market offerings and terms used. For breads, specifications should include size or weight of loaf,

number of slices, and enrichment. Although federal laws require enrichment of some bread products sold interstate, some states do not require enrichment of breads produced and sold within their boundaries. Frozen bread and roll dough have become popular because they provide the desirable fresh-baked characteristics with greatly reduced labor and equipment requirements. The quality of products from various vendors and cost should be evaluated before purchasing decisions are made.

Their consistent quality and labor-saving advantages make baking mixes an important staple in many foodservice operations. Cake mixes, pudding mixes, quick bread mixes, and other dessert mixes are just a few examples of the products available that can add variety to the menu at a low labor cost. When purchasing such products, the food buyer should compare the product quality and yield from various brands and calculate the cost per serving.

Nuts

"Nuts are good for you," as an FDA-approved package label "qualifies" the health claim for nuts: "Scientific evidence suggest but does not prove that eating 1.5 ounces per day of most nuts as part of a diet low in saturated fat and cholesterol may reduce the risk of heart disease." The FDA label is eligible for almonds, hazelnuts, peanuts, pecans, pine nuts, pistachios, and walnuts. For the label to go on the package, the product cannot exceed 4 grams of saturated fat per 50 grams of nuts.

Nuts frequently used in a foodservice operation include: almonds, cashews, hazelnuts, peanuts, pecans, pine nuts, and walnuts. Nuts are a welcome addition to salads, cereal, pasta, cooked vegetables, yogurt, cakes, pies, pancakes, waffles, and muffins. For specifications check with a vendor as nuts may be salted, blanched, roasted, or in shells or hulls.

Edible Flowers

Flowers can add beauty to a presentation, flavor and variety. When considering using flowers **know** your flowers, because not all are edible and some are poisonous; be aware that some people are allergic to flowers. Lists of "DOs-and-DON'Ts" and of the most common edible flowers follow.

DON'T	DO
Use flowers gathered from the roadside	Eat only when positive they are edible
Use flowers that have been sprayed with pesticides	Wash thoroughly before eating
	Introduce into diet slowly
	Eat only the portion of the flower that is edible
Eat flowers from florists, nurseries, or garden centers	In most cases eat only the petals of flowers

Edible flowers			
Nasturtiums	Carnations	Day lilies	Hibiscus
Impatiens	Pansies	Violets	Lavender
Mimosa blossoms	Marigolds (petals only)	Rose petals	
Squash blossoms	Chrysanthemums	Clover	

HERBS AND SPICES

Herbs add to and bring out the flavor of food. See Chapter 20 for a list.

BEVERAGES

Popular beverages include coffee, tea, cocoa, and carbonated potables. Customer preferences, food cost, and available equipment are factors to consider when selecting these products.

Coffee

Coffee is a popular beverage among the young and baby boomers and is the most common menu item. Coffeehouses are everywhere, and a variety of coffees are available in many health care facilities. The trend is for the following new coffee drinks: espresso, a shot of hot strong caffè served in a small cup with hot cream and sweetener; cappuccino, a blend of espresso and steamed and foamed hot milk; caffè latte, same ingredients as cappuccino but with more steamed and less foamed milk; and cafe mocha, mostly steamed milk with a shot of espresso and mocha syrup. All these coffees may have cinnamon, chocolate, plus additional flavors added.[△]

There are more than 6,000 variations of coffee beans worldwide, but only 25 are considered as major types; of these 25 major types only three are important and common types used by customers.

Kona, *Robusta*, and *Arabica*. Kona has the smallest production and is the most expensive. Kona is grown in Hawaii. It has a powerful aroma, pleasant taste, and is rarely blended with other kinds of drink flavorings.

Robusta makes up more than 40 percent of the coffee production worldwide. It is the least expensive of the three. It can be blended with other coffee because of its strong flavor and does not vary in flavor. Arabica covers 60 percent of the coffee production worldwide. Due to pest, disease, and frost Arabica beans are expensive. Its flavor is delicious and may be used in other coffees for flavoring.

Different blends of coffee beans result in the unique flavor characteristic of various brands. Much of the flavor of coffee beans comes from growing conditions and production methods. A coffee bush takes a minimum of five years to yield its first crop. Each bush produces one pound of coffee or approximately 3,500 hand-picked coffee cherries annually during its productive years. Coffees may also be a blend of several types of beans. Coffee may be categorized by roasting methods. Some varieties and origins of coffee beans include:

- *Armenia:* Full bodied (Colombia)
- *Blue Mountain:* Full bodied (Jamaica) and the most expensive
- *Coatepec:* Full bodied (Mexico)
- *Java:* Full flavored with exotic elements (Indonesia)
- *Maracaibo:* Light, rich, evenly flavored (Venezuela)
- *Santo:* Somewhat acidic, high quality (Brazil)
- *Kona:* Only coffee grown in the United States, mild, favorable, expensive (Hawaii)

Coffees from east Africa have a unique flavor and are typically medium to full bodied.

Coffee can also be *decaffeinated*. Decaffeinated coffee is made by using a chemical solvent or the Swiss water method to remove most of the caffeine from the green coffee bean. The FDA sets limits on the amount of solvent that can be used.

Instant coffee is a concentrated extract of the coffee bean in powder form. Coffees, including decaffeinated, may also have flavors added. Some flavors include hazelnut, almond, chocolate, apricot, raspberry, and vanilla. Alcohol may also be added, such as cordial, brandy, or whiskey.

Liquid coffee is a freeze-dried instant coffee where water is added and brewed, the temperature lowered, then it is packaged and sent through a freezer tunnel for three to four hours. It takes a special machine to dispense this coffee.

Selection should be based on consumers' preference and the amount they are willing to pay per cup. Specifications for coffee should include roast, grind, and percentage of types desired in the blend, plus packaging. Because the volume of coffee purchased by most foodservice operations is significant, the food buyer should order several brands "in the bean" and send them to the coffee brewing center for quality evaluation. Results should be used in writing coffee specifications.

Tea

All teas come from the same tea plant, a shrub (*Camellide sinenis*) of the Theaceate family. The difference between black tea, green tea, and oolong results from the way tea leaves are processed after they are plucked. Black tea makers air-dry newly harvested tea leaves and then crush them in a natural process that turns them to a pleasing coppery color. Then the leaves are dried at a high temperature, which causes them to turn black.

Oolong tea undergoes the same process as black tea, but the air-drying time is shorter, resulting in less natural fermentation and a flavor and aroma between a black and green tea.

Green tea makers steam the leaves within 24 hours of harvest to prevent fermentation and change in character. The tea has a delicate greenish yellow color and a fruity, slightly bitter flavor.

There are three basic types as listed above and more than 3,000 varieties. Factors such as where grown, weather, and altitude affect the flavor. Tea leaves can also be mixed with fruits, nuts, and vanilla to give a pleasant taste. Hot tea can be served with sugar, cream, or lemon, or just as tea.

Tea may be purchased for an individual cup of tea, loose for institutional use, or in larger bags that can be used in institutions. Flavored teas are popular, with raspberry and peach the most accepted. Iced tea is served sweetened or unsweetened and with or without lemon.[△]

Herbal Tea

Herbal teas do not come from tea plants but from any part of herb and spice plants, including the leaves, flowers, bark, seeds, stems, or roots. Herbal teas are not teas but are naturally caffeine-free blends of dried herbs. Herbal teas may also have flavors added, such as orange and raspberry. The most popular herbal teas are chamomile and rosehip.

Decaffeinated Tea

Caffeine is removed in most instances naturally through a process of pure water. Tea has about half the caffeine of coffee. Tea may be decaffeinated, instant, or flavored.

There are several new tea types available, such as Rooibos, a caffeine-free herb indigenous to South Africa and known as red tea.

Yerba maté comes from a South American plant and, when harvested, tastes similar to pan-fired green tea. It is also caffeine free.

Cocoa

Cocoa is processed by roasting, grinding, and defatting the niles of cocoa beans. Cocoa must have at least 22 percent but not more than 35 percent cocoa butter. The higher the cocoa butter content, the richer the product. Cocoa that has been treated with an alkali during processing is darker, has a less acidic flavor, and is more soluble.

Specifications for Other Staples

When writing specifications for other miscellaneous items, such as spices, condiments, sweeteners, and specialty beverages, the various brands available should be considered and the quality of each evaluated. Prices for various package sizes should be compared, and the food buyer should keep up to date on price trends. Package sizes, particularly for spices, should be considered. Some may be used in much larger quantities than others and should be purchased in 1-pound or larger units; those used only occasionally should be purchased in smaller retail market packages so that they retain their quality until used. If available, federal standards and grades should be used. Federal grades have been defined for honey, maple syrup, nuts, olives, pickles, and catsup. Federal standards of identity also are available for many products.

The following specifications for some food staples may be useful in developing others:

- Walnuts, U.S. No. 1, small pieces, latest season's crop, six 5-pound boxes per case, priced per case
- Olives, green, giant, U.S. Grade A or Fancy, six No. 10 cans per case, priced per case

- Pickles, dill, thin, cross-cut, fresh pack, U.S. Grade A or Fancy, six plastic jars per case, priced per case
- Honey, light amber from orange blossoms or clover, pasteurized, U.S. Grade A, extracted, six 5-pound containers per case, priced per case

SMALL EQUIPMENT AND UTENSILS

Adequate and appropriate equipment and utensils are required for maintaining control in preparation and service. These items are not classified as equipment, and there is no depreciation account for their replacement. This class of equipment includes measuring devices, pans, knives, cutting boards, scales, thermometers, and portioning utensils. Careful selection of utensils can influence work efficiency, product quality, portion control, and initial cost. Ergonomically designed equipment should be purchased to reduce the risk of musculoskeletal problems.

General selection factors include appearance, durability, cost, and satisfaction for specific use. Most utensils are made according to standard manufacturers' specifications. The item may be selected from a manufacturer's or equipment supplier's catalog rather than by writing a detailed specification.[△]

Measuring Devices

Liquid and dry measuring devices range in size from a cup to a gallon. Liquid measurers should have a pouring lip, and dry measurers should have a level top. Measurers should be made of durable materials because accuracy can be affected by dents and bends in lightweight metals. Both measurers and measuring spoons are available in either stainless steel or heavy-duty aluminum. Although aluminum may be satisfactory, the extra cost of stainless steel may be balanced by its longer life. For safety reasons, glass measurers should not be used in institutional foodservice departments.[△]

Pans

Preparation equipment should be standardized as much as possible. Perhaps the most important application of that principle is in the selection of pans. Most standard recipes are based on the standard pan that measures about 12 by 20 inches—the size that fits the openings in the hot-food serving table or cart. Standard pans, used for many purposes such as cooking, holding, and storing foods under refrigeration, are available in 2½-, 4-, 6-, and 8-inch depths. Smaller pans of several sizes are based on the 12-by-20-inch serving table opening, half-sizes measuring 12 by 6⅔ inches (three to fill an opening), and other smaller sizes.

Considerations other than size that apply to pan selection are type and weight of the metal and design. Both stainless steel and aluminum pans are available. For stainless steel pans, 18- to 22-gauge metal usually is used. Standard pans have either solid or perforated bottoms.

Pan design is important for storage reasons. Pans that taper slightly from top to bottom nest well and can be stacked without becoming wedged together. Covers come in several designs: flat, hinged, and domed.

Besides the serving table pans, sheet pans (*bun pans*) also are needed. Sheet pans are 18 by 26 inches or 20 by 24 inches, with a depth of ¾ to about 2 inches. Sheet pans are usually made of 16-gauge aluminum.

If pots, kettles, saucepans, and stockpots are needed for food preparation, heavy-gauge metal pans are more durable and help prevent scorching and sticking. Saucepans and stockpots are available in various thicknesses of aluminum and stainless steel as well as other metals. Although the bright appearance and durability of stainless steel are desirable, this material does not conduct heat as evenly as heavyweight aluminum when used in surface cooking. Handles should be sturdy, and large saucepans should have an additional bracket handle on the side opposite the long handle to make lifting easier and safer.

In selecting pan sizes, keep in mind the kind of cooking to be done, burner sizes on ranges with circular heating units, and the weight of the pan when filled with product. Employees' safety when lifting these pans must be considered. Four-quart saucepans are useful for many purposes; however, the capacity of small pans should be based on portion sizes and the total quantity needed of any product. Lids should be purchased for pans to be used in surface cooking because they help to reduce the cooking time needed for some products and thus save energy.$^{\triangle}$

Knives

The quality of a knife is determined by the material of the blade and handle and its shape and construction. Most knife blades are made of carbon steel. A high-carbon-steel blade has the finest cutting edge when it is properly cared for and sharpened. When chrome is added to the alloy, the result is stainless steel. When vanadium is added, the blade is stronger and tends to hold its cutting edge longer.

Knife handles can be made of wood, plastic, wood and plastic combinations, and bone. Possibly more important than the material used in the handle is how the handle is attached to the blade. High-quality knives have a continuous piece of metal extending from the knife tip through the handle. In such knives, the handle is usually made of two pieces that are attached to the blade with heavy rivets. The blade must be well fastened into the handle or it will loosen with use. Several types of knives are needed, including French cooks' knives that have a 10-inch blade for chopping, paring knives, utility or boning knives with slim 5- or 6-inch blades for trimming, and carving knives for slicing.$^{\triangle}$

Cutting Boards

Cutting boards$^{\triangle}$ must provide sanitary cutting surfaces that are made of hard rubber or plastic. Cutting boards need to be scratch resistant, thoroughly cleanable, and will not absorb juices from foods or allow food particles to collect. Hard-composition rubber or plastic cutting boards are superior to the wooden variety and are frequently required by local or state health departments. Small 10-by-12-inch boards are convenient for employees to use in cutting small amounts of food. In the cooking or salad preparation areas, 18-by-24-inch boards are adequate. Cutting boards should be colored to specific areas of use. Cutting boards are highly susceptible to bacteria growth and transferring food-borne pathogens as they come into contact with a variety of foods and surfaces. Cutting boards that are scratched or scored need to be replaced immediately. Cutting boards need to be cleaned and sanitized after each. Do not use the same cutting board for meat, and then raw vegetables.

Scales

Scales are needed for checking deliveries, weighing ingredients in food preparation, and controlling serving portions. Scales must be accurate, easy to use and read, durable, and easy to clean. Types used in foodservice facilities include floor scales; suspended platforms; overhead tracks (in large facilities); built-ins; and portion, counter, and table scales. Some of the new models can generate a printout with the date, time, and weight of the product.

The capacity of bakers' scales ranges from 5 to 20 pounds. For all-purpose use in preparation areas, a 25- to 50-pound capacity scale that will weigh in fractions of an ounce is ideal. For controlling portion sizes, a scale with quarter-ounce gradations and a capacity of up to 2 pounds should be available.

Thermometers

Thermometers$^{\triangle}$ are essential in the control of food quality. Oven thermometers should have a temperature range of 200°F to 600°F (93°C to 315°C). Several bimetallic thermometers with a tubular metal stem equipped with a dial or digital temperature indicator should be available to monitor temperature of food products (see a more extensive discussion on thermometers in Chapter 14).

Thermometers for refrigerators, freezers, and dry storage areas also are needed. In newer models of cold storage equipment, they are built in and can be read without opening the door. Periodic checks using a freestanding shelf thermometer will validate their accuracy. Deep-fat thermometers are essential for frying equipment that is not thermostatically controlled.

Portioning Utensils

Portioning equipment$^{\triangle}$ such as scoops, ladles, and spoons should be available in both the production and service areas. Scoops are numbered from 6 to 60, the number referring to the number of scoops it takes to equal 1 quart. Equivalent measures of scoops in cups, tablespoons, and teaspoons are printed in most quantity food cookbooks and manufacturers' catalogs.

Portioning ladles, usually made of 18-gauge stainless steel, are available in sizes of 1, 2, 4, 6, 8 ounces, and larger. Most are labeled with the number of ounces they hold or color-coded for the number of ounces. Large ladles, which hold 1 to 4 quarts, may be needed to transfer foods from steam-jacketed kettles or stockpots to serving pans. These ladles may also be color-coded.

In addition to scoops and ladles, stainless steel and heavy-duty plastic spoons are needed. The spoons are made with various handle lengths and with solid, slotted, or perforated bowls and may also be color-coded for the number of ounces.

SERVICE SUPPLIES

The selection of appropriate service supplies$^\Delta$ (trays, dinnerware, tableware, hollowware, glassware, and disposables) is important for presenting meals attractively. The initial investment; the replacement cost; labor, water, and energy costs; and waste-disposal costs are essential factors to consider. The kind and size of trays required for patient and resident service depend on the delivery system used (described in Chapter 22). Whatever system is used, preserving food quality is of prime importance. Trays should be made of durable materials that will not bend, dent, warp, or lose their shape over continuous use. Trays of hard rubber, plastic, and molded fiberglass in a variety of shapes and sizes are designed to withstand repeated washing. Attractively colored trays that are plain or have designs molded under a protective surface layer eliminate the need for place mats at all meals.

The type of dinnerware chosen may be reusable, *single-service disposable*, or a combination of these. *Reusable ware* should be durable, easy to clean, stain resistant, and attractive. Its colors and designs should be compatible with the trays and the food items served. If reusable dinnerware is purchased, vitrified china is recommended. Three weights are available: thick, hotel, and medium. However, weight does not necessarily indicate strength; only the quality of materials and the manufacturing methods determine durability.

Foodservice directors who prefer china because of its appearance but also want to minimize breakage have found that dinnerware made from glass components and modified to resist breakage, crazing, chipping, and staining is satisfactory. Many sizes and shapes, plain white or with designs, are available. Foodservice departments that use microwave ovens for heating foods before service find these dishes useful.

Another type of dinnerware, light in weight and easy to handle, is made of melamine plastic. *Melamine* costs less than conventional dinnerware and is more resistant to breakage. However, melamine dishes lose their finish with use, thus are susceptible to stains and scratches, and are difficult to sanitize.

The tableware (flatware and hollowware) chosen for institutional use should be designed for durability and attractiveness. Eating utensils made of stainless steel meet both these criteria because they have the added advantages of being tarnish-proof and easy to clean. The size of flatware selected for tray service should be based on ease of handling and size of the tray. Choosing the same size and pattern for both patient and nonpatient service reduces sorting and washing time and replacement cost. China and flatware for pediatrics and disabled persons are available for purchase. Several sets of these products should be kept in stock at all times.

The types and sizes of beverage service ware needed vary among foodservice departments. Service requirements and available labor and ware-washing equipment influence the type of material selected (glass, plastic, or single service). Whichever type of service ware selected should be durable, easy to clean, and suitable for the portion sizes served.

Single-service disposable dinnerware and tableware are used in part or exclusively by some foodservice departments. Customer acceptance; local regulations; temperature-retention capability; and supply, labor, storage, and disposal costs should be analyzed before selection. Disposables, available in a variety of materials, colors, and designs, should be selected for their strength and rigidity on the basis of service needs. Attractive geometrical, floral, or modern patterns can enhance tray or cafeteria service. Plates used for entrées should resist cutting, sagging, and soaking. Beverage containers should be appropriate for maintaining the temperature of either cold or hot liquids. Eating utensils must be sturdy enough not to break.

SUMMARY

Foodservice purchasers must be familiar with current quality standards established by the USDA, FDA, national and local legislation as they pertain to wholesomeness and quality of all categories of food and ingredients (especially meats and meat products, given that they comprise the biggest cost outlay).

Foodservice department managers need to ensure proper production scheduling, storage times, and shelf life of products—without overstocking or understocking inventory. This balancing act must be done in keeping with meeting customer expectations while staying within a prescribed budget. A key component of this effort is writing up purchase specifications, which depend on USDA mandates as well as IMPS, NAMP, and MBG standards (for meat and meat product purchases). The federal grade stamps and inspection marks used for meat, poultry, and eggs have been described in this chapter, as well as the USDC standards and PUFI mark for seafood.

Even the most nutritionally sound and carefully prepared foods will not meet customer expectations in the presentation area without tastefully selected service supplies. Making appropriate tray, dinnerware, tableware, hollowware, glassware, and disposable ware purchases also is a key responsibility. Therefore, texture, color, and durability of service equipment must be coordinated as closely as possible with the aesthetic features of menu offerings.

Acidophilus-cultured milk
Aquaculture
Arabica coffee
Beef grades
Bun pan
Cheese
Eviscerated
Exotic fruits and vegetables
Fowl
Game meat
Genetically engineered
Herbal tea
Institutional Meat Purchase Specifications (IMPS)
Irradiation
Kosher

Lactose-free milk
Melamine
Mercury
Olive oil
Oolong tea
Organic
Packed Under Federal Inspection (PUFI)
Reusable ware
Robusta coffee
Single-service disposable
Shochet
Standard of fill
Standard of identity
Standard of quality

DISCUSSION QUESTIONS

1. Relate the procurement system to the overall system in a food-service operation.
2. What is the role of irradiated, genetically engineered, organic, and cloned food in a foodservice establishment?
3. What are some methods to recognize the grade stamps and inspection marks used for meat, poultry, eggs, and seafood?
4. Distinguish between the various grades of food products.
5. What is the role of the foodservice director in developing specifications that will provide the vendor the necessary information to meet the needs of the establishment?
6. Why is it important to know where fish and seafood is harvested, processed, and delivered?
7. How would you avoid overuse of tuna on children, pregnant women, and nursing mothers?
8. Why do poultry and eggs need to be handled in a safe and sanitary manner?
9. How could you use soy, almond, or goat milk on a menu?
10. What are the various methods of incorporating a variety of cheeses in a menu?
11. How are fruits and vegetables classified?
12. If your customers would eat and enjoy the addition of various exotic fruits and vegetables on a menu, what should you consider in purchasing these foods?
13. Why it is important to wash all fruit and vegetables before serving?
14. How is olive oil used in food production?
15. List the variety of flours and their various uses.
16. Why are flours, rice, pasta, cornmeal, and cereals enriched?
17. What are the differences between the three coffees—Kona, Robusta, and Arabica?
18. Write specifications for china to replace disposable ware and give advantages and disadvantages of using each.

CHAPTER 18

PURCHASING

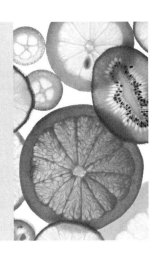

LEARNING OBJECTIVES

- Determine the amount of food, supplies, and equipment to purchase by using specifications and ethical practices.
- Evaluate purveyors and the service they offer.
- Explain the various methods used to purchase goods/services.
- Demonstrate whether it is best to purchase or make various products on-site.
- Know the advantages and disadvantages of various purchasing methods.
- Follow all applicable laws, regulations, and rules related to purchasing products.
- Develop a sustainable program for a foodservice operation.

FOOD PURCHASING PLAYS an essential role in meeting customers' needs and ensuring the success of the health care foodservice operation. Aside from being well versed in product selection and food-quality standards as discussed in the preceding chapter, the purchasing agent (or buyer) should be knowledgeable about product availability, trends directing customer expectations, the purchasing process, market conditions, production demand, and purchasing methods. The buyer or purchasing agent provides leadership in establishing partnerships with distributors and serves on the product evaluation team. Knowledge of the food distribution system, the structure of wholesale markets in which purchasing occurs, and ethical issues that arise in purchasing also are important to the buyer's role. (The term *buyer* is used throughout this chapter to describe the individual primarily respon-

sible for acquiring food products, equipment, and services for a health care foodservice department.)

In this chapter, trends that influence purchasing decisions and the purchasing process are discussed. Specific trends explored are continuous quality improvement, technology, distributors' changing product line, and the changing role of distributors' sales representatives.

Food marketing and wholesaling are examined within the context of a larger food distribution system that tracks the flow of food from a raw product grown by a farmer to an item for consumer consumption in the health care environment. The intermediate points—food assembly, grading, storing, processing, transport, and the like—are translated to the foodservice area and expedited to buyer and distributor.

A 10-step procurement model is broken down into its component parts and examined, starting with assessing needs for a new product, service, or piece of equipment, and ending with receipt and distribution of items throughout the production area in a foodservice operation. Buyers and department directors will be able to adapt the model to suit their individual needs. The buyer's responsibilities and optimum qualifications needed to perform the functions of procurement are delineated.

"Power-purchasing" strategies are described, some of which are group purchasing organizations, just-in-time purchasing, one-stop purchasing, and prime vendor agreements. Their advantages and disadvantages are explored, along with other distinctions—such as centralized versus noncentralized and contract versus noncontract purchasing.

Issues examined in-depth are how vendors are selected, the buyer-vendor relationship, and ethical issues that can arise in the purchasing process, and a brief how-to list of computer-assisted procurement is given.

GENERAL PURCHASING GUIDE FOR FOOD SUPPLY BUYER

Purchasing is a functional subsystem of the system model. Purchasing is one of the four interlocking processes in transformation and must be carefully managed to meet the fiscal responsibilities of the department.

The goal of purchasing is to secure the products needed at the best price, of the best specified quality, and delivered as needed, in refrigerated/freezer trucks, or enclosed trucks, that are sanitary; products are handled in a safe and sanitary manner during the delivery process. Every effort must be made to purchase food that has been processed under safe and sanitary conditions. The following precautions should be considered:

- Purchases should be made only from licensed food-processing and supply sources that comply with all laws relating to processing and labeling. A note of caution—when buying locally be sure you know the source and the conditions under which the food was grown and processed; if buying organic know the source and the "type" of organic.
- Fluid milk and fluid milk products must be pasteurized and meet Grade A quality standards. (Be aware of raw milk and raw milk products that may be local and have not undergone inspection of the milk herd or the processing plant.) Dry milk products should be made from only pasteurized milk.
- Only meat and meat products inspected by USDA or state regulatory agency should be purchased. The USDA should have inspected poultry, poultry products, and eggs products. Fishery products inspected by the U.S. Department of Commerce should be purchased and certificate of proof may be requested.
- Shellfish should be purchased from reputable dealers that comply with state and local agencies guidelines. Certificates of proof may be requested.
- Only clean eggs with uncracked shells or pasteurized liquid or frozen or dried egg products should be used. Commercially prepared hard-cooked peeled eggs may be used. Eggnog must be pasteurized.
- Food products that have been contaminated by insects, rodents, or water and fire and food in cans that bulge or are severely dented should not be accepted at delivery or be discarded if the damage occurs between delivery and use. Eggs that are delivered with cracked, discolored, or dirty shells need to be rejected. Avoid the use of any food that is delivered where the packing has been compromised.
- All incoming food supplies should be inspected for evidence of damage to the cartons, packages, or containers, from filth, water, insects, or rodents. Damage or spoiled products and frozen foods that show evidence of thawing or refreezing should be rejected.
- All products and packing should be carefully examined for tampering—if noted, do not touch but call security, administration, and the facility emergency preparedness director.

REGULATION

Throughout history, societies have attempted to control the quality and safety of the food supply. The advent of extensive urbanization in the twentieth century brought with it significant improvements in this area. Food laws go hand in hand with urbanization because in urban areas, most people do not grow their own food. However, the fact that today's foods go through many hands—growers, processors, wholesalers, distributors—increases the possibility of mishandling, fraudulent practices, and misrepresentation. Advances in science and technology have also contributed to the need for the regulation of the food supply system. Although the use of chemicals in food production and processing has increased crop yields, improved shelf life and product quality, and created new products, the dependence on chemicals has also created serious problems. To prevent the overuse and misuse of chemicals, government controls have been established.

Food laws protect both consumers and the food industry. Consumers are assured of receiving safe and nutritious food supplies. In addition, responsible growers, processors, and distributors are protected against unfair competition from irresponsible competitors. Food laws have several purposes:

- To ensure the nutritional value of all foods
- To maintain the integrity of all foods
- To protect the quality and quantity of all basic foods
- To promote honesty among producers, processors, and distributors
- To provide evidence-based informative, accurate labeling for consumers

The first pure-food law passed in the United States was the Pure Food and Drug Act of 1906. This act played a significant role in decreasing the misbranding and adulteration of foods. When the act became outdated with advancing technology, the more comprehensive Food, Drug, and Cosmetic Act of 1938 replaced it. The act, amended several times since its passage, accomplishes the following:

- It prohibits the shipment of misbranded food products in interstate commerce.
- It prohibits the shipment of adulterated foods (containing harmful substances) in interstate commerce.
- It gives the Food and Drug Administration (FDA) the authority to regulate the use of food additives.
- It gives the FDA the authority to establish standards of identity, standards of fill for food products marketed in containers, and standards of quality.

The FDA has established *standards of quality* for a number of canned fruits and vegetables to supplement the standards of identity by limiting and describing the number and kinds of defects permitted. These standards of quality are minimum standards. To be sold, products that do not meet the standard must be labeled substandard. However, few, if any, substandard products are available on the market. All of the FDA standards are **mandatory** and apply to all food manufacturers, packers, and processors.

Two major amendments to the federal Food, Drug and Cosmetic Act are the Food Additive and Color Additive Amendments of 1958 and 1960. These amendments safeguard consumers against adulteration and misbranding of foods. *Adulteration* is defined as food that contains a substance injurious to health; it was prepared or held under unsanitary conditions; or any part is filthy, decomposed, or contains portions of diseased animals. Food is also considered to be adulterated if (1) damage or inferiority is concealed, (2) the label or container is misleading, or (3) if a valuable substance is left out.

The Fair Packaging and Labeling Act of 1966, which supplements the Food, Drug, and Cosmetic Act, requires complete information in labeling and nondescriptive packaging. The following kinds of information are required on labels:

- Common or unusual names of all ingredients, listed in descending order of predominance by weight
- Name and address of manufacturer, processor, packer, or distributor
- Statement of the quantity of the contents in weight, measure, or numerical count
- Names of added artificial flavorings, colorings, or chemical preservatives

The processor may voluntarily add descriptive information such as brand names, recipes, and the number of servings.

Requirements for nutrition labeling are in the regulations issued in late 1992 by the FDA and the USDA Food Safety and Inspection Service. FDA regulations meet the provisions of the Nutrition Labeling and Education Act of 1990, which requires nutrition labeling for most foods, except meat and poultry, and authorizes the use of nutrient content claims and appropriate FDA-approved health claims. The current label is identified as "nutrition facts." It lists the fat, cholesterol, sodium, carbohydrates, fiber, and protein content as a percentage of the recommended daily allowance. The amount is shown in grams or milligrams per serving of the nutrients listed. The "% of daily value" is based on a 2,000-calorie diet.

The FDA also has developed specific definitions for products that are described as "free," "no amount," "trivial amount," "low," "lean," and "extra lean." The FDA also regulates food irradiation, genetically modified foods, and nutrition labeling.

Meat, poultry, and other animal products are regulated by the USDA's Food Safety and Quality Service by authority of the 1906 Meat Inspection Act, the Poultry Products Inspection Act of 1959, and the Wholesale Meat Act of 1967. The Poultry Products Inspection Act was amended in 1968 to the Wholesome Poultry Products Act. This act requires inspectors to check on the cleanliness of processing plants and the maintenance of processing equipment. Labels on poultry and poultry parts must be approved. The Egg Products Inspection Act of 1970 allows the inspection of processing plants that break and further process shell eggs into liquid, frozen, or dried egg products. Monetary and technical assistance is provided to help plants meet federal requirements.

The purpose of these laws is (1) to control the sanitary conditions of slaughtering and processing facilities; (2) to ensure that animals and birds are healthy and free from harmful disease before slaughter; and (3) to set standards of identity that specify the kinds and proportions of ingredients in meat, poultry, and egg products.

The labeling of animal products is also controlled by USDA regulations. The regulations require that federal inspectors check all meat, poultry, and egg products moving in interstate commerce and that state inspectors check such products provided by companies only within a single state. A round inspection stamp placed on the product itself or printed on its label or package means that basic requirements were met and that the product is wholesome and truthfully labeled.

Although no federal law requires grade standards, the USDA on a voluntary basis provides such measures of quality. The number of grades varies with the particular products and indicates the eating quality, the absence of defects and other characteristics of appearance, uniformity, and size. Although manufacturers are not required to grade products, when a grade shield appears on a product or when a grade name is used, federal inspectors must actually have graded the product. Grade standards have been developed for more than 300 farm products and are revised periodically to reflect changes in production, use, and marketing practices. Whenever a producer or processor wants a product graded, a fee must be paid for the service.

TRENDS INFLUENCING PURCHASING DECISIONS

Like all other functions of the foodservice department, purchasing is influenced by, and must respond to, changes in the internal and external environments. The changes in menu items or type of menu change the needs for purchasing. If changes are made in the menu, recipes need to be developed, and the inventory of supplies on hand will need to be taken to determine if supplies are needed or if there is an overstock of certain items. Plans need to be made to use the inventory on hand before the "use by date" expires. Trends that affect the purchasing function include:

- Continuous quality improvement (CQI)
- Technology
- Distributors' changing product lines
- Changing role of distributors' sales representatives
- The increased use of preprepared food items
- Concerns for the environment, use of locally grown food, and the move to sustainability

An overview of some of these trends was presented in Chapter 1. Specific effects of these trends on the purchasing function are discussed below.

Continuous Quality Improvement

Purchasing is an area that should be integrated with CQI. Because CQI is designed to be customer driven, it has a direct link with product selection. If foodservice is to provide products and services to meet the demands of different customers, it is imperative that feedback be obtained from the patients, employees, administrators, and guests. Foodservice staff who think they know better what customers need or deserve often ignore data collected on what customers really want. Instead of using information collected to identify new products and develop or modify specifications, the information is ignored.

CQI can be used to enhance the relationship between the foodservice department and brokers and distributors. This is particularly critical in a prime vendor arrangement. Open communication, sharing of information, and being customer focused are essential elements of the CQI process. Benefits include faster introduction of new products, provision of product information that will meet a specific operation's needs, and enhanced training on product use and marketing. (Vendor relations are discussed in detail later in this chapter.)

In addition to selecting and evaluating products using can-cutting techniques and sensory focus groups, a product evaluation team should be empowered to identify the need for new products, select them, evaluate their acceptability, and recommend purchases. The team may be composed of food production employees, the production manager, the buyer, tray line and cafeteria employees, and customers.

Group purchasing organizations (GPOs) can implement CQI in providing services to their members. The process should help overcome some of the barriers described later in this chapter.

Technology

The most rapidly changing trend that affects foodservice distributors and health care operations is to be observed in technological developments, which influence distributors' interactions with customers, order placement, and inventory control. Electronic data interchange (EDI) will replace face-to-face meetings and other modes of communication such as the telephone, fax machine, and written messages. Described as a totally automated process where data are transmitted, received, and processed by computers without direct interaction between sender and receiver, EDI already is processing orders. In larger establishments, 90 percent of all ordering is done directly by the buyer using personal computers with software distributed by a specific distributor or generic direct-order-entry software application that processes purchase orders. EDI is used to monitor customers' buying habits and provide nutritional breakdown of all products in the distributor's line, as well as assess market outlook and menu suggestions.

Advantages to using EDI systems for placing foodservice orders include immediate order confirmation; notification of out-of-stock items, with a list of suggested substitutions; automatic price updates; menu analysis; inventory control; and portion control. The expansion of cost-effective EDI communication systems will provide at least three benefits: immediate customer access to the distributor's computer while decreasing telephone expenses, the transfer of inventory data to a personal computer within the foodservice operation, and bar-code scanning that can facilitate deliveries and receiving. Some systems allow any member of the management team to use electronic databases from the distributor to obtain product information including a color photo of the product, unit cost, and other data needed in planning menus and analyzing cost implications of different menu items and menu mixes.

Distributors' Changing Product Line

Distribution will continue to be a people business in which service is the way to distinguish one distributor from another. The move toward "full-line" foodservice distribution is predicted to continue, with distributors' product mixes expanding and the number of items available greater than ever before. Food distributors not only are the main source for food but are becoming the primary source for supplies and equipment to foodservice operations. Specialty distributors in meat, poultry, paper products, and so on are being forced to expand their product lines to compete with full-line distributors for national accounts. The specialty distributor of the 1980s has become the broad-line distributor of the 2000s. Distributors are placing more emphasis on packaging relative to its effect on the environment and the "green" movement. They are working in partnership with foodservice organizations and the packaging industry to develop packages that are less dense and contain recycled materials.

To become more competitive, distributors are offering *value-added service*, those services that go beyond simply completing the delivery accurately and on time. Value-added services to providers include:

- Computerized services that incorporate EDI and advanced technology
- Advice on new products, nutrition information, food cost, and so on
- Continuing education seminars
- Menu development, merchandising, and marketing services
- Floral service
- Consulting services on design, layout, and equipment
- Coordination of a good service operation's recycling efforts
- Cash discounts for early payment of invoices
- Promotion of products at a reduced introductory offer
- Reduced price for quantity purchasing
- Coupons and *rebates*

Today's competitive environment requires distributors and their sales representatives to continue to provide and expand value-added services to retain customers and acquire new ones.

Perhaps the change that most affects the product line is the move to buying locally and directly from the "farmer" who produced the products from field to table—to be *sustainable*. The American Dietetic Association Task Force identified sustainability as "the capacity of being maintained over the long term in order to meet the needs of the present without jeopardizing the ability of future generations to meet their needs." An undercurrent of mistrust of foods mass-produced with the use of pesticides, fertilizers, antibodies, sewage sludge, or ionizing radiation and transported for long distances without supervision drives this trend.

There continue to be major concerns that food production is one of the largest producers of human-induced greenhouse gas (GHG) emission. GHG is only one of the concerns concerning the environment; other concerns include the use of water, biodiversity, and other forms of air, soil, and water pollution, animal welfare, international development, and food security.

The Green Seal™ Environmental Standards for Restaurants and Foodservices, GS-46 has many programs and hand-out information to help an establishment become aware of how to become more sustainable. Their handout for purchasing describes three important points and how to accomplish them. The three points include:

1. Buy food from responsibly produced sources and aim to increase amounts purchased over time.
2. Make it a priority to buy animal products more responsibility.
3. Start tracking the transport of your food.

The trend toward organic and sustainable foods has some merits. Organic food is procured according to legally regulated standards (Chapter 17). There is evidence that organic farms are more sustainable and environmentally sound. Such benefits include the use of less energy and production of less waste materials, less use and release of pesticides and herbicides into the environment, and support of a diverse ecosystem benefiting population of plant and animals. Additionally, locally grown foods do not incur large transportation costs to the source of consumption and in many cases retain more nutritive values due to a shorter time from field to plate.

Downsides of organic and sustainable foods are the high overall cost and lower yields due to not using pesticides and artificial fertilizer. Many scientists believe that organic food is related to the anti-technology, and antimodern science movement and is not beneficial to society as a whole.

Whether you believe that organic and sustainable foods are good, bad, or neutral, the fact remains that the trend is here to stay and that culinary professionals, dietitians, and the entire food industry must become familiar with these concepts and trends.

Changing Role of Distributors' Sales Representatives

Distributors' sales representatives (DSRs) have become consultants and problem solvers rather than mere order takers. Because purchase orders are processed using EDI, DSRs are trained to be customer-oriented and to provide information on products, packaging, economics, environmental issues, commodities, market trends, inventory control, conditions influencing costs, availability of products and supplies, and promotional and recipe ideas. All DSRs have a thorough knowledge of their accounts and of their company's product lines. In effect, they provide value-added services as a strategy to increase customer loyalty.

Food Marketing and Wholesaling

The food distribution and marketing system is part of the food and fiber system, the largest industrial system in the United States. Using inputs of technology, capital, machinery, fertilizers, chemicals, petroleum, and labor, farmers produce the nation's supply of raw food and fiber products. They then wholesale these basic raw products to the marketing sector of the food and fiber system.

Transporting is a vital link from farm to table. The use of modern transportation systems and the continuing application of new transportation systems play vital roles in meeting the volume and quality demands of foodservice operations and customers. Transportation cost is added to the overall cost of the product. It is important for the foodservice director to know the distance the food has traveled until it reaches the establishment's dock. The director needs to ask questions about the delivery vehicle—does it use alternative fuel, and fuel efficiency vehicles. Can the same food product be purchased locally or within 100 miles of the establishment?

Another factor in food marketing involves *processing*. Today many of the major food manufacturers are subsidiaries of large industrial corporations that deal in many industries other than food. Because of this factor, the level of concentration in any particular industry has been reduced. Other major industries have become more concentrated through the horizontal integration of their activities. *Horizontal integration* occurs when a large corporation purchases a company that manufactures and distributes products that often are totally unlike those of the larger company. Modern food-processing companies have also become *vertically integrated* into a wide range of activities other than processing. Contract production for processors is a more common means of integration than ownership of production facilities.

Marketing System

The U.S. food-marketing system serves the country's population by supplying farm products in the desired forms and at the appropriate times. The system assembles, grades, stores, processes, packages, transports, wholesales, retails, prices, takes risks on, controls the quality of, merchandises, exchanges ownership of, brands, regulates, develops, and tests most of the food products—old and new—consumed in the United States.

Food processors and manufacturers are a direct-market outlet for vast quantities of raw farm products and the source of supplies for hundreds of thousands of distributors. This large, complex system must mesh smoothly to overcome problems of food perishability, seasonal availability, volume, and logistics. To remain dynamic and responsive, the system must provide not only a means for product flow from producer to consumer, but also a communication system for the flow of information about consumer preferences and demands from consumer to producer.

The food-marketing system includes more than half a million businesses that employ the equivalent of more than 5 million full-time employees. Persons employed by restaurants and other food-service facilities make up almost half of that total. The output of

FIGURE 18.1 Food Distribution System

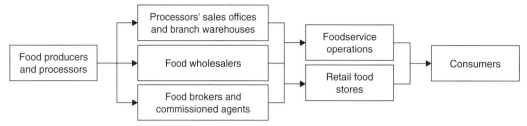

Source: Developed by Ruby P. Puckett©.

farms in the United States, combined with food products from other countries around the world, is gathered by wholesalers and distributors within the marketing system and processed to various degrees by the nation's food manufacturers and processors.

Wholesaling

Wholesaling is the link in the marketing system responsible for distributing food from the producer or processor to the retailer. The principal wholesaling activities involve gathering foods from many sources and distributing them to retailers, hotel and restaurant operators, and other institutions.

Because of the extensive number of products available and the variety of items stocked in relatively small amounts in foodservice operations, foodservice managers could not possibly search out and deal with the producers and processors of all the food products needed. Conversely, processors could not (in many instances) profitably provide the limited quantities needed by individual foodservice units. The job of a food wholesaler is to set up an efficient system for gathering the various products in sizable quantities from various producers and processors and then to sell them in smaller quantities to direct users of the materials.

As shown in Figure 18.1, the structure of a typical food distribution system, the food wholesaler (who buys and assembles the needed products) is the central figure in the distribution process. Some processors can perform the function of wholesaling through their sales offices and branch warehouses. The fact that processors' sales agents specialize in a limited product line means that they can concentrate their expertise and sales efforts on fewer products. These agents do not take title, submit bills, or set prices for the goods sold. Some processors distribute a limited product line or a limited volume of products through food brokers and commissioned agents who act as their sales representatives. This group of intermediaries in the distribution system helps the processors by keeping them informed of current trade conditions and requirements of the market. In turn, the broker's sales staff provides goods and services for the retail and foodservice trade without taking actual possession of the products for sale. Brokers and commissioned agents are paid by the food processors for their services.

Food wholesalers are classified on the basis of their position and their activities in the marketing system. One category includes full-function wholesalers. *Full-function wholesalers* perform all the marketing functions in varying degrees. Their knowledge of the market, buying methods, and techniques for merchandising items to the best advantage is their strongest asset. Because wholesalers must be able to supply their customers with relatively small quantities at frequent intervals, they purchase large quantities of food and store the food and other goods in the form of stock in inventory. Full-function wholesalers extend credit to the customer and deliver goods when ordered. This type of wholesaler is the one most commonly used by foodservice operations.

In contrast, *limited-function wholesalers* carry a limited product line, may or may not extend credit, and establish order-size requirements for delivery. Processors' sales forces usually fall into this category.

Wholesalers also can be classified according to the types of products they handle. For example, wholesalers that stock a wide variety of goods so that the buyer can obtain a significant percentage of the items needed from one source are known as *general-line wholesalers*. There has been a trend toward expansion of the types and lines of products and services handled by institutional wholesalers so that volume-feeding establishments can purchase virtually all their supplies from one wholesaler. This strategy is sometimes called *one-stop shopping*. (More information about this trend is provided later in this chapter.)

In contrast to general-line wholesalers, *specialty wholesalers* handle only one line or a few closely related lines of products. For example, some specialize in perishable products, such as fresh produce; they may handle some frozen fruits and vegetables and other related products as well. The number and economic importance of specialty wholesalers are declining in the U.S. food distribution system.

Make or Buy

Because of recent changes in the health care industry, including reductions in the length of stay and increased operating costs, foodservice directors more than ever must seek ways to contain or reduce costs at the same time they continue to provide high-quality foodservice. Food products can be purchased in ready-to-eat or ready-to-bake form. Alternatively, they can be made from "scratch," that is, by beginning with basic raw ingredients and completely preparing the item in the foodservice department, this process is known as "make." However, fewer and fewer foodservice departments prepare items from scratch because of the time and labor involved. Making the decision whether to make or to buy particular food items requires that the director spend time investigating the level of quality received for the price when items are purchased ready-made. (Providing high-quality food is always the primary goal for a foodservice operation.) The foodservice director must determine the best method for the quality and quantity and economic concerns for the production of a menu item. This may mean that the foodservice director will need to produce the menu item by starting with the raw items, purchase the same items and assemble, and/or purchase ready prepared items and serve.

When making the decision to make or to buy a particular item, the foodservice director should consider:

- The smell, taste, and appearance of the item made from scratch in the facility compared with the item purchased ready-to-cook or ready-to-eat. (Use objective written score cards—File.)
- The labor costs involved in making the item from scratch. (Labor hours need to include regular pay plus fringe benefits, which vary from 25 to 35 percent for all personnel involved in the preparation for both and compare the purchase versus determining the difference in labor costs.)
- The storage space required for the purchased items. (If frozen, is there adequate space for additional items?)
- The quantity of the item that can be prepared at one time.
- The time needed for preparing the item and skills of personnel. (Do employees have the skills to produce the same product?)
- The availability of equipment. (Will the product require the use of equipment that will interfere with other production items?)
- The quality of vendor service. (Deliveries on time, runout of products?)
- The administration's policy on the facility's quality of foodservice.
- Budgetary constraints. (Will the convenience save money, considering labor as well as food cost?)
- Customer satisfaction survey results.
- Clean-up and sanitation of equipment and work area.

For example, determine price difference between purchasing lasagna, a labor-intensive product, and making it:

Purchase:
    48 pounds of lasagna to serve 4 oz. per person.
    Total cost = $56
Make:
    Labor cook $15 per hour × 2.0 hours = $30 plus benefits
        factor of 22%
    Labor cost $30 × 1.22 cost per hour = $45
    Supplies cost (meat, noodles, sauce, and cheese) = $40
    Total cost = $40 + $45 = $85 for 48 pounds
Purchase is $29 less than make.

When product labor cost is high it is usually better to purchase the convenience item.

Value Analysis

A formula to determine the best value in service and price is known as *value analysis*. The formula is:

$$V = QP, \text{in which}$$

V represents value,
Q represents quality, and
P represents price.

If the quality (**Q**) increases and price (**P**) remains constant, the value (**V**) increases. Although the formula can express the concept of value analysis, it is hard to use quality entirely. Price is not the only factor and may not be the most important one. Many factors affect value and quality. The product and service must meet the customer needs. Standards of quality vary from one operation to another.

PROCUREMENT PROCESS

The purpose of *procurement* (buying or purchasing) is to:

- Procure the products needed at the most economical price, quality, quantity, and value
- Have the products delivered in a safe and sanitary condition
- Have the products delivered as scheduled
- Have the products transported in the appropriate vehicle

Procuring products and services for the foodservice department is a complex process involving much more than the buyer simply acquiring products and services from reputable distributors and organizations. The term *procurement* involves a broad range of product selection and purchasing activities required to meet the needs of the foodservice department.

The process depends on a complex decision-making process that includes determining quality and quantity standards for the facility; specifying and ordering foods that meet those standards; and receiving, storing, and controlling the food supply inventory (Figure 18.2). (Inventory control, receiving, and storage are discussed in detail in Chapter 19.) Effective procurement requires that buyers have immediate access to a great deal of current and accurate information so as to make the best decision given the resources at their disposal.

Buyer's Responsibilities

Responsibility for the *procurement process* varies depending on the size and philosophy of the health care institution and on available expertise in the foodservice department. In smaller facilities, the foodservice director or manager often performs or coordinates

FIGURE 18.2 Procurement Process

1. Complete needs assessment

   - Evaluate menu
   - Standardize recipe
   - Gather input from product evaluation team
   - Gather input from management staff
   - Forecast production demand

2. Select purchasing method(s)

   - Consider size and philosophy of operation
   - Determine purchase volume
   - Determine frequency of delivery
   - Consider distributor location
   - Evaluate department storage facilities
   - Determine available personnel

3. Develop approved vendor or distributor list

   - Decide whether to use a prime vendor

4. Establish and maintain inventory system

   - Just-in-time purchasing
   - Perpetual inventory
   - Physical inventory
   - Consider value of inventory
   - Determine frequency of delivery

5. Determine order quantity

   - Forecast menu portions
   - Determine standard portions
   - Determine serving supplies
   - Assess food on hand

6. Obtain bid or price quotes

   - Develop specifications for each item
   - Obtain best prices and terms

7. Place order

   - Specify price
   - Specify quantity
   - Specify payment method
   - Distribute copies of order

8. Receive order

   - Request minimum number of shipments

9. Store order

   - Consider type of food

10. Issue items

Source: Developed by Ruby P. Puckett©.

procurement activities. Large organizations may employ an individual with special training or expertise in procurement. The buyer may be a foodservice employee if decentralized purchasing is used or an employee of the purchasing department if the facility has centralized its purchasing activities. Responsibilities of the food buyer include:

- Determining foodservice department needs in terms of product, equipment, and services
- Selecting the method(s) of purchasing
- Selecting vendor(s)
- Soliciting and awarding bids or contracts

- Placing and following up on orders
- Training and supervising employees in receiving, storage, and issuance of food and supplies
- Establishing and maintaining an inventory control system
- Conducting research, including evaluating new products and conducting value analyses and make-or-buy studies
- Participating on the product evaluation team
- Maintaining effective vendor relations
- Assessing cost benefit of value-added services provided by the distributor
- Providing product information such as cost data and nutrition information to others in the foodservice department
- Tracking changes in the market and economic conditions through open communication with DSRs, attending trade and food shows, and keeping abreast of trends by reading trade and professional publications
- Utilizing current technology to facilitate the procurement process
- Maintaining open communication lines throughout the foodservice department and the larger institution
- Maintaining ethical conduct above reproach as defined by the National Association of Purchasers, the Academy of Nutrition and Dietetics, Association of Nutrition and Foodservice Professionals, Association of Healthcare Foodservice, and Foodservice Consultants Society International

Buyer's Qualifications

Ideally, a buyer's educational and experiential qualifications should encompass the following areas: (1) food quality; (2) product specifications; (3) computer skills, especially in spreadsheet applications; (4) marketing and distribution channels in the food distribution system (see Figure 18.1); (5) accounting and other business activities associated with purchasing, such as soliciting and awarding bids; (6) contracts, performing make-or-buy analyses; and (7) setting up "can-cutting" demonstrations with the foodservice department and the wholesale company. Experience in food production and service also is beneficial. In addition, the buyer should possess certain managerial, interpersonal, and personal attributes. Some of these are organizational skills and a penchant for detail and accuracy, a team mind-set, initiative, good human relations and communication skills, and high ethical standards. Because of the complexity of activities performed, the buyer must be organized and follow through on tasks. Good human relations and communication skills are essential because he or she must meet the needs of several individuals in the foodservice department and communicate these needs to DSRs, members of GPOs, and all other parties with whom the buyer interacts. Not only must the buyer demonstrate initiative in continuously assessing opportunities to increase or maintain food quality, but he or she must do so while decreasing cost whenever feasible. Attention to detail is critical because accuracy in purchase orders and inventory affects operating costs and service delivery. The buyer must maintain high ethical standards at all times—avoiding conflict of interest and kickbacks, for example.

No matter who has ultimate authority for the procurement function, a procurement specialist or the foodservice manager, the individual must maintain high standards in product quality. The buyer must continuously assess how to obtain products, equipment, and services to meet the needs of various components of the food-service department while remaining within the financial constraints imposed on the operation.

Steps in the Foodservice Procurement Process

As illustrated in Figure 18.2, the procurement process in a food-service department is a 10-step sequence of activities. This process may be adjusted as needed to accommodate a particular facility or organizational structure. The process includes not only the 10 steps but three other points to consider:

1. Food must be purchased from an approved source. An approved source is one that is inspected based on federal, state, and local laws and has appropriate HACCP procedures in place.
2. Purchasing must meet quality, quantity, price, and schedule.
3. Needs assessment is essential.

The following sections discuss the procurement-process steps, and more information on receiving and storing is provided in Chapter 19.

Needs Assessment

The purpose of a needs assessment is to determine the operation's requirements for food, supplies, equipment, and services, including quality, quantity, and required time frame. Information sources the buyer should rely on in completing the needs assessment include menu(s), standardized recipes, production demand forecasts, input from the product evaluation team and management staff, customer surveys, and the image the operation wants to project. Current and projected needs should be determined such as a change in menu or type of service. Maintaining a master calendar of catered functions and other special activities that would influence the procurement process is strongly recommended.

Food Budget　By estimating the cost of food items as each menu is planned, the overall cost can be kept within the limitations of the budget. Before food is purchased, the estimated costs should be checked against current food prices. The foods purchased should make the best possible contribution to the consumers' nutrition for the money spent.

Availability of Food Items　Food items appearing on the menu should be available to the department in the desired form, quantity and quality. The seasonal availability of various fresh foods affects their quality and price. The choice among fresh, canned, and frozen items varies, depending on the season. Weather conditions can affect the movement of food supplies, especially fresh fruits and vegetables, through market channels and sometimes may necessitate

changes in the menu. Adverse weather can also cause shortages and increased prices. This is extremely important if using "local" sources.

Labor Budget　The number and skill levels of production workers and the cost of their labor should be considered in relation to the cost of purchasing certain food items in a partially or fully prepared state. If the number of labor hours will not be reduced, the higher cost of convenience foods may not fit within the total budget.

Equipment and Space　The availability of both equipment and space for the preparation and storage of food directly affects menu planning. If the production area is adequately equipped, the facility's menu planner should make good use of what is available by including a variety of items to be prepared on-site. If the production area is poorly equipped, however, the menu planner should include enough prepared food products to ensure adequate variety on the menu. The type and amount of storage space affect the type and amount of foods that can be purchased and, therefore, the kinds of items that can be included on the menu. When ample storage space is available, some foodservice directors maintain large inventories because they think that they can save money by buying large quantities. However, the savings advantage gained by buying large quantities may not equal the institution's cost of having money tied up in large food inventories. The best size for the inventory varies among foodservice departments and depends on the size of the institution, the institution's inventory policies, the amount of space available, and the location of suppliers. In addition, carrying more inventory than necessary can result in a loss of food quality and poor use of funds.

Selection of Purchasing Method

The next step in the process is to select the procurement method(s) most appropriate for a particular facility. Factors that influence the decision may include the decision to make or buy a product, the size and philosophy of the foodservice operation, purchase volume, frequency of delivery desired, distributor's location, department storage facilities, available personnel and their skill levels, and type of purchasing system—centralized or decentralized, for example. The two basic methods are formal and informal.

Approved Vendor or Distributor List

Identifying the vendor, distributor, or suppliers with whom the organization will conduct business is a critical step in the procurement process. Specific factors to consider, which are discussed more fully later in this chapter, also may influence the selected method(s) of purchasing. These factors also may determine whether a distributor would meet a particular organization's needs or even conduct business with the facility.

Inventory System

The inventory system established helps determine whether to implement just-in-time purchasing, a perpetual inventory, or a physical inventory (among other choices). It also determines the quantity of supplies maintained on hand, value of the inventory (in other words, how much money is tied up in inventory and unavailable for other uses), and frequency of delivery.

Order Quantity

The planned menu and past statistical data tell the buyer what kinds of food are needed, but only careful planning can ensure a supply of food sufficient for producing the anticipated number of meals with a minimum amount of leftovers. The quantities of food needed can be calculated by following four steps:

1. Forecast as accurately as possible the number of serving portions required for each item on the menu. When a selective menu is used, the forecast can be based on records of the number of selections previously made when the same combinations were served. Forecasting is more difficult when other types of menus are used. *Forecasting* is estimating needs for specific items using past data to determine future needs. It is the basis of procurement.

2. Determine a standard portion size for each food item. The standard portion size should correspond to the portion size stated on the standardized recipes to be used. Standardized recipes also should state the amount of each ingredient to be purchased for the stated yield.

3. Determine the quantities of food supplies required for the number of serving portions needed.

4. Check the amount of food on hand in refrigerated, frozen, and dry storage areas and subtract that amount from the quantity needed for the planned menus. Prepare a list of supplies that must

be purchased and a list of those to be requisitioned from the storeroom.

Regardless of the purchasing method used, order quantities should be large enough to make transactions economically worthwhile for vendors. The advantages of price comparison and product choice are lost if small orders are split among several vendors because of price.

Bid and Price Quotes, Order Placement, and Record Keeping

If purchasing is centralized, the foodservice department usually completes a purchase requisition form like the one shown in Exhibit 18.1 to inform the purchasing agent (centralize purchasing) of the quantity and quality of specific foods to be ordered. The *purchase requisition* should contain complete specifications for each item, the unit of purchase (dozen or case, for example), the total quantity of each item, and the requested delivery date. In addition, a vendor and a price may be suggested; however, the purchasing agent is responsible for obtaining bids and awarding the purchase to the supplier quoting the best prices and terms. This approach works best when the director of the foodservice department and the central purchasing agent can pool their knowledge and communicate freely. Administrative policy usually requires that purchase requisitions be approved by a designated person in the foodservice department before being sent to the purchasing department. The purchase requisition should be prepared in multiple copies, the number depending on the organization's record-keeping system. At least one copy should be kept on file in the foodservice department.

EXHIBIT 18.1 Purchase Requisition

PURCHASE REQUISITION

To: Purchasing Office   Requisition No.: _____

Date: _____   Purchase Order No.: _____

From: _____   Date Required: _____

Item	Unit	Total Quantity	Description	Suggested Vendor	Unit Cost	Total Cost

Requested by: _____ Approved by: _____ Date Ordered: _____

Source: Developed by Ruby P. Puckett©.

Whether a purchasing department or the foodservice department does the purchasing, a *purchase order* should always be used to inform the vendor of specific requirements. A purchase order is a legal document authorizing a supplier to deliver merchandise in accordance with the terms stated on the form. Purchase order forms, such as the example shown in Exhibit 18.2, are standardized by the institution and used by all departments.

The information contained in these forms includes the name and address of the supplier; a complete specification for each item, unless the vendor already has the specification on file (in which case the specification number can be used along with a brief description); the total quantity of each item ordered; the price per unit quoted by the vendor; the total price for the amount ordered; the terms of delivery; and the method of payment. This process is known as *closed bidding* and is not as formal as *contract bidding*, which is discussed later in the chapter. The bid process should also make sure that all bidders receive the same bid packet. In addition to the information described above the bid to purchase the sealed packet should also contain:

- That the price quoted must remain the same for the entire period of the contract (except in rare instances when the price increases to a point the supplier is not making a profit or cannot secure the item due to crop failure, weather conditions, and so forth. The foodservice director and/or the purchasing agent will meet with the supplier and renegotiate the price).
- All bidders **must** bid on the specification for all products listed.
- Designate by a ☺ what items offer a manufacturer's rebate and if the supplier or the foodservice director will request the rebate.
- All suppliers who request a bid must be allowed to receive one.
- The date the bids will be opened and if the opening is a closed or open meeting for all bidders to attend.
- Before the result of the bid is made public, the foodservice department reserves the right to request from bidders samples of "questionable" bid items or new products, for quality and quantity evaluation.
- Once all testing is completed the bids will be awarded—again if appropriate during an open meeting where bidders, foodservice personnel, and purchasing personnel are in attendance.

The number of copies of the purchase order to be made varies among institutions, but because it is the record of merchandise ordered and the form used to check the receipt of deliveries, all departments dealing with supplies or with payments need copies.

EXHIBIT 18.2 Purchase Order Form

PURCHASE ORDER

To: _____

_____

Purchase Order No.: _____

Date: _____

Requisition No.: _____

Department: _____

Date required: _____

Ship to: _____ F.O.B. _____ Via: _____ Terms: _____

Item	Unit	Total Quantity	Description	Price per Unit	Total Cost

Approved by: _____

Source: Developed by Ruby P. Puckett©.

Obtaining Bids and Price Quotes

Once the requisition is approved, the purchasing department or foodservice director develops a *bid packet* to be sent to or picked up by a number of suppliers that will compete over price quotations that meet the specifications, time frame, and quantities as stated in the bid. Once all suppliers return their bids, the bids are opened, and a flow sheet is made for comparing prices, discounts, delivery schedules, and other pertinent data. After the suppliers' data are compared, the bid is awarded and purchase numbers given. Choices for awarding the bid are based on all-or-nothing or line-item bidding, sometimes referred to as *cherry picking*. In an *all-or-nothing bid*, the supplier bids on all items and offers a price per line and the best price for the complete bid. *Line-item bidding* is selecting items that meet the lowest price and quality per item. With this method, a number of suppliers are awarded items. If the quantity award is not sufficient for the supplier to realize a return on his or her investment, the supplier may not accept the bid. Line-item bidding is more time-consuming than *all-or-nothing bidding*.

Price quotes are used for perishable goods and are usually made by telephone, e-mail, or fax. The buyer, usually someone in the foodservice department, requests price quotes on specific food items from approved providers for a specific amount of goods and quality. Prices are secured from one or more vendors, and price and quality are compared after all quotes are received. The lowest price may not be the best bid, depending on the use of the product. After the decision is made, the buyer contacts the supplier by telephone, fax, or e-mail and places the order.

In some cases, the quote sheet may be used as the purchase order. If a purchase order is needed it can be prepared by using the information from the quote sheet.

All bids and price quotes need to include the shipping terms, method of delivery, and terms for payment. A common shipping term, *free-on-board* (FOB), means that the products are delivered to a specific location (preferably the foodservice loading dock) with all transportation paid. *FOB origin* refers to the place from which the product is originally transported, and *FOB destination* refers to the place the product is going to be received. FOB origin is stipulated when the order is placed, and the buyer selects the transport company and pays the freight company, owns the title, and files the claims for bad or damaged goods. If FOB destination is stipulated, the buyer pays the freight charges, but the supplier owns the title and files any claims.

After bids and quotes are received, orders are placed with the suppliers. A purchase order number may be issued for a certain period and for certain items (milk, bread) is used for each order, and these are filed in sequential order blanks. The order may be placed face-to-face (buyer to supplier), by fax, or electronically.

Record keeping of all purchases is vital to the foodservice department and organization for paying invoices and an audit trail.

EVALUATING PRODUCTS

Before awarding a bid, some operations may request that the suppliers provide samples of their products for taste and test evaluation. It is important to taste the products on the bid list to determine if the quality requested is being offered and to compare prices.

One method to use to evaluate products is *can cutting*. A number of suppliers provide the products, and foodservice personnel, the purchasing officer, and others as appropriate receive the products and carefully evaluate against written specifications. A rating sheet is used, and each person involved should objectively and independently rate the products (see Exhibit 18.3). Once all independent evaluations are completed, they are tallied, the results of the evaluation discussed, and the decision made on which product to select.

EXHIBIT 18.3 Sample Score Sheet for Can-Cutting

Measurements	Sample A	Sample B
Head space	_____	_____
Drained weight	_____	_____
Count	_____	_____
Brix	_____	_____

Maximum points: 20

Color	Sample A	Sample B
Bright	_____	_____
Uniformity of color	_____	_____
Free from skin pigment	_____	_____

Maximum points: 20

Uniformity of size	Sample A	Sample B
Symmetry	_____	_____
Shape	_____	_____

Maximum points: 20

Absence of defects	Sample A	Sample B
Free from blemishes and peel	_____	_____
Free from trimmed or crushed portions	_____	_____
Free from loose seed, stem, and core material	_____	_____

Maximum points: 30

Character	Sample A	Sample B
Uniformly ripened	_____	_____
Fleshy tender texture	_____	_____
Reasonably well-drained edges	_____	_____
Intact and pliable flesh	_____	_____

Maximum points:

After testing each sample, check which sample is preferable in:

	Sample A	Sample B
Texture	_____	_____
Flavor	_____	_____

In general, which sample is preferable? Why?

100–90 points	Grade A Fancy
86–80 points	Grade B Choice
76–70 points	Grade C Standard

Yields

The weight of a product should be evaluated to determine yield. A *product yield* tells how much usable food is obtained from each product.

There is a difference between package weight and net weight, for example, for cereals. *Net weight* is the weight of the product once it is removed from all packing. When dealing with canned fruits and vegetables, the drained weight is also important. *Drained weight* is the amount of usable product once all the liquid has been removed. For example what is purchased may not be the useable amount:

> Product A:
>   Canned sliced peaches #10 can weighs 105 ounces
>   AP Cost per can $3.25/can
>   Drained weight 90 ounces EP
> Product B
>   Canned sliced peaches #10 can weighs 105 ounces
>   AP Cost per can $3.20/can
>   Drained weight 85 ounces EP
> Which is the best buy?
>   Product A: $3.25 ÷ 90 = $0.0361 per ounce
>   Product B: $3.20 ÷ 85 = $0.0371 per ounce

Another important method of evaluation is to determine the *as purchased* (AP) weight, which is the amount of food purchased before processing to give the number of edible portions required to serve a specific number of customers. The *edible portion (EP)* is the amount of weight or useable product is left after the removal of such—skin, bones, outside leaves, stems, peels, and so forth—are removed and discarded and are unusable to produce or serve. During the cooking process the shrinkage of meat product varies from 35 to 60 percent. In purchasing it is important to know the amount of shrinkage to ensure enough product is ordered. To determine the *edible price* (EP price) use this formula:

$$AP \text{ price} \div EP \text{ yield} = EP \text{ price}$$

Edible yield factor (EYF) is the figure that assists in the calculation of how many products will remain after preparation. The EYF is expressed as a percentage and equals the EP divided by the AP.

Usually a difference exists between raw quantities and final quantities after preparation.

As purchased (AP) includes

- Bones in chicken and meat
- Peels on potatoes, cores and seeds in certain fruits, outer leaves of lettuce, cabbage; celery bottoms, green stalks on cauliflower, stems on broccoli, hulls on beans/legumes
- Total weight of cereal, canned fruits, vegetables

It is vital that the AP and EP and the EYF be known when purchasing. Price may not always be the best factor especially if the EP is less per ounce, piece, or pound. One way of predicting the proper amounts of food to purchase is to produce a given number of servings, such as 10 4-ounce beef patties.

Common Mistakes Made in Purchasing

The foodservice director and purchasing agent are responsible for cleanly and objectively developing specifications and guidelines for purchasing. The following are mistakes that are frequently made.

- Using "or equivalent" on a bid. The buyer is responsible for determining the equivalency, such as price, quality, package size, grade, and so forth (many state-supported facilities require this). The specifications should be clearly defined and accurate and specify who will determine what product is equivalent (can cutting, taste panels, and the like) (Chapter 16).
- Being unaware of rebates, discounts, and promotions and how these pricing arrangements from manufacturers will affect a firm bid price. Determine if the suppliers or the foodservice director (or both) will apply for these discounts and how they may be applied back to the total food cost.
- Failing to add quality assurance and food safety to the specifications. Hazard analysis critical control point programs should be in place from farm to delivery site, the type of delivery trucks, and the method used to monitor temperature from warehouse to facility dock.
- Failing to clearly state how often deliveries are to be made, the approximate day and time of deliveries, and what role the delivery person will have in off-loading products.
- Not being aware of selecting line items versus all categories, especially for price and quality. When suppliers think they may be awarded only one to three items, they may inflate costs.
- Failing to respect the manufacturer. It is important that all persons involved in the purchasing process realize that the manufacturer must make a profit and that the buyer must receive the quality of the food that has been specified.
- Failing to specify how the FOB will be handled.

Order Receipt, Storage, and Issuance of Items

Delivery schedule requests should be considered carefully. Increased transportation costs will affect food costs if deliveries are requested at the last minute or for only one or two items. The delivery schedule required depends on the size of the institution, its geographical location, its storage facilities, and the size of the foodservice staff. In general, however, economy of food delivery and storage can be achieved as follows:

- Meat, poultry, and fish delivered once a week or less frequently, depending on whether the products are chilled or frozen
- Fresh produce delivered once or twice a week, depending on the storage space available and the quantities needed
- Canned goods and staples delivered weekly, semimonthly, monthly, or quarterly, depending on the storage space available, quantities needed, and price quotes for specific volumes

- Milk, milk products, bread, and baked goods delivered daily or every other day
- Butter, eggs, and cheese delivered weekly or as needed
- Frozen foods delivered weekly or semimonthly, depending on the storage space available, usage rate, and price quotes for the quantities needed

On-delivery and acceptance items should be stored in the appropriate area until requisitioned for use.

PURCHASING METHODS

The purchasing method used by the buyer varies depending on the organization's size, philosophy and policies, purchasing volume, and financial stability, and the distributor's location and current environmental trends. The most common methods of purchasing used by health care foodservice facilities include group purchasing, consortium purchasing, prime vendor, one-stop purchasing, just-in-time purchasing, and formal (competitive) and informal (off-the-street) purchasing.

Group Purchasing Organizations

Some institutions are combining their buying power by forming purchasing cooperatives, or GPOs, to save costs. These units are also known as *cooperatives*, buying groups, and purchasing support groups. Generally, the term *cooperative* is used to describe nonprofit organizations, whereas the term *group purchasing* describes the relationship among for-profit organizations that pool their purchasing power. Regardless of which term is used, about 90 percent of all health care organizations belong to one or more of these groups. Compared with other health care departments, purchases by foodservice departments account for less than 10 percent of purchases made by the largest national and regional GPO.

The concept of group purchasing is based on the premise that several organizations have more purchasing power when negotiating collectively than any one entity alone. Purchasing groups can be organized on a local, state, regional, or national level. The requirements for membership and services provided vary. In most instances, members of a GPO pay a membership fee that is often based on bed count, dollar value of operating budget, or some other scale based on the volume of purchases. These fees provide capital for operating the central office and employing procurement personnel, consultants, and legal services attendant to negotiating contracts. Some GPOs require members to purchase a specified volume of products, whereas others expect members to use their contractual agreements to their fullest potential.

Most GPOs have several characteristics in common, including:

- At least one full-time procurement person/consultant works with members to identify their needs and to negotiate contracts.
- Members usually meet formally to establish or update policies and operating procedures, establish specifications, evaluate products, share information, provide educational programs, and assess the GPO's function.

- GPOs frequently function as agents for the members, acting on members' behalf when negotiating contracts.
- A membership fee is required.
- Many GPOs are currently establishing prime vendor programs requiring committed-volume contracts. Members are **required** to purchase a minimum of 80 percent of their products from prime vendors with whom the GPO has contracts. Produce is rarely included in group purchasing. In some instances, members are prohibited from joining other GPOs with prime vendor arrangements.
- Competitive bidding is the primary procedure used for determining pricing, terms, and contract conditions between the GPO and the supplier.
- Value-added services such as product quality testing, value analysis, computer systems and software, employee development seminars, recipe ideas, and menu planning may be provided to GPO members. Working with suppliers to offer rebates and discounts.

Savings in excess of 20 percent is the primary reason foodservice directors use group purchasing. Other benefits include product standardization, increased quality, decreased administrative cost for processing multiple purchase orders, and less time spent in purchasing products and supplies. Members also cite improved knowledge of new and existing products and enhanced networking as a result of participation in GPO meetings. Membership commitment and support of the GPO's philosophy are essential for success of the group.

Some barriers that influence the effectiveness and cost savings of participating in a GPO include difficulty in obtaining consensus on product specifications; loss of control over supplier selection, product variety, quality, and contract awards; and unwillingness of representatives of competing health care organizations to work as team members. Group members who join multiple GPOs decrease the negotiating power of the group because the volume of purchasing is diminished. The group's purchasing power is increased only when volume is significantly more than it would be for each foodservice department.

When selecting a GPO, the buyer and foodservice director should adhere to certain guidelines, such as the following:

- Select a group composed of members from foodservice organizations sharing similar characteristics such as size, philosophy, teaching/university hospitals, and so on.
- Interview current members and the GPO's employees to assess potential savings in excess of required fees.
- Answer the following questions:
  What are membership requirements? Is a guarantee to purchase a specified quantity (percentage) or dollar volume through the GPO required?
  How does the GPO operate?
  What value-added services are provided to members?
  Is a prime vendor contract used? If so, what product lines are available?
  What is the GPO doing to obtain data on current market prices, new products, and trends?

- Discuss findings with foodservice management staff and members of the quality product evaluation team.
- Consult with the financial officer when evaluating the cost-benefit ratio of membership.
- Present a proposal for joining a GPO to the administration.

One-Stop Purchasing or Single Sourcing

One-stop purchasing or single sourcing is defined as the strategy of selecting and using a single supply source. This purchasing method is used by large and small health care facilities (including long-term care facilities). The method is based on a cooperative relationship between the foodservice department and the vendor.

One vendor (a full-line distributor) provides the buyer with most of the food and supplies needed. The efficiency of food purchasing is improved by eliminating the time-consuming processes of placing bids and getting quotations. A substantial reduction in warehousing costs is possible if deliveries are made frequently. Lower net costs of products can result because the supplier knows relatively far in advance that certain foodservices will be needing specific products; thus, the vendor can buy from wholesalers in larger quantities.

Certain disadvantages can arise from relying on one vendor exclusively. For one thing, backup suppliers might be difficult to find should the single-source vendor fail to deliver the supplies ordered. For another, the quality of available foods might be inferior or inconsistent. For larger foodservice departments, the number of distributors able to supply one-stop services may be limited; nonetheless, the supplier pool for this service provision is definitely growing. The effectiveness of one-stop purchasing is directly related to the efficiency and credibility of the supplier. Most foodservice departments generally have found this method to work satisfactorily.

Prime Vendor Agreements

The *prime vendor* method involves a formal agreement between the foodservice department (buyer) and one vendor (supplier) whereby the buyer contracts with the vendor to supply a specified percentage of a given category (or categories) of product. The percentage ranges from 60 to 80 percent, with 80 percent being more common today. The prime vendor contract, also referred to as a *systems contract*, includes an agreement to purchase certain items for a specified time period and frequently specifies a minimum quantity of any or all items to be ordered during the contract period.

The steps involved in establishing a prime vendor relationship are outlined below. The bidding system is similar to contract purchasing, which is discussed later in this section.

- The buyer completes an ABC analysis of purchases to determine which items make up the majority of purchases (see Chapter 20).
- The foodservice department solicits bid proposals from several distributors for an estimated committed volume (annual or monthly usage); product specification; and designated delivery, services, and inventory.

- The foodservice director (or other buyer) reviews the bid and determines the lowest bidder that meets all criteria.
- The buyer negotiates and awards a contract.
- The foodservice department (through the director or other channel) provides feedback to the vendor on quality of service, delivery, and products. The foodservice representative can require the vendor to "open the books" and provide information on the structure of its cost and pricing data if this privilege is a condition of the contract. It is imperative that the purchasing agent continue to track prices and market conditions.
- The buyer develops secondary sources for products and supplies.

The benefits of a *prime vendor agreement* are increased competition and lower prices; reduced cost of inventory, space, and order processing; and availability of value-added services. One value-added service that many health care foodservices use is computer systems provided by the prime vendor that allow the foodservice operation to place orders, obtain current price information and availability of products and supplies and product information (including nutrient analysis), and implement menu-planning and merchandising ideas. Some prime vendors provide a variety of software programs to their customers.

Disadvantages include potential gradual price increases, a decrease in competition, and a limited number of vendors with whom the operation conducts business. A reduction in service level can occur, especially in areas where only a limited number of vendors are available to conduct business. For the concept to be effective, continued enhancement of the vendor-buyer relationship is essential. The buyer must treat the DSRs and individuals delivering the product as partners rather than adversaries. Prime vendor contracts are also used in group purchasing.

Just-in-Time Purchasing

Just-in-time (JIT) *purchasing* is a production planning strategy adopted by many manufacturing firms. The process involves purchasing products and supplies in the exact quantity required for a production run or limited time period and only as they are needed ("just in time"). Distributors deliver small quantities of supplies more frequently, and deliveries are timed more precisely based on production demand. Thus, JIT purchasing has an effect on both purchasing and inventory. Three goals are achieved with the JIT purchasing process: inventory is decreased significantly, as are related costs; space management is simplified; and problems must be resolved immediately as they occur. Unlike the manufacturing industry, each day foodservice operations produce a large number of perishable products in smaller quantities. The effectiveness of JIT purchasing warrants investigation because of potential cost reductions. JIT is an excellent method of purchasing disposables, cleaning, and ware-washing supplies.

The ability to implement this method depends on several factors. These include complete support and cooperation of suppliers, the commitment of all employees (including top administrators), accurate production demand forecasts, and changes in most aspects of the operation from menu planning through final service.

Locating foodservice distributors willing to provide frequent deliveries may be a challenge to some buyers, given that most distributors are requesting that customers accept fewer deliveries so as to decrease costs. Like the prime vendor concept, JIT purchasing requires building partnerships with distributors, and the adoption of the JIT-purchasing philosophy could require a change in attitude regarding quantity of supplies to maintain in inventory. JIT-purchasing practices emphasize ordering small quantities rather than storing large quantities just in case additional product is needed.

Centralized Purchasing

With *centralized purchasing*, the most common method of purchasing used in health care institutions, a separate department in the institution specializes in purchasing the materials and supplies needed by the institution's various services and departments. In this system, the foodservice director (like all other department heads) requisitions supplies from the purchasing department. Only representatives from the purchasing department deal directly with outside vendors and suppliers. Vendors have direct contact with end users of the supplies only if new products or services are being brought into the purchasing system. In many institutions that use centralized purchasing, the purchasing department also handles receiving, storage, and issuing rather than the individual departments that use the supplies. This system has a number of disadvan-tages, which include the "lack" of knowledge of the needs of the foodservice department, especially for quality ED portions and special needs such as medical nutrition needs and keeping suppliers from interacting with foodservice personnel. It is important that suppliers and foodservice personnel keep the line of communications open in order to find out about trends, rebates, and other helpful information the company offers.

Contract and Noncontract Purchasing

Two other general methods of buying are contract purchasing and noncontract purchasing. *Contract purchasing* (sometimes called formal buying and/or closed bidding) involves a binding agreement between vendor and purchaser. With this process, foodservice directors develop written specifications for each product and an estimate of the quantity needed for the designated bid period. A written notice of requirements, or a bid request (Exhibit 18.4), is made available to vendors, who are invited to submit price bids based on the quality and quantity needed. The bid request includes instructions about the method of bidding, delivery schedule required, and frequency of payment; the date bids are due; the basis for awarding contracts; and any other information needed by buyer and seller. This process may be formal, with notices of intent to bid published under "legal notices" in the local newspaper. Alternatively, it may be informal, with copies of the bid distributed widely through the mail or by other means.

EXHIBIT 18.4 Bid Request

Bid Request

Bids will be received until _____ for __[indicate type of]__ delivery on the date indicated.

Issued by: _____   Address: _____

Date issued: _____   Date to be delivered: __[5–10 days after bid is awarded]__

Increases in quantity up to 20 percent will be binding at the discretion of the buyer. All items are to be officially certified by the U.S. Department of Agriculture for acceptance no earlier than two days before delivery; costs of such service to be borne by the supplier.

Item No.	Description	Quantity	Unit	Unit Price	Amount
1.	Chickens, fresh-chilled fryers, 2.5 to 3 lb., ready-to-cook, U.S. Grade A	500	Pound		
2.	Chickens, fresh-chilled hens, 4 to 5 lb., ready-to-cook, U.S. Grade A	100	Pound		
3.	Turkeys, frozen young toms, 20 to 22 lb., ready-to-cook, U.S. Grade A	100	Pound		
4.	Eggs, fresh, large, U.S. Grade A, 30 dozen cases	150	Dozen		
5.	Eggs, frozen, whole, inspected, six 4-pound cartons per case	60	Pound		

Vendor: _____

In addition to specifications for each item to be purchased, the bid request may include general provisions, for example:

- A performance bond by the seller
- Errors in the bid
- Alternate or partial bids
- A discount schedule
- Definition of the terms of the contract
- Time frame for performance
- Requirements for the submission of samples
- Requirements for delivery points
- Inspection provisions
- Provisions for certification of quality
- Packing requirements
- Billing instructions
- Payment methods
- Requirements for standard package size
- Cancellation clause

Obtaining firm, fixed prices for the specified bid period is desirable. However, when product prices fluctuate frequently or rise steadily, vendors may be unable (or unwilling) to quote firm prices for an extended period. Bid requests that state a maximum amount required and a minimum quantity to be purchased from the suc-cessful bidder allow some flexibility for both buyer and vendor when prices of the product needed are likely to fluctuate considerably, for example fish and seafood, which depends on the market price. Although price is a major consideration in awarding the contract, the buyer should carefully consider quality of the product and ability of the vendor to meet the delivery schedules specified in the contract. In addition, the vendor's reputation, previous performance, and compliance with specifications and government regulations are important considerations. All bidders, including those not awarded the contract, should be informed when the contract has been awarded.

Standing order purchasing is made for such items as bread, milk, eggs, and other products that have daily deliveries. Bids are requested for these items usually for a year at a time. The bid will state a firm price or market price of a specific geographical market. Once the bid is awarded, the delivery person will build the stock to meet the level required for a specific time period (daily, twice a day, weekly, and so forth). Stock needs will fluctuate during holidays, weekends, and increased patient census. The foodservice director and delivery person must maintain ongoing communication to avoid an oversupply or undersupply of goods. Who is responsible for the rotating of stock must be clearly defined.

Noncontract purchasing (sometimes called informal buying) is done through verbal and written communications between buyer and vendor through telephone sales representatives. However, it may be handled without direct contact with the sales representative through the open market. Price quotations are obtained from two or more suppliers. Quotation sheets, or call sheets, such as those shown in Exhibit 18.5, are useful. A quotation sheet provides spaces for the name and description of food items, amount of food needed, and prices quoted by various suppliers. After the price quotes have been received, the service and quality record of the supplier that gave the lowest quotation is checked. If the supplier has a history of providing good-quality products on schedule, the order usually is placed there. Although small institutions may use this method to purchase most of their foods, larger ones may use it only for perishable fresh products or foods needed in limited quantities. One disadvantage of noncontract purchasing is the amount of time required to check and compare prices, interview sales representatives, and place orders. Problems also can result from verbal commitments to buy. Some of these problems can be avoided, however, by providing vendors with a list of accurate product specifications as a communication aid.

SUPPLIER SELECTION AND RELATIONS

Supplier selection may be the single most important decision made in the purchasing process. Few distributors or vendors can meet the needs and expectations of all foodservice operations. Thus, it is imperative to select:

- One compatible with a specific operation
- One with which the buyer can work cooperatively to obtain products that meet established standards and the operation's financial constraints
- Quality of the vendor's products and service
- Negotiate a fair price
- Receive consistent quality and quantity as specified
- Receive order on time, willingness to schedule convenient deliveries for organization

- Willingness to have deliveries inspected
- Willingness to refund monies for products rejected at delivery
- Warehouse, delivery trucks are clean and sanitized, products and facilities are free of pest infection, products are FIFO
- Vendor and buyer practice ethical policies
- Allows visits to warehouse, posted inspection codes
- Develop relationships with vendor based on trust
- Avoid internal conflicts over vendor relations
- Build relationships with local vendors to develop goodwill within the community

Achievement of these objectives is essential to the overall success of the procurement process.

Selection

Supplier selection involves a four-stage process, which is best remembered by the mnemonic SINE:

1. **S**urvey: Explore all possible sources of supply.
2. **I**nquiry: Compare and evaluate prospective vendors to identify qualifications, such as size, capacity, or both; financial strengths; technological services; geographical locations; labor relations; and advantages and disadvantages.
3. **N**egotiation and selection: Enter into effective and clear dialogue with candidates to secure the best price, quality, and delivery commitment.
4. **E**xperience: Monitor vendor service and product quality to ensure that what is promised is delivered, delivery is provided in emergency situations, prices do not suddenly change, the number of rejects is kept to a minimum, and the sanitary condition of the warehouse and the hygiene of personnel are appropriate.

EXHIBIT 18.5 Quotation Sheet

Type of product: __Fresh produce__ Day: __Monday__ Date: __2/xx/xxxx__ Approved by: __DL__

Amount on Hand	Quantity	Unit	Description and Specifications	Supplier and Quotations per Unit			
				Smith	Brown		
21	23	50-lb. bag	Carrots	11.40	13.85		
0	1	40-lb. bag	Bananas, #4	12.00	13.40		

The *survey stage* is devoted to identifying the need for new products, investigating new suppliers, or reevaluating current suppliers. Questions in this regard include:

- What is available on the market?
- Who can supply the product(s) or service(s)?
- Who can supply it (them) most (or more) economically within the required time period?
- Who are the distributors that service this area?

This stage results in a list of potential suppliers. The goal is to use the management information system described in Chapter 11 to identify as many sources as possible. A buyer who is new to an area must also network with other foodservice directors or buyers to assemble the list. Additional sources of information include past experience, interviews with DSRs, trade journals and shows, yellow pages, and buyers' guides.

In the *inquiry stage*, after identifying all potential sources, the buyer must compare and analyze sources that appear capable of meeting the needs of the foodservice department. Criteria for evaluation include price, quality, service, delivery schedule, and available quantity. Also during this phase, the buyer should contact other buyers or managers for their feedback and experience with the suppliers from which they purchase. Sample questions that could be asked include:

- Is the firm reliable?
- Is quality consistently excellent? Do they carry national brands or "local/state" types of brands?
- Are deliveries accurate and on time? Delivered using appropriate delivery vehicles?
- How would they rate DSRs and other vendor employees with whom they have interacted?
- What additional value-added services do they use?
- How would they evaluate these services?
- What do they like most about this distributor? Would they recommend them? Why? Why not?
- Have you visited the supplier's warehouse? Was it clean, showed no signs of pest infestation, sanitary procedures followed, refrigerators and freezer temperature monitored, did it meet *Food Code* temperature standards, was the warehouse temperature at least 70°F?
- What problems, if any, have they experienced in conducting business with this vendor?

Another factor that must be evaluated is whether to use local or national vendors, each of which offers advantages and limitations. Additional criteria for comparing distributors are financial stability of the firm, technical expertise of the distributor's staff, and compatibility of business practices with regard to ethical standards. Business practices include strict adherence to delivery schedules, credit terms, minimum order requirement, lead time, return policy, and product-line variety. It is recommended, when possible, to make an appointment to visit the vendor's facility, especially if there has been no prior business relationship. After comparing all the potential distributors based on these criteria, the buyer narrows the options and prepares a second list called a qualified supplier list.

During the *negotiation and selection stage*, the buyer uses information obtained during the inquiry stage to issue an initial purchase order. Before doing so, however, he or she should meet with the suppliers to discuss payment, delivery, and contract terms, if applicable.

During the *experience stage*, the buyer follows up to ensure that the chosen vendor is providing the type of service and quality of products previously agreed on. If problems occur, the buyer should record them and provide immediate feedback to the distributor so that corrective action can be taken. Any problems (and their resolution) should be recorded for future reference and evaluation.

The goal of the supplier selection process is to establish several product, supply, and equipment sources that can consistently provide the quantity and quality of products required at the right price and the right time. Communication and feedback are critical ingredients for a long-term and effective buyer-vendor relationship.

Buyer-Supplier Relations

Sound business practices and well-stated purchasing policies are the bases for good purchasing decisions. Careful planning and an accurate statement of food needs are the starting points in building good buyer-supplier relations. As always, fairness and honesty are essential. Product requirements should be specified, and complete information as to availability and prices should be obtained. The buyer or foodservice director should make visits to the warehouse to observe pest control, safe handling of food and supplies, and overall sanitation. The buyer should establish an appointment schedule with sales representatives and adhere to it. At no time should one supplier's price information be discussed with another supplier. Accepting gifts, favors, coupons, and other promotional offers can create a potentially unhealthy obligation to a vendor that can adversely affect the buyer's freedom to make objective vendor selections. Buyers should be familiar with and follow the fair business policies of their institutions. Special services that ordinarily would not be available from vendors should not be requested.

BASIC PURCHASING GUIDELINES

As a quick reference tool, the following purchasing guidelines are summarized. They provide the fundamental how-tos of purchasing:

- Develop a specification for each food item. Government and industry specifications can provide a starting point to help foodservice managers and buyers develop their own. For some products, specifications can be brief, whereas others will require substantial detail (Chapter 16).
- Make sure that a copy of the specifications developed by the foodservice department is available to and used by the buyer. Many departments find it convenient to provide a complete set of their specifications (classified by commodity group and number) to vendors with whom they routinely

do business. This decreases the time required to get a price quotation.

- Compare food quality and yield in relation to price. A food of higher quality and a higher unit price may yield more serving portions of better quality and at a lower cost per serving than the same food of lower quality and price. Frequent studies of the net yield in serving portions and of the cost per serving of various brands make it possible to base buying decisions on cost per serving rather than on unit purchase price.
- Use bid requests or quotation sheets to get price quotations.
- Purchase only the types, quality, and quantities required for the planned menu or production forecasts. However, if a special buy becomes available and the quality is acceptable, a surplus of the product may be purchased if adequate storage space and conditions permit. For example, prices on the previous year's pack of canned or frozen fruit or vegetable items may be reasonable just before the new pack reaches the market.
- Purchase foods only from vendors known to maintain approved levels of sanitation and quality control in accordance with government regulations and recommended practices of food handling and storage.
- Purchase foods by weight, size, or count per container. The minimum weights acceptable for purchase units should be stated in the specifications.
- Establish a purchase-and-delivery schedule based on the storage life of various foods, the location of vendor in relation to the buying facility, delivery costs, storage space, inventory policies, and the food needs specified in the menu(s).
- Ensure that all purchases are inspected on delivery. An item should be rejected at the time of delivery unless there is a prior agreement that the vendor will give credit for any defective products or gross errors. Delivery sheets or invoices should not be initialed or signed until the quality and quantity of foods delivered have been checked against the purchase order.
- Maintain written purchase and receiving records for all foods and supplies ordered and received.

Purchase of Food Supplies

Every effort must be made to purchase food that has been processed under safe and sanitary conditions. Toward this end, certain precautions should be considered.

- All produce should follow Good Manufacturing Practices (MP) and Good Agricultural Practices (GAP). These programs need to be documented and audited each season. GAP audits measure critical areas in which food safety could be compromised.
- With the ongoing move to be more sustainable and use "local produce, meat, eggs, milk" the foodservice director must know the source of all products, the rowing/harvesting

conditions and delivery methods. Check with local authorities concerning using these products, especially raw milk and other dairy products. Chapters 19 and 20 contain more information concerning purchasing and storage.

COMPUTER-ASSISTED PROCUREMENT

Technology's effects on foodservice distributors and health care foodservice operations have already been discussed. Predictions of the role EDI will have on the procurement process also have been described (see Chapter 10).

This section provides a brief footnote to the earlier section so that buyers understand the fine points of *computer-assisted procurement* from actual practice. The steps enumerated below are intended as another quick reference tool that explains computerized purchasing by buyers whose computer terminals are connected to a central processing unit.

1. The buyer calls up from the computer's files a listing for the product to be purchased. The computer record shows the specification for the product, its unit price, and a list of vendors who can supply the product.
2. The buyer selects the vendor, the quantities needed, and the desired delivery date and time.
3. After the products have been delivered and accepted, delivery confirmation is entered into the computer record and conveyed (or telecommunicated) to the vendor's computer.
4. The vendor's computer sends an invoice directly to the institution or to the institution's bank for payment for the products delivered. The invoice may be communicated by computer or with hard copy of the invoice printed out from the computer record.
5. For an invoice communicated directly to the bank, the institution's bank automatically credits the vendor's account and debits the institution's account for the purchase.

In addition to the system described above, a number of spreadsheet applications might facilitate record keeping and provide current cost information. Examples include vendor evaluation, bid analyses, usage reports, and inventory analysis and valuation. Point-of-sale systems can be directly linked to a perpetual inventory.

ETHICS

About $40 billion each year is lost through nonviolent crimes. These crimes include employee theft, shoplifting, kickbacks, promotional expenses, and other forms of cheating in the marketplace. No business, regardless of its size, is immune to this problem. About 18,000 businesses go bankrupt every year because of a combination of employee and management thievery. All managers must have their own code of *ethics* and be able to live with the consequences of their code. If a superior asks a manager to falsify an invoice, accept gifts, and the like, and the manager agrees, even though he or she feels it is wrong, then the manager must live with his or her conscience and the decision to do as requested, or else quit the job.

All foodservice personnel must be sensitive to ethical problems and all times avoid *conflict of interest*. An example of conflict interest would be doing business with a company/vendor in which you or your family have an interest/ownership or with a vendor that is a family member or a close friend.

It is vital that foodservice personnel know what they will and will not do in various situations. Will they tolerate exceptions, half-truths, or omissions? Is profit in business more important than morality?

The buyer's basic requirement is to remain loyal to his or her employer and to the ethical standards established by the organization. This means avoiding conflicts of interest whereby personal gain could be derived from conducting business with a specific vendor.

The food buyer must be alert to temptations. He or she is in a position to influence the purchasing decision; he or she must be honest. Purveyors may offer any of the following to retain the business:

- Entertainment, including sexual favors, "free" tickets to sporting events, and so forth
- Golf games, including membership fee, green fees, and entertainment
- Use of a cabin or condominium for a weekend
- Membership in an exclusive club
- Credit cards
- All-expenses-paid trips or cruise with the "guys" for an extended weekend
- A percentage of the total bid amount refunded in "real" money to the buyer
- Loans for the business
- Overcharging on a food item, with the amount of the overcharge going to the buyer
- Conflict-of-interest buying, such as purchasing from friends and from family-owned businesses
- Personal gifts of food and so forth

The management of the facility is obligated to set the standards and the code of ethics when it comes to purchasing. Rigid policies and procedures must be developed and followed. Management must be honest and demand honesty from its personnel. Management should maintain open, honest communications with the employees and be available for advice by involving everyone in the facility in discussing situations. The buyers should be thoroughly investigated before being given the authority to spend the facility's funds. Personnel should be paid well enough to reduce the temptation to steal. An outsider should audit all financial records, inventories, and specifications. Internal controls should be clearly defined. Accepting bribes, kickbacks, and gifts in exchange for special ordering consideration, then, is not only unethical but illegal. Money dilemmas will occur for which there is no one "right" or "wrong" action. When this happens, a buyer's personal ethical imperative and organiza-tional policies must provide a framework for action. For example, the following sensitive issues have occurred in foodservice and interfered with fair and honest business practice:

- Gaining confidential information about a competitor from a supplier
- Accepting free trips, entertainment, and gifts beyond the dollar amount set by the organization
- Purchasing from suppliers favored (requested) by the administration
- Disclosing one supplier's quote to another supplier
- Using the organization's economic clout to force a supplier to lower prices

The best way to avoid these situations is to adhere to defined policies and procedures for conducting good and ethical business practices with vendors. A good way to minimize product and mon-etary theft is to implement a buddy system. For example, the person ordering product/equipment should not receive the product (see Chapter 19). The foodservice director may consider adopting the National Association of Purchasing Management's Principles and Standards of Purchasing Practices as a guide for everyone involved in the procurement process (available from the National Association of Purchasing Management, P.O. Box 22160, Tempe, AZ 85285–2160).

SUMMARY

Whether a health care facility hires a procurement specialist or charges the task of purchasing to the foodservice director or a cen-tralized purchasing department, procurement activities ultimately have one objective. That objective is to ensure that everything needed to produce menu items is in place, on time, and within budgetary boundaries.

To accomplish this massive objective, buyers must survey sup-plier sources, inquire about prospective suppliers, negotiate for the best selection at the most favorable price, and monitor selected sup-pliers to make sure they deliver what they promised when they promised it. Buyers must do this while minimizing leftovers, plate waste, and rampant overstocking.

Certain trends affect these efforts significantly. For example, distributors no longer can rely on the traditional "sales call." Their service representatives—DSRs—now must promote value-added services to retain a buyer–client base they once could take for granted. Thus, technology such as direct computer linkups between buyers and distributors' product and service line can expedite the buyer's ordering process and inventory control methods. Such ser-vices provided by distributors create distributor-buyer alliances whose common goal is customer retention. Moreover, this interac-tion can be accomplished without either party leaving his or her office. Foodservice buyers must practice ethical behavior at all times, following the policies of the facility.

Adulteration of food
As purchased (AP)
Centralized purchasing
Computer-assisted procurement
Contact/noncontract purchasing
Drained weight
Edible portion (EP)
Edible yield factor (EYF)
Ethics
Full-function wholesaler
General-line wholesaler
Group purchasing
Horizontal integration
Just-in-time (JIT) purchasing

Limited-function wholesaler
One-stop purchasing
Prime vendor agreement
Procurement process
Purchase order
Purchase requisition
Rebates
Standard of quality
Supplier
Sustainable foods
Value analysis
Vertical integration
Wholesaling

DISCUSSION QUESTIONS

1. What are the regulations that govern the quality and safety of food supplies?
2. Which methods would you use when working with vendors and the information technology department to utilize electronic data interchange (EDI)? What are the advantages and disadvantages to the supplier and the foodservice operation?
3. Review the distributors' changing product line; include the impact of the "move to be more sustainable." Will it increase cost, improve quality and safety of the food supply, increase prices in the cafeteria and will funds be available?

4. Describe how to develop/maintain the buyer/supplier relations, include ethical behavior on the part of the buyer and supplier.
5. Select menu item and demonstrate "the make or buy" concept. Include quality, taste, appearance, and cost—develop and use and objective from for evaluation.
6. What is the role of the foodservice buyer? Is it better to use a central purchasing system—why or why not?
7. Differentiate between price quote, cherry-picking items from a bid, and various bidding processes.

ENDNOTE

The National Agricultural Library publishes a Purchasing and Procurement Resource List updated in January 2007. The list cites 14 books published between 1994 and 2007 and describes their contents. The list was compiled by Desire Stapley, MEd, RD, Nutrition Specialist, and Jamie Rasmussen, Student Nutrition Specialist, with acknowledgment of the assistance of two other RDs and a student.

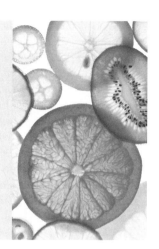

CHAPTER 19

RECEIVING, STORAGE, AND INVENTORY CONTROL

LEARNING OBJECTIVES

- Identify various methods used in receiving goods.
- Explain the ways security can be breached when receiving goods.
- Outline the temperature requirements for dry, refrigerated, and freezer storage.
- Describe how the supplier can assist with receiving.
- Use appropriate storage and issuing procedures.
- Apply efficient inventory controls to keep inventory at an appropriate levels.
- Trace the steps in the documentation and accounting procedures from purchasing through receiving, storage, issuing to invoice payment.

THE PROCESS OF receiving, storing, issuing, and inventory control influences not only a health care foodservice's cost but also the quality of the food served to its customers. Critical steps in each process should be monitored as a part of the department's continuous quality improvement efforts.

These processes and how they are related to and influence the health care foodservice operation are examined in this chapter. How to receive goods, inspect them for correlation between the quality and quantity specified in the purchase order and those of the materials delivered, and maintain receipt documentation are also discussed.

Once shipments are accepted (and rejections returned immediately), they must be stored properly. Procedures and conditions for dry storage items and low-temperature storage items are delineated. Conditions for proper storage area upkeep (cleaning and sanitizing) are outlined. For example, floor, window (if applicable), wall, and ceiling maintenance recommendations are provided, along with suggestions for shelf height, shelf-wall clearance, lighting and light fixture, and ventilation. Ideal storage temperatures and humidity levels for specific foods also are detailed. Ancillary storage equipment—refrigerators and freezers, thermometers, and mobile equipment, for example—are described.

Because foodservice inventory represents the bulk of a department's financial investment, inventory control, cost containment, and continuous quality initiatives are critical factors that department directors and buyers must always keep in mind. Therefore, significant attention is given to how foods and supplies are issued throughout the production and service areas. Specific inventory control tools are provided; these include perpetual inventory calculations and physical inventory taking. Other techniques (all oriented to the accounting concept of "first-in, first-out" [FIFO]) are described as well.

THE SUPPLIER

The *supplier* needs to be honest in all his dealings, operate a sanitary and pest-free warehouse, and abide by all applicable laws. The supplier receives goods at the warehouse that meet quality and quantity standards, rejects those that are unacceptable. All the employees (warehouse employees, drivers/delivery personnel, sanitation personnel, office management) are trained in safe food handling.

The delivery personnel are key to proper receiving; the driver is responsible for the condition of the delivery vehicle, (temperature control/monitoring), meeting the delivery schedule and delivering the correct products to the right location, at the right time, and in the right condition. Through the delivery route the driver needs to monitor the temperature of the vehicle, especially when delivering refrigerated/freezer products and contact the wholesale warehouse manager for assistance if there is a problem. The delivery personnel may also be responsible for off-loading product to the loading dock. This individual **must** use appropriate body techniques when unloading product, always using safety first. The supplier needs to always be concerned for food safety (temperature maintenance), cross-contamination (wet, leaky, thawed products dripping on potentially hazardous foods during the delivery process) and personnel hygiene of **all** personnel.

RECEIVING PROCEDURES

The receiving area should be located near the loading dock, storeroom, refrigerators, freezers, and ingredient control area to facilitate the movement of products into proper storage. This is a security and food safety measure.

An effective procurement system requires adequate receiving procedures to ensure that the food and supplies delivered match the quality and quantity of the items ordered. The economic advantage gained from competitive bidding based on well-written specifications easily can be lost as a consequence of poor receiving practices. Acceptance of poor-quality products or incorrect amounts can mean financial loss to a foodservice department. This risk can be eliminated or minimized if sound receiving procedures and properly trained personnel are in place.

Receiving procedures vary among institutions, but some basic rules apply to all facilities. Responsibility for checking quantities should be assigned to receiving or storeroom personnel who have been trained. In small organizations, this may be one of several tasks assigned to production personnel. Inspection and evaluation for quality should be the responsibility of someone who knows the specifications or at least is qualified to judge the quality of the goods being delivered. Whoever is charged with inspecting shipment deliveries should prepare ahead of time for each one. They should understand the process by which products are received and know what to do if a problem occurs with an incoming shipment. Deliveries should be made at scheduled times and days. This means knowing the delivery dates and approximate times so personnel are available, that space and equipment are clean and uncluttered to receive the products, and receiving personnel know how to complete receiving records. Because most deliveries are made on a regular schedule, this should be relatively easy.

When receiving products be aware of possible injuries due to:

- Loose staples on boxes
- Broken glass containers
- Metal wires on cases
- Insects and rodents
- Excessive weight of product
- Dripping water, juices from products (could cause falls)

Receiving staff should immediately check the merchandise against the purchase order and specifications, perishable items first, while the delivery person is still present. Temperatures of potentially hazardous foods, inspection stamp (meats, poultry, etc.) and date, expiration date, and the "use-by date." The count, weight, quality, color, texture, odor (especially of fish), and condition of the merchandise should be compared with the purchase order or quotation sheet before delivery is accepted (Chapter 18). If there is a description it should be noted on the invoice and a credit memo (Figure 19.1) attached to the supplier's copy of the invoice as well as the foodservice and accounting invoices. Scales should be available for checking items ordered by weight. Any cases or cartons that appear damaged but not tampered with should be opened right away and the contents carefully examined. The quality of fresh produce should be inspected at the top and the **bottom** of each container. The inter-

FIGURE 19.1 Credit Memo

Credit Memo

Number _____   Date _____

XYZ Hospital

Foodservice

123 First Street

Any State, AB 12345

To: DFG Supplier

Address: 456 N. 55th Place

City, State: Any State, AB 12357

On April 19, xxxx there was a problem with a delivery from your company. We are requesting a credit be made to the XYZ Hospital, Foodservice

Invoice No.	Item	Quantity	Unit of Product	Unit Cost	Extension

Reason for request:

1. Wrong quality   2. Wrong weight   3. Product thawed   4. Did not order

5. Short count   6. Recalled item   7. Broken/open case   8. Dented can

9. Incorrect price   10. Other _____

Delivery Person: Name Smith Foodservice Receiving Person: Name Jones

Delivery Person Signature: Foodservice Person Signature:

Triplicate form: White copy: supplier, Pink copy: Foodservice, Yellow copy for accounting. Attach to invoice

FIGURE 19.2 Receiving System

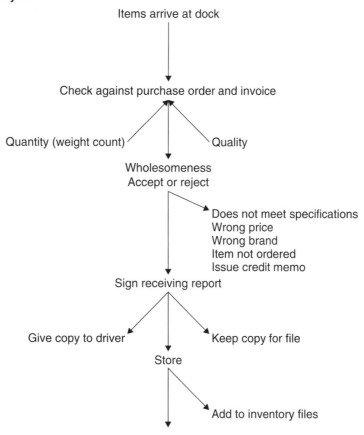

```
                        Items arrive at dock
                               │
                               ▼
              Check against purchase order and invoice
                          ↗    ▲    ↖
         Quantity (weight count)     Quality
                          Wholesomeness
                          Accept or reject
                               │        ↘
                               │          Does not meet specifications
                               │          Wrong price
                               │          Wrong brand
                               │          Item not ordered
                               │          Issue credit memo
                               ▼
                        Sign receiving report
                          ↙    │    ↘
          Give copy to driver  │   Keep copy for file
                             Store
                               │        ↘
                               │          Add to inventory files
                               ▼
```

Source: Developed by Ruby P. Puckett©.

nal temperature of all frozen foods should be 0°F (−18°C). If the temperature exceeds 0°F, the foods should be rejected. If such a detailed check is not possible, the receiving staff should inspect packages for signs indicating that the product may have been subjected to undesirably high temperatures. Wet or dripping packages should never be accepted.

Next, the staff should tag all chilled, frozen, and nonperishable foods as they are received to ensure their use on a first-in, first-out (*FIFO*) basis, which means that the older products should be rotated to the front of the shelf, and the newer products placed **behind** the older products. Such foods should be stored immediately. (The price per unit can be recorded on frozen and nonperishable items at this point.)

Meat tags are a good idea for tagging all large pieces of meat (Exhibit 19.1). These tags can be purchased from large supply companies. Use meat tags to assist with inventory, to label FIFO meat, and to assist in avoiding theft. This is a two-part tag that is attached to the product before it is placed in storage; the duplicate copy is filed, and when the product is issued from storage to production, the tag is compared with the copy on file. This method helps in the rotating of stock and in determining daily food costs. This method may not be useful in small institutions because it is time-consuming.

Invoices or delivery slips are stamped with an invoice stamp (Exhibit 19.2), and the receiving clerk initials the appropriate line. Information is then entered into a computer file and sent to the finance and accounting department.

Only after foods have been inspected, dated, tagged, stamped, and approved should the staff sign the delivery slip from the vendor and fill out the required receiving report. Unordered or rejected merchandise should be returned immediately and noted on the invoice. Rejection of products should be made at the time of delivery to avoid excessive paperwork, possible misunderstanding, and assurance of credit for the unacceptable product. Nonperishable foods and supplies should be transferred to appropriate storage areas as soon as possible (nonfood items should always be stored separately from food supplies).

Receiving and issuing staff should be provided needed equipment to perform their functions. This includes hand trucks or forklifts that can move pallets. *Pallets* are portable wooden or metal platforms for handling by a forklift truck and can be used for storing products in the storeroom. Scales that weigh items up to 200 to 500 pounds, desks, chairs, computers, calculators, crowbars, and short-blade knives for opening containers and packages are also needed. Digital computerized thermometers to check chilled and frozen foods, clipboards, pens, pencils, marking pens, and meat tags should also be available. Electronic receiving tools such as those that read bar codes and tabulator scales that weigh and automatically print the weight on paper are used in large-scale foodservice operations. The use of bar code readers and the ability of the receiving personnel to read the 12-digit Universal Product Code (UPC) are valuable tools for receiving and taking a physical inventory. A major problem in reading bar codes is poor eyesight.

EXHIBIT 19.1   Meat or Storage Tags

Tag Number: _____	Tag Number: _____
Date of Receipt: _____	Date Received: _____
Weight Cost: _____	Weight: _____
_____ × _____ = _____	Price: _____
No of #s Price Cost	Cost: _____
Name of Supplier: _____	Supplier: _____
Date of Issue: _____	Date Issued: _____

Source: Developed by Ruby P. Puckett©.

EXHIBIT 19.2   Invoice Stamp

Date Received: _____

Quantity: _____

Price Correct: _____

Extension Correct: _____

Entered in Computer: _____

Sent to Finance and Accounting: _____

Receiving department, whether foodservice or centralized, must have a written report for all merchandise received. The foodservice director and the buyer should have copies for their files.

Two receiving methods are used most often in foodservice operations. These methods are invoice receiving and blind receiving.

Invoice Receiving

Invoice receiving involves having a receiving clerk check the items delivered against the original purchase order or telephone order (documented in writing) and note any discrepancies. This method makes it easy for the clerk to check the quantity and quality of the materials delivered against the specifications. Invoice receiving is quick and economical, although it loses its advantage if the clerk fails to compare items delivered with the specifications and simply uses the delivery invoice as a reference.

Blind Receiving

With *blind receiving*, the clerk uses an invoice or a purchase order that has the "quantity ordered" column blacked out. The clerk records the quantity actually received for each item on the invoice or purchase order—not on the supplier's invoice. This method takes more time than invoice receiving because it requires that the clerk prepare a complete record of all merchandise delivered. Even so, blind receiving is the more reliable method of the two.

Record Keeping

Maintaining *records* of all merchandise delivered is as important as inspecting deliveries for quality and quantity. The methods and forms used for this purpose may be simple or complex, depending on the level of documentation required. A *receiving report* must be kept so that all personnel involved in purchasing, using, and paying for supplies are informed of what was received. Depending on whether receiving is centralized or takes place in the foodservice department, one or more of the following records may be used.

Product Receipt   A *product receipt* like the one shown in Exhibit 19.3 may be required for each shipment received. A receiving clerk in the central storage area, who sends copies to appropriate department staff members in purchasing, foodservice, accounting, and so forth to inform them that the goods have been received, completes this type of form. Notations of items ordered but not delivered or items returned may be included on this form or on a separate form (called a *credit memo*) used for this purpose. The merchandise receipt and the credit memo should be signed by the person taking delivery and either attached to the invoice or sent separately, depending on the department's policy. (The procedure for routing receipts and credit memos should be clearly stated in the department's policy and procedures manual.)

Receiving Record   A *daily receiving record* similar to the one shown in Exhibit 19.4 may be required, in addition to the merchandise receipt. Alternatively, it may be the only form used to record incoming goods. Either or both records can be used to verify receipt of merchandise. The forms also are a source of information for processing payments in the accounting department or for updating inventory records.

EXHIBIT 19.3   Product Receipt

PRODUCT RECEIPT		
	Date: _____	
	No: _____	
Received from:		
_____		
Purchase Order No: _____		

Quantity	Description	Distribution

Products received and inspected by: _____

EXHIBIT 19.4   Daily Receiving Record

Receiving Record								
Merchandise received and inspected by: _____ Date: _____								
							Distribution	
Quantity	Unit	Description of Item	Name of Vendor	Quantity Verified by	Unit Price	Total Cost	To Kitchen	To Storeroom

SECURITY

Security concerns become important during the receiving process because there are many opportunities for employee and supplier theft. Some of the more common methods include:

- Receiving the wrong item and paying a higher price for lower-quality products (6 to 10 sliced peaches in light syrup rather than 6 to 10 peach halves in heavy syrup). This would be a major cost and quality difference.
- Receiving products that have been thawed and represented as fresh.
- Receiving short weight or count (or both): paying for products not received.
- Grinding ice or adding dry milk or soy products as extenders.
- Including weight of ice in fresh chicken and being charged for ice.
- Duplicate invoices, especially to fictitious companies.
- Errors in arithmetic.
- Padding the invoice.
- Delivery and receiving personnel are family members or good friends.
- Allowing the supplier to stock goods without any foodservice supervision (i.e., milk, bread, canned sodas).

The foodservice director or manager should monitor and check security in the receiving area on a random basis to ensure that procedures are followed. It is important to recheck weights, quality, and quantities. Persons responsible for purchasing should not be responsible for receiving. There should be scheduled days or dates for deliveries. Products should be moved to storage immediately.

There are many more ways to be dishonest. Cameras, locks on doors, allowing only authorized personnel in the area, and well-written policies and procedures that are strictly followed help to deter some of this behavior. Doorbells can be installed to permit delivery personnel to signal their arrival. Salespeople should not enter the department through the loading dock, receiving room, or storeroom.

STORAGE PROCEDURES

Once foods have been received they must be protected from contamination, spoilage, and other damage during storage in the dry, refrigerated, or frozen state. Once the products have been accurately received they should be stored immediately to ensure the quality and wholesomeness of the product, to prevent theft, and to update inventory records. These products need to be stored in dry, refrigerator, or freezer stores, or issued for immediate use.

Dry storage and low-temperature storage facilities should be accessible to both the receiving and food preparation areas so that transport time and corresponding labor costs can be kept to a minimum. Ideally, these facilities should be on the same floor as the production area, but if this is not possible, space should be allocated in the production area for one or more days' supply of foods. The storeroom should be equipped with a scale that is capable of weighing items up to 200 to 500 pounds, along with a smaller scale for weighing smaller items.

Refrigerated Storage

Recommended storage temperatures and durations are listed in Table 19.1.

Dry Storage Maintenance

The amount of space required for dry storage depends on the types and amounts of foods needed, the frequency of deliveries, the facility's policies and procedures on inventory size, and the amount of money invested in inventory. These factors vary from one institution to another.

Storage areas should be dry and easy to keep free of rodents, birds, and insects. Walls and ceilings should be constructed of nonporous materials, and ceilings should be free from water and heating pipes. Any windows should be screened and equipped with an opaque security sash to protect supplies from direct sunlight. Floors, preferably made of quarry tile, terrazzo, or sealed concrete, should be slip-resistant. All components—walls, ceilings, shelves, and floors—should be easy to clean and kept clean, free from debris, and dry at all times.

All parts of a storage room should be well lighted so that supplies and labeling are visible and housekeeping can be achieved properly. Light fixtures covered with wire mesh help protect against breakage and shield employees from falling glass should breakage occur. About two or three watts of light per square foot of floor area is recommended, with fixtures centered over the aisles.

Ventilation and temperature control are critical to dry storage rooms for retarding deterioration of food supplies. A temperature range of 50°F to 70°F (10°C to 21°C) is recommended. A thermometer placed in a highly visible location (for example, at the entrance) is essential. Fans or other specially designed systems should provide ventilation.

Food should not be stored under exposed or unprotected water or sewer lines except for automatic fire protection sprinkler heads, which is required by law.

To promote security, it is preferable to have only **one** entrance to the storage area so that deliveries and supplies can be monitored. Access should be limited to foodservice or employees responsible for inventory control and receiving. Secure locks should be installed on all doors, and keys should be carefully safeguarded (for example, by a key sign-out system). A door width of at least 42 inches allows easy movement of supplies into and out of the area.

All foods should contain a *label* and be marked with the date received. Labels should be turned face out. When this system is used it allows for FIFO, thereby using the oldest product first. All foods that have passed the manufacturers' expiration date should be discarded according to local regulations. Store food and single-service items in a designated area, never in toilet rooms, locker rooms, and mechanical rooms or directly on the floor.

TABLE 19.1 Recommended Storage Temperatures and Times

Food	Refrigerator Storage (32°F to 40°F) ([0°C to 4°C])	Freezer Storage (0°F [−18°C]) (or Below)	Dry Storage (50°F to 70°F) ([10°C to 21°C])
Roasts, steaks, chops	3–5 days	Beef and lamb: 6 months Pork: 4 months Veal: 4 months	Never
Bacon	7 days	Bacon: 2 months	
Sausage raw from chicken, turkey, pork, beef	1–2 days	1–2 months	Never
Ground meat, stew meat	1–2 days	3–4 months	Never
Ham, baked whole	1–3 weeks	4–6 months	Never
Hams, canned	12 months	Not recommended	Never
Chicken and turkey	1–2 days	Chicken: 6–12 months Turkey: 3–6 months Giblets: 3–4 months	Never
Fish or shellfish	30°F to 32°F (−1°C to 0°C) (lean 6 months) on ice, (fatty 2–3 months) 1–2 days	3–6 months	Never
Shell eggs	3–5 weeks	Not recommended	Never (Check carton for expiration date)
Frozen eggs	1–2 days after thawing	9 months	Never
Dried eggs	6 months	Not recommended	Never
Fresh fruits and vegetables	5–7 days	Not recommended	Never
Frozen fruits and vegetables	—	Variable, depends on kind	Never
Canned fruits and vegetables	—	Not recommended	12 months
Dried fruits and vegetables	Preferred	Not recommended	2 weeks
Canned fruit and vegetable juice	—	—	Satisfactory
Regular cornmeal	Required over 60 days	Not recommended	2 months
Whole wheat flour	Required over 60 days	Not recommended	2 months
Degermed cornmeal	Preferred	Not recommended	Satisfactory
All-purpose and bread flour	Preferred	Not recommended	Satisfactory
Rice	Preferred	Not recommended	Satisfactory

Source: Adapted from Nebraska Extension and FSIS Fact Sheet 2007. Most complete information was developed by the Virginia Cooperative Extension: Food Storage Guidelines for Consumers 2009.

Miscellaneous supplies and broken (open) case lots can be stored on adjustable metal shelves installed at least 2 inches from the walls. Specific guidelines for shelving and spacing between shelves are discussed in Chapter 22. The aisles between shelves and platforms should be wide enough to accommodate mobile equipment. (Check with The Joint Commission (TJC) and the Center for Medical Services (CMS) concerning cardboard boxes.) All boxes need to be removed from the storage area as soon as possible; remove corrugated cardboard. Canned fruits and vegetables and other canned items need to be removed from boxes and placed on shelves/cart. There should be **no** corrugated boxes in the foodservice area. Check out TJC and CMS for specific standards on the storage and use of cardboard boxes in the storeroom. The 2009 *Food Code* states the following: 3–202.15 "Food packages shall be in good condition and protect the integrity of the contents so that food is not exposed to adulteration or potential contamination"; and 3.350.12 states that food cannot be stored in locker rooms, toilet areas, dressing rooms, garbage rooms, mechanical rooms; under sewer lines that are not shielded to intercept potential drips; under leaking water lines, including leaking automatic fire sprinkler heads or under lines on which water has condensed; under open stairwells; or under other sources of contamination.

Metal or plastic containers with tight-fitting covers should be used for storing dry foods such as bulk cereals, cereal products, flour, sugar, and broken lots of bulk foods. Containers, which should be legibly and accurately labeled, can be placed on dollies for ease of movement from one place to another. Foods packed in glass should not be exposed to direct sunlight or any other strong light. When possible, purchase and store products in plastic containers rather than glass, as glass can easily be broken and could cause an accident.

Toxic materials used for cleaning and sanitation should be clearly labeled and kept in a locked storage area away from food and paper supplies. Empty food containers must never be used for storing broken lots of toxic materials, nor must empty cleaning and sanitation containers be used to store food. Food should be stored only in food-grade containers.

A worktable should be provided near the entrance of the storeroom for unpacking supplies, putting up small orders of bulk products, and assembling orders. Large and small scoops should be on hand for each food container in use, such as bins for flour, sugar, cereal, and so forth. Scales need to be accessible for weighing small and large quantities of food. Several types of mobile equipment, such as platform dollies and shelf trucks, may be needed for delivering supplies to the various work areas. Hand-washing facilities are essential and should be located near the storeroom entrance.

A regular cleaning schedule should be developed and a staff member or crew assigned to the tasks of cleaning the floor, walls, ceiling, light fixtures, shelves, and equipment in the storeroom. Routinely, the foodservice director or a supervisor should inspect the area. Any violations of sanitation standards and facility policies should be corrected immediately.

Fire extinguisher(s) need to be place in the area of the storeroom that is most vulnerable for a fire. Fireproof refuse containers that are located in conformance with local public health laws should be emptied at least daily. Leaking or bulging cans of food and spoiled foods must be disposed of promptly. The storeroom should be treated regularly for the control of rodents and insects. Further information on safe and sanitary preservation of food and supplies in dry storage areas is available from local and state public health departments.

The items most frequently issued should be located near the storeroom. Heavy cases/packages should be stored on lower shelves. Stock should be systematically arranged, and inventory records should follow the same system to save time when stock is issued or inventoried. New stock should be placed behind like items so that the older stock will be issued first, again using the FIFO method. As mentioned, each item should be marked or stamped with its date of delivery and unit cost as it is placed on the shelf. The cost can thus be noted on the inventory sheets as the actual count is taken in the physical inventory. This method permits rapid computation of the cash value of inventory on hand. Price marking also is an effective way of familiarizing production personnel with the cost of foods:

1. Quantity lots of bagged items, such as flour and sugar, should be cross-stacked on slatted platforms or racks raised high enough above the floor to permit air circulation.
2. Store baking powder, soda, spices, and herbs and tea in tightly covered containers at 70°F or below and away from heat.
3. Check herbs and spices frequently for pest infestation.
4. Bulk cereals, rice, grits, cornmeal, dried vegetables, and dry milk should be refrigerated if the storeroom temperature cannot be maintained below 70°F.
5. Once the original container or package of bulk foods (flour, sugar, and so forth) has been opened, the remaining product should be emptied into good quality plastic or metal containers with tight fitting lids. The containers should be labeled clearly and stored on dollies or shelves that are six inches above the floor. (Check your local health department.)
6. Quantity of cases and boxed foods are more stable for handling when they are stacked in alternating patterns on dollies or pallets.
7. Smaller lots of canned or packaged foods may be stored on metal shelves in or out of the case.
8. A stock numbering or dating system is recommended so that all stock may be rotated.
9. When cases of canned foods are stacked, their labels should be exposed for easy identification.
10. Cartons of foods packed in glass jars should be kept closed because light tends to change the color and flavor of some foods.
11. Dried fruits can be stored satisfactorily for a limited time in their original boxes if the storeroom temperature can be kept below 70°F and the humidity below 55

percent. If refrigerated space is available, storing dried fruits at lower temperatures will retard mold growth.

12. Spices should be stored away from heat. They should be checked regularly for pest infestation.

Bananas should be kept in the dry storage area or at a temperature of 60°F to 65°F (15°C to 18°C). To prevent bruising, they should be left in the delivery boxes. Because a temperature of 58°F (14°C) or below darkens the flesh of bananas, they should not be refrigerated. Unripened fruit and vegetables should be placed in dry storage until they become edible (unripe melons, peaches, pears, pineapples, plums, avocados, and tomatoes ripen at 65°F to 70°F [18°C to 21°C]; colder temperatures, however, can damage these products so that they will not ripen).

Potatoes should be stored away from light, if possible, in a dry, well-ventilated room at a temperature of 40°F to 55°F (4°C to 14°C). If peeled potatoes are purchased, they should be refrigerated and held no longer than the number of days suggested by the processor. Sweet potatoes and winter squash keep best in a well-ventilated room at a temperature of 50°F to 60°F (10°C to 15°C). Sweet potatoes spoil more quickly under refrigeration than in dry storage. Onions keep best in dry storage at a temperature of 40°F to 60°F (4°C to 15°C). Store away from other vegetables that might absorb odor. Store rutabagas, turnips, hard rind squash, whole citrus, eggplants, root vegetables in a dark place, with good air circulation and at room temperature. It is important to avoid indiscriminate overbuying because food quality can deteriorate even under the most ideal storage conditions. Products should be stored 6 to 10 inches above the floor, 2 inches from the wall, and 18 inches from overhead sprinklers.

Don't wash berries, cherries, peaches, plums, or fresh vegetables **before** storing. In high-risk operation avoid the use of raw seed sprouts. Avoid the use of sulfides and other products to preserve freshness.

Low-Temperature Storage Maintenance

Enough conveniently located refrigeration should be provided to ensure the proper maintenance of food at 41°F (5°C) or lower during storage. Each refrigerator should be equipped with a numerically scaled indicating thermometer that is accurate to plus or minus 3°F (1.5°C). The thermometer should be located in the warmest part of the unit and placed where it can be easily read, preferably outside of the refrigeration unit. Temperature records must be maintained. Recording thermometers accurate to plus or minus 3°F may be used in lieu of indicating thermometers.

To preserve their nutritional value and appeal, perishable foods should be placed in refrigerated or frozen storage immediately after delivery and kept there until they are to be used. The type and amount of low-temperature storage space required varies with the facility's menu and purchasing policies. Some foodservice operations are fortunate to have separate refrigerated units for meats and poultry, fish and shellfish, dairy products, and vegetables and fruit, with separate freezers for ice cream and other frozen foods.

Separate facilities are desirable because each kind of food has its own ideal storage temperature. However, satisfactory storage conditions can be maintained with fewer units following these temperature guidelines:

- Fruit and vegetables (except those requiring dry storage): 40°F to 45°F (4°C to 7°C)
- Dairy products, eggs, meats, poultry, fish, and shellfish: 32°F to 40°F (0°C to 4°C)
- Frozen foods: −10°F to 0°F (−23°C to −10°C)

If separate refrigerators and freezers are available, foods should be stored at the following temperatures:

- Fruit: 45°F to 50°F (7°C to 10°C)

Most fruits and vegetables spoil rapidly. Fruits continue to ripen after being harvested. Vegetables and fruits have different temperature in transportation and storage. Products should be stored 6 to 10 inches above the floor, 2 inches from the wall and 18 inches from overhead sprinklers.

- Poultry, eggs, processed foods, and pastry: 40°F to 45°F (4°C to 7°C)

Fresh poultry is stored at an internal temperature of 40°F (5°C) or below for 2 to 3 days. (Check for dehydration, odors, or slimy feel to touch; it may be necessary to throw out. If product must be discarded a record must be kept for inventory control and daily food cost.) Store in the coldest part of the refrigerator. Store wrapped in airtight wrapping to prevent dehydration, contamination, and loss of quality. If whole remove the giblets and neck before storing. Store eggs in the original carton or closed carton in refrigerator that can maintain constant temperature and humidity. Use by the date stamped on the carton. Store at 41°F (5°C). Check eggs before cracking for cleanliness of shell or cracks. If eggs are dirty or have cracks **do not use. Discard.** Do not wash eggs and do not store them near strongly flavored foods such as onions.

- Dairy products: 38°F to 40°F (3°C to 4°C)

Milk is one of the most perishable foods used in foodservice. Always check the date on the carton. Use the FIFO system; it may be necessary to discard milk if this is not followed. Store milk away from strongly flavored foods. Cover all open cans/cartons of milk stored in refrigerators. Refrigerate all cheeses. Place all open packages of cheese in airtight bags or wrap tightly in foil. Store unripe cheese, cottage cheese, cream cheese, sour cream, half-and-half, and yogurt in the refrigerator and use by the date on the product. Store ice cream, sherbet, and sorbet in the coldest part of the freezer. Do not purchase or use raw milk. Do not leave dairy products out of the refrigerator/freezer for long periods of time. Use care in storing and handling soft cheese.

- Fresh meats: 34°F to 38°F (1°C to 3°C) with a relative humidity between 85 and 90 percent

Store all meats loosely wrapped, other than bacon and cured ham that needs to be tightly wrapped. Do not wash meat before storing. Do not store ground meat more than one to two days, unless frozen.

- Fish and shellfish: 30°F (−1.1°C) to 34°F (1.1°C)

Store fish at an internal temperature of 41°F (5°C) or lower. Store in wrapped heavy waxed paper. Handle carefully. Store fresh shellfish at 30°F to 34°F (−1.1°C to 1.1°C). Use fresh fish and shellfish within 24 hours unless they are stored in crushed ice that is drained from the product as it melts. Place products that are in ice **under** cooked or ready-to-eat food to avoid cross-contamination. Do not store shrimp or crab for more than 24 hours unless frozen. Cook and refrigerate if storage is needed for a longer period of time. Do not bruise or puncture the flesh or skin of fish as doing so causes the fish to deteriorate rapidly.

- Potentially hazardous food (PHF) requiring refrigeration after preparation should be cooled to an internal temperature of 41°F (5°C) or lower within a cooling period of not more than four hours. Using shallow pans, agitation, quick chilling, or ice-water circulation external to the food container should rapidly cool PHF-prepared foods in large quantities. Do not consume or reuse ice that has been used for cooling stored food, food containers, or food utensils.
- In walk-in refrigerators, all foods should be covered and stored above the floor on easily cleaned metal shelves or on moveable equipment. Shelves should be uncovered to allow full air circulation around food and to facilitate shelf cleaning.
- Cooked food should be covered and positioned on shelves above raw food to avoid contamination from dripping and spills.
- Food stored in refrigerators should be covered, labeled, and dated. The maximum time to store open containers of food is **two to three days.**
- The cleaning of refrigerated storage rooms and reach-in should be scheduled at regular intervals, and a preventative maintenance program for all refrigeration equipment should be followed.
- Refrigerator storage rooms (walk-ins) must be equipped with latches inside to allow exit, and an ax should be available for emergency if someone is locked in. (Some walk-ins are equipped with alarm bells.)
- Frozen foods should be kept frozen and stored at temperatures of 0°F (−18°C to −10°C). The freezer thermometer should be checked frequently and the temperature recorded and filed with any notes that describe the problem and the resolution.
- All frozen food packages should be labeled and dated and well wrapped in moisture-proof and vapor-proof material to prevent freezer burn.
- Do not store wet, dripping packages of frozen foods. Use FIFO to ensure a quality product.

- The shelves, walls, and floors should be kept clean at all times, with defrosting done as often as necessary to eliminate frost and ice build-up. Contents should be moved to another freezer during the defrosting process.
- Frozen foods should be thawed in a refrigerator at a temperature not higher than 41°F (5°C) or under clean potable running water not higher than 70°F (21°C). Keep food in original waterproof packages. Frozen foods may be thawed as part of the cooking process.
- Frozen foods can be thawed in a microwave oven **only** when the foods will be transferred immediately to conventional cooking equipment or when the entire uninterrupted cooking process will take place in the microwave.
- Thawed food should be used immediately or stored in the refrigerator for a short period before use. Refreezing of thawed foods should be avoided because of the possibility of spoilage and loss of flavor and nutritional value.
- Partially thawed frozen foods may be safely refrozen **if** they still contain ice crystals, but their quality will be reduced. Do not refreeze foods that have completely been thawed. The quality of fruits, vegetables, and red meats usually is not as severely affected by temperature changes as that of fish, shellfish, poultry, and cooked foods.

In large institutions, walk-in refrigerators and freezers are common. In smaller operations, the trend is away from walk-ins and toward "reach-ins" because available storage space is used more efficiently, less floor space is required, and cleaning is easier. Regardless of the type of refrigeration available, location is the key for saving labor and avoiding nonproductive work. Walk-in refrigerator doors should be flush with the floor so that movable racks or shelves can be wheeled in and out with ease. Employees should be trained to obtain all supplies needed at one time to eliminate the constant opening of doors, which increases energy usage.

Refrigerators and freezers should be provided with one or more thermometers, such as a remote-reading thermometer, a recording thermometer, and a bulb thermometer. The remote-reading thermometer, placed outside the refrigerator, shows the temperature inside. The recording thermometer, also mounted outside the refrigerator, has the added feature of continuously recording the temperature in walk-in, low-temperature storage. One can see at a glance any fluctuations in temperature. The bulb thermometer probably is the most common one used for refrigerators and freezers that do not have a thermometer built into the door. The warmest area of the unit should be determined and the thermometer placed there. Whichever type of thermometer is used, a staff member should be assigned to check the temperatures in all units at least once a day, preferably in the morning and in the evening, and to record the data on a chart.

Humidity also is important for maintaining food quality because perishable foods contain a great deal of moisture, and evaporation will be greater when the air in the refrigerator is dry. Evaporation causes foods to wilt, discolor, and lose moisture. Food held at low humidity shrinks considerably and requires extra trimming. Although a humidity level as low as 65 percent is suggested for some products, a range between 80 and 95 percent is recommended for most foods.

Good air circulation should be provided throughout the refrigerators and freezers at all times, with foods arranged so that air can circulate to all sides of the pan, box, or crate. For sanitary reasons, foods should not be stored on the floor. All foods are to be covered and labeled with the receiving date. Most foods should be left in their original containers—mandatory for frozen foods—to reduce the possibility of freezer burn and drying. Fresh produce should be examined for ripeness and spoilage before it is stored and may be transferred to specially designed plastic containers if it passes inspection. The paper wrappings on fruit should be left on to help keep them clean and to prevent spoilage, moisture loss, and bruising.

INVENTORY CONTROL PROCEDURES

Inventory represents money in the form of food, supplies, and small equipment. Efficient inventory control keeps the size of inventory at a level appropriate for the facility and ensures the security of goods on hand. Foodservice inventory management starts with the menu-planning process. The quantities of food supplies needed to produce the menu items are projected on the basis of how frequently individual items appear on the menu and on the probable demand for each item as determined from records of its past popularity. Once appropriate inventory levels have been established for various food supplies, they should be monitored continuously and adjusted periodically to correct for any shortages and overstocks.

Issuing of Food and Supplies

Issuing is the process of providing food and nonfood supplies to other areas within the foodservice department, including the production and service units. Products such as milk, bread, and other bakery items, and fresh produce may be issued directly from the receiving area to the appropriate production units without the products ever going into storage. Referred to as *direct issuing*, this method bases the quantities of items issued on records of past usage. Most food and supplies, however, are issued from dry, refrigerated, or frozen storage. Issuing is essential to control the quantity of food removed from storage and to provide cost-accounting information to the accounting department and to the storeroom clerk if the foodservice operation uses a perpetual inventory system. In addition, usage data are required for budgeting.

Many facilities have two or more types of storage areas for dry goods: one for bulk supplies and the other for supplies used daily. The main storage area for bulk supplies is kept locked, and goods are issued by a stock clerk after the clerk receives a *stores requisition* like the one shown in Exhibit 19.5. To secure food from the main storeroom and ingredients control area, the requesting units fill out a food requisition form the day before and take or send it by electronic process to the storeroom. The storeroom clerk fills the order, delivers it, and has the requisition employee sign the form to ensure that the order has been property filled. The needed products and quantities are based on the menu and forecast needs for the area. Using requisition forms and specifying times for issuing allow controlled access to the storage area. Any unused product is returned to the storeroom for credit to the specific unit. The issue requisitions and returned credits are used for determining the cost of the daily raw food. The issuing sheets are also used to maintain a perpetual inventory.

EXHIBIT 19.5   Stores Requisition Form

	Stores Requisition	
	_____ Hospital	

Day to be used: _____   Day issued: _____

Ordered by: _____   Issued by: _____

Stock Number	Total Quantity	Order Unit	Item Description	Issued to	Price per Unit	Total Cost

In some large institutions, nursing stations have nourishment carts that may be built to par level (described in more detail later in the chapter) or the nursing unit may electronically requisition items from food stores for use on the patient unit.

Some foodservice operations use an *exchange cart process* of issuing. All products needed for the day's menu are placed on the cart following a list from previous same-day menus. The cart is loaded the day before and wheeled to the production area the following morning. At night the cart is wheeled into the storeroom, and any unused food items are credited.

Another method of issuing is the *computerized issuing process.* The products issued are optically scanned by reading the bar codes, and data are automatically entered in the database; this method allows a constant running inventory to be kept.

To increase control of the issues, requisitions should be prenumbered to permit tracking of lost or duplicate forms. The type of information to include on the form is determined by whether the cost-accounting system is manual or computerized. For a manual system, information should include the unit requesting supplies, date, product description, quantity, supply unit, unit price, and total cost. For a computerized system, the above information (excluding unit price and total cost) and an inventory number for the item should be included. Some computerized systems generate requisitions. Requisition forms should provide for the initials or signatures of the person completing the requisition and the storeroom clerk (or other employee) responsible for filling the request.

In operations too small to justify a full-time clerk to issue food and keep records, other systems can be considered. For example, one staff member can be designated to issue food and keep records during a specified time of day. Alternatively, a sign-out sheet can be placed in the storeroom so that the staff members responsible for

food production can prepare a list of the kinds and amounts of foods they used that day. At the end of each day, the lists are given to a manager who records on the inventory record the supplies used each day. The last two methods, however, can create security and control problems in the department.

Some larger foodservice operations issue ingredients from an ingredient control room. If this system is used, the personnel in this unit requisition supplies from the different storage areas. Ingredients are weighed and measured before being issued to the production area at specified time periods. Some ingredient control rooms maintain a limited inventory of frequently used nonperishable products and supplies such as flour, sugar, and shortening.

Record Keeping

In addition to effective receiving and issuing procedures, good inventory records are essential for providing management with the information needed to calculate and monitor food and supply expenses. Four reasons have been cited for maintaining accurate inventory records:

1. To provide data for cost control
2. To assist in identifying purchasing needs
3. To provide accurate information on type and quantity of food and supplies on hand
4. To monitor usage of products and prevent theft and pilferage

The actual quantity of each item in inventory is another important aspect of an inventory control system. Two basic methods are used to determine the quantity of goods on hand: a perpetual inventory system and a physical inventory system.

Perpetual Inventory

The process of recording all purchases and food issues is known as *perpetual inventory*. This system contains five steps. Under this system:

1. A continuous record of the quantities of supplies on hand at any given time, as well as their value, is created—this is called a *balance on hand*.
2. When new products are received they are added to the existing inventory balance.
3. When products are issued they are subtracted from the total amount on hand. (On hand + received goods –issues = amount on hand at that point in time.)
4. At this point the inventory balance can be evaluated to determine if additional products need to be purchased.
5. At a predetermined date the perpetual inventory balance is reconciled by taking a physical inventory. The balance on hand should equal what was physically counted. When there is a discrepancy it should be investigated. Depending on the size (product and dollar value) of the discrepancy administration, security, and others, as advised by administration, will need to be involved. The result may be termination and possible jail time for a number of employees. To avoid this occurrence, policies and procedures may need to be revised or new ones put into place. Security will need to be involved to assist with methods to secure all foodservice products.

Perishable foods delivered directly to the production area are not usually kept on the perpetual inventory because they are usually consumed shortly after they come in. Perishable supplies may require only a monthly consumption record compiled from purchases.

Maintaining a perpetual inventory system is time-consuming. Therefore, small institutions may not have the staff or the need for such detailed records. For them, a physical inventory and a record of purchases are sufficient, especially when limited amounts of supplies are kept on hand.

To estimate the amount of time required to maintain a perpetual inventory system, the following formula can be used:

Number of items purchased per week × 4 weeks per month
  = number of purchases per month

Number of items issued per day × 30 days per month
  = number of issues per month

Number of items counted to verify perpetual system
  = number of items counted per month

(Purchases per month + issues per month + number of items counted per month) ÷ time required to enter each item

For example, if a foodservice purchased 500 items per week and issued 1,000 items per day and it took the storeroom clerk 30 seconds to enter each item, a total of 270.83 labor hours per month would be required to maintain a perpetual inventory system in this operation.

500 items per week × 4 weeks per month = 2,000 items

1,000 items issued daily × 30 days per month
  = 30,000 items issued per month

500 items counted × 1 time per month = 500

The labor cost required to maintain a perpetual inventory must be justified. Before an operation can justify using a perpetual inventory system, data calculated and maintained must be used frequently by management and be essential to cost control.

Physical Inventory

Periodic physical counts of all stock are necessary even when a perpetual inventory is maintained. Regardless of how well systems and personnel perform, errors can be made in recording transactions, food can spoil, and pilferage can occur. In small operations in which the labor involved makes keeping a perpetual inventory impractical, physical inventories can be taken monthly to determine the cost of foods team during the preceding month.

Physical inventory is conducted by a team of at least two employees, who survey and count, document, and sign off for the verification of the count. If there are discrepancies in the count from one person to the other a third party will need to recount products where the discrepancies occurred. To help with security of the inventory the supervisor should make spot checks. The installation of security cameras is an added protection, as it will record unauthorized persons in a secure area. When unauthorized employees/vendors are recorded in a secure area corrective action needs to be taken.

Taking a *physical inventory* is simplified when the storeroom is organized by food categories and the foods in each category are stored alphabetically. A form for recording goods on hand should be developed to correspond to the storeroom's organization. Each item on the inventory form should be listed on a separate line. If more than one package size of an item is stocked, it still should be listed separately. The form should include space for the product description, the unit size, the quantity on hand, the unit cost, and the total value of the amount on hand.

After a physical inventory has been conducted, the cost of the food used can be calculated in the following manner. The value of the beginning inventory plus the cost of the foods purchased equals the value of the food on hand. When the value of the final inventory is subtracted from the value of the food on hand, the result is the cost of the food used between inventories. In other words,

Beginning inventory + purchases = food on hand

Food on hand − final inventory = food used

An example of a physical inventory record is given in Exhibit 19.6. Inventory records are essential not only for calculating costs but also for managing purchases and making the best use of available funds. With continued emphasis on cost containment in today's health care industry, foodservice directors must stay on top of inventory distribution and cost control in their departments.

EXHIBIT 19.6   Physical Inventory Record

Physical Inventory

Date: _____   Taken by: _____   Beginning inventory: $ _____

Quantity on Hand	Order Unit	Article	Description	Unit Cost	Total
	#10	Apples	Sliced, 6 #10/case		
	#10	Apples	Dehydrated, low moisture, 6 #10/case		
	#10	Apple rings	6 #10/case		
	#10	Applesauce	6 #10/case		
	#10	Apricots	Unpeeled halves, 6/case		
	#10	Blueberries	Water pack, 6/case		
	#10	Cherries	RSP, water pack, 6/case		
	1 Gallon	Cherries	Maraschino halves, 4/case		
	#10	Cranberry sauce	6/case		
	1 Pound	Dates	Pieces, 25-pound box		
	#10	Fruit cocktail	6/case		
	#10	Fruit for salads	6/case		
	#3	Grapefruit sections	Whole, 12		
	#3	Grapefruit-orange sections	Whole, 12 cylinder; 46 ounces/case		
	#10	Mincemeat	Solid pack, 6/case		
	#10	Mandarin oranges	6/case		
	#10	Peaches	Halves, 6/case		
	#10	Peaches	Sliced, 6/case		
	#10	Pears	Halves, 6/case		
	#10	Pineapple	Crushed, 6/case		
	#10	Pineapple	Sliced, 6/case		
	#10	Pineapple	Tidbits, 6/case		
	#10	Plums	Purple, 6/case		
	#10	Prunes	6/case		
	1 Pound	Raisins	Dried, seedless, 24 16-ounce/case		
	#10	Rhubarb	5/case		

Inventory Turnover

Slow inventory turnover may indicate an excessive amount of food on hand and money tied up in inventory that could be used elsewhere. Inventory turnover can be calculated as:

$$\text{Inventory turnover} = \frac{\text{Cost of food consumed}}{\text{Inventory value}}$$

Most foodservice operations try to turn over inventory from two to eight times per month. The use of technology helps track inventory and provides reports on slow-moving products. Some of the slowness may be due to a change in the menu where the item is no longer used but the item is still in inventory. Once slow-moving products have been identified, if possible, they should be incorporated into the menu as "specials of the day."

Shrinkage

It does not matter what type of inventory is used unless all records concerning the products are maintained. When records are not maintained it may appear that there is a theft problem (see earlier). It is for these reasons that records need to be kept on what may be labeled **shrinkage,** which means loss of inventory. The following are examples of shrinkage:

- The stores clerk drops a glass jar of cherries when filling a requisition, it breaks, another jar is issued, but there is no record to show two jars were issued.
- Due to the lack of policies and procedures "unauthorized" employees go into the storeroom and pocket coffee for their personal use. There is no record of the missing coffee.
- Chicken is left in ice for more than a day and half and becomes unusable and needs to be replaced. No record of the discarded chicken.
- A good deal goes bad—a sale on a product to buy one get one free sounded good, the deal was made, and the menu changed; the product spoiled and was discarded and no record was kept.
- There are two major problems—the delivery person and the receiving person are family, and apples and heads of lettuce were not counted, meat was not weighed or tagged, but all items were received as stated on the invoice even when there was a shortage of products.
- Suppliers entered the storeroom and "made a decision" that stock needed to be increased—due to an increase in much of the stock being spoiled.

Inventory Control Tools

Several types of inventory records are maintained in an effort to monitor food cost, determine purchase quantity, and identify inventory levels to maintain. Six of them are outlined in the following subsections: valuing inventory, the "ABC method," fixed-item inventory, par stock system, "mini-max system," and economic order quantity.

Valuing Inventory

One of the most common records foodservice departments keep is the dollar value of the assets in inventory. The first step in calculating the inventory value is to count the number of each type of item on hand. This value is computed by multiplying the quantity of the item by a predetermined cost. The following three methods are used most frequently to determine cost:

1. *Last-in, first-out (LIFO):* All products counted are valued at first price paid during the accounting period.
2. *First-in, first-out (FIFO):* Products are valued at the last price paid during the accounting period. This method is used by operations that attempt to ensure that the oldest items in inventory are used first.
3. *Weighted average:* The actual price paid for an item is multiplied by the number of units on hand for a specific order. The sum of the total actual dollar value is divided by the number of units on hand to compute the average cost per item.

The method selected for valuing the inventory influences the calculation of cost of goods sold in the operation's financial statement. This value influences the profit or loss status of the foodservice department.

ABC Method

The concept of the *ABC* is based on the premise that a small number (15 to 20 percent) of the items purchased accounts for most of the inventory value. Items in the inventory that constitute the greatest value are the ones on which management should spend most of its tracking effort. These items are often referred to as the "A" items, and they represent about 20 percent of all inventory items but account for about 80 percent of inventory value. Only the minimum quantity required to meet current demand should be maintained in inventory. The "B" items represent 10 to 15 percent of the inventory items and 20 to 25 percent of the total inventory value. The low-value items, the "C" items, contribute only 5 to 10 percent of inventory value and consist of 60 to 65 percent of the total number of items in inventory. Examples of each class of items are:

- **A items**: Meat, frozen convenience entrees, seafood
- **B items**: Dairy products, china
- **C items**: Staples (beans, flour, and sugar), breakfast cereals, paper products

Fixed-Item Inventory

The *fixed-item technique* for monitoring inventory is similar to the ABC method except that the foodservice director selects only a limited number of items to track the usage. Order quantity and flow of these products are carefully monitored. Steaks would be an example of one meat item that might be included on an operation's fixed-item inventory list.

FIGURE 19.3 Comparison of Par Stock and Mini-Max Inventory Systems

Par Stock System

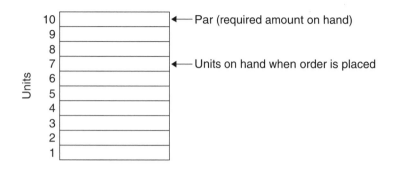

Mini-Max System

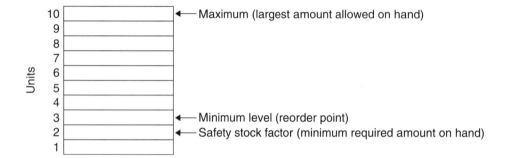

Par Stock System

The *par stock system* requires that a certain quantity level be established for each item that must be kept on hand to meet the needs of the planned menu and any unusual circumstances that might occur. Orders are placed at regular fixed intervals over a specified period. Each time the ordering date comes around, enough stock is purchased to replenish the supply to the predetermined level. The usage rate of each item must be carefully planned between order dates.

Mini-Max System

The *mini-max system* involves establishing both a minimum and a maximum amount of stock to have on hand. Minimum quantity is the minimum amount of products that must be on hand and inventory levels should not fall below this level. Maximum quantity is the amount of products that should be on hand at all times; inventory levels should not exceed this amount. Goods are ordered whenever the minimum is reached and only in the quantity needed to attain the maximum level. With this system, the amount of each food ordered would be the same each time, but the time when it is purchased varies. Again, the *usage rate* (the amount of product used over a defined period of time) of each item must be carefully scrutinized so that the determined minimum and maximum levels remain appropriate. For example the *maximum level* for canned peas is 10 cases of 6 #10 cans. On hand in *inventory* are 4 cases 6 #10 cans of peas.

To bring the inventory to maximum level 6 cases need to be *ordered* (10 − 4 = 6). This is referred to as *purchase quantity* or the *amount ordered.* It may be necessary to order the 6 cases of peas as soon as possible as the usage rate may change and time needed to place the order, receive order, process order for inventory and issuing. This process is called *lead time.*

Figure 19.3 compares the par stock and mini-max systems. Both approaches work to help prevent overstocking and avoid shortages of frequently used foods.

Economical Order Quantity

Economical order quantity is a method to calculate reorder points to ensure that the best price is obtained after taking into consideration the carrying cost or the cost of maintaining the item in inventory for an extended period of time. This method is not used frequently by foodservice directors but may be a helpful tool in operations that order large quantities at one time or for GPOs. Unless the inventory system is computerized, the calculation of economical order quantity is time-consuming and cumbersome.

COMPUTERIZED INVENTORY MANAGEMENT SYSTEM

Technology is available for computerizing receiving, storage, and issuing. Some systems link inventory files with recipes, ingredient files, and forecasts. With this system, the storeroom manager can monitor stock levels, assess reorder points, calculate actual product usage, and calculate daily cost. These systems can calculate variance between actual usage and expected usage based on production and number of servings. Most computer systems can operate on the basis of perpetual inventory system, minimum-maximum, par level, or any variety of methods. Some systems can track products through purchase, storage, issuing, and usage. As technology improves, the procurement system will be simplified.

Accounting Process

Once all the products have been purchased, received, stored, and issued, the suppliers must be paid. Verification that what is being paid for is actually what was received is usually the role of the finance and accounting department; however, they must have correct documentation before payment can be made. The flow of documents between foodservice and accounting may be paper based or computerized. The flow of documents where payments are made by a central accounting office follow the path shown in Figure 19.4.

Paperwork and payment practices may be audited internally and by an outside auditing company. Paperwork may be delivered daily to the accounting department or held in file in the foodservice department by supplier name, in date sequence, and sent to the accounting department at the end of the month. The accounting department checks invoices against statements, and if there are any discrepancies, the department, supplier, or both

FIGURE 19.4 Accounting Process

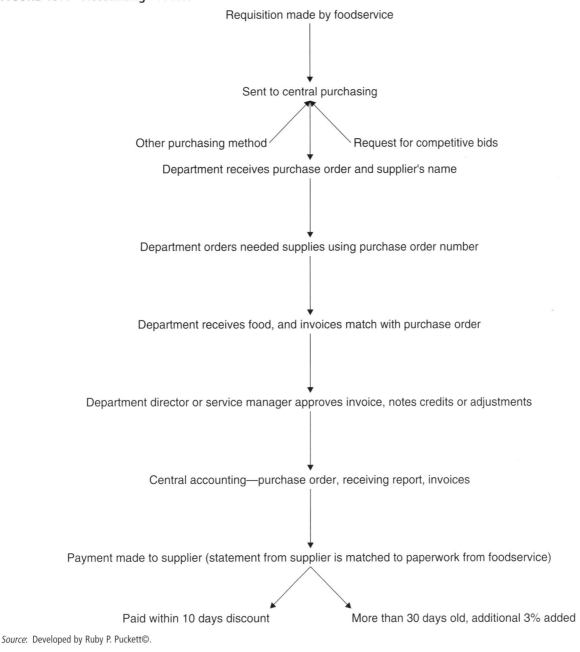

Source: Developed by Ruby P. Puckett©.

are contacted. Once these are cleared, the statement is processed for payment.

Other Payment Methods

Depending on the credit standing of the organization, the following other payment methods may be used:

- *Cash on delivery:* Products are paid for at the time of delivery or in advance of delivery.
- *No cash discounts:* A specific time frame exists for payment.
- *Penalty for late payments:* Usually the penalty for late payments (after 30 days) is 1 to 2 percent per month, or 18 to 25 percent annually.
- *Cash discounts:* A percentage reduction may be given if invoice is paid within a specific time, such as 2 percent discount if paid within 10 days.

affected by menu planning. Inventory control is vital to department survival because it represents money in the form of food, supplies, and small equipment. Enough food should be kept on hand to ensure that the menu can be prepared and that emergency situations can be handled. On the other hand, food spoilage, theft, and pilferage as a result of overstocking must be avoided. A periodic count of items on hand determines whether the proper controls are in place.

Receiving procedures must ensure that the quantity and quality of food and supplies ordered match those of the materials received. On receipt, inspection, and approval, goods should be date-stamped, the cost determined, and the items stored in the proper area. Invoices of goods received should be checked for accuracy.

Items should be stored appropriately, always using the FIFO method. Storage areas should be clean, have proper temperature controls and adequate maintenance, and be monitored by efficient security systems. Toxic chemicals used for cleaning and sanitizing should be stored away from food products.

SUMMARY

Receiving, storage, and inventory control are critical aspects of the foodservice department's procurement system that are directly

KEY TERMS

ABC method	Mini-max system
Blind receiving	Pallets
Credit memo	Par stock
Daily receiving record	Perpetual inventory
Direct issuing	Physical inventory
Exchange cart	Receiving process
FIFO	Receiving reports
Inventory	Shrinkage
Invoice receiving	Stores requisitions
Invoices	Supplier
Lead time	Usage rate
LIFO	Weighted averages
Meat tags	

DISCUSSION QUESTIONS

1. How would you develop a good relation with the supplier?
2. Differentiate between blind receiving and invoice receiving.
3. Explain the advantages and disadvantages of the four major inventory control procedures.
4. Discuss the importance of keeping accurate records when receiving, storing, inventorying, issuing, and paying invoices.
5. Describe the accounting process.

CHAPTER 20

FOOD PRODUCTION

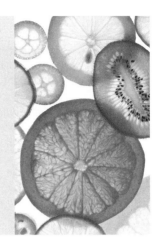

LEARNING OBJECTIVES

- Develop standardized recipes using the HACCP principles, and set up a recipe file.
- Compare the advantages and disadvantages of the four major food production systems.
- Describe various methods to forecast production needs.
- Communicate with production staff through production schedules, meetings, and quality monitoring.
- Explain how ingredient control is a component of the total system.
- Define various cooking methods for the production of meat, fish, poultry, eggs, vegetables, soups, sandwiches, salads, desserts, and beverages, and enhancement of flavors by using a variety of herbs and spices.
- Develop evaluation forms to monitor food production for quality, proper production methods, portion control, and customer satisfaction.
- Describe the appropriate equipment to use in food production.

FOOD PRODUCTION PLAYS a critical role in meeting the objectives of the health care foodservice department and satisfying the expectations of its customers. This system is responsible for translating the menu into food of the highest caliber possible in the required quantities. Nutritious, carefully prepared, flavorful, and attractive foods are vital tools for restoring or maintaining the health of patients or residents and in satisfying the wants of nonpatients.

Two of the most important management decisions that affect the system's success are which food production systems to use and

which production forecasting methods to apply. Several alternatives have evolved for both of these functions. A health care operation considering a change or evaluating the effectiveness of these functions should study closely the factors described in this chapter, because they affect food quality, microbiological safety, customers' expectations and needs, and the operation's financial status.

The foodservice director is responsible for developing food quality standards (as described in Chapter 4), implementing those standards, and following procedures to control the quality and quantity of food provided. Production controls vital to this process include standardized recipes, ingredient and portion standards, and production schedules. Well-trained production workers should strive to maintain the nutritional value and the natural flavor, color, and appeal of the foods they prepare.

In this chapter, four food production systems—cook and serve, cook and chill, cook and freeze, and assembly and serve—are described and compared. Next, production forecasting techniques—that is, determining what menu items need to be prepared, in what quantities, and over what time frames—are outlined.

Because a foodservice department manager must balance the production schedule with workload, food quality standards, and employee skills (among other demands), the chapter delineates the elements that make up a workable production schedule, and details methods and devices for portion control, recipe standardization (including techniques for testing recipes), ingredient control, and the benefits of a centralized ingredient room or area.

The chapter gives an in-depth breakdown of food production processes for the key food groups. For example, optimal cooking procedures for various meats and meat products (dry heat, roasting, broiling and grilling, and so forth) are suggested. The same is done for poultry, fish and shellfish, eggs and egg products, and the dairy group (including milk and milk products). Storage guidelines for these food groups are provided as well. Similar selection, preparation, and storage pointers are presented for fresh and frozen fruits and vegetables; for starches (potatoes, pasta, rice, and cereals); for breads (yeast and quick varieties specifically); and for beverages.

FOOD PRODUCTION SYSTEMS

Food production is the second functional subsystem in system management of a foodservice department. Once the food has been procured, it needs to be *transformed* into edible and serviceable food for the customer; this is considered the *output*. The food production systems used most commonly today are classified as cook and serve (conventional), cook and chill, cook and freeze, and assembly and serve (convenience) (Figure 20.1). The systems differ in several areas: in the market form in which foods are purchased, in the amount and type of labor required, in the timing of production relative to service, in the holding methods used before serving, and in the types of equipment required. Although each system has certain strong and weak points that have been identified by researchers and acknowledged by users (Table 20.1), all the systems successfully provide food of acceptable quality in operational situations. The key to their success lies in adequate managerial control of the critical control points in each production system (as described in Chapter 14) and in thorough employee training.

Cook-and-Serve System (Conventional)

In a *cook-and-serve system*, most menu items are prepared primarily from basic ingredients on the day they are to be served. Most cook-and-serve systems incorporate ingredients with some degree of processing. The prepared items used most frequently are bakery goods, canned and frozen vegetables and fruits, and ice cream. Portion-cut chilled or frozen meats have replaced the traditional meat-cutting operation. Bread products and dessert items are still baked on-site in some cook-and-serve systems. Baked items are made by starting from scratch with basic ingredients or by using standard production methods along with some mixes and frozen pies, bread dough, and desserts. Vegetables are purchased in many forms: canned, frozen, fresh, prewashed or prepeeled, and dehydrated.

The number of different food supply items kept in inventory for cook-and-serve systems is relatively high. The availability and cost of labor, the equipment available, and the facility's supply sources affect purchasing decisions, but rising labor costs have accelerated the trend toward purchasing more extensively processed foods.

The cook-and-serve system can be further categorized based on the amount of holding required between production and service of food items to customers. These subcategories include limited holding and extended holding of finished food products.

FIGURE 20.1   Flow of Products in Foodservice Production System

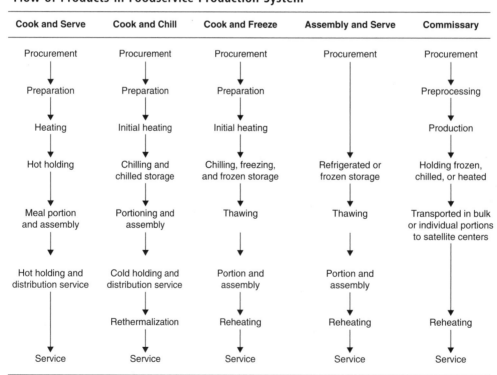

Source: Adapted from Boberg and David, 1977, and revised by R. P. Puckett, 2003, reviewed 2010.

TABLE 20.1 Advantages and Disadvantages of Food Production Systems

Conventional (Cook and Serve)		Cook and Chill or Cook and Freeze		Commissary (Control Production)		Assembly and Serve	
Advantage	Disadvantage	Advantage	Disadvantage	Advantage	Disadvantage	Advantage	Disadvantage
1. Quality control	1. Stressful workday due to peak demands	1. Reduction in "peaks and valleys" workload	1. Need for large cold and freezer space	1. Cost savings due to large-volume purchasing	1. Food safety and distribution of food	1. Labor-saving	1. Limited to good selection of menu items, regional food items
2. Individual for operation	2. May have lower productivity due to change daily in menu	2. One shift (40 hours weekly, 8 hours a day)	2. Food safety	2. Reduced labor	2. Need to employ a food microbiologist for constant testing	2. May not need experienced or highly skilled personnel	2. May have higher costs of menu items
3. Control of menu, recipes, and quality of ingredients	3. May not use talents of skilled employees due to task assignment	3. Decreased employee turnover	3. Need to modify recipes and ingredients	3. Quality control more effective	3. Temperature maintenance during loading and transporting	3. Lower procurement cost	3. Quality
4. Meets standards of quality	4. Need for two shifts of employees	4. Reduction in production cost	4. Equipment needs for rethermalization	4. Less supervision	4. Specialized equipment and trucks needed for delivery	4. Less waste	4. Customer acceptance
5. Not dependent on commercially prepared items		5. Improved quality	5. Location of equipment		5. May be delays in delivery due to weather, breakdowns, and accidents	5. Better portion control	5. Portion sizes may not meet protein requirement
6. Adaptable to regional, ethnic, and individual preferences of customers		6. Improved nutrient retention			6. High cost of equipment and maintenance and repair of specialized equipment	6. Reduction in purchasing time	6. Need constant evaluation of quality, portion size, and customer satisfaction
7. Flexibility in menu changes		7. Control over equipment				7. Less pilferage	7. Additional freezer space needed
8. Needs less storage space for freezers		8. Close control over menu selection, quality of ingredients, and quantity				8. Equipment and space minimal	8. Equipment and energy cost may increase
9. Reduced or minimal distribution cost						9. Reduced costs of water, gas, and electricity	9. Disposition of packaging materials

Cook and Serve with Limited Holding

Cook and serve with limited holding, often referred to as *à la carte cooking*, is used extensively by full-service and quick-service restaurants. Because customers dine at varying times and usually select items from a written menu, individual food items are cooked to order rather than cooked ahead. This type of system, as opposed to the other types of food production systems, minimizes the holding time between food preparation and service to customers. However, this system requires rather extensive prepreparation of ingredients so that food preparation can be expedited once the customers have placed their orders. This type of system is appropriate if the health care organization operates a full-service or quick-service restaurant.

Cook and Serve with Extended Holding

Cook and serve with extended holding is the traditional system of food production for health care operations. It differs from the previous system in that most menu items are held hot or cold until they are served. Production may take place in a kitchen located in the facility or in a separate kitchen or commissary that supplies several sites. Foodservice directors who use a system of cook and serve with extended holding believe that they have better control over menus, recipes, and overall quality. Menus can reflect changes in seasonal supply and marketplace conditions and the food preferences of patient and nonpatient markets. Also, menus can be tailored to the specific standards of the facility. In some cases, however, menu variety may be more limited than in other systems because of the amount of production time allowable, the skill levels of employees, or the availability and capacity of equipment.

A 12- to 15-hour production and service day is common for facilities using cook and serve with extended holding, because foods are produced just before assembly and service. Periods of increased activity are necessary because the quality and nutritional value of some foods are adversely affected by extended holding. However, it is difficult to produce all the foods on the menu within the ideal period, and the holding that becomes necessary often results in having to serve lower-quality food.

Both skilled and semiskilled employees are needed in this type of system, and the need for skilled employees often leads to higher labor costs than is the case with other production systems. In addition, the availability of skilled employees may be limited because of the location of the facility or because of the undesirable working hours characteristic of the system of cook and serve with extended holding.

Production is scheduled on a seven-day workweek. The level of productivity in these systems may not be as high as in other systems because it is difficult to schedule a balanced daily workload that covers service time peaks and yet minimizes the number of employees on duty during slow periods. As a result, skilled employees are frequently assigned routine cleaning jobs to equalize the workload even though less-skilled employees could perform these tasks.

Many types and sizes of equipment are needed in a system of cook and serve with extended holding. More total capacity may be needed for certain pieces of equipment because of the volume demand and same-day service that characterize the system. Poor utilization of equipment can occur, depending on the menu item mix, because both hot-holding equipment and cold-holding equipment are needed. However, cook and serve with extended holding can require less energy than other systems because chilling and freezing of hot foods are not necessary. Another shortcoming of the system is evident when foods must be prepared well in advance of service time, because it is difficult to maintain proper temperatures during extended holding. Food perishability increases with overcooking, and foods held at a high temperature for a long period lose their palatability and some of their nutritional value. This system is used for selective and nonselective menus as well as employee meal service.

Cook-and-Chill and Cook-and-Freeze Systems

Cook-and-chill and *cook-and-freeze systems* do not have the labor, productivity, and cost problems associated with the cook-and-serve system or the problem of diminished food quality associated with extended holding. In a cook-and-chill system, prepared menu items are chilled and ready for assembly and reheating one or more days after production. Foods can be purchased at any stage of processing as basic ingredients for recipe preparation, as partially prepared recipe components or as fully prepared items. After initial preparation, menu items may be individually portioned or stored in bulk. These food production systems require two stages of heat processing—initial cooking and reheating before serving.

The quality of food can and should be high in cook-and-chill and cook-and-freeze systems because chilled or frozen food is less perishable and retains its nutrients longer than food cooked and held in the cook-and-serve system. Menu selections can be more varied, particularly when menu items are individually portioned before chilling or freezing. It is possible to offer a restaurant-style and spoken menu when production does not take place on the same day as service. These foods smell, look, and taste good because they are not overcooked during holding, as in the cook-and-serve system. This is because the cooking process is finished during reheating. However, an internal temperature of 165°F for 15 seconds must be reached during the initial partial cooking process to ensure that foods are not contaminated by bacterial growth.

Recipe quantities may need to be increased for large-volume production runs for frozen items. In such cases, the traditional steps in preparation are often changed to accommodate the expanded volume and to save time.

Not all foods can be held successfully in cook-and-chill or cook-and-freeze systems without extensive modification of the ingredients, recipes, or both. Special ingredients, such as thickening agents, are needed for some recipes. Foam and sponge products, gels, coatings, and emulsions pose other problems. When foods are frozen, structural and textural changes occur because of cell damage and protein coagulation. As a result, odd flavors can develop in some vegetables and meats.

The extended period between initial preparation and consumption of the food in cook-and-chill systems creates many opportunities for the mishandling of food. Foodservice directors are responsible for controlling potential microbiological hazards at critical control points. This process involves monitoring equipment sanitation and time-temperature conditions at all stages from food procurement through service. During the production stage, quick-chilling procedures are essential to bring the temperatures of cooked foods to 41°F (5°C) or lower in less than four hours after initial cooking. Factors that influence the cooling rate of foods include the initial internal temperature of the food, size or depth of the batch, dimensions of the food mass, density of the food, and temperature and load of the refrigerator.

Similar quick freezing is necessary in a cook-and-freeze system to optimize the taste and smell of the frozen food and to ensure a product free of contamination. It is recommended that a temperature of 0°F (−18°C) or lower be reached within 90 minutes after initial cooking. Frozen food should be stored at 0°F or lower and must be properly packaged to prevent dehydration. Entrées should be thawed in a refrigerator and used within 24 hours after thawing. In all cook-and-chill and cook-and-freeze systems, the temperature of the entrées should be kept at 41°F (5°C) or lower during portioning, assembly, and distribution.

As in cook-and-serve systems (and all food production activities), good personal hygiene for food handlers is a critical control point at all stages—initial preparation, portioning, assembly, and service—of processing food in cook-and-chill and cook-and-freeze systems. Employees can directly and indirectly contribute to microbiological contamination through poor personal hygiene and work habits (see Chapter 13).

In both cook-and-chill and cook-and-freeze systems, production usually can be scheduled into a 40-hour workweek with regular 8-hour shifts. For this reason, these systems (because they have already incorporated production tasks that require high skill levels) usually require fewer skilled employees. In cook-and-chill systems, the plating of food can be spread over a longer period because all items are held cold during plating and tray assembly. This system can reduce the number of employees needed and possibly increase their productivity and satisfaction.

More balanced and efficient use of equipment is possible in cook-and-chill and cook-and-freeze systems because production can be distributed over the entire work shift rather than being done in the limited time just before service. Total equipment requirements may be lower than in a cook-and-serve system, but the types of equipment and capacities needed depend on whether a cook-and-chill or a cook-and-freeze system is being followed. For example, specialized quick-chill refrigerators are needed for both systems, but blast or cryogenic freezers also are needed for a cook-and-freeze system.

Adequate refrigerated space must be available for storing foods and holding them during the assembly process. Also, the amount of refrigeration space needed for preplated items is greater than for bulk storage items. The acquisition of needed equipment adds to capital investment costs. Research also indicates that more energy is used in the cook-and-chill and cook-and-freeze systems than in the cook-and-serve system because of the significant amount of energy required to chill or freeze, thaw, and reheat foods.

Cook-and-chill and cook-and-freeze systems may operate in an on-premises kitchen, or they may be located in a commissary separate from the service area. Many commissaries use these systems because the scheduling and control of production and service are easier for chilled and frozen foods than they are for hot foods. This method or production is a good system for spoken menu or room service. Individual portions of various products can be blast frozen for future use.

Assembly-and-Serve System

With an *assembly-and-serve production system* (sometimes called a *convenience system*), most or all foods are obtained from a commercial source in a ready-to-serve form. This includes entrée items that are purchased frozen, canned, or dehydrated; ready-to-serve dessert and bakery products that are purchased fresh, frozen, or canned; salads and salad ingredients that are purchased ready to assemble; canned, frozen, or dehydrated sauces and soups; frozen concentrated, portion-packed, canned, or dehydrated fruit juices and beverages; and individual portion packets of condiments such as sugar, jelly, syrup, salad dressing, and cream.

Menu variety can be wider in assembly-and-serve systems than in cook-and-serve systems, but it depends on the facility's access to suppliers that can provide a wide range of products. However, the variety of preplated items is not as large as that offered in bulk-packaged products. Inconsistent quality among different products and among different lots of the same products has been observed. Because of this inconsistency, it is desirable to try several potential vendors before implementing an assembly-and-serve system. Also, the geographical location of the foodservice operation and small purchase volumes may intensify problems in obtaining products of the same quality from one purchase period to another.

An assembly-and-serve system requires minimal use of skilled labor. Labor costs should decrease if the foods used in the system are at a maximum convenience level. However, labor savings must compensate for the higher food costs characteristic of an assembly-and-serve system.

The system should eliminate the need for most standard production equipment, but in many cases it does not. Many operations are reluctant to abandon the option of on-premises production in case the quality, availability, or cost of the prepared items fails to meet expected standards. Thus, a primary economic advantage is lost.

Questions related to the feasibility of implementing an assembly-and-serve system include:

- Do available products meet the operation's nutrition standards for normal and modified diets?
- Are enough products available to provide variety throughout the menu cycle?
- Do products meet the quality standards of the operation and its customers?
- Is the cost per serving within an acceptable range?
- Is the operation's storage space sufficient for handling disposable ware?
- Will changes be required in the type and amount of equipment needed for reheating foods?
- Is the facility's refrigerator and freezer space adequate?
- How many labor hours can be eliminated with this system?

- How will tray assembly and delivery be performed?
- Will additional packaging materials create waste disposal problems?

In an assembly-and-serve system, attention must be paid to preventing microbiological contamination at critical control points. Some of the hazards present in other systems are eliminated because there is little or no on-premises food preparation. The amount of freezer and refrigeration space needed for storing and thawing frozen foods before final heating exceeds that needed in cook-and-serve systems. Thawing or tempering frozen products must be carried out under refrigeration, and storage times for purchased chilled foods should be kept to a minimum. Perishable foods must be maintained at 41°F (5°C) or lower during portioning, assembly, and distribution. In the reheating stage, foods must reach temperatures of at least 140°F (60°C) as rapidly as possible. For maximum safety and palatability, an end-point temperature of 165°F (74°C) is recommended for most hot foods. Food temperatures should be routinely checked before service. As in other systems, personnel and equipment sanitation are essential to control microbiological hazards. When room service is the primary patient food delivery system, this method of production is best, as requested individual items may be thawed and rethermalized as requested. This system works well with room service.

PRODUCTION FORECASTING

In addition to determining the type of food production system (or combination of systems) to be implemented, the foodservice director must decide which forecasting technique is appropriate for the foodservice operation. *Forecasting* is the process of estimating future events based on past data; it is also determining how much of which product to produce. It also includes future purchasing, inventory, and service needs. Forecasting tells how much food to produce and how much to order. Each operation will need to know how far in advance to forecast; some organizations use from 4 to 7 days. How a menu is served—set versus room service; the purchasing system—buying group or local distributor; inventory system, storage system—on-site versus off-site warehouse; skills of personnel; leadership of managers and supervisors; and the wants and needs of the customers all come into play. For patient foodservice, these records will be needed: previous census records, tallies, and special orders and modified diets. Records need to include weather conditions, holidays, and unused foods and underproduction. Where employee feeding is the responsibility of the department, point-of-sale (POS) information, which gives numbers of servings and what time various products ran out or were returned to the production area, is valuable information to be used in forecasting. Using this information, the manager can forecast needs for the next menu cycle that the data had been collected for and make any needed adjustments.

Because most food production systems require extensive advanced preparation of menu items, *production-demand forecasting* is critical to satisfying customer expectations. Some operations now use a computer-based information system to forecast production levels. In selecting a system for forecasting, it is important to choose a system that is user friendly, whose cost is within budget allocations, and that can be programmed for the facility's foodservice department for its specific production system.

Forecasting Techniques

Data will need to be available to develop a forecasting system for each individual organization. Even though the system must be specific to the organization, census figures from the past time period, the menu cycle, and the number of portions for each item can be compared to today's data. Forecasting techniques can be divided into three categories: subjective, time-series, and causal models. A *subjective technique* is the simplest model. This technique uses information, experience, and intuition to determine the amount of product to produce. This technique works well in small operations, but it is not sophisticated and is only as reliable as the person doing the forecasting. Therefore, it is not a good technique, and its use should be discouraged.

Time-Series Forecasting Techniques

Time-series forecast techniques rely solely on historical data about the demand for menu items. These techniques, which assume that the demand for menu items follows a pattern over time, are appropriate for short-term forecasting, such as the demand for menu items. They are the forecasting techniques most frequently used by health care foodservice operations.

Examples of time-series techniques include simple moving average and weighted moving average. Both combine data about the demand for menu items over several periods and menu cycles. They result in an average, or the forecast, for the number of servings to prepare during the next menu cycle. *Exponential smoothing* is another time-series technique that is available in computer software packages. It differs from the averaging techniques in that it does not weigh data from the past menu cycles equally.

Causal Forecasting Techniques

In addition to historical data, *causal techniques* use other types of data as well. These techniques might relate the demand for menu items to other variables thought to influence demand, such as patient census or the number of patients on regular and modified diets. Causal techniques generally are more costly to implement than time-series techniques. For short-term forecasting, these techniques do not result in increased accuracy over the time-series techniques.

Regression analysis is the causal technique used most commonly. It draws on past data to establish a relationship between two variables, such as the number of patients on a normal diet and the number of servings of a particular entrée, and point-of-sale data to forecast the number of servings to prepare.

Several operations depend on a *tally* technique for forecasting needs for the next meal and the entire day. With tally techniques, orders (such as patient selections) are counted to determine production needs. This technique has several drawbacks, such as patient discharges and changes in diet orders; the delivery system such as room service plus the technique is labor-intensive. This technique should be used only for items not on the master menu, such as special requests and write-in items. Some computer systems can tally menus and provide the production staff with the number of orders to prepare. Accurate historical data are needed to provide a good usable forecast.

Another practice that is not a real forecast technique is what is termed *padding*. This is a technique of adding additional portions for a product to avoid a shortage of food products. Different food-service operations specify the number or percentage to pad for each item. If this technique is used, a person who has the experience, authority, and knowledge to add more portions should be the one to do it. This method needs constant monitoring to avoid overproduction. Special orders and write-ins should not be padded.

Designing a Forecasting System

An effective forecasting system is key to health care foodservice operations. A number of factors must be considered when designing or redesigning a forecasting system. Messersmith and Miller, in *Forecasting in Foodservice* (1992), indicate that the nature of the information to be forecast and the availability of data essential to generate the forecast are key concerns. Before a specific forecasting technique is selected, each technique should be evaluated on the basis of the accuracy of the forecast and the cost of implementing and operating the technique. Implementation issues include personnel training, modification of operational procedures, and consideration of computer-assisted applications. In addition, a strategy should be developed to evaluate the technique after it has been implemented.

PRODUCTION SCHEDULES

Daily schedules for food production can be valuable management tools for controlling the use of labor while ensuring food quality. A *daily production schedule* assigns specific tasks to each production employee. The workload is balanced according to the assigned duties and the specific skills of individual employees, and management establishes a time sequence for all production activities. In a cook-and-serve food production system, efficient production timing is perhaps the greatest benefit of following a daily production schedule. It can ensure that foods will not be cooked too far in advance of service and yet can allow adequate time for preparation.

For each item to be prepared, daily food production schedules should state the name of the item; the name of the employee assigned to prepare the item; preparation start and completion times; and specific details regarding ingredients, portion control, assembly, and so forth. In smaller operations, one production schedule for the entire kitchen staff may be sufficient. Larger operations with several employees in each specialized unit may require separate schedules for each work group. When work assignments are not highly specialized, production schedules can eliminate the confusion about which tasks are to be performed by each employee.

Daily food production schedules should be developed concurrently with menu planning. This prevents a workload imbalance from day to day and allows adequate time for preparation of foods

for later service. During scheduling, the equipment to be used for preparing each food item is considered so that all necessary equipment will be available when needed.

Sequencing

The sequence in which food is prepared, from purchasing → issuing → thawing → preparation → production → and serving is important because it ensures all items are on hand and available to meet the menu items and all food is ready at the same time. Preparatory work—thawing, cleaning, chopping, weighing, and measuring—is vital to ensure that needed items are available for production. Production sequencing means all food items are cooked in the amount required and at the time of service. This means that all items are finished on time for service or else the tray line will start late or the employee cafeteria will not have all the foods that have been advertised for the meal.

Production Meetings

Production meetings are an excellent method of communicating with the staff. One meeting should be held before service of the meal and another at the end of the meal. Monthly production meetings should also be conducted to discuss productivity, menus, recipes, safety, sanitation, and other concerns. The manager of production should conduct this meeting.

The daily production service meeting should be held in the main preparation area and include a tray setup depicting how the food should be placed on the plate and the appropriate garnish. A *taste test tray* should also be available. If a special menu or menu item has been prepared, it should be carefully evaluated for quality, time, skills of personnel, and acceptability.

After the meal has been served, a short meeting should be conducted to discuss any problems with the forecast, the quality of the prepared food, overdemands or underdemands for food and equipment used, and whether the production schedule was balanced among the employees. The disposition of leftovers should be decided because they should be used within 24 to 48 hours (Exhibit 20.1). It may be necessary to dispose of some leftovers immediately. Leftovers increase the food cost and the possibility of bacterial contamination if proper sanitation and safety principles are not followed. At this same meeting, the incorporation of the leftovers for the next meal or next day should be decided and any foreseeable problems with the next meal should be discussed. The objective of all the production forecasting and scheduling is to reduce the amount of overproduction or underproduction.

Production Monitoring

Production monitoring is a part of the manager's job. It involves monitoring during production and after it has occurred to determine whether the production plan was met for quality, over/underproduction, acceptance, skills of production, and equipment use. If the plan was not met, then the plan should be evaluated to determine if it was unreasonable and needs to be changed to a more reasonably achievable plan. Communication and input from the staff are needed to develop a new plan. When the staff is involved, a new plan will be more readily accepted. If the plan needs only small adjustments, these should be made immediately so that the production goals can be reasonably achieved.

Overproduction the results in *leftovers*. The disposition of these products must be carefully handled and methods established on how to use them. The following points are suggested:

- Discard food that that has been at room temperature for more than two hours.
- Quickly chill or separate food into smaller portions before refrigerating (check Food Code for various methods).

- If any potentially hazardous food (PHF) has been prepared and held below or at 41°F, *label* with the date when the food should be used or discarded. It is suggested that these prepared foods be used within seven days if stored at 41°F or less.
- When using leftovers in their original form, reheat to at least 165°F for at least 15 seconds.
- Do not heat leftovers more than once. Discard remaining leftovers after the first heating.
- When adding leftovers to a new food product, such as soup, do not add until the soup is almost ready—heat entire product to at least 165°F.
- If leftovers have been frozen, thaw using correct procedure.

EXHIBIT 20.1   Leftover Report

Menu Cycle:		Date:	Meal:	
Item	Amount	From Area	Disposition	Suggestions

Source: Developed by Ruby P. Puckett©.

PORTION CONTROL

Each foodservice department should determine the appropriate portion size its facilities can accommodate for each category of food served. In setting portion sizes, the type of customers and their nutritional needs, the type of menu served, and the food budget should be considered. In most situations, evaluations solicited from patients, residents, or nonpatient customers help in judging the acceptance of portion sizes and the overall quality of the food produced. *Portion control* is another procedure that is used as a production control.

Many measures can be taken to ensure that equal portions of food are served. For example, purchased supplies should meet well-defined specifications, recipes should be standardized, and the right utensils should be used for portioning and serving (Table 20.2). Slicing machines can ensure that equal portions of meat, cold cuts, and cheese are cut. Gram scales can also be used for the accurate portioning of meats and other entrée items. Dough cutters and pie or cake scorers can be used to portion breads, rolls, biscuits, and desserts. Portion control of other items is done by count, such as the number of slices of bread, packages of crackers or cookies, pats of margarine, and so forth. Ladles, scoops, and spoons are color coded to reflect the yield. Table 20.2 lists the approximate yield from scoops and ladles. The number of portions in canned foods also can be estimated from the size of the can. A daily production sheet (Exhibit 20.2) should also give portion sizes.

TABLE 20.2   Approximate Yield from Scoops and Ladles

Size	Use	Cup Equivalent
Scoops		
No. 6	Main dishes (casseroles and salads)	$2/3$
No. 8	Main dishes	$1/2$
No. 10	Cereals and meat patties	$3/8$
No. 12	Salads, vegetables	$1/3$
No. 16	Muffins, small desserts	$1/4$
No. 30	Drop cookies, large	$1/8$[a]
Ladles[b]		
1 ounce	Relishes, sauces	$1/8$[a]
2 ounces	Gravy	$1/4$
4 ounces	Vegetables	$1/2$
6 ounces	Chili, soups[c]	$3/4$
8 ounces	Stew, chili, soups[c]	1

[a]Equivalent to 3½ tablespoons.

[b]Ladles also come in 12-, 24-, and 32-ounce sizes.

[c]A cup of soup is usually 6 ounces, and a bowl of soup or chili may be 8 to 12 ounces. A bowl of chili, stew, or soup is usually a main entrée.

Note: For medical metric conversion tables go to www.simetric.co.uk/si_medical.htm.

STANDARDIZED RECIPES

Standardized recipes are followed in the ingredient control area (discussed later in the chapter) and in the production area to control the quality, quantity, and cost of the menu items prepared. A *standardized recipe* is one in which the amounts and proportions of ingredients, as well as the method of combining them, have been developed and tested for a particular foodservice operation. The ingredients needed and the preparation procedures to be followed must be stated accurately so that a high-quality product and an exact number of portions can be produced every time the recipe is used. Substitutions for specified ingredients and changes in procedures must be avoided.

When standardized recipes are used, changes in personnel should not affect food quality because each ingredient and prepara-

tion detail is precisely stated in the recipe. Purchasing is simplified because the exact quantities and forms of food needed for each food item were established when the recipe was tested. Job satisfaction is increased because employees know they will produce a successful product when they follow directions carefully. In addition, new employees can be trained much more rapidly when they have standardized recipes to follow.

The use of standardized recipes helps to control cost when the recipe is followed exactly as printed. This means that a cook may not add additional ingredients; it also means correct measuring of ingredients, and portioning the finished product into the correct number of portions. When these procedures are not followed, the cost of the finished product increases and the food budget will not be met.

EXHIBIT 20.2   Daily Production Sheet

Day _____   Meal _____

Meal Times: 7:30 A.M.—Breakfast

                   12:00 Noon—Lunch

                   6:00 P.M.—Dinner

Menu Item	Recipe Number	Amount Needed		Total	Name of Cook	Starting Time	Production Time	Equipment	Garnish	Serving Utensil	Portion Size
		Cafe.	Pts.								
Frozen seasoned green beans	V-10	50	75	125	Jones	11:15	20 min	Stack steamer	Almonds	Slotted spoon	4 oz

Although recipes are available from many sources, each food-service department should reevaluate and test all new recipes used to ensure that the quantities produced, the portion sizes stated, and the overall quality meet customer needs and are suited to the equipment available. When reviewing new recipes, the director should compare the stated portion size with the portion size established for the operation.

Recipe Files

A master and working file should be maintained of all recipes used in the foodservice operation. The master file may be stored on a computer disk in the director's office. Computerized copies with noted changes should be provided to the ingredient control staff, storeroom, and production personnel. Recipes can be filed by classification, code number, and alphabetically under the appropriate headings, such as bread, meat, salads, and so forth. Evaluation dates and changes to the recipe should be maintained, noted on the recipe card, and filed for future use.

Elements of Recipe Standardization

Before a recipe can be standardized, a number of factors should be analyzed, as discussed in the following sections.

Proportion of Ingredients

Each recipe should be read carefully, particularly if it has not yet been tried, because it may prove to be inappropriate or the number of ingredients used or the complexity of the procedures may make it impractical to use. The *proportions* of ingredients should be analyzed in relation to one another. For example, in a cake recipe, the sugar, flour, and shortening ratios should be appropriate for the

product. Finally, the new recipe should be compared with other tested recipes for similar products.

Quantity of Ingredients

The quantities of ingredients should be listed in the recipe in both weight and volume measures. Because weighing ingredients is more accurate than measuring them by volume, volume measurements should be converted to weights. However, small amounts of spices and seasonings can be measured by volume rather than weighed.

Form of Ingredients

The *form* of ingredients should be described in the recipe. Descriptive terms placed before the name of the ingredient designate the kind and form of food purchased or the cooking or heating required before the food is used, such as *canned* tomatoes, *fresh chopped* spinach, *cooked* chicken, and *hard-cooked* eggs. Descriptive terms are placed after the ingredient name to indicate the preparation necessary to make the form of the ingredient different from the form as purchased or cooked: for example, onions, *chopped*; canned carrots, *diced* and *drained*; and apples, *pared* and *sliced*. If waste is likely to occur in the initial preparation steps for some ingredients, the quantity should be listed as *edible portion* rather than as *amount purchased*. The purchase amount should be recorded in a separate section on the recipe card.

Order of Ingredients

Ingredients should be *listed in the order* in which they are combined. Ingredients requiring pretreatment before they are combined should be listed first or specially marked to indicate that advance preparation is needed.

Procedures

If possible, *preparation procedures* should be simplified or some steps eliminated to save time, equipment, and ware washing. For example, in a kitchen equipped with steam-jacketed kettles, the easiest way to prepare a cooked pudding is to place measured cold milk in the kettle, combine all dry ingredients, blend them into the milk with a wire whip, and then heat the entire mixture. The procedure for combining ingredients should be stated clearly. Specific terms—such as *blend*, *whip*, *cream*, and *fold*—tell the cook exactly what to do. Mixing speeds and times and the type of beater to be used should be stated in recipes to be prepared in the mixer. When batch size is increased or decreased, mixing times may need to be adjusted accordingly. If chilling is required before the entire recipe can be completed, the chill time should be stated.

Recipe Format

Standardized recipes may be written in a variety of ways. A standard format for all recipes should be developed for ease of use. (A sample format is shown in Figure 20.2.) Spaces for recording calculations of portion cost, for other batch sizes and as applicable nutritional analysis, also can be included. Recipes can be filed according to the types of items in a standard recipe box, a file drawer, a notebook, or on a computer system. Transparent plastic envelopes or laminated cards can be used to protect the recipes in the kitchen. Figure 20.2 provides details that can be used by any production personnel.

Batch Size Adjustment

The *batch sizes* for tested recipes often need to be altered to make handling easier or to suit the capacity of the facility's equipment. To adjust the total recipe yield, the number of servings needed is determined first. That number then is divided by the number of servings stated in the original recipe to arrive at a factor for adjusting the ingredient quantities. To increase batch size, the amount of each ingredient is multiplied by the factor and rounded off to the nearest convenient weight or measure. To decrease batch size, the amount of each ingredient in the original recipe is divided by the factor to arrive at the appropriate quantity for the reduced recipe. It is important that ingredient proportions never be changed when recipes are increased or decreased, although mixing and cooking times should be adjusted as necessary.

Adjusting Recipes for Portions

Recipes for portions often need to be changed because of many factors: holidays, the number of patients or residents, employees' days off, and so on. Because of these influences, it is important to

FIGURE 20.2   A Standardized Recipe Format

Recipe: Pizza Casserole (Casserole Recipe #25)		
Portions: 96 Pans: 3 Pan size: 12 × 20 × 2.5	**Cooking temperature: 350°F (177°C)** Cooking time: 20–25 minutes Portion size: 8 × 4 inches Portion utensil: Spatula	**Total recipe cost:** Cost per portion: Date calculated:

Ingredients	Amount	Procedure
Ground beef, 85/15 Pork sausage, bulk		1. Sauté beef and sausage until cooked. 2. Drain excess fat.
Spaghetti, thin Salt Cooking oil		3. Cook spaghetti in boiling salted water in steam-jacketed kettle. Add 2 tablespoons oil to water to prevent boiling over. 4. Drain. 5. Put in pans.
Canned tomato sauce		6. Pour equal amounts of sauce over spaghetti. 7. Sprinkle cooked meat over sauce.
Oregano, leaves Sweet basil, leaves Mozzarella cheese, grated Onions, chopped Green peppers, chopped Mushroom pieces, drained Ripe olives, sliced		8. Sprinkle oregano and basil over meat. 9. Sprinkle cheese over oregano and basil. 10. Top with chopped onions, green peppers, mushrooms, and ripe olives. 11. Bake.

This recipe in the HACCP format is Recipe Casserole 25 HACCP
Nutritional information:

know how to *adjust or scale* (the act of adjusting a recipe to meet the needs of the department; this may mean increasing or decreasing the number of portions) a recipe and still maintain food quality and appearance. There are four ways to adjust a recipe: adjusting the number of portions yielded, changing the size of the portions, yielding a specific number of portions of a specific size, or changing the amount of an ingredient.

Number of Portions   To yield a specific *number of portions*, divide the portions needed by the portions given in the recipe to obtain the ingredient ratio. Then multiply the specified quantity of each ingredient by the ingredient ratio to obtain the quantity needed. For example, 120 portions are needed, but the recipe yields only 25 portions. Divide the portions needed (120) by the portions given (25) to obtain the ingredient ratio of 4.8.

Next, multiply the specified quantity of each ingredient by the ingredient ratio to obtain the quantity of the ingredient needed. For example, the recipe calls for 3 pounds of ingredients to yield 25 portions:

$$3 \text{ pounds (specified quantity)} \times 4.8 \text{ (ingredient ratio)}$$
$$= 14.4 \text{ pounds, or 14 pounds 6 ounces (quantity needed)}$$

Size of Portions   To obtain a *portion size* other than the one specified in the recipe, divide the desired portion size by the specified portion to obtain the portion ratio. Then multiply the specified quantity of each ingredient by the portion ratio to determine the quantity needed.

For example, to *reduce size of each portion* from 7 ounces to 4.5 ounces, divide the desired portion size (4.5 ounces) by the recipe's specified portion size (7 ounces) to obtain the portion ratio of 0.64. Multiply the specified quantity of each ingredient by the portion ratio to determine the quantity needed:

$$3 \text{ pounds (specified quantity)} \times 0.64$$
$$= 1.92 \text{ pounds, or 1 pound 15 ounces (quantity needed)}$$

Specific Number of Portions of a Specific Size   To adjust a recipe to a specific number of portions of a *specific size*, multiply the portions needed by the portion ratio to obtain the conversion factor. Next, divide the conversion factor by the number of portions given to obtain the ingredient ratio. Then multiply the specified quantity of each ingredient by the ingredient ratio to obtain the quantity needed.

For example, the recipe will serve 80 portions, each portion consisting of 4 ounces. The forecast technique indicates that 120 portions of 5 ounces each are needed.

To obtain the *portion ratio*, divide 5 ounces (desired portion size) by 4 ounces (specified portion size) to obtain a portion ratio of 1.25. Multiply the portion ratio by the portions needed (120) to obtain the conversion factor of 150. Divide the conversion factor by the portions given (80) to obtain the ingredient ratio: 1.9. Multiply the specified quantity of each ingredient by the ingredient ratio to obtain the quantity needed:

$$20 \text{ pounds} \times 1.9 = 38 \text{ pounds (quantity needed to serve 120}$$
$$\text{portions of 5 ounces each}$$

An example of scaling is as follows: To increase the production from 6 portions to feed 200 people, divide the number of servings needed by the number of servings yield in each batch: $200 \div 6 = 35$.

All ingredients would need to be multiplied by 35, with the exception of condiments, sugar, and spices.

Amount of an Ingredient   To adjust a recipe to accommodate the *amount of an ingredient* in inventory, first obtain the ingredient ratio, and then multiply it by the specified quantity.

For example, the recipe calls for 10 pounds, but only 8 pounds are on hand.

To obtain the ingredient ratio, divide the amount specified (10 pounds) into the amount available (8 pounds), yielding an ingredient ratio of 0.80. Multiply the amount specified by the ingredient ratio of each ingredient to obtain the quantity needed:

$$10 \text{ pounds (amount specified)} \times 0.80 = 8 \text{ pounds (quantity needed)}$$

To *convert decimal fractions* to the next smallest weight unit, use the following as a guide.

- To obtain ounces from pounds, multiply by 16. Example: 6.7 pounds is calculated as follows: $0.7 \times 16 = 11$, or 6 pounds 11 ounces.
- To obtain *cups* from *quarts*, multiply by 4. Example: 3.29 quarts is equal to: $0.29 \times 4 = 1.16$, or 3 quarts 1.16 cups or about 3¼ quarts.
- To obtain *cups* from *gallons*, multiply by 16. Example: 2.85 gallons is equal to: $0.85 \times 16 = 13.6$ cups, or 2 gallons 13½ cups.
- To obtain *tablespoons* from *cups*, multiply by 16. Example: 2.6 cups is equal to: $0.6 \times 16 = 9.6$ tablespoons, or about 2 cups 9½ tablespoons.

Convert measurement ingredients from volume measurement to weight. Weight is usually quicker and also involves fewer calculations.

Many institutions use a computer to adjust recipes. Using computers for this function eliminates mathematical errors. Some food companies also have a ready supply of recipes that have been adjusted for various portion sizes. Computer-calculated nutrition also helps to eliminate errors.

When adjusting large-quantity portion-size recipes to smaller sizes and vice versa, it is extremely important to *test* the recipe before the final product is served to customers. Be extremely careful when decreasing or increasing condiments in a recipe—less is better than more. Taste test the product as each additional condiment is added; when satisfied the amount is satisfactory, note it on the recipe card. When decreasing the portion size of a recipe, add only half to three-fourths of the required amount of spices (especially sugar or

FIGURE 20.3 Product Evaluation Check Sheet (Another Example of Continuous Quality Improvement)

Name of panel member: _____ LPW _____   Date: _____ March 17, xxxx _____

Name of product: _____ Beef stew

Please rate, using 6 as best to 0 as unacceptable

	6	5	4	3	2	1	0
Aroma			X				
Color				X			
Texture				X			
Appearance					X		
Taste			X				
Salty				X			
Sweet				X			
Bitter					X		
Savor					X		
Portion size					X		
Garnish							X
Appropriate temperature			X				
	Excellent	Very Good	Good	Fair to Poor	Fair	Poor	Unacceptable

Comments:
Meat hard to chew, sauce tasted like it had sugar added, yet it had a metallic taste. Overall, I would rate between fair and poor.

Note: Using the Likert scale for this could provide percentages for each of the rating numbers.

---

salt). Then taste it (see "Two-Spoon Tasting Technique" later in this chapter); if more is needed, add a little more. Make corrections on the recipe card for the next use.

Other Details

The recipe should specify small equipment needed and cooking container (such as pan type, size, and method of pretreatment). To get an accurate yield of uniform portions, the weight or volume of the mixture to be placed in each pan must be stated in the recipe and followed. It is helpful to note the total weight or volume of the batch as well. Cooking times and temperatures should be double-checked because those in the original recipe may not be suitable for the type of equipment available. For example, baking temperatures and times for standard ovens may have to be reduced for convection ovens. Portioning instructions should be stated, as well as any instructions for cooling or holding before portioning. The portioning tools to be used may be stated in certain recipes. Suggested garnishes also may be listed.

New recipes should be prepared exactly as the procedure states. It often is tempting to begin modifying ingredients, quantities of ingredients, or preparation steps before discovering what kind of product would have been produced by the original recipe. Measurements should be checked for accuracy. If the original recipe does not list weight and volume measures, quantities should be weighed as the recipe is prepared and the actual yield carefully noted to determine whether it is the same as the stated yield. The finished product should be evaluated for eye appeal, quality, and acceptability. Exhibit 20.3 and Figure 20.3 are examples of recipe and product evaluation sheets. Because products fully acceptable to foodservice department personnel may be less appealing to customers, in most operations, seeking evaluations from customers is helpful in determining the level of acceptance.

If careful evaluation indicates that changes are needed in the recipe, they should be made and carefully noted on the recipe. It is important to have the cooks' cooperation because they may find it hard to resist asserting their individuality by changing the ingredients or procedures without authorization.

EXHIBIT 20.3   Recipe Evaluation Sheet (Another Example of Continuous Quality Improvement)

Product name: _____

Date of evaluation: _____   Recipe No.: _____

Style of preparation: _____   Quantity prepared: _____

Number of portions: _____   Size of portions: _____

Did the end product yield the number of servings as stated in recipe? <u>Y N</u> _____

If not, was it less? <u>Y N</u> How much? _____   More? <u>Y N</u> How much? _____

What quantity was obtained? _____   Are the portion sizes adequate? <u>Y N</u> _____

If not, what size do you suggest? _____   Did product look like photo? <u>Y N</u> _____

Was product accepted? <u>Y N</u> _____   Were the condiments too much or too little? _____

Comments of evaluation: _____

_____

_____

Comments of production staff: _____

_____

_____

Accept   Reject

Source: Developed by Ruby P. Puckett©, revised 2010.

INGREDIENT CONTROL

The preparation of high-quality food is the most important task of the foodservice department. *Ingredient control* is a vital component of the total system, as illustrated in Figure 20.4.

Traditionally, each person responsible for food preparation performed all the tasks, from collecting and weighing the ingredients to portioning the final product. Because of the need for greater control over quality and costs, some foodservice operations have centralized the preparation of recipe ingredients in *ingredient areas* or a *single ingredient room*. Centralized ingredient control frees skilled cooks from performing repetitive tasks that do not require their level of skill. Eliminating the possibility that production workers might alter the ingredients or batch size, ingredient control operations can control food quality and quantity. In some operations, only dry ingredients are weighed or measured. (Table 20.3 lists standard weights and measurements.) In others, all the steps necessary to weigh recipe ingredients accurately are performed in a central location. The latter system achieves the greatest degree of control but requires more labor and equipment.

In the ingredient area, the quantities of ingredients stated in the standardized recipe are weighed, measured, and collected for each menu item. The worker weighing the ingredient uses a production forecast that indicates the batch size needed for each recipe. Premeasured ingredients that bear labels listing the recipe name, ingredient name, and quantity are delivered to the cooks in the kitchen at the appropriate point in the production schedule.

The physical layout of the ingredient room can take many forms. When enough space is available, an area within the storeroom itself can be equipped to handle this function. Otherwise, a location close to the storeroom and refrigerators can be used. Regardless of the physical layout, the equipment needed includes large and small scales, measuring spoons, cups, a sink, large storage bins for large amounts of product such as 100 pounds of flour, medium and small containers for measured ingredients such as a pound of sugar, trays or baskets, carts, tables, knives, potato peelers, and vegetable choppers. In addition, there should be a hand-washing sink, clean dishes, computer recipe files, menus, and storage for spices. Even without a separate ingredient area, some of the advantages of this system can still be realized. During slow periods in the workday, employees can be assigned to weigh ingredients for the next day's production.

Accurate measurement is important for consistent results with standardized recipes. Measuring tools and scales must be easily accessible in all work areas when centralized ingredient control is not used. It is quicker and more accurate to weigh ingredients when the right kinds of scales are provided. Standard measuring spoons and measuring cups for both dry and liquid ingredients are needed. In each work center, measuring equipment should be stored in an easily accessible place.

Standardizing a recipe is of little value if the item has not been carefully portioned before serving. All items served should have a standard portion. All employees should know the number of portions to be expected from each item as well. It is a good idea to post this information in each work area.

The use of scoops and ladles standardizes the measurement of many items. Individual molds standardize portions of gelatin. Some cuts of meat are purchased in standard portion-size cuts, and others (such as meatballs) can be measured to standard size during preparation (Table 20.4). Slicing on a meat machine is another method of portion control. Foodservice staff may be able to think of other methods to help serve equal portions to their patrons.

It may become necessary to substitute one ingredient for another. This may happen due to late arrival of the needed item, needed item spoiled or contaminated, or a new item not yet ordered.

FIGURE 20.4   Production System Based on Ingredient Control

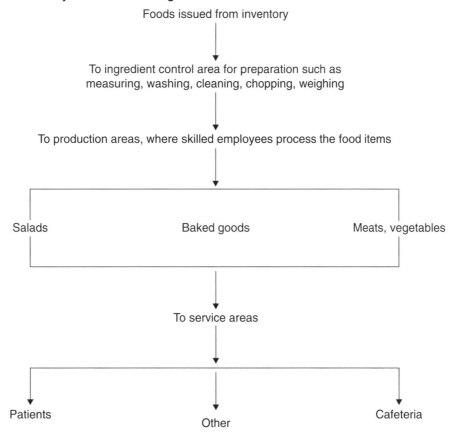

Foods issued from inventory

To ingredient control area for preparation such as measuring, washing, cleaning, chopping, weighing

To production areas, where skilled employees process the food items

| Salads | Baked goods | Meats, vegetables |

To service areas

Patients   Other   Cafeteria

Source: Adapted from R. P. Puckett, 2009. Used by permission.

When substitutions are necessary, choose an ingredient as close to the original item as possible. Post a list of approved substitutions in the production area. Some substitutions are simple: butter or margarine, bread crumbs or cracker crumbs, and so forth.

FOOD PRODUCTION SYSTEM

The objectives of food production are to destroy harmful bacteria (food safety); increase digestibility; change and enhance flavor, form, texture, aroma, and color; and protect the nutritive value of the food, following all policies and procedures to maintain quality.

The preparation of food in a foodservice department is referred to as the *production system*. This means that there are menus, recipes, purchasing, and inventory of a tangible product: food. This food would remain forever—or until ruined—in storage if some action were not taken to change it into another, perhaps more usable, product.

The production system must include safe handling of food products. The USDA Food Safety and Inspection Service (FSIS) provides safe food handling tips. The program titled Fight BAC™ provides four guidelines to keep food safe:

1. Clean—Wash hands and work surfaces often.
2. Separate—Don't cross contaminate.

3. Cook—Cook to proper temperature.
4. Chill—Refrigerate promptly.

FSIS also suggests that:

- Purchasing procedures are developed (see Chapter 18).
- All foods are properly received and stored (See Chapter 19).
- Proper preparation methods are used to cook specific food items (Chapter 20).
- Proper techniques are used: thawing (refrigerator, cold water, or microwave); cooking (to correct internal temperature) (Chapters 13 and 14).
- Serving—patients and nonpatients (Chapter 21).
- Sanitation (Chapters 13, 14, and 15).

To produce cooked food for service, skilled employees use equipment and techniques to make the transformation (to produce). There are a number of transformation systems—meat preparation, salad preparation, vegetable cooking, and baking. Many foods have to be preprepared before production takes place. Prepreparation includes washing, cleaning, peeling, chopping, slicing, grinding, measuring, weighing, greasing pans, mixing, beating, and heating. The last step in preparation is combining the foods to make a final product. In graphic form, this system is depicted in Figure 20.5. In

TABLE 20.3 Weights and Measurements and Conversion Chart*

Weights and Measures				
16 drams	dr	=	1 ounce	oz
16 oz		=	1 pound	lb
100 lb		=	1 hundredweight	cwt
2,000 lb		=	1 ton	

Principal Liquid Weights				
3 teaspoons	tsp	=	1 tablespoon	T
4 T		=	1/4 cup	
8 T		=	1/2 cup	
16 T		=	1 cup	
2 cups		=	1 pint	pt
2 pt		=	1 quart	qt
4 qt		=	1 gallon	gal

Principal Dry Measures				
2 pt		=	1 qt	
8 qt		=	1 peck	pk
2 pk		=	1 bushel	bu

Conversion of Weights and Quantities				
Granulated sugar	2¼ cup	=	1 lb	
Bread flour	4 cup	=	1 lb	
Pastry flour	4½ cup	=	1 lb	
Grated cheese	4 cup	=	1 lb	
Butter, fats	2 cup	=	1 lb	
Average large eggs, shelled	10 eggs	=	1 lb	

Metric Conversion

1 tsp = 5 grams (g) or 5 milliliters (mL)

2 tsp = 10 grams or 10 mL

1 T = 15 grams or 15 mL

2 T = 30 grams or 30 mL

1 oz (2 T) = 28.35 grams

1 lb = 454 grams or 0.45 kilogram (kg)

2 lb 2 oz = 34 oz = 1 kilogram

1 cup = 230 mL or 0.24 liter (liquid)

1 qt = 0.94635 mL or almost 1 liter

*Container size and yields can be found in Chapter 17 under Consideration in Buying Fruits and Vegetables—Container Size

TABLE 20.4 Pan Size Yield

Pan Size, Inches	Depth, Inches	Portions
12 × 20	2.54	7
	6	13
	8	18.5
		27
12 × 10 (½ size)	2.5	3.5
	4	6.5
	6	9
	8	12
6 × 12	2.5	2.5
	4	4
	6	6
Roasting pans		
18 × 24	4.5	24
16 × 16	4	8

a production system, there must always be input (raw materials, resources); transforming (action); and output (results, finished product). Food production closely resembles any other manufacturing system, such as an automotive plant (Input → Transformation → Output with controls, feedback, policies and procedures, and following applicable laws, regulations and rules, and records). (See Chapter 6.)

For this system to function properly, there must be an organization, policies, procedures, direction, controls, and coordination. There must also be a means of evaluation and feedback to determine if the system is achieving its goal, which is to deliver quality food and service to clients within budget limitations. Feedback can be by word of mouth, plate-waste study, formal questionnaires, and so forth.

Some foods are Potentially Hazardous Foods (PHF) and others are Time Temperature Control for Safety (TCS). These types of foods require control of time and temperature. The temperature should be measured as the "endpoint temperature," the temperature reached at the end of cooking.

Four basic methods of production use a form of heat. They are conduction, convection, radiation, and induction. *Conduction* is the transfer of heat through direct contact from one item or substance to another. Conduction is used in grilling, frying, boiling, and to some extent in roasting and baking.

Convection is the distribution of heat by the movement of liquid air or steam. In convection ovens and steamers, a fan circulates heat, which is transferred more quickly, causing faster cooking.

Radiation is where energy is transferred by waves from the source to the food. The waves do not pass energy but induce heat by molecular action entering the food; microwave is a type of radiation.

Induction is the use of electromagnetic fields to cause the molecules of metal cooking surfaces to produce heat.

FIGURE 20.5   Food Production Process

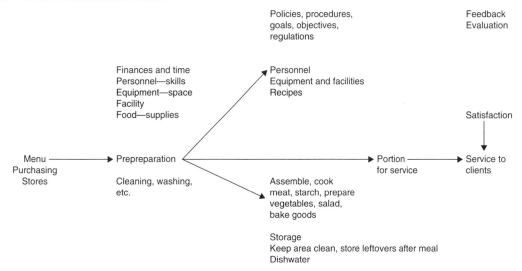

Source: Developed by Ruby P. Puckett©.

TABLE 20.5   Cooking Terms

Term	Heat Source	Equipment	Food Item
Baking	Dry heat	Variety of ovens	All food items
Barbecuing	Dry heat	Grills, ovens	Meat, poultry
Blanching	Moist heat	Steam kettles	Vegetables, fruit
Boiling	Moist heat	Steam kettles, stockpot	Pasta
Braising	Dry or moist	Fryer, steam-jacket kettle	Cereal, rice
Broiling	Radiant heat	Specially designed equipment	Meat, poultry, tender cuts of meat
Deep-fat frying	Dry heat	Deep-fat fryer	Fish and poultry
		Pressure fryer	Fish, shellfish, chicken,
		Convection oven	vegetables
Griddling	Dry heat	Griddle	Meat, eggs, pancakes, sandwiches
Grilling	Dry heat	Grill, gas, electric, charcoal	Meat, fish, vegetables
Oven frying	Dry heat	Oven	Chicken, fish, meat
Panfrying	Dry heat	Skillet, fryer, steamer, oven	Chicken, eggs, onions
Poaching	Moist heat	Shallow pan on top of range	Fish, eggs, fruit
Roasting	Dry heat	Variety of ovens	Poultry, tender cut of meats, vegetables
Searing	Dry heat	Skillet, fryer	Meat
Sautéing	Dry heat	Skillet, fryer	Poultry, fish, tender cuts of meat, vegetables
Simmering	Moist heat	Steamer, stockpot	Soup, sauce, meat, poultry
Stewing	Moist heat	Steamer, fryer, pot on top of stove	Vegetables, fruits, poultry, dumplings, pasta, rice, cereal
Stir-frying	Dry heat	Fryer, skillet, wok	Vegetables, chicken, pork, shrimp, tender beef

Basic cooking methods apply to all food products. These methods use either *dry* or *moist heat*. Table 20.5 lists the terms used in food preparation.

Meat

The flavor, tenderness, juiciness, and color of cooked meat are the primary measures of quality in meat products. In addition to maintaining these sensory qualities of meat, the food production director must know the total quantity and number of servings obtainable after the meat has been cooked. Cooking methods that produce the highest yield of palatable, edible meat must be selected to control the cost of each serving. Cooked yields are reduced by shrinkage caused by excessive evaporation of water from the surface of meat and through drip loss of fat, water, and natural flavoring substances from the tissue.

The control of cooking temperatures and times is critical in minimizing *shrinkage* (loss of weight) of meat during preparation. Research has shown that low temperatures consistently produce higher meat yields that are more evenly cooked. The other basic factor that affects shrinkage is length of cooking time. As cooking time increases, losses from evaporation increase, with undesirable changes in meat texture, flavor, and carvability.

Several factors affect cooking time. Among these are the size of the cut and uniformity of its shape. Usually, the larger the roast, the longer the cooking time required. If the cut is not uniform in shape, one end of the cut can become overcooked before the rest is done. A large flat roast cooks faster than one of similar weight that has been rolled and tied.

Cooking time also is affected by the composition of the meat itself. The more plentiful the fat covering and marbling, the less cooking time is required because fat is a better heat conductor than muscle. For roast meats, cooking times are also increased by multiple oven loads and by the degree of doneness desired. Overcooking is a particularly wasteful practice because not only does it cause higher losses in yield, but it also diminishes tenderness and palatability.

Cooking methods for meat usually are designated as dry-heat or moist-heat methods, depending on the atmosphere surrounding the meat. The differences are in the rate of heat transfer to the meat and in the temperatures to which the meat surface is exposed. Water vapor, used in moist-heat cooking, is a more efficient heat conductor than air, so it helps supply heat energy more rapidly to the meat. The temperature to which meat is subjected in moist-heat cooking should be no higher than the boiling point of water. In dry-heat cooking, the heat transfer is slower, but the meat surfaces are subjected to much higher temperatures.

Dry-Heat Methods

Dry-heat methods cause the *caramelization*, or *browning*, of meat surfaces, which makes meat more palatable but does not provide additional moisture to soften the collagen in the meat. Naturally tender meats need to be prepared by the dry-heat methods of roasting, panfrying, grilling, and deep-fat frying. Muscles that received relatively little exercise during the meat animal's life, such as rib and loin cuts of beef and pork and cuts that come from higher-grade animals, usually are suitable for dry-heat cooking. Meat from young animals, such as veal and lamb, also is tender but often is cooked by moist-heat methods to develop its flavor.

Because of changes in methods of beef production as well as in consumer preferences over the past decade, other exceptions apply to these general recommendations. Less-tender chuck and round roasts may be cooked by dry heat to the rare (not recommended) and medium-rare states and then thinly sliced to yield a flavorful, tender, finished product. Other methods are used by foodservice operations to tenderize less-tender cuts enough to allow dry-heat cooking. Meat processors also use some of these treatments. To physically break down muscle fibers and connective tissue, mechanical means—such as cubing, dicing, grinding, and chopping—often are used. Marinating less-tender cuts in oil and acid mixtures can break down muscle fibers as well. Tomato juice, vinegar, lemon

juice, wine, and sour cream commonly are used in marinades. Enzymatic tenderizers, which often contain papain (a protein from papaya), can be applied to meat surfaces, used as a marinade, or injected into the muscle. Surface applications of such tenderizers are most effective on thinner cuts of meat.

Roasting Meats can be *roasted* in several different types of ovens (conventional, convection, deck, range, conveyor, microwave, smoker, low-temperature holding oven, and combination oven), but the cooking procedure is similar in each. The meat is placed on a rack in an open pan with no moisture added. The heat in a regular oven or the heated moving air in a convection oven helps produce surface browning. It was once common to sear roasts in a hot oven for 20 to 30 minutes and then reduce the temperature to about 300°F (149°C) for the remainder of the cooking time. Searing, or coagulating the surface proteins, was supposed to prevent loss of juices and nutrients. However, studies have shown not only that this is not the case but that searing can increase total cooking losses from the surface. Without searing, there is no hard outer crust, and slicing is easier. Repeated studies have shown that roasting at low, constant temperatures ranging from 225°F to 250°F (107°C to 121°C) decreases the amount of shrinkage and produces meat that is juicier, more uniformly cooked, and more tender. The lower temperature is recommended for convection ovens.

A *meat thermometer* should be used to determine the interior temperature and doneness of meat. The thermometer should be inserted so that the tip is in the center of the largest muscle and is not touching bone or embedded in fat. Because the internal temperature of meat continues to rise after it has been removed from the oven, the meat should be taken out of the oven slightly before the desired temperature has been reached. If a roast is allowed to stand in a warm place for 10 to 15 minutes, its texture will become firmer, and it will slice more easily.

Tables that list roasting times in minutes per pound at best provide only a guide to help estimate total cooking time. It is essential to use meat thermometers to determine doneness and to keep careful records of the actual cooking times needed to reach that state of doneness for each quality, style, and size of roast prepared.

Minimum temperature and time for meat production are detailed in the *Food Code*; oven temperatures by oven types are also found in the *Food Code* (discussed in various chapters; see Index).

Broiling and Grilling *Broiling* and *grilling* are dry-heat cooking methods in which direct or radiant heat from gas flames, electric coils, or charcoal briquettes provides the heat source. This method is most successful for relatively tender cuts between 1 and 2 inches thick. Thinner cuts tend to dry out, and thicker cuts are difficult to broil to the more well-done stages. Cuts should be turned only once during broiling and should not be seasoned until cooking is complete. Adding salt tends to draw moisture from the meat surfaces and delays browning.

Many kinds of equipment can be used for broiling and grilling, such as char broilers, rotisseries, and smokers, so cooking times vary from one unit to another. Timetables for broiling and grilling are not particularly useful because the thickness of the cut, distance of the meat from the heat source, and degree of doneness affect total cooking time. Frozen cuts can be broiled with consistent results, but they should be placed farther from the heat or cooked at a lower temperature to reach uniform doneness. Broiling time is almost doubled for most frozen steaks. Cuts more than 1½ inches thick should be thawed before broiling.

Panfrying   In *panfrying*, heat is conducted from the surface of a grill, braising pan, or skillet to the meat surface. The metal surface should be oiled before very lean cuts are placed on it, but most meats generate enough melted fat to prevent sticking. Moderate temperatures should be used to avoid overbrowning and crusting the meat surfaces. Excess fat can be removed as it accumulates, and care should be taken to avoid temperatures high enough to cause smoking, which make the meat taste off flavor. Many meat cuts (such as hamburger, steak, liver, cube steak, ground lamb, lamb chop, ham steak, Canadian bacon, and other similar thinner cuts) can be completely cooked by this method. Many recipes combine an initial sautéing or grilling with moist-heat finishing.

Panfrying large quantities of the cuts mentioned is often too time-consuming to be practical. For this reason, oven frying is substituted. With this method, meat is placed in well-greased, shallow pans with or without additional fat dribbled over it. Meats may be dredged in seasoned flour or crumbs and cooked at temperatures ranging from 375°F to 400°F (190°C to 204°C). The pan is left uncovered, and no liquid is added.

Deep-Fat Frying   *Deep-fat frying* is not a primary method of cooking meats but rather is usually the initial step for browning meats that will be finished by another method. For example, round steaks or pork chops may be browned in deep fat and then finished in the oven. Meats should be coated or breaded before deep-fat frying; the fat temperature should be kept at 350°F (177°C), high enough to avoid overabsorption of fat and yet low enough to produce a tender product and avoid breakdown of the fat. Meat that is to be deep-fat fried should be free of excessive moisture and loose particles of breading. Moisture will cause the fat to spatter or bubble and will speed fat breakdown.

When meat is deep-fat fried, uniformly sized pieces should be loaded into the fryer basket and lowered slowly into the hot fat. The fryer should not be overloaded, because this will reduce the fat temperature and increase the amount of fat absorbed into the meat (particularly important when frying frozen meat). The meat should be cooked until the outside is properly browned or until the cut is completely done. Cutting into a sample piece from the batch should check the degree of doneness. When the meat is removed from the fat, the fryer basket should be lifted and allowed to drain over the dryer kettle, and care should be taken to avoid shaking excess crumbs from the coating into the fat. Because salt hastens the deterioration of fat, the meat should be salted *after* its removal from the fryer basket. Additional fat should be added during the cooking process to maintain the correct frying level and extend the life of the fat. The fat should be brought up to proper cooking temperature before more meat is fried. Frying fat should be filtered at least once daily—more often if the fryer is used extensively or if breaded foods are cooked in it.

Frying   Fats used for *frying* (deep-fat or pan) should have a high *smoke point* (the temperature at which fat begins to break down, indicated by smoking). Fat is used in panfrying to keep the particles of food from sticking to the pan. In deep-fat frying, foods are submerged in a vat of fat and are totally surrounded by the cooking medium. Fat used for deep frying should be kept clean and handled carefully. It should be filtered after each use and kept covered in a cool place. Fresh fat may be added periodically. Kettles should be washed and dried. Fat that bubbles excessively before food is added or that produces a gummy substance that collects on the frying basket and heating elements should be discarded.

Use and Smoke Point of Fats   The quality of fat used for cooking influences the results of the cooked product. The fat chosen should have a *high smoke point* and little or no flavor. Each time the fat is heated, the smoke point is lowered. The use of high temperatures, especially holding fats at high temperatures, reduces the life of the fat. Shortenings and vegetable oils that do not contain an emulsifier have the highest smoke points. The best temperature for deep-fat frying is 350°F to 375°F (177°C to 190°C). The highest temperature that should be used is 390°F (199°C). Olive oil, butter, and margarine are not suitable for frying because of their low smoke points. Table 20.6 shows the smoke points of various fats.

Fats used in preparing baked items should be free of strong flavors or odors and should combine readily with ingredients in the flour mixture. These fats include:

- Lard is used for making pastries and some Southern-style biscuits.
- Vegetable shortening is used for cakes.
- Other shortenings may be used for baking and panfrying.

Emulsions   An *emulsion* is a dispersion of one liquid in a second liquid in which it is not soluble. One such solution is oil and vinegar. The oil may be dispersed in the vinegar by shaking, but it takes only a minute or two for the separation to reappear. This type of emulsion is called a temporary emulsion. In contrast, mayonnaise is a permanent emulsion.

TABLE 20.6   Smoke Points of Various Fats

Fat	Smoke Point
Bacon fat	290°F–300°F (143°C–149°C)
Olive oil	300°F–315°F (149°C–157°C)
Shortening with emulsifiers	300°F–350°F (149°C–177°C)
Lard	340°F–350°F (171°C–177°C)
Vegetable oil	410°F–430°F (210°C–221°C)
Shortening with no emulsifiers	420°F–440°F (216°C–227°C)
Hydrogenated vegetable compound	440°F–460°F (227°C–238°C)

Note. Several factors affect the smoke point: the presence of food particles and sediment, salt in food, repeated use of the fat, too high a temperature, the presence of emulsifiers, and surface of the fat exposed to heat.

Vegetable, seed, and nut oils are generally used in salad dressings. The oil should be bland in flavor and be able to withstand cold temperatures.

Moist-Heat Methods

Steam or *hot liquid* surrounds meats cooked by moist heat. The external surface of the meat is exposed to temperatures no higher than that of boiling water, except when the meat is cooked under pressure. Moist-heat methods are used to tenderize tougher muscles and cuts that contain larger amounts of collagen. In general, the cooking times for moist-heat methods are considerably longer because the temperatures are lower than in dry-heat cooking. Many cuts that could be cooked by dry heat are cooked in moist heat to add greater variety and appeal to entrée selections. For example, certain tender cuts such as pork or veal steaks, chops, and cutlets, and beef and pork liver are cooked this way. Slow cooking develops flavor, tenderizes meat, and reduces handling time.

Braising   Braising (also called *pot roasting*, *Swissing*, and *fricasseeing*) is one of the most frequently used moist-heat cooking methods. Meat cuts are cooked slowly in a covered utensil in a small amount of liquid. The meat may be browned first in a small amount of fat, in which case the cut can be dredged first in seasoned flour to enhance browning. After the browning, the meat or vegetables are cooked in bouillon or wine until gravy is formed.

In foodservice facilities, several different pieces of equipment can be used to braise meat. Steam-jacketed kettles or tilting braising pans are ideal because they speed the cooking process, create uniform cooking temperatures, and make handling the cooked meat easier. Covered shallow heavy-duty pans also can be used for braising on the range top or in an oven at 300°F to 325°F (149°C to 163°C).

Stewing   Stewing meat involves cooking in a *large amount of liquid* at temperatures just below the boiling point. Although the method is sometimes described as boiling, temperatures between 185°F and 200°F (85°C and 93°C) are better than boiling temperatures (212°F [100°C]) because they produce a more flavorful and tender product. Boiling makes meat stringy and difficult to slice, and it causes more shrinkage.

Stewing is suitable for less-tender cuts of meat, such as fresh or corned beef brisket; beef, lamb, or veal cubes for stews or casseroles; and any meats, such as shank and neck, being used to make soup stock. For additional flavor and color, some meat may be dredged in seasoned flour and browned before stewing. Although stewing can be done in many different types of equipment, it is important to select pots, kettles, and pans that are large enough to accommodate efficient handling of batches.

Steaming   Meat can be steamed by using pressure steamers or by wrapping it in heavy foil. This moist-heat method tenderizes less-tender cuts, but shrinkage and drip loss may be greater than with other cooking methods. Many foodservice operations use compartment steamers to reduce the cooking time required for meat that will be used in salads, creamed dishes, and sandwiches. However, the flavor and color of steamed meats usually are less attractive than the flavor and color of meats cooked by other methods. Experiments with the heavy foil wrapping of beef roasts have shown that cooking time is increased, cooking losses are higher, and the meat is less tender.

Preparing Frozen Meat

More and more foodservice operations are moving toward purchasing more types of frozen meat items. Most frozen meats can be cooked with essentially the same yield and quality as fully or partially thawed meats. The same cooking procedures and temperatures apply, but additional cooking time and energy are needed to reach the desired degree of doneness. In roasting meat from the frozen state, the cooking time should be increased about one and a half times. This additional time and the cost of fuel for the extra roasting must be considered in production scheduling. A meat thermometer should be inserted midway in the cooking process so that accurate end-point temperatures can be determined.

Some cuts of meat, such as fabricated veal and pork cutlets, should not be thawed before cooking. Thawed cuts of these kinds are difficult to handle, and when they are breaded, there is a tendency for the breading to fall off when the cuts are thawed before cooking. Also, browning may be uneven when these cuts are thawed before cooking.

According to the *Food Code*, food should be thawed under refrigeration that maintains the food temperatures at 41°F (5°C) or lower. Other methods include (1) completely submerging under potable running water at a temperature of 70°F (21°C) for a period of time that does not allow the thawed portion of ready-to-eat foods to rise above 41°F (5°C); (2) as part of the cooking process; and (3) in a microwave oven, immediately transferring to conventional cooking equipment with no interruption in the process.

Slacking is the process of moderating the temperature of frozen foods before preparation such as deep fat frying. For example, if you are deep fat frying an item that is frozen you should bring the item up from 0°F to approximately 32°F. (Check your location for rules.) The *Food Code* states, "If you practice slacking you should maintain the temperature of food you are slacking at or below 41°F, under refrigeration or maintain the product at any temperature as long as the product remains frozen."

In a cook-and-chill production system, a specially designed quick-chilling refrigerator should be used to bring hot foods containing meat down to 41°F within four hours. After chilling, the foods should be stored at 32°F to 38°F (0°C to 3°C) and used within 48 hours to avoid safety risks and loss of palatability.

Portioning Meat

Standard portion sizes for each type of meat served must be determined to ensure adequate cost control and consumer satisfaction. A chart giving individual portion sizes can be developed in the department and made available to the workers responsible for portioning. For roasts and other large cuts, electric slicing is the most efficient way to produce uniform portions. The sliced meat should be weighed for the desired individual portion size, and an equal number of portions should be placed in each pan (covered to prevent moisture loss). For fully cooked meats, such as hams, rolled meats, and beef roasts, the meat should be sliced and put in a pan before heating. The manufacturer's instructions for handling should be followed.

Electric slicers must be carefully cleaned immediately after each use and maintained in a sanitary condition. In operations that do not have electric slicers, sharp knives and properly sanitized cutting boards are needed. The work area used for portioning cooked meats also should be kept in a sanitary condition. Knives and boards used in preparing raw meat or poultry products must always be sanitized before they are used with cooked products.

Holding Cooked Meat

Cooked meats must be held at temperatures of 140°F (60°C) or higher. Before holding, bring the meat to a safe temperature of at least 140°F or higher as needed for palatability and safety. Most holding equipment is designed to maintain these temperatures and not to reheat cold foods. Ideally, meat and menu items containing meat should be held for as short a time as possible and never for more than two hours. In many situations, however, holding for transport or an extended service period is necessary. Meats cooked by moist heat are more suitable for extended holding, but medium-rare beef roast can be held for a short time without becoming over-done. Pork should be brought to a temperature of 170°F (77°C) before holding.

In many foodservice operations, staggered production schedules reduce the necessity for extended holding and decrease the probability of quality loss, shrinkage, and lower acceptability. Batch production is almost always necessary for fried and breaded items because they do not hold well on a steam table.

Storing Cooked Meat

Regardless of how accurately a department forecasts production, unused cooked meat items occasionally may remain at the end of the service period, as well as meat items that were cooked in advance of the service time. Despite care in preparation and holding, the risk that these foods have been exposed to microbiological contamination is always present. For that reason, cooked meats must be stored carefully to prevent the possibility of causing food-borne illness in consumers.

Cooked meat and foods containing meat must be quickly chilled to temperatures below 40°F (5°C) within two hours. For some items, cooling will be more rapid if the hot food is placed in shallow pans about 2 inches deep and refrigerated immediately. The food should be covered after it has cooled. For dense foods, such as lasagna, quick cooling can be accomplished by placing the pan of food on ice or in a sink containing ice and water. Stews, soups, and other semiliquid foods should be treated similarly and be stirred frequently during the initial cooling period. Hot foods should not be placed in deep pots, jars, or pans because doing so slows the cooling rate. Store in a container that facilitates heat transfer. Hot stock, gravy, and other liquid products should not be added to a pan that contains leftovers. The risks in doing so are twofold: the entire batch may be warmed to temperatures that can support bacterial growth, and the safe storage life of the newly cooked food will be shortened. Large roasts of meat and poultry should be separated into smaller or thinner portions. Cooked potentially hazardous foods must be cooled within two hours from 135°F (60°C) to 70°F (21°C) and then within an additional four hours from 70°F to 41°F (21°C to 5°C) or lower.

In a cook-and-chill production system, a specially designed quick-chilling refrigerator should be used to bring hot foods containing meat down to 41°F within four hours. After chilling, the foods should be stored at 32°F to 38°F (0°C to 3°C) and used within 48 hours to avoid safety risks and loss of palatability.

Using Leftover Meat

Leftovers should always be stored separately, dated, and kept for no longer than 48 hours. If it is known that the products will not be used within that period, they should be frozen immediately after service in a freezer that has adequate air circulation. Pans of food should not be stacked, and refrigerator shelves should not be covered with foil or trays because this can block the flow of cold air around the foods.

Leftovers should not be combined with fresh products; for example, leftover beef stew should not be added to a fresh batch of beef stew. However, many kinds of leftover meat can be used in casseroles, salads, sandwich fillings, and soups. When devising ways to use leftovers, department managers must consider the cost of additional labor needed to make the items usable. If considerable labor will be expended in reworking the item, it may be more economical to serve it with fewer changes or to freeze it until it appears again in the menu cycle.

Leftover meats to be frozen should be packaged in moisture-proof and vapor-proof materials such as freezer wrap, freezer bags, and heavy-duty foil. Plastic or foil containers are suitable for casseroles, stews, and other semiliquid products that can be thawed in the refrigerator before reheating. These products should be reheated to at least 165°F to 170°F (74°C to 77°C) so that all parts of the food reach an internal temperature of 165°F for 15 seconds. Reheating for hot holding should be done quickly, and the time the food goes from 41°F (5°C) to between 140°F (60°C) and 165°F (74°C) may not exceed two hours. After one reheating, leftovers should be discarded.

Poultry

Most poultry purchased today is ready to cook either fresh chilled or frozen. Many forms of cooked poultry are also available to food-service facilities. The most widely marketed poultry—broiler-fryer chickens, turkeys, Cornish game hens, ducks, and geese—are all young, tender birds. For that reason, broiling, frying, and roasting are the preferred preparation methods. Moist-heat cooking methods offer wide menu variety and appeal, and today's poultry does not need long cooking in moisture to yield a tender product.

Poultry must be properly handled during preparation, cooking, holding, and cooling to prevent contamination that might cause food poisoning. Chilled fresh poultry should be stored at 28°F to 32°F (−2°C to 0°C) for not more than two or three days. If poultry must be purchased more than two or three days before service, it should be purchased frozen.

Poultry should always be thawed in the refrigerator. For large birds, this can mean up to four days. Frozen whole turkeys, ducks, and geese can be thawed more rapidly by placing them, in their original wrappers, fully submerged under cold running water. Defrosting at kitchen temperature or in warm water is hazardous because this can promote growth of bacteria on the surface of the poultry. The body cavity is especially rich in Salmonella bacteria, which are capable of causing food poisoning. Thawed poultry should be washed inside and out in cold water, drained, refrigerated, and cooked within 24 hours. Breaded or battered chicken pieces, either cooked or uncooked, should not be thawed before cooking or reheating. Fully cooked frozen turkey rolls, frozen diced turkey and chicken, and other similar forms may be thawed in the refrigerator before use. Knives and cutting boards used to prepare uncooked poultry should be sanitized before they are used to prepare other food products.

Dry-Heat Methods for Cooking Poultry

There are also dry-heat methods for cooking poultry. These are discussed in the following subsections.

Roasting   One of the most common methods of preparing poultry uses the dry-heat method of oven roasting. Turkey can be roasted whole or cut in half or in pieces. The results are similar in all cases, but the decreased oven space and roasting time required may make the cut forms more efficient to use. Overcooking white meat can be avoided by roasting the white pieces in a separate pan and allowing a shorter cooking time. A turkey to be roasted whole should not be stuffed, and roasting should be done in one continuous period. Raw turkeys can be cooked from the frozen state or partially thawed and then cooked.

Whole turkeys and chickens should be placed on a rack in a shallow pan and roasted at 325°F (163°C). Low oven temperatures ensure higher yields of edible meat, with better flavor and succulence. The skin can be brushed with margarine, oil, or shortening. If desired, the body cavity of whole birds may be seasoned with salt, pepper, and herbs. A meat thermometer can be used to determine the degree of doneness. For turkeys, the thermometer should be inserted in the thigh muscle adjoining the body cavity or in the thickest portion of the breast. The minimum internal cooking temperature needs to be 165° (74°) for 15 seconds for all parts of the cooked poultry. Doneness also is indicated when the thigh or breast meat feels soft or when the leg moves readily at the thigh joint and the juice is clear with no pink color.

A tent of aluminum foil placed loosely over the breast of a whole turkey will delay browning and excessive drying of the breast meat, but it should be removed for the last 30 minutes of roasting. (Wrapping the whole bird in foil or cooking it in a covered pan results in steam cooking, and the rich browning and true flavor of roasted poultry does not develop.) Basting should be done as needed during cooking. All poultry products should be cooked until well done.

In roasting ducks or geese, no basting is needed. Fat should be poured off as it accumulates in the roasting pan. A small amount of water may be added to each pan to reduce spattering, but the birds should be roasted uncovered, following the same procedures as described for turkey and chicken.

For easier slicing, roasted poultry should be allowed to stand for 15 to 20 minutes after removal from the oven. This permits the hot juices to be absorbed into the meat so that they flow less freely during slicing. Also, the flesh will be firm and will slice with less tearing and crumbling.

Darkening of bones and meat around the bones occurs primarily in young broiler-fryer chickens (6 to 8 weeks old). The bones have not calcified or hardened completely, so pigment from the bone marrow seeps through the bones and into the surrounding area. Freezing also contributes to this darkening. This is an aesthetic issue, not a safety one.

Oven Frying   Fried chicken has long been a favorite entrée, and an easy way to prepare it in quantity is to oven-fry it. Chicken pieces are washed and dried, dredged in seasoned flour, and placed in a single layer on a well-greased sheet pan or in a 12-by-20-inch pan. The chicken is then cooked in a 400°F (204°C) oven for 45 to 50 minutes. Variations on the basic oven-fried chicken recipe are almost unlimited. The chicken may be dipped in milk, buttermilk, undiluted cream soup, or margarine before coating. Coatings include bread crumbs, cornflake crumbs, and cracker crumbs seasoned with herbs, paprika, and Parmesan cheese. Instant potato flakes make a crunchy coating, and commercial coatings can provide further variety for this popular menu item.

Deep-Fat Frying   Deep-fat frying produces chicken pieces with a uniform golden color. This method, however, requires more attention than oven frying. To ensure that the chicken is thoroughly cooked, many foodservice operations fry it until it is golden and then place it in a 325°F (163°C) oven to complete the cooking. The temperature of the fat should be 350°F to 365°F (177°C to 185°C), and the same procedures described for frying meat apply. Deep-fat frying can be used for reheating the breaded or battered chicken pieces that are used in many foodservice operations, although oven frying yields a product lower in fat. The poultry processor's instructions for cooking time and temperature should be followed.

Broiling and Grilling   Tender young chickens can be broiled or grilled if the foodservice operation's equipment capacity is sufficient for the quantity needed. Halves or parts may be brushed with melted fat, seasoned, and placed skin side down on the broiler rack about 6 inches away from the heat source or directly on the grill. The chicken parts should be turned after 10 or 15 minutes and brushed with fat. Total broiling time will be 35 to 50 minutes, depending on the size of the pieces. For calorie-restricted or fat-restricted diets, brushing the chicken with fat should be eliminated. Also popular for both modified and normal diets are recipes for boneless, skinless chicken breasts, which can be marinated for flavor enhancement and then broiled or grilled to the proper degree of doneness.

In extended-care facilities, an outdoor chicken barbecue can provide a welcome change from the regular summer meal routine.

Several times during cooking, chicken quarters, halves, or pieces may be brushed with oil, a mixture of equal parts of oil and vinegar, or a seasoned barbecue sauce. Seasoned barbecue sauces should not be added until the last 15 or 20 minutes. The chicken pieces should be turned every 10 or 15 minutes during the 45 to 60 minutes required for doneness. Check the internal temperature with a meat thermometer. To shorten the cooking time, the pieces can be partially cooked in a steamer or oven just before barbecuing.

Moist-Heat Methods for Cooking Poultry

Several moist-heat methods may be used for cooking older, less-tender poultry or for menu variety. These methods include braising, stewing, simmering, and steaming and may be used for cooking whole or split poultry to be sliced, creamed, or made into soups and stews. The flavor that develops depends on the concentration of the broth. In braising, only enough liquid is used to cover the bottom of the pan; in stewing and simmering, the meat is fully covered with liquid. In all moist-heat methods, the pan or kettle is covered tightly, and the temperature is kept at about 185°F (85°C). Cooking time depends on the age and size of the bird and the quantity in the pan. The poultry should be cooked until fork tender. Poultry parts also may be steamed in low- or high-pressure steamers according to the manufacturer's instructions.

If moist-heat methods are used to produce cooked boneless meat for use in other recipes, the poultry should be removed from the cooking liquid as soon as it is done. The pieces should be placed in a single layer on a flat pan and allowed to cool only enough to ensure safe handling. The meat should be quickly boned by using a fork, tongs, and nonlatex disposable gloves. The boneless meat should be placed in a shallow layer on a flat pan, refrigerated immediately, and kept refrigerated until used. The broth should be cooled separately by adding ice, if the broth is concentrated, or by placing the hot broth in a pan in a sink filled with ice water and stirring until cold. Cooked poultry meat should be stored in the same manner as other meat products.

Fish and Shellfish

Good-quality fish that is well prepared can compete with the finest meat or poultry. Fish flesh is delicate and contains some connective tissue and variable amounts of fat. Fat content is one of the characteristics that determine the best cooking method for a particular species of fish, although almost any cooking method will produce a tender product. Most finfish and all shellfish are lean, with less than 5 percent fat. This means that they are susceptible to drying by exposure to either air or heat. Other considerations are the size, texture, form, and strength of the fish's flavor.

Well-done (the point at which the flesh becomes opaque, flakes easily, and is moist) is always the stopping point when cooking fish. High cooking temperatures or overcooking yield a hard, dry, pulpy fish that breaks up easily. Table 20.7 lists recommendations for cooking methods for several common species of freshwater and saltwater fish. Fish should be served as soon as possible after cooking, because holding makes unbreaded products dry and breaded products mushy.

Handling and Storage of Fish and Shellfish

Proper handling and storage are necessary to protect the quality of fresh and frozen fish. Ease of handling, product quality, and microbiological safety are all primary concerns. Fresh fish and shellfish should be stored in the refrigerator at about 35°F to 40°F (2°C to 4°C) for no longer than two days.

Unbreaded frozen fish products should be thawed in the refrigerator; 24 to 36 hours should be allowed for thawing 1-pound packages and 48 to 72 hours for 5-pound, solid-pack packages and 1-gallon cans. If faster thawing is necessary, sealed containers can be thawed under cold running water. This is not a recommended practice, however, because soluble flavors will leach out into the water if the fish pieces become waterlogged. Breaded products should not be thawed before cooking.

Methods for Cooking Fish and Shellfish

No matter what recipe is used, certain basic principles and procedures should be followed when cooking fish and shellfish. Some of these are discussed in the following subsections.

Baking   One of the easiest ways to prepare fish in quantity is to bake fillets, steaks, or unbreaded pieces. Pieces of uniform size should be placed on a well-oiled pan and baked in a 350°F to 400°F (177°C to 204°C) oven for the shortest time that will produce a cooked product. Herbs, lemon juice, paprika, chopped parsley, chives, dill, or seasoned salts can add flavor and appeal to baked fish. In baking already breaded and cooked pieces of fish, the manufacturer's instructions should be followed.

Broiling   Broiling requires careful watching and thus increases labor time. However, broiled fish adds variety to menus and, if prepared properly, is well accepted by many people. It is best to thaw frozen unbreaded fish to reduce cooking time. Lean fish should be brushed with melted margarine; fish containing more fat may not need the added fat. The fish should be placed on an oiled broiler pan, with skin (if any) away from the heat source, and broiled 2 to 4 inches away from the heat for 5 to 15 minutes, depending on the thickness of the fillet. The fillets may be brushed with melted margarine as needed to keep them moist.

Panfrying   If small quantities of fish are prepared, panfrying, or sautéing, may be a suitable method. Thawed dried fish should be dusted with seasoned flour or coated with breading and fried in an eighth inch of hot oil over moderate heat, first on one side and then the other, until each side is browned. Breaded frozen fish should not be thawed before panfrying.

Oven Frying   A simple procedure that requires little direct labor time is oven frying. A standard oven should be heated to 500°F (260°C) or a convection oven to 450°F (232°C). Thawed fish fillets may be dipped in beaten egg or milk and then in flour or breading. Frozen breaded portions or sticks should not be thawed. The fish should be placed on a well-greased baking pan, and some added fat may be poured over the fish. Fat should not be added to cooked

TABLE 20.7   Recommended Cooking Methods for Fish

Species of Fish	Fat or Lean	Broil	Bake	Simmer, Steam, Poach	Fry, Panfry
Alewife	Fat		Best	Good	
Barracuda	Fat	Good	Best		Fair
Black bass	Lean	Good	Good		Good
Black cod (sablefish)	Fat		Best	Good	
Bloater	Fat				Best
Bluefish	Fat	Good	Best		Fair
Bonito	Fat	Good	Best		Fair
Buffalo fish	Lean	Good	Best		Fair
Bullhead	Lean		Fair	Good	Best
Butterfish	Fat	Good	Fair		Best
Carp	Lean	Good	Best	Good	Fair
Catfish	Lean			Fair	Best
Cod	Lean	Best	Good		
Croaker (hardhead)	Lean	Good	Fair	Good	Best
Drum (redfish)	Lean		Best	Fair	
Eel	Fat		Good		Best
Flounder	Lean	Good	Fair		
Fluke	Lean	Good	Fair		Best
Grouper	Lean		Best		Best
Grunt (hog snapper)	Lean	Good	Best		Best
Haddock	Lean	Best	Good	Fair	Best
Hake	Lean	Fair	Fair	Good	
Halibut	Fat	Best	Fair	Fair	
Herring (lake)	Lean	Good	Best		Best
Herring (sea)	Fat	Best	Good		Good
Jawless fish	Lean	Good	Best		Best
Kingfish	Lean		Good		
King mackerel	Lean	Best	Fair	Fair	
Lake trout	Fat	Best	Fair		
Ling cod	Fat	Fair			
Mackerel	Lean	Best	Best		Good
Mango snapper	Fat	Best	Good	Fair	
Mullet	Lean	Good	Good	Fair	Best
Muskellunge	Fat	Best	Best		Fair
Perch	Lean	Best	Good		Fair
Pickerel	Lean	Good	Good		Best
Pike	Lean	Fair			Best
Pollock	Lean	Fair	Good		Best
Pompano	Lean	Fair	Good	Best	
Porgy (scup)	Fat	Best	Fair		Fair
Redfish (channel bass, rosefish)	Fat	Good	Good		Best

TABLE 20.7 (*Continued*)

Species of Fish	Fat or Lean	Broil	Bake	Simmer, Steam, Poach	Fry, Panfry
Red snapper	Lean	Good	Good	Good	
Rockfish	Lean	Good	Good		
Salmon	Lean		Fair	Best	
Sardines	Fat	Good	Best	Fair	
Sea bass	Fat		Good		
Sea trout	Fat	Best	Good		Good
Shad	Fat	Best	Best		Fair
Shark (grayfish)	Fat	Good			Fair
Sheepshead (freshwater drum)	Fat		Best	Good	
Sheepshead (saltwater)	Lean		Fair	Best	
Smelts	Lean	Best	Good		Fair
Snapper	Lean	Good	Best		Best
Snook (robalo)	Lean	Good	Best	Fair	
Sole	Lean	Good	Good		
Spanish mackerel	Lean	Good	Good		Best
Spot	Fat	Best	Good		Fair
Striped bass (rockfish)	Lean		Good	Best	
Sturgeon	Fat	Good	Best	Fair	Best
Sucker	Fat	Good	Fair		Best
Sunfish (pumpkinseed)	Lean	Good			
Swordfish	Lean	Best	Good	Fair	Fair
Tautog (blackfish)	Fat	Best	Good		Best
Trout	Lean	Good	Fair		
Tuna	Lean	Fair	Best	Good	
Walleye (pike, perch)	Fat			Best	
Weakfish (sea trout)	Lean	Best	Good		Fair
Whitefish	Fat	Good	Best		Fair
Whiting (silver hake)	Lean			Best	
Yellowtail	Fat		Good	Best	

Note. Fish may be harvested from freshwater or saltwater, or be farm raised. Fish may contain low, medium, or high levels of mercury. Pregnant women, nursing mothers, women who intend to have children, and children younger than 15 years should not eat fish more than once a month if it is harvested from contaminated waters. Fish with the highest levels of mercury include fresh and canned tuna, swordfish, king mackerel, marlin, amber jack, Chilean sea bass, and shark.

breaded portions. Precooked items will reheat rapidly, so the cooking time should be watched carefully.

Deep-Fat Frying If properly prepared, fried fish and shellfish have good visual appeal, flavor, and texture. To obtain an attractive brown, crispy crust, the oil for deep-fat frying should be heated to a temperature of 350°F to 365°F (177°C to 185°C). Fish or shellfish should be dipped in batter, milk, or egg and breading; excess breading should be shaken off. The pieces should be placed carefully in the fryer without overloading and fried about 4 or 5 minutes, depending on thickness, until the coating is golden brown and done. The fish should then be drained and served as soon as possible. If

necessary, fish can be held for a short period uncovered in proper hot-holding equipment or in open pans under infrared food warmers. For breaded products, the manufacturer's instructions should be followed.

Batter ingredients are a critical factor in producing a good deep-fried product that is crisp, is not greasy, and maintains the characteristic flavor of the specific fish. Common batter ingredients are flour, egg, baking powder, salt or other seasoning, and a liquid. Although baking powder helps produce a fluffier, lighter batter, it increases fat absorption. Many batter recipes use a carbonated beverage instead of baking powder to avoid this problem. Egg also increases the tendency for fat absorption but helps the batter adhere to the product. Some experimentation may be needed to develop and standardize a suitable batter recipe or to find an acceptable commercial batter mix.

The frying oil should be kept in good condition by periodically filtering it, adding more oil as needed, and controlling the temperature. Oil that has begun to break down will cause the food to overbrown, absorb more fat, and take on strong off flavors. Too high a temperature, as well as the presence of food particles, moisture, and salt in the oil, will hasten fat breakdown. When the fryer is not in use, the thermostat should be set at 200°F (93°C) or the fryer turned off.

Steaming, Poaching, and Simmering Steaming and poaching are good ways to prepare fish or shellfish without adding fat or calories. In steaming, the fish is placed on a rack in a shallow pan with liquid on the bottom, covered tightly, and cooked in the oven or on the range top until the fish is done. A low- or high-pressure steamer also may be used following the manufacturer's instructions.

In poaching, the fish is placed in a shallow pan containing a small amount of seasoned hot liquid such as water, water and lemon juice, or milk. The pan is covered, and the fish is simmered gently at about 185°F (85°C) until it flakes easily. Portions should retain their shape.

For chowders and stews, the fish is cooked at simmering temperatures in a larger amount of liquid used as stock. Shellfish such as shrimp, lobster, and crab also should be cooked in large amounts of seasoned water at temperatures between 185°F and 200°F (85°C and 93°C) only long enough to cook through. However, for most operations, it is more economical and efficient to purchase such fish in a partially prepared form to eliminate the labor involved in shelling and handling.

Eggs and Egg Products

An egg is one of the most versatile and valuable foods available. Served at breakfast, lunch, or dinner, in appetizers, soups, entrées, salads, sandwiches, or desserts, eggs are a good source of many nutrients. In addition to regular shell eggs, a number of processed egg products are available and appropriate for use in health care foodservice operations.

Using Processed Egg Products

The term *egg products* refers to liquid, frozen, dehydrated, and freeze-dried eggs produced by breaking and processing shell eggs. These products include separated whites and yolks, mixed whole eggs, and blends of the whole egg and yolk. Using egg products can save labor time, effort, and storage costs; furthermore, there is less waste than with shell eggs (refer to the *Food Code* for additional data).

Chilled or Frozen Egg Products Chilled or frozen egg products are available in 4- or 5-pound paper cartons and in 30-pound containers. The products are suitable for use in almost any menu item. Handled properly, they are even safer to use than fresh shell eggs because they are pasteurized at temperatures high enough to destroy bacteria. Additional ingredients and special production processes improve and preserve the performance characteristics of many egg products.

Chilled egg products should be stored at 38°F (3°C) or lower. These products have a longer shelf life than thawed frozen eggs and usually can be held at least five days. Manufacturers usually list recommended storage conditions and times on the product labels.

Frozen egg products should be stored at 0°F (−18°C) or lower. They should be thawed in the refrigerator for two or three days or placed under cold running water for quicker thawing. Once thawed, they should be refrigerated and used within four days.

Other available convenient frozen egg products include omelets, scrambled eggs, and hard-cooked eggs. These products should always be handled according to the manufacturer's instructions.

Dehydrated Egg Products New processes that remove the small amount of glucose in eggs have permitted the development of improved dried egg products. Glucose removal is necessary for longer shelf life. The products are treated at temperatures high enough to destroy pathogenic organisms.

Dried egg solids are available in several forms: egg white, whole egg, egg yolk, and fortified products. For quick breads, yeast breads, cookies, and cakes, the dry egg solids can be blended with the other ingredients, and the water required for reconstituting is added to other liquids in the recipe. For other recipes, dried eggs are reconstituted before they are combined with the other ingredients. Table 20.8 lists the conversion factors to use in substituting one form of egg for another.

Most quantity recipe files and manufacturer's labels provide information on reconstituting dried whole eggs. However, as a general rule, equal measures of dried egg and water are used. If products are weighed, one part dried whole egg to three parts water should be used.

Egg Substitutes Cholesterol-free egg substitutes are useful in some modified diets. Individual manufacturers use different formulas, but in general the natural egg white is retained, and a substitute for the yolk is added. Yolk substitutes contain vegetable or other oil carotenoids as coloring and nutritional additives. Although manufacturers suggest various uses, egg substitutes do not have all the

TABLE 20.8 Conversion Factors for Substituting Egg Products

	Frozen	Shell Eggs Equivalent	Dried Egg Solids
Whole	1 pound	9 eggs	4½ ounces plus 11½ ounces of water
Yolk	1 pound	23 yolks	7¼ ounces plus 8¾ ounces of water
White	1 pound	15 whites	2¼ ounces plus 13¾ ounces of water

functional properties of eggs, their satisfactory performance being limited to scrambled eggs, omelets, and binders in other recipes. The manufacturer's directions should be followed for storage and preparation of egg substitutes.

Methods for Cooking Eggs and Egg Products

Eggs should not be served raw or undercooked as there is a possibility of food-borne illness. Pasteurized eggs should be used to reduce the risk of food-borne illness, especially when being prepared for an at-risk population, such as long-term facilities.

In preparing eggs, it is important to remember these two principles: use low temperature, and minimize cooking time. Eggs may be cooked either in or out of the shell. Shelled eggs that are cooked for immediate service should be cooked to a minimum internal temperature of 145°F (63°C) for 15 seconds. Typical breakfast fare includes hard-cooked, poached, fried (the white is set and the yolk begins to thicken), scrambled, and baked eggs. For variety, they can be served as omelets or soufflés, or they can be incorporated in other meal components. Whatever the method of preparation, prolonged cooking and high heat are to be avoided.

Some general suggestions that apply to cooking eggs follow:

- Only eggs that are free from dirt and cracks should be purchased or used.
- Eggs should be kept refrigerated (45°F [7°C] or less) until preparation time unless they are being prepared for egg foam. In that case, they should be allowed to stand at room temperature for 30 minutes before use.
- Eggs and egg combinations should be cooked at moderate to low temperatures. High temperatures and prolonged cooking should be avoided.
- Commercially pasteurized eggs or egg products can be substituted for raw eggs in such items as Caesar salad.
- Appropriate techniques should be used when beating eggs. For a binding or coating mixture, whole eggs should be beaten lightly with a fork or wire whip. For lightness and volume, they should be beaten thoroughly with an electric mixer until they are thick and light yellow. For stiffness, they should be beaten until peaks form that fold over slightly as the beater is withdrawn.
- Egg whites should be combined carefully with other ingredients by folding (rather than stirring) with a wire whip or an electric mixer at low speed.
- Hot liquids should be added to eggs slowly and beaten constantly.

Medium and Hard Cooking Eggs can be cooked in the shell to various degrees of doneness by using any one of several different pieces of equipment. However, regardless of the equipment used, time and temperature are the critical factors. Medium- and hard-cooked eggs can be prepared in a compartment steamer, a steam-jacketed kettle, or a pan on the range top. Eggs at refrigerator temperature are more likely to crack when placed in hot water if the pan method is used. Placing them in warm water for a few minutes before cooking can prevent this.

Medium-cooked eggs require cooking for 5 to 7 minutes in water brought to a boil (212°F [100°C]) and then reduced to a simmer. Small-batch cooking is necessary when serving medium-cooked eggs. Holding for even a short time will cause them to overcook. Hard-cooked eggs need 15 to 20 minutes when cooked by this method. Excessive temperatures and prolonged cooking cause hard-cooked eggs to toughen, and a greenish black ring forms around the yolk, the result of hydrogen sulfide in the white combining with iron in the yolk to form ferrous sulfide.

Hard-cooked eggs placed in cold water immediately after cooking will be easier to peel. Quick cooling also helps prevent formation of the ring around the yolk. Hard-cooked eggs should be thoroughly cooled before being mixed with other ingredients, particularly in salads.

A time-saving method for making hard-cooked eggs that are to be chopped is to cook them out of the shell in a shallow, greased pan. The pan is placed either uncovered in a steamer for 20 minutes or covered in an oven at medium temperature for 30 to 40 minutes. After cooling, the eggs can be removed from the pan with a spatula and chopped with a French knife or food chopper. With this method, however, timing is critical because overcooking results in a product of inferior quality.

Poaching In poaching eggs, the addition of 1 tablespoon of salt or 2 tablespoons of vinegar to 1 gallon of water will help reduce spreading of the egg whites. Fresh Grade AA or A eggs and simmering water should be used to retain the eggs' shape. A 4-inch-deep, full-sized pan filled with about 2 inches of water should be used. The eggs should be gently slipped into the water and cooked for 3 to 5 minutes until the whites are coagulated and yolks are still soft. In a cafeteria, eggs can be poached in a counter-insert pan in the hot-holding counter. Whichever method is used, small-batch cooking is recommended.

Frying Fried eggs lend variety to the menu, particularly for residents in long-term care facilities. However, more labor time may be needed to produce good-quality fried eggs than eggs prepared by other methods. Careful handling during the preparation and holding processes is necessary. Small-batch or continuous preparation during the service period is suggested. A grill, griddle, tilting braising pan, or large skillet can be used to fry the eggs, depending on the number of servings needed and equipment available. Fresh Grade AA or A eggs should be fried in ample fat heated to about 275°F (135°C). The fried egg should have a firm white that is free from browning or crispness, and the yolk should be set but not hard or dry. (Regulations require that the yolk of fried eggs be cooked. Do *not* serve raw or undercooked eggs. Check your local and state guidelines.)

Scrambling Scrambling is one of the easiest ways to prepare eggs. Large quantities can be cooked in a short time by using a griddle, tilting braising pan, oven, steamer, or large skillet. Eggs lower than Grade A quality result in a high-quality product when scrambled. High cooking temperatures and long cooking and holding times in a heated serving unit will cause scrambled eggs to curdle. An undesirable flavor and greenish color also may result.

If scrambled eggs must be held at a serving temperature for an extended period, a buffer such as powdered citric acid should be added at the ratio of 0.1 percent (3 grams per gallon of egg). Cream of tartar also may be used at 0.5 percent (5 grams or ½ teaspoon per gallon of eggs). Today, many foodservice operations purchase frozen blended egg products to use in scrambling. The buffers in these products enable them to hold well for extended periods. Frozen egg mixtures require less preparation time and provide a consistent product. Frozen or chilled eggs in a waterproof pouch may be used for scrambled eggs. If mixtures are prepared on the premises, milk, cream, or medium white sauce can be used to make the egg mixture; the ratio is ½ cup (4 ounces) liquid to 1 pound of whole eggs.

For the best appearance, eggs for scrambling should be beaten just enough to blend the yolk, white, and liquid. They should then be cooked over low heat or in the oven, with occasional stirring, to form a tender, moist food.

Baking   Eggs for baking are broken into individual greased baking dishes or greased muffin tins. An attractive way to serve baked eggs is to remove the crusts from a bread slice, butter it, press it into a greased muffin tin, and drop a shelled egg in the center. It should then be baked in a slow oven (325°F [163°C]) for 12 to 20 minutes, depending on the firmness desired.

Making Omelets   Omelets require greater skill and time in preparation than many other egg products. For this reason, it is not feasible to serve them to a large number of patients or residents. However, frozen prepared omelets are currently available from several food processors. If menu variety is desired and the facility's resources of time, personnel, and equipment are limited, omelets should be considered.

Making Soufflés   Soufflés add interest and consumer appeal to menus. They are similar to fluffy omelets but have a thickening agent (such as a thick white sauce or tapioca) added to the beaten egg yolks before the whites are folded in. The soufflé mixture is placed in a well-oiled pan that is set in water and baked at 375°F (190°C). A lower temperature (300°F [149°C]) can be used if the pan is not set in water, although more cooking time is required. Soufflés should be light, fluffy, tender, and delicately browned.

Cheese

Flavorful and rich in nutrients, cheese is a good source of complete protein that can substitute for meat and add variety to menus. Like other protein-rich foods, cheese must be cooked at a low temperature. A high temperature or prolonged heating causes stringiness and fat separation, which give a curdled appearance to the product. Cheese blends into most recipes more smoothly if it is first grated or chopped.

Some recipes use several varieties of cheeses, each with its own distinctive flavor and characteristics. Processed cheese and cheese foods often blend into recipes more smoothly because they have already been heated during processing and contain an emulsifier. However, processed cheeses lack the distinctive flavor of natural aged cheese. If a strong cheese flavor is desired, a combination of the two can be used. Dried cheeses also are used to heighten the cheese flavor in some products.

Milk

Milk, an important component of many prepared foods, requires careful preparation procedures to prevent curdling and scorching. High temperatures and prolonged cooking coagulate and toughen milk protein, change milk flavors, and cause caramelization of the lactose in milk. But the curdling and coagulation of the milk protein can be caused by other factors as well. For example, table salt and curing salt such as that used in ham and bacon can cause milk to curdle, as can tannins, found in many vegetables such as potatoes and in chocolate and brown sugar. Strong food acids can cause almost immediate curdling. Because milk scorches easily, it should be heated over water or in a steam-jacketed kettle with low steam. Prolonged heating at low temperatures may darken milk (by caramelization of the lactose) or cause it to lose some of its flavor.

Several techniques can be used in preparing foods that contain milk to decrease the risk of curdling. For example, the milk can be thickened with flour or cornstarch, as in white sauce and puddings, to stabilize the milk protein during the cooking process. Salt should not be added early in the cooking process. Acid ingredients, which should be at the same temperature as the milk, should be added in small amounts toward the end of the cooking time.

Evaporated milk is whole milk with 50 percent of the water removed. Diluted with an equal quantity of water, it can be substituted for fresh whole milk in most recipes with good results because it is more heat stable and resistant to curdling. It produces smooth, even-textured puddings and white sauces.

For reasons of economy and convenience, nonfat dry milk can be used for many cooking purposes. Fourteen ounces of nonfat dry milk and 1 gallon of water produce the equivalent of 1 gallon of fresh skim milk. Adding 5 ounces of margarine or other fat to this recipe makes the equivalent of 1 gallon of fresh, whole milk in fat and calorie content. In many recipes, ½ to ¾ cup of nonfat dry milk can be added for each cup of liquid to supplement the nutritional value and protein content of the food.

Dry milk can be combined into food products by several methods. In cakes, cookies, quick breads, and instant mashed potatoes, milk solids can be added to the other dry ingredients, and the water needed to reconstitute the dry milk is added with the other liquid ingredients. For custards, puddings, and similar dishes, dry milk solids should be combined with the sugar. The water required for reconstitution is added separately. If the milk is to be reconstituted and used in liquid form, the amount of dry milk specified by the manufacturer's instructions should be weighed and the water carefully measured. Once reconstituted, the milk should be refrigerated immediately and protected from contamination.

Dried cultured buttermilk also is available and convenient to use in many recipes. It is combined with recipe ingredients in the same manner as nonfat dry milk. Dried cultured buttermilk should be refrigerated after the container has been opened.

Many desserts use dairy product foams. When air is beaten into cream or evaporated milk, semistable foam is produced. Cream that contains less than 30 percent milk fat will not whip without the use of special methods or ingredients. Whipping cream foams to about twice the original volume and evaporated milk to about three times the original volume. The cream or milk must be cooler than 40°F (4°C), and bowl and beaters should be thoroughly chilled. One tablespoon of lemon juice per cup of evaporated milk will help stabilize the foam produced. The lemon juice should be added after whipping.

If substituting nondairy whipped toppings for whipping cream in recipes, remember that the nondairy products whip to larger volumes. Therefore, substitutions should be made according to the quantity of whipped material required by the recipe, rather than by equal volumes of unwhipped liquid.

Vegetables

With the abundant variety of vegetables in every season and every region, good vegetables that are well prepared should have an almost universal appeal. *Well prepared* means that the texture, flavor, and appearance are up to standard; the serving temperature is right; and the vegetable harmonizes with the rest of the meal. The nutritional value and quality of vegetables depend on the nutrient content of the fresh vegetables, storage and preparation methods, and the length of time between preparation and service.

Preparation of Vegetables

Because many nutrients are concentrated under the skin of raw vegetables, care must be taken in their preparation to minimize nutrient loss. Ideally, vegetables should be prepared just before cooking or service. However, this is not always possible because of limited personnel and time. Vegetables that are cleaned, peeled, chopped, or sliced in advance must be refrigerated in covered containers or tightly sealed plastic bags until needed. Vegetables that darken when peeled and are exposed to air must be treated with an antioxidant before storage. To avoid severe losses of vitamins and minerals, peeled or cut vegetables should not be stored in water.

Vegetables should be washed thoroughly in cool water before further processing. Leafy green vegetables should be rinsed several times. Long soaking periods in salted water are no longer necessary to remove insects from broccoli, cabbage, Brussels sprouts, and cauliflower because commercial vegetable growers now wash produce before it is shipped. However, these vegetables still need thorough washing in plain water. Many vegetables may be purchased raw sliced, diced, shredded, or mixed with other vegetables for salads or coleslaw or for stir-fry. These vegetables do not need any additional washing. Use the vegetables by the use date marked on the package.

Many kinds of equipment can be used to reduce the labor required to prepare raw vegetables. Shredders and mixers with grater and slicer attachments are frequently used. More sophisticated food cutters, choppers, slicers, and vertical cutter-mixers have been designed to uniformly process large quantities of vegetables in a short time. If machine peeling is used for vegetables, the time should be carefully controlled to reduce loss and control cost.

The overall purpose of preparing vegetables is to make them more digestible and to give them a more desirable flavor. Cooking may be needed to soften cellulose or to make the starch more digestible. Cooking methods for various vegetables differ in some respects, but several general principles apply. A cooking method that best preserves nutrients by a short cooking time and use of a limited amount of water should be chosen. It is not always possible to achieve optimum nutrient retention. For example, steaming under pressure reduces nutrient losses that occur when vegetables are cooked in water, but the higher cooking temperature may increase loss of heat-sensitive vitamins. However, shorter cooking times in low- or high-pressure steam equipment reduce this kind of loss. Flavor enhancement also should be a guide in selecting a cooking method. In most instances, the best method for nutrient retention also produces the most desirable flavor. To preserve nutrients as much as possible and make them aesthetically pleasing, vegetables should be cooked only until they are fork tender or slightly crisp.

Although general charts listing cooking times for various types of equipment are available, each facility should use the information provided by equipment manufacturers. The times given should be tested and posted on a chart beside pieces of equipment used for vegetable preparation. Cooking times vary according to steam pressure and design of equipment. A timer should be used no matter what equipment is used. It is difficult to obtain the desired quality of vegetables in large-batch cooking either in a steam-jacketed kettle or on the range. Production workers may need to be retrained to use the batch method and to time batches to match the demands of the serving period.

Methods for Cooking Vegetables

Cooking methods for vegetables vary depending on a number of factors. Some of these—color, flavor, canned versus fresh, and the like—are discussed in the following subsections.

Color The vibrant colors of properly cooked vegetables add greatly to their appeal, but an unattractive color can cause a vegetable to be rejected even before it has been tasted. For that reason, color preservation and enhancement are primary objectives in vegetable cooking. The pigments that create vegetable colors are affected in different ways during cooking—by heat, acid, alkali, and cooking time.

Chlorophyll, the pigment in green vegetables, is slightly soluble in water and is changed to olive green by acids and heat when the vegetables are cooked in a covered pan or are overcooked. Although alkalis such as baking soda intensify the bright green color, they should not be used because they destroy some vitamins and alter the texture of the vegetable. Steam cooking is ideal for green vegetables because the continuous flow of steam around the vegetable carries off the mild acids that cause undesirable color changes, and vitamin losses into water are eliminated. When steam equipment is not available, green vegetables should be cooked uncovered in a small amount of rapidly boiling water for as short a time as possible.

Yellow and orange vegetables, tomatoes, and red peppers contain the *carotenoid pigment*, which is insoluble in water and unaffected by acid and alkali. Overcooking affects the texture of yellow and orange vegetables and can dull the color. Because corn and carrots contain relatively large amounts of sugar, overcooking or extended holding can cause the sugar to caramelize and the vegetables to turn brown. Yellow vegetables may be cooked in a steamer or in a covered or uncovered pan with a small amount of boiling water.

Anthocyanin pigments color beets, red cabbage, and eggplant. Anthocyanins are extremely soluble in water; they turn blue in alkaline solutions but become brighter red in acid solutions. Adding a small amount of mild acid is an acceptable way to maintain the color of red cabbage. However, it usually is unnecessary to add acid to beets while cooking. Cooking times for these red vegetables should be short. With long cooking, anthocyanin pigments turn greenish and eventually lose most of their color.

Light-colored vegetables contain pigments that are colorless, slightly colored, pale yellow, or brown. Heat and alkali adversely affect this group of flavonoid pigments. In mild acid solutions, they remain white. In the presence of alkali, as in hard water, they become yellow or gray. Although the color change to yellow may not detract from the appearance of cooked onions, the graying that can occur in cauliflower and turnips is unattractive. Adding a small amount of cream of tartar to the cooking water or cooking in a steamer can prevent this color change.

Strong-Flavored Vegetables   Onions, cabbage, cauliflower, broccoli, Brussels sprouts, rutabagas, and turnips all have strong flavors. Members of the onion family contain *sinigrin*, which is driven off when onions are cooked, leaving a sweet flavor. The cabbage family develops *sulfide* compounds during cooking and becomes sulfur flavored if cooked too long. Cooking methods for these vegetables differ. Onions should be sautéed in fat or cooked in relatively large amounts of water for the best flavor. Members of the cabbage family are best cooked in a steamer for short periods. However, when a steamer is not available, they can be cooked in a small amount of water on top of the range, in shallow pans, uncovered or loosely covered. Rutabagas and turnips should be cooked in a moderate amount of water, uncovered, and only until tender to keep the flavor as sweet as possible.

Canned Vegetables   Canned vegetables offer several real advantages in foodservice operations: moderate cost, year-round availability, consistent quality, reduced energy use, and good variety. However, poor handling can yield cooked products that have lost much of their appeal and nutrient content. Canned vegetables are fully cooked and should be reheated only enough to meet immediate needs, with batch heating throughout the serving period. They can be reheated in a steamer, a steam-jacketed kettle, or a kettle on the range top. For best results, heat the drained liquid from the vegetable to about 200°F (93°C), add vegetables, and heat to 150°F to 160°F (65°C to 71°C). The vegetable should be cooked only long enough to heat through, with little stirring. A No. 10 can of any vegetable reheats to 150°F (65°C) in about 5 minutes. However, the vegetable should not be reheated on a steam table because reheating will take too long and spoil the quality. If cooked vegetables will not be used for extended lengths of time, they should be refrigerated and reheated before use to keep the product in good condition. Imaginative seasoning can greatly enhance the appeal of canned vegetables. Herbs, small amounts of meat, nuts, mushrooms, lemon juice, sauces, and cheese can be used for variety.

Frozen Vegetables   In many instances, frozen vegetables are fresher than fresh vegetables and have a more uniform color and size, having been blanched and flash frozen within an hour or two of harvesting. High-quality frozen vegetables provide freshness, beautiful color, and portion control and save labor time and waste. Small-batch cooking is essential for top-quality cooked products.

Many products are available in individually quick-frozen forms that make it convenient to cook only the amount needed immediately. Most frozen vegetables should be cooked from the frozen state. Only a few, such as spinach, need tempering in the refrigerator before cooking to allow more uniform heat transfer. Frozen vegetables should be cooked in shallow layers in half- or full-sized steamtable pans to eliminate handling time and damage in transferring from cooking to serving container. A full-size (12-by-20-by-2½-inch) pan will hold three 2- to 4-pound packages of vegetables. As with any other form of vegetable, frozen vegetables should be undercooked if they are to be held hot for more than 15 or 20 minutes.

Steam is the best method for cooking frozen vegetables. The manufacturer's directions for the type of steamer to use should be followed. Range-top cooking time should be carefully watched to avoid overcooking, and serving pans should be used rather than large kettles.

Frozen vegetable combinations add interest to vegetable offerings. In such combinations, blanching times are adjusted to produce a uniform cooking time for the mixture. Package directions indicate the cooking time.

Starches

Foods that are composed primarily of starch serve an important role in meals from both an aesthetic and a nutritive perspective. High-carbohydrate foods, or starches, appear at almost all meals. The most popular starches are potatoes, pasta, rice, and cereals, with potatoes being the number one choice.

Potatoes

Potatoes can be cooked in many ways (in water or in sauce, steamed, fried, or baked) and are one of the most versatile and well-liked vegetables. The sugar, starch, and moisture content vary with the variety of potato and method of preparation. New potatoes and red-skinned potatoes, which often have a higher moisture content, are suitable for boiling, steaming, and serving whole.

All-purpose potatoes are especially useful for mashing, although a number of highly acceptable dehydrated products also are available. In addition, this type of potato can be used in many recipes that require baking in a pan or casserole, such as potatoes au gratin.

Russet or Idaho potatoes produce a more desirable baked product, with a fluffy, mealy texture. Baked potatoes should not be wrapped in foil because foil slows down the cooking process, adds to the cost, and produces a steamed product. The potato skin should be oiled or perforated with a fork before baking to allow steam to escape. Specially designed racks for baking potatoes are used in many foodservice operations. The metal pins on the racks allow potatoes to be placed vertically in the oven and promote faster cooking.

French-fried potatoes are popular among certain customer groups. Although most French fries served are made from frozen products, some are made from fresh potatoes. The steps for deep-fat frying presented earlier in this chapter should be followed for this menu item. Frozen French fries that can be oven-cooked also are available.

Pasta

Macaroni, noodles, and spaghetti form the basis of many combination entrées. Pastas enriched with B vitamins and iron should be used. Those made from *durum wheat* remain firmer and do not stick together as much as other pastas after cooking. Pastas are cooked in a large volume of rapidly boiling salted water in a kettle or steam-jacketed kettle until they are tender and yet firm or al dente. A compartment steamer also could be used. Adding oil to the cooking water keeps the pasta from sticking together and helps keep the water from boiling over. If the pasta is to be combined with other ingredients for further cooking, it should be slightly undercooked. Durum wheat pastas usually do not need rinsing after cooking. However, any pasta can be rinsed in a colander under either hot or cold water to remove excess starch. If pasta is to be served hot, it should be rinsed with hot water; cold water should be used if the pasta is to be included in a combination salad. Pasta served from a steam table should be tossed with a small amount of fat (such as olive oil) before placing it in the pan.

Rice

Rice is available in brown, milled, parboiled, and partially cooked forms. Rice combinations with seasonings also are available but are more expensive. The amount of water and cooking time vary according to the type of rice, so it is necessary to follow the preparation methods recommended for the specific form used. Rice can be cooked in a tightly covered pan on the range, in the oven, in a compartment steamer, or in a steam-jacketed kettle. Rice held for later service should be kept in shallow pans to prevent packing. To avoid losing the vitamin B content, enriched rice should not be rinsed either before or after cooking. Long-grain rice should be used when the rice is to be served plain or in combination with entrées. When cooked, the grains remain firm, fluffy, and separate. Leftover rice can be refrigerated or frozen. Half a cup of water is added for each quart of rice when it is reheated for service.

Cereals

When dry cereal is added to water, the starch granules absorb moisture, become greatly enlarged, and thicken after heating. Instant and quick-cooking cereals have been further processed by various methods that allow them to cook within a few minutes. The manufacturer's directions should be followed in preparing cooked cereals. The amount of liquid needed and cooking times vary according to the type of cereal being prepared. The cereal should be kept covered until served to prevent drying. If a dry crust forms on the cereal, remove it. Do not mix it with the remaining cereal, and do not serve it to a customer.

Sandwiches

Sandwiches are popular in any season and with nearly everyone. Sandwiches add variety and interest to menus and provide the needed nutrients alone or in combination with other foods.

Sandwich Ingredients

Sandwiches can be made from any number of ingredients. They can be open- or closed-faced, cold or hot, and served in a variety of shapes and forms. The essential things to remember are that they should have good flavor, texture, and appearance and that they should be served fresh at the appropriate temperature.

So many varieties of specialty breads, rolls, and buns are available from commercial sources today that the problem is which one to choose. Using bread with a close-grained, firm texture is desirable to prevent the sogginess caused by moist fillings. Spreads such as salad dressings, butter, mustard, mayonnaise, and combinations of these with other ingredients can be used for flavor. Sandwich fillings should contain a combination of ingredients with some contrast in flavor, color, and texture. Mixed fillings, especially those that contain meat, fish, poultry, or eggs, must be handled in accordance with safe food preparation practices. Cheese and meats for sandwiches can be purchased already sliced for uniformity. Some meats—ham, roast beef, corned beef, and turkey—can be machine sliced paper thin and stacked high for appeal and easy eating.

Foodservice magazines are helpful for new ideas that can appeal to patients and staff. Attractive sandwiches can be convenient and profitable items in employee and visitor cafeterias and can add interest to traditional menu patterns.

Sandwich Assembly

Assembly lines should be used to streamline sandwich making. After the steps for sandwich assembly have been determined, the ingredients should be arranged in the proper order. To save steps, time, and motion and to be efficient enough to meet production schedules during sandwich assembly, employees should:

- Cover head with bonnet or hair net; wash hands.
- Wear disposable gloves, use both hands, and arrange the slices of bread in two or four rows on a clean, sanitized cutting board or a clean, sanitized worktable.
- Distribute the spread on the bread with a spatula and cover each slice with a circular motion.
- Use both hands to place slices of meat, cheese, poultry, or tomato on the bread slices in alternate rows.
- When making sandwiches using a mixture of ingredients, scoop mixture portions onto the center of bread slices and spread with a spatula, using one stroke moving in and one stroke moving out.
- Use both hands to place lettuce on top of the filling.
- Close sandwiches by turning a slice of bread over the filling-covered slices.
- Stack sandwiches two or three high and cut through the entire stack.

- Wrap sandwiches individually in plastic bags or film before refrigerating.
- When storing sandwiches, do not cover with a damp cloth.

If a large volume of sandwiches is to be made, these steps can be divided between two or more employees.

Sanitation and safe food-handling procedures must be followed when making cold sandwiches because of the amount of handling and because they are not cooked. Mixed filling containing poultry, eggs, fish, meat, or mayonnaise should be prepared the day they are to be served and only in quantities that will be used during the one serving period. Fillings should be refrigerated until needed. Do not add lettuce or tomatoes if sandwiches are to be stored for some time in the refrigerator, because the lettuce will wilt.

Salads

Well-prepared salads add appeal and flavor variety to any menu. They are an excellent means of serving nutrient-rich vegetables and fruits and provide good sources of fiber. Careful handling and imagination in combining flavors and colors make the difference between appealing and mediocre salads. Using well-designed recipes and careful preparation methods, anyone trained in food preparation can achieve attractive results.

The colors, flavors, and textures of salad ingredients should be balanced. Salad *underliners* of lettuce, endive, or other greens can complement and enhance the appearance of almost any salad. Garnishes and dressings accent salad flavors and add color and eye appeal. There are several basic types of salads, such as mixed-green and combination salads, main-dish salads, and molded salads, but almost endless variables are possible.

Salads are made up of the following four parts:

1. *Salad base.* The salad base or undergarnish is usually lettuce or some form of greens. The base helps to shape or hold the salad together; it is the frame for the salad. The salad base should never flow off the salad plate. The base must be thoroughly cleaned and chilled.
2. *Salad body.* The body is the main ingredient of the salad, such as meat, vegetables, or fruit. Ingredients in the body of the salad should never be overchopped. The body needs to be thoroughly chilled.
3. *Salad dressing.* Dressing may be added to greens just before serving time, or as an accompaniment on the side of the salad, and should be served chilled, except for oil and vinegar or hot bacon dressing.
4. *Garnish.* All garnishes must be edible and should accent or complement the color, flavor, shape, and lettuce of the body.

Combination Salads

The simplest salad is lettuce torn, not chopped, into bite-size pieces tossed with a savory dressing; a combination of greens can be used for variety in color, texture, and flavor. Salad recipes that specify weights of ingredients are useful when substituting one green for another as availability or cost changes. The wide variety of salad greens available allows plenty of latitude for varying basic combination salads. Iceberg lettuce, leaf lettuce, Bibb lettuce, Boston lettuce, endive (chicory), escarole, romaine, spinach, watercress, and Chinese cabbage can be used in various combinations. Other ingredients such as radishes, tomatoes, cauliflower, red cabbage, fresh mushrooms, green onions, red onion rings, cucumber, broccoli, croutons, and hard-cooked eggs can be added with appealing results. Shapes should be varied. Color should be contrasting, and flavor should combine mild and strong flavors and salty with bland, tart, or sweet flavors.

All salad ingredients should be clean, crisp, and mixed lightly to avoid breaking or crushing. To keep the greens from wilting, dressings should be added just before service, or the customers can add them. Whenever possible, a choice of dressings, either prepared on the premises or selected from a wide variety of commercial dressings, should be offered.

Main-Dish Salads

A salad served as the main course of a meal should contain some protein-rich food, such as chicken, seafood, eggs, cheese, ham, turkey, or other meat, usually combined with raw or cooked vegetables. For added flavor, meat and vegetable pieces may be marinated in a tart French dressing or vinaigrette, drained, and combined with mayonnaise or a cooked dressing before serving. Such mixtures can be used to stuff tomatoes or served with tomato wedges as garnish. Care in handling the meat or other protein food is essential to maintain safety. Marination in the acid salad dressing provides some protection from bacterial growth, but clean utensils and refrigeration are still required.

Julienne strips of poultry, meat, and sliced cheese or cottage cheese can be used to top combination green salads for main-dish entrées. Salad plates offering a salad mixture accompanied by cold cuts, cheese slices, and fresh fruits are attractive and appealing year-round. In cold seasons, a cup of hot soup or consommé provides a good accompaniment.

In arranging main-dish salads, different shapes should be used to make an interesting pattern. The food shapes can be varied for contrast and accented with contrasting and complementary colors. Visual appeal is just as important as substantial character and a pleasing blend of flavors and textures. Salads should be kept thoroughly chilled at all times.

Relishes

Relishes may be used as a garnish or body of a salad. All relishes must be thoroughly clean, fresh, crisp, and chilled. Relishes include:

- Celery, carrots, and zucchini sticks
- Cherry or grape tomatoes
- Cucumbers, peeled or unpeeled, sliced
- Whole small radishes
- Green, red, or yellow pepper rings
- Mushrooms, sliced, or some may be left whole, depending on size
- Cauliflower and broccoli buds

Molded Gelatin Salads

Molded gelatin salads usually are sweetened mixtures made with flavored gelatin mixes or plain gelatin. Water, fruit juice, and vegetable juice can be used as the liquid. For fast congealing, only enough hot water to dissolve the gelatin should be used before adding cold water, ice, or other liquid for the remaining quantity. In hot weather or when unrefrigerated holding is necessary, the amount of liquid used should be reduced slightly. Before other ingredients (such as chopped vegetables, fruit pieces, and cottage cheese) are added, the mixture should be cooled until it has the consistency of unbeaten egg whites. This step will keep the added ingredients from sinking to the bottom of the pan.

For quantity service, standard 12-by-20-inch pans should be used so that the gelatin can be cut for serving. Individual molds are attractive, but they are more time-consuming to prepare. Molded salads should be made the day before service.

Preparation of Salad Ingredients

Efficient salad preparation and assembly calls for good tools, equipment, and work procedures. Some basic rules should be followed in preparing all salad ingredients. All ingredients should be of top quality and should be kept in the refrigerator except during actual preparation. Salad greens should be thoroughly washed, dried, and stored in vapor-proof containers until used. Trays of finished salads should be refrigerated until they are served. All salads can be attractively arranged and garnished by using the natural color and shape of each ingredient to advantage. For example, the contrasting colors and shapes supplied by purple onion slices, tomato wedges, and ripe olives can enhance a salad composed of salad greens. Maximum sanitation control in work methods and equipment should be observed. Automated equipment should be used whenever possible to reduce labor time and to produce uniform results. When cutting boards are used, they should be used only for raw vegetable preparation. Cutting boards should be sanitized and air-dried after each use. Colored boards are a good way to ensure that the correct board is used for raw vegetable preparation.

Assembly of Salad Ingredients

Most individual salads can be assembled in advance, put on trays, and refrigerated until they are needed. To save time and steps in assembly, all equipment and ingredients should be arranged within easy reach of the employee. Mobile carts can be used to extend the workspace and to store salad trays. Trays should be stacked on the work counter, and each tray should be stacked with all the plates or bowls it will hold. Both hands should be used during assembly, and appropriate portion utensils or disposable nonlatex gloves should be used to handle ingredients.

Salad Bars

Salad bars are often a part of the nonpatient foodservice and are self-serve. The bar may contain salad greens, a variety of dressings, fruits, vegetables, cheese, meat, chopped hard-cooked eggs, cottage cheese, coleslaw, potato and pasta salads, crumbled bacon, croutons, gelatin, and other vegetable or fruit salads. The bar should be attractively laid out, and all ingredients and serving dishes should be cold. The bar should be kept clean at all times and items replenished as needed.

Fruits

Fresh, canned, dried, and frozen fruits, either plain or in combination, are often served as a salad, dessert, or snack and with breakfast foods. Fresh fruit in season, carefully selected for quality, can be a regular and popular menu item. When selective menus are used, fresh fruit should be offered daily. Bowls of whole fresh fruit can be used on cafeteria lines as an attractive merchandising tool and as a simple serving method.

All whole fresh fruits should be thoroughly washed before they are served, including bananas, citrus fruits, melons, and cantaloupes. (Melons and cantaloupes may need to be cleaned with a soft vegetable brush.) Cutting clusters of grapes makes them easier to serve, but many fresh fruits need almost no preparation before service. Cut-up fresh fruits can be combined in a virtually infinite number of variations or combined with canned fruits. Peeled and cut fresh fruits should be stored in fruit juices to maintain their juiciness and flavor. Due to oxidation, some fruits turn brown when cut. To maintain their color, these fruits should be dipped into an acid solution such as lemon or orange juice. Various shapes and sizes of fruits should be used to enhance flavors and colors.

Breads

Whole-grain and enriched breads, cereals, and cereal products are a significant part of the daily diet because they supply carbohydrates, protein, B vitamins, and iron. The wide range of bread and cereal foods offers many opportunities for menu variety.

Yeast Breads

To save time and labor, most institutions purchase commercially based bread and rolls, supplementing them with mixes for quick breads or frozen dough products for yeast breads. Quick-bread mixes also can be prepared on-site and kept on hand for many uses. Facilities that have adequate equipment and labor time can prepare yeast bread products on site. The use of standardized recipes and procedures makes it possible for any experienced person to produce high-quality yeast breads.

Two basic methods are used for mixing yeast breads: the *sponge method* and the *straight-dough method*. The sponge method includes two mixing processes and two fermentation processes in alternating sequence. Part of the flour, water, yeast, sugar, and shortening is mixed and allowed to ferment. This mixture is then combined with the remaining ingredients, mixed again, and allowed to ferment a second time. In the straight-dough method, all ingredients are mixed at one time before any fermentation takes place. This latter method is the most practical and saves time.

Bread structure depends on developing the gluten by mixing and kneading. If bread flour is used, more kneading is needed to develop the gluten than when all-purpose flour is used. Over-kneading is preferable to under-kneading.

During fermentation (rising), a humid atmosphere prevents dehydration or crusting of the dough surface. A temperature of around 85°F (29°C) is ideal to ensure adequate yeast growth; a proof cabinet that controls moisture, temperature, and time is used to provide the correct atmosphere for the bread to rise. After the first rising, the dough should be punched down, scaled, shaped, and put in pans. The second rising will be more rapid because more yeast cells are present in the dough. The bread is ready for baking when the dough has doubled in size. A relatively high baking temperature is used to allow the gas in the dough to expand further, to firm the bread's structure, and to develop a golden brown color.

After baking, the loaves should be removed from the pans and placed on racks to allow steam and alcohol to escape. Bread can be held for long periods if frozen in moisture-proof and vapor-proof material. For freezing, it is recommended that baked bread be wrapped while it is still warm to reduce moisture loss in the freezer.

Unbaked dough also can be refrigerated for at least 12 hours or overnight. The first rising will occur during refrigeration. By refrigerating dough in this manner, the traditional early-morning baking schedule can be avoided. Dough will be ready to shape and bake when employees arrive at standard starting times, and yet the products will be ready for the main meals of the day. Although dough can be frozen immediately after mixing and before fermentation, the frozen bread dough must contain enough yeast to perform effectively after thawing.

Quick Breads

Quick breads leavened with baking powder, baking soda, or steam can add appeal to any meal with a minimum of labor. Prepared mixes for muffins, cornbread, biscuits, pancakes, popovers, and other items require only the addition of liquid, eggs, or both to produce high-quality products. Mixes purchased or made on the premises minimize the skill and time needed for preparation.

Two basic methods are used in mixing quick breads: the *muffin method* and the *biscuit method*. In the muffin method, dry ingredients are mixed together. Then liquids, including oil or melted shortening, are added. Mix ingredients only enough to thoroughly combine. Overextended mixing will overdevelop the gluten and cause toughness, tunnels, and holes in the finished product. For uniform-size muffins, use a portion scoop when filling the muffin tin.

The biscuit method, which is used for *soft dough*, also involves a minimum of mixing. Solid fat is cut into the combined dry ingredients. Liquid is then added and mixed just enough to moisten the ingredients. Then the dough is rolled out on a floured board and cut or rolled directly on the baking pan. The labor-saving method of rolling directly on the baking pan may make it possible to serve freshly made biscuits more often. The dough can be cut into squares or triangles before or after baking. All the dough can be used without the reworking involved in traditional methods of cutting.

Frozen biscuits, yeast breads, and muffins are available, their quality is good, and they do not take a highly skilled employee to prepare them for baking.

Soups

Soups are classified as clear, unthickened, cream, or thick. Clear and unthickened soups are broths to which vegetables, pasta, rice, meat, or poultry are added. Bouillon is clear soup without solid ingredients such as chicken or beef. Consommé is a concentrated broth or stock (chicken, fish, or meat) that has been clarified to make it clear and transparent. Broth or *stock* is the basic ingredient for all clear soups. Broth is made by simmering meat, poultry, seafood, or vegetables in water to extract flavor.

Stock may be *brown*, from browned cracked bones and meat that has been browned before simmering with vegetables and seasonings, or white, made from rinsed beef and veal bones with added vegetables and seasonings. *White* stock may also be made from chicken or fish.

Cream soups or *thick soups* are made with a thin white sauce combined with mashed, strained, or finely chopped vegetables, meat, chicken, or fish. *Chowders* are unstrained thick soups prepared from vegetables, chicken, seafood, or meat. *Bisques* are a mixture of chopped shellfish, stock, milk, and seasonings that has been thickened. *Purees* are soups that are usually a thin white sauce that is thickened by pureeing one or more ingredients. Puree soups are usually vegetable. *Gumbos* are made from a *roux* (flour and fat that has been slowly browned), vegetables, spices, and seafood or chicken (or both). Okra and tomatoes are major components of gumbos.

Soups that may be served as an appetizer include thin, clear soups and light cream and puree soups. Main-dish soups are more generous in size of serving and nutrition. Main-dish soups include bisques, chowders, cream soups, gumbos, and mixtures of meat, vegetables, and pasta.

Sauces

Roux, the basis of most sauces, is equal parts by weight of fat and flour that is slowly cooked. A roux may be blonde, white, or brown, depending on the cooking time to change color. The most common sauce is the *white sauce* that is made with a roux of fat, usually butter or margarine, and flour, with milk as the liquid. *Béchamel sauce* and its variations use milk and chicken stock as liquid and are generally served with added seafood, eggs, poultry, or vegetables. *Brown sauce* is made from a brown roux and beef stock and is used mainly with meats.

Other sauces include:

- *Simple sauce:* Such as au jus
- *Butter sauce:* Butter with added seasonings
- *Sauce thickened with eggs:* Hollandaise
- *Tart sauces:* Barbecue sauce, ketchup
- *Starch-thickened sauces:* Use of different thickening agents

Desserts

Imaginative dessert planning and thoughtful preparation can complement the rest of the menu, balance cost, and add nutritional value to the entire meal. Dessert choices balance the satiety level of a menu—for example, a fruit or light dessert with a hearty meal and a cool, delicately flavored dessert after a spicy main dish or salad.

Foodservice operations with limited resources can increase the variety of desserts they offer by using mixes and other convenient dessert products. Cake mixes in particular yield consistent, uniform results when directions are followed carefully. Manufacturers provide recipes for variations on the basic cakes, which can be substituted for many cakes requiring on-site skilled labor for preparation. Frozen dessert products such as cakes, cheesecakes, pies, and other pastries are also widely accepted. When deciding to use a convenience dessert, foodservice managers must evaluate the cost of the convenience item compared with the skills of the employees, the cost of ingredients, and labor for in-house preparation. In addition, the product's quality should be evaluated objectively to determine which approach will yield the most flavorful, attractive product.

Few institutions use convenience desserts exclusively. For high-quality preparation in the facility, standardized recipes, appropriate tools, scales, and standard-size pans are needed. As always, employees should be trained in the correct use of recipes and equipment. Cooks and bakers need to understand the preparation principles for different kinds of desserts and the functional properties of the various ingredients.

Cakes

Cakes are flour-mixture desserts that contain a leavening agent to incorporate air into their structure. In butter cakes, the shortening, sugar, and eggs are creamed to incorporate air. Pound cakes are leavened almost completely by creaming. Angel food and sponge cakes are leavened by egg-white foam. Sifting ingredients and beating or manipulating the batter also incorporate air. When experienced employees are required to make cakes, it may be more profitable to purchase frozen cakes for consistency and quality.

Butter Cakes Four common mixing methods are used for butter cakes. One is the *conventional method*, in which the thorough creaming of the fat and sugar is the first step. Eggs or egg yolks are added next. All dry ingredients are sifted together and added alternately with the liquid. If only egg yolks are used, beaten whites may be folded in last. Although more time-consuming and complicated than the others, this method is widely used because it produces good cakes with a light, fine, velvety texture.

The *muffin method* is quick and easy. In this method, dry ingredients are weighed, sifted, and mixed together. All the wet ingredients—liquid, eggs, and melted shortening—are stirred into the dry ingredients. Although the muffin method is easy and fast, it tends to produce a coarse-textured cake that quickly becomes stale.

The *quick method* or *one-bowl method* is sometimes called the high-ratio method because it has increased proportions of both sugar and fat. The dry ingredients, shortening, and part of the milk are combined and beaten at medium speed for 2 minutes. The rest of the milk and the eggs are blended into this mixture for another 2 minutes. High-ratio cakes have good volume, are tender, and have a moist and flavorful texture.

Many commercial bakers use a fourth method, known as the *pastry-blend method*. In this method, fat and flour are blended before other ingredients are added in two stages. First, half the milk and all the sugar and baking powder are combined and blended into the fat-flour mixture, after which the eggs and remaining milk are added.

All four methods are suitable for quantity recipes. As new recipes are tried and evaluated, it is helpful to see which method is specified. The method determines the characteristics of the end product.

Panning is an important aspect of making cakes. Uniform and appropriate amounts of batter per pan are essential to produce uniform portions. If possible, the batter that goes into each pan should be weighed. If there is no scale available for this purpose, the same amount of batter should be measured into each pan by using a measuring cup or similar item. Butter cakes are baked in greased and floured pans, either in the standard 12-by-20-by-2-inch pan or in an 18-by-26-by-2-inch pan for sheet cakes. More variety is possible when the shape of the baking pan is varied. Layer cakes are easy to make by stacking two 12-by-20-inch cakes or by stacking quarters of a sheet cake baked in an 18-by-26-inch pan.

The oven temperature specified in the cake recipe should usually be used. Baking temperatures for conventional ovens should be lowered by 25°F (14°C) for convection ovens. Excessive temperatures cause cakes to peak and crack on top; deficient temperatures cause them to fall. Cakes should be cooled before frosting. Staleness will occur more rapidly if the cake is refrigerated, but some frostings make refrigeration necessary. Freezing retains quality in cakes for a long time and allows advance production for service on days when production loads are heavy. Cakes should be frozen unfrosted.

Foam Cakes Angel food cakes that have added ingredients to produce better foaming properties should be considered. Batch size should not be so large that uniform mixing is impossible. Dry ingredients may be combined by hand with egg-white foam using a wire whip; machine blending can be done at low speed just until all ingredients are combined.

Sponge Cakes Sponge cakes are similar to angel food cakes except that whole-egg foam is used, with lemon juice added to stabilize the foam. In either type of cake, overbeating must be avoided. Superfine granulated sugar will produce a cake with a finer grain. Accurate time and temperature control are needed to produce a light brown crust. Cakes should be cooled thoroughly in pans before they are removed for icing and portioning.

Cookies

The methods of preparing cookies are similar to those used for butter cakes: sugar, shortening, and eggs are creamed; any other liquids are added; and dry ingredients are blended in last. Labor time for portioning cookies is greater than for cakes but can be decreased by using scoops to portion, by avoiding cookies that have to be rolled and cut, and by making larger cookies. Bar cookies cut labor time significantly.

Cookies should be baked on bright aluminum baking sheets or pans with low sides. Pans should be oiled with unsalted fat unless the cookies are rich in fat and the recipe specifies no pan greasing. Baking sheets should be cooled between each use. Most cookies freeze well after they are cooled. When time permits, several varieties should be baked at once to handle the projected needs over several weeks or months. Cookie dough may be purchased frozen, preformed, or chilled.

Pies and Pastries

Piecrust has few ingredients but must be in just the right proportion to produce a tender, flaky, and flavorful crust. Pies can be made in round pans or, for greater simplicity, in 12-by-20-inch or 18-by-26-inch pans. If large pans are used, a single-top crust makes handling easier during service. These pies save assembly time and baking space. If individual round pans are used, pie making can be handled in an assembly-line process.

Pastry dough should be weighed before rolling to achieve uniform crusts with minimum waste. Various kinds of pastry rolling or forming machines can be used to eliminate hand labor. If hand rolling is necessary, a lightly floured board should be used, and the dough should be rolled evenly. Pie dough should not be stretched to fit the pan; some slack should be provided to offset shrinkage during baking. Shells baked unfilled should be pricked with a fork and chilled before baking to cut down on shrinkage. Double-crust pies should have cuts in the top crust to allow steam to escape during baking. Brushing the top crust with milk or beaten egg produces a golden brown color. Frozen preformed pie shells in pie tins save time and failure of the product.

A wide variety of pie fillings can be made from traditional recipes or from prepared mixes and canned fillings. Broken or irregular pieces of fruit of good quality and flavor can be added to prepared pie fillings to give them a fresher taste.

Pastry and pies can be frozen. The quality of most pies will be better if the pie is frozen unbaked. Most custard- or pudding-filled pies should not be frozen unless special starches for thickening have been used in the fillings.

Fruit Desserts

Fruits make an excellent dessert offering. Cut fresh fruits can be combined in almost endless variations to produce fresh-fruit desserts. They can also be combined with canned fruits. Varied shapes and sizes of fruits and complementary flavors and colors should be used. Fresh-fruit desserts should be garnished attractively, and the fruits should be kept chilled until service.

Thoroughly chill canned fruits that are served as a dessert. Adding a garnish such as whipped cream, mint leaves, or an edible flower can dispel the right-out-of-the-can look. Frozen fruits should be thawed in the refrigerator before serving.

Canned or frozen fruits can be used in crisps (that is, with crumb topping) or served warm and with a whipped topping or a hard sauce. A fruit cobbler can be made by spreading sweetened biscuit dough over layers of canned or fresh fruit and baking until the top is browned. Shortcakes are another simple yet attractive fruit

dessert, made in the same way as baking-powder biscuits but using a richer and sweeter dough. Preparation can be streamlined by rolling the dough directly onto 18-by-26-inch pans, baking, and then cutting into squares. Two squares, with fruit in between and on top, are stacked to build the shortcake. Whipped topping or whipped cream is added as a garnish.

Other Desserts

Light and nutritious desserts can be made from various egg and milk combinations: puddings, dessert soufflés, and cornstarch puddings. They are easily prepared in quantity and are relatively inexpensive compared with many other desserts. Mixes and frozen egg products can simplify the production of these items. (The principles and techniques for the preparation of these foods are described in the sections on eggs and milk earlier in this chapter.) All desserts in the category should be stored in the refrigerator until they are served.

Fruit-flavored gelatins are the basis for many easy and attractive desserts. For an appealing look, plain gelatin can be congealed in shallow layers and cut into cubes. Cubes of various colors can be combined for serving, with or without the addition of whipped topping. Partially congealed gelatins can be whipped and poured over a layer of clear gelatin for other simple yet attractive layered desserts.

Beverages

Most customers enjoy a beverage with their meals or to accompany a snack. Two of the most popular beverages for these purposes are coffee and tea.

Coffee

Although making coffee is a relatively simple task, a number of principles apply for producing good coffee. The process must begin with clean brewing equipment. Next, the quality and freshness of the coffee, water, and filters must be considered. Ground coffee must be stored tightly sealed in a cool, dry place usually under refrigeration or freezing; usually regular tap water is preferred. The correct grind, proportion, brewing time, and brewing as specified by the coffee brewing equipment should be followed. Finally, holding of brewed coffee must be monitored carefully so that it is held at 185°F to 190°F (85°C to 88°C) for no longer than one hour. Flavored and specialty coffees are popular. Some foodservice directors have found that offering these types of coffees along with espresso and cappuccino from take-out counters can be both popular and profitable.

Tea

Tea is a popular beverage served either hot or iced. A simple beverage, it does not require the equipment or labor needed for coffee service. For hot tea, fresh hot water should be poured directly into a heated pot and served with an individual tea bag. The customer can then brew the tea to the preferred strength.

Larger tea bags can be used for brewing iced tea. Fresh, hot (not boiled) water is poured over the tea bags and allowed to steep for five minutes. The tea bags should then be removed and cold water added to achieve the correct strength. The tea should be held at room temperature for no more than four hours. Specialty teas, particularly herbal blends, have also become popular as a beverage with dessert or at break time.

Two-Spoon Tasting Technique

Tasting a product before it is served helps to control flavor and food quality. Tasting does not mean eating a meal to satisfy hunger.

The following is an acceptable antiseptic method for tasting foods:

- Secure two clean spoons for each item to be sampled.
- With the first spoon, take a sample from the pot that is to be tested.
- Remove the spoon from over the food.
- Transfer the sample to the second spoon.
- Move to the side of the pot before tasting.
- Taste the food.
- Be sure the second spoon is not returned to the pot.

Spices and Herbs

What is the difference between a spice and an herb? There are several ways to define the two words. *Spices* are often defined as the flowers, fruits, buds, bark, roots, leaves, or seeds of certain plants and herbs. Another definition is that spices are parts of aromatic plants grown in the tropics, whereas *herbs* refer to leaves and soft portions of aromatic plants grown in the temperate zone. (Thus, *spice* can be used to mean either an herb or a spice.)

Spices are divided into three categories:

1. *Aromatic:* Anise, caraway, cardamom, cinnamon, cloves, cumin, ginger, mace, nutmeg, rosemary
2. *Stimulants:* Mustard, pepper, turmeric
3. *Sweet herbs:* Basil, marjoram, oregano, sage, savory, thyme

Cooking with herbs and spices is an ancient and universal art. When used well, these are the ingredients that distinguish a master chef from a mundane cook.

When cooking with herbs and spices, the eye and the nose are almost as important as the tongue when it comes to judging the relative age and quality of a dried herb or spice. The greener the herb (such as parsley) or the redder the spice (such as paprika), the more likely it has kept its best flavor traits.

The freshness and quality of spices may be tested by briskly rubbing a small amount between the palms, then smelling. Experiment with cinnamon first and leave cayenne until later.

Store dried herbs in covered glass jars or tightly closed containers. Keep the jars and containers away from heat or steam. Purchase in small quantities that can be used within a year. Spices and herbs depend on certain oils formed during growth for their flavor.

Improper storage will damage these natural oils. Constantly check for pest infestation.

Herbs

Herbs are plants that do not have permanent woody tissue and dry down at the end of the growing season, although a plant may have a biennial or perennial life span. The whole plant or plant parts are used medicinally or for their flavor or aroma in food preparation. The following are tips for using herbs and spices:

- Dried herbs are far more potent than fresh; ¼ teaspoon of dried herb is about as strong as 1 teaspoon of fresh herb.
- There are no set rules for using herbs and spices. To experiment, one could start with ¼ teaspoon dried herbs in a recipe to serve four.
- Use a light hand. The goal should be just enough flavor to complement a dish, but not enough to crowd out the flavor of the food. To season with herbs and spices, the cook must taste frequently.
- Blends should be so subtle that only the cook, or perhaps an expert, can tell what herbs have been used.
- If fresh herbs are used, they should be chopped finely. The more finely they are chopped, the more the herb oils can escape. The flavor of the herb depends on the presence of these oils.
- Blending or heating with butter, oleo, or salad oil is the best way to draw out and extend the flavor of herbs.
- Dried herbs should be soaked in a teaspoon of water, lime juice, or both for 15 minutes before using.
- For soups, sauces, or vegetable juice cocktails, sprigs of fresh herbs should be tied in bouquets or dried herbs put in a small cloth "bag" and added. They should be removed from soups or other hot dishes after 15 minutes and after 1 hour from chilled juices.
- Leaving herbs in any dish too long will cause strong flavors to develop.
- For casseroles or à la king dishes, finely chopped fresh or dried herbs should be added directly to the mixture, with the admonition that a little does a lot!

Spices

Spices are vegetable substances with a distinctive flavor and aroma, such as cloves and pepper, used in food preparation to add zest, piquancy, or interest to any food. Unlike herbs, which are frequently used fresh, spices are usually dried.

Cooking with Herbs and Spices

The following list offers suggestions on when to use which herb or spice (see Appendix 20.1 for other terms):

- Allspice: Soups, stews, pot roast, sauces, marinades, fish, shellfish, cakes, candies, cookies, spaghetti, sweet potatoes, squash

- Anise: Leaves: salads, especially apple; seeds: cookies, candy
- Balm, lemon (leaves): Steep for a delicate aromatic drink or add to hot or cold tea; use lemon and sugar
- Basil (leaves): Tomatoes, cucumbers, eggplant, squash, green salads, eggs; can be grown in a kitchen window box or garden
- Bay (leaves): Meats, potatoes, soups, fish, casseroles, marinades
- Caraway (seeds): Boiled with potatoes in jackets, potato salad, sauerkraut, cream or cottage cheese, cookies; partly matured green caraway seeds are delicious to munch
- Chervil (leaves): Salads and salad dressings, soups, omelets; chief ingredient in what the French call *fines* herbs
- Chili powder: Used in Mexican dishes such as chili, tamale pie, enchiladas; tomato and barbecue sauce; dips; egg dishes; corn; cheese; bean casseroles; eggplant; and Spanish rice
- Chives (leaves): More delicate than onion; blend with any herb mixture; used in salads, omelets, potatoes, and with cream and cottage cheeses; can be grown in a kitchen window box or garden
- Cilantro (Chinese parsley): Leaves of the coriander plant; used in burritos, tacos, enchiladas, Mexican salsas, and guacamole; in dry form, used in Spanish, Asian, and Mexican foods
- Cinnamon: Used whole in pickling, preserving, hot chocolate, coffee, mulled wine, stewed fruits, and compotes; used ground in cookies, cakes, French toast, bread, dessert sauces, sweet potatoes, squash, lamb roast, stew, ham glaze, apple sauce and butter, pudding, and custard
- Cloves: Whole: used as garnish for ham, fruit peels, onions, pork, beef, beverages, pickling, and soups; ground: used in fruit cakes, spice cakes, cookies, bread, fruit salads, green vegetables, and mincemeat
- Coriander (seeds): Cookies, French dressing
- Dill: Leaves: broiled or fried meats and fish (especially salmon), fish sauces, creamed or fricasseed chicken, potato salad, cucumbers; seeds: pickles and bread; can be grown in a kitchen window box or garden
- Fennel, sweet: Leaves: fish, salads; stems: blanched stems of Florence fennel may be eaten raw like celery, added to salads, or braised in meat stocks
- Garlic (bulb): Italian foods, kosher foods, salad dressings, cocktail sauces, barbecue sauce, beef, pork, and lamb roasts
- Ginger (root): Preserves, chutneys, curries, carrots, tea, cookies, and fruit compotes
- Marjoram: Cold meat sandwiches, meat and poultry stuffing, gravies, soups, and sausage; can be grown in a kitchen window box or garden
- Mint (leaves): Lamb, peas, cream of pea soup, tea, fruit drinks, and candies; can be grown in a kitchen window box or garden
- Nutmeg: Cakes, cookies, pies, pastries, meat, vegetables (especially green beans), poultry, seafood, eggnog, fruits, puddings, and soups

- Oregano (leaves): Used in Italian dishes, especially pizza, ravioli, lasagna
- Parsley (leaves and stems): Sauces, meat loaves, soups, casseroles, cocktails, garnish, and sandwiches; can be grown in a kitchen window box or garden
- Rosemary (leaves): Use rosemary sparingly for special accent in cream soups made of leafy greens, poultry, stews, sauces; blend chopped parsley and a little rosemary with sweet butter and spread under the skin of the breast and legs of roasting chicken; can be grown in a kitchen window box or garden
- Sage (leaves): Use sparingly with onion for stuffing pork, duck, and geese; pound fresh leaves and blend with cottage and cream cheeses; steep for tea
- Savory (leaves): String beans, soups, veal and poultry stuffing and sauces, egg dishes, and salads
- Tarragon (leaves): Leading accent in green salads, salad dressings, salad vinegar, fish sauces, tartar sauce, and some egg dishes
- Thyme (leaves): Meat and poultry stuffing, gravies, soups, and egg dishes; can be grown in a kitchen window box or garden
- Winter savory (leaves): An important accent in chicken and turkey stuffing, sausage, and some egg dishes; combine with parsley and onion juice for French omelets in winter

SUMMARY

The selection of a food production and forecasting system should be carefully considered because each health care operation presents its own unique demands. A variety of food production equipment and forecasting techniques have been developed to help operations meet their specific needs. The foodservice director must become familiar with all of these options and their cost and versatility. The selection of a food production and forecasting system appropriate for a particular operation also requires a thorough study before a decision can be made. Patients' food preferences, the availability of a skilled workforce, the quality of food products available, budget resources, and cost of the equipment needed for a food production system must all be analyzed.

In this and preceding chapters, procedures for planning the menu; purchasing, receiving, and issuing the ingredients; and measuring and preparing the ingredients in accordance with standardized recipes for a specific number of portions have been discussed in detail. Now it is time to transform the raw materials into finished products, with the objective of producing high-quality products at allowable costs.

High-quality food production depends on the use of appropriate preparation methods and equipment by skilled foodservice workers. Fulfilling the objective of destroying harmful microorganisms and at the same time producing nutritious, appealing, and affordable food is the responsibility of the foodservice director and the production workers. The success of every foodservice department depends on the quality and cost of the food served.

Assembly and serve
Béchamel sauce
Biscuit method
Bisque
Chowder
Conduction
Convection
Cook and chill or freeze
Cook and serve
Emulsion
Fricasseeing
Herbs/spices
Induction
Ingredient control
Muffin method
Padding
PHF

Portion control
Production forecasting
Production monitoring
Production system
Quick method
Radiation
Roux
Slacking
Smoke point
Standardized recipes
Stock
Subjective technique
Tallying
TCS
Time-series forecasting
Two-spoon tasting

DISCUSSION QUESTIONS

1. Analyze the various food production methods to determine the advantages and disadvantages of each.
2. What are the best, most efficient, and less time-consuming forecasting methods? Discuss in order.
3. How would you improve communications with the production and service staff?
4. Demonstrate how to take a household recipe and enlarge for use in a 150-bed facility.

5. How would a computer system improve the review of all recipes used by the department, including evaluating for a consistent format, updated cost, and nutritional information.
6. Explain the concept of an ingredient control program for cost-saving, equipment, space, and labor needs and consistency of product.
7. Discuss various cooking terms used in foodservice, equipment needed for each method, type of heat source, and what food would be best cooked by each term.

APPENDIX 20.1
A Culinary Glossary

à la carte   On the bill of fare, prepared as ordered

à la king   Served in cream sauce containing green pepper, pimento, and mushrooms

à la mode   "In the fashion"; when applied to desserts, they are served with ice cream

al dente   Cooked just enough to have a little resistance to the bite

anchovies   Small fish found in the Mediterranean; salted and pickled, they are used as appetizers or mashed as a spread for bread and crackers

antipasto appetizer   A course consisting of relishes

aspic   A clear savory jelly, usually made with gelatin and seasoned with meat juice; used as a garnish for entrées, tongue, and salads

au gratin   "Scalloped"; meat, poultry, fish, or vegetables in cream sauce sprinkled with cheese

au jus   Served in its natural juice or gravy

bard   Wrapping meat in fat before cooking

béchamel   White sauce made by stirring equal portions of chicken stock and light cream into a white roux (flour and butter mixture)

Benedictine   A religious sect; a liqueur made principally at the time of knighthood, at the Abbey Fecamp in Europe

bisque   A thick soup made from fish or shellfish; may also refer to a type of frozen dessert, sometimes defined as ice cream to which finely chopped nuts have been added

blacken   Cajun style of cooking, food is heavily seasoned, cooked over high heat until charred

blend   Combining ingredients until a smooth texture and consistency is reached

borscht   A vegetable soup made primarily of beets; a native dish of Russia

bouillon   A clear soup made by cooking meat, fish, or vegetables in liquid

canapé   An individual appetizer served either hot or cold, usually fried or toasted bread spread with or supporting any of a wide variety of highly seasoned foods; generally served as the first course of a meal as an hors d'oeuvre and eaten with the fingers (unless accompanied by a sauce or otherwise made impossible to eat this way); often served on a doily

caper   The bud of a southern European plant; it is pickled and used as a flavoring or garnish

caviar   The salted roe (eggs) of the sturgeon (or other fish) that is served as a sandwich spread or as an appetizer

chantilly cream   Sweetened, flavored whipped cream

chicory   A green of the endive family; the leaves are used for salad, and the root is used as a cooked vegetable or sometimes roasted and ground and used as an additive for coffee

chiffonade   With or of finely shredded vegetables

chitterlings   Pig intestines used as food or as sausage casings

chop   Cutting into smaller pieces by using a knife, food processor, or major piece of chopping equipment

chowchow   A relish of chopped vegetables in a strong mustard sauce

chutney   An Indian relish frequently made of fruits, spices, vinegar, and sugar

clarify   Skimming the surface of a food to remove fat

compote   A dish of stewed fruits, usually retaining their natural shapes

consommé   A highly seasoned clear soup usually made from two or three kinds of meat, fowl, veal, and beef

crepe   A thinly rolled pancake of egg and flour batter served filled with a meat, fish, or vegetable mixture, covered with sauce, and served as an entrée; made with sweeter batter, the crepe may be served with a fruit or liqueur sauce as dessert

croutons   Diced pieces of thin, toasted bread served with soup or salads

curry   An East Indian dish originally meaning a stew, characterized by the pungent flavor of curry powder; the finishing, or seasoning, of the dish is frequently done at the table

demitasse   A small "half" cup of black coffee usually served after dinner

dredge   To coat a food item with flour, bread crumbs, cornmeal or other product—usually done before frying

eclair   A pastry with a cream or custard filling

eggs à la Benedictine   Poached eggs served on broiled ham placed on split, toasted muffins and garnished with hollandaise sauce

endive   A curly salad green

entrée   A subordinate dish served between the main courses at a dinner, usually a "made" dish of unusual food or food prepared in an unusual manner; it is garnished and may be accompanied by a sauce; an entrée should be easy to eat and pleasing to the appetite but not satisfying; the term originally referred to dishes accompanying the first course, but in the United States, it now refers to the main dish of the main course

fillet   Strips cut from the underside of the loin of beef or mutton or from the boned sides of fish

fines herbs   A combination of chives, tarragon, chervil, and parsley chopped finely for flavoring soups, sauces, omelets, and fish

flambé   To flavor food with an alcoholic liquid, such as rum, by igniting the liquid; the alcohol burns off, but the flavor remains

flan   A dessert of baked custard covered with a burnt-sugar syrup

frappé   A mixture of fruit juices frozen to a mush and eaten with a spoon

fricassee   Veal, rabbit, or fowl cut in pieces, browned, and stewed in gravy

gherkin   A small warted pickle

glacé   Iced, frozen, glassy, glazed, frosted, candied, crystallized; glacé fruit is fruit dipped in hot syrup that has been cooked to a hard-crack stage

goulash   A Hungarian hash of diced meats, onions, tomatoes, potatoes, and seasonings

gratin   See au gratin

grenadine   Pomegranate syrup used for beverages

gumbo   A thick, rich creole soup containing seafood, okra, and other ingredients

hollandaise   A sauce of butter, vinegar, egg yolks, and seasonings; much used with broiled fish, vegetables, and the like

hors d'oeuvre   Side dish or relish served before the meal; used for luncheons but not for dinners in France; usually served cold and made of salty, tart, or crisp materials, such as canapés, radishes, olives, pickles, fish, sausages, and the like

jardiniere   Something prepared with a variety of vegetables

julienne   Vegetables or meat cut into fine strips or shreds; named for the famous chef Jean Julienne, who invented clear vegetable soup with the vegetables cut into matchlike strips

jus   See au jus

kosher   A term applied to food prepared with special precautions; kosher meat from strictly healthy animals that have been slaughtered and prepared with the Jewish requirements

knead   To work dough by pressing it with the palms of the hands, folding, turning, and pressing it until it has been worked to a contained, elastic texture

lyonnaise   A sautéed dish seasoned with onions and parsley

marinade   Usually a French dressing in which salad foods, such as cooked vegetables and meats, are allowed to stand to render them more palatable; it is also used for uncooked meats to soften tough fibers and to keep meat fresh; in the latter case, the marinade may be simply a brine or pickling solution

marinate   Soaking food in a liquid to flavor or tenderize it

marzipan   A confection made from almond paste, egg whites, and sugar; it is frequently molded into special shapes and decorated

meringue   A combination of beaten egg whites and sugar; it may be formed into small cakes and baked or used as a pie topping and baked until brown

monosodium glutamate (MSG)   A white crystalline substance added to food to bring out and enhance natural flavors, usually meaty flavors

mousse   A delicate mixture containing whipped cream or beaten egg whites; mousses with pureed meats, fish, poultry, or vegetables as a base are usually bolstered by gelatin and served cold; dessert mousses contain flavored whipped cream and eggs and are either frozen or chilled; also used to describe hot dishes that have a particularly smooth texture

mulligatawny   Derived from two East Indian words signifying "pepper water"; a highly seasoned thick soup characterized chiefly by curry powder; meats, vegetables, mango chutney, coconut flesh, rice, cayenne, and so forth are used to suit the taste of the cook

neapolitan   A molded dessert of two to four kinds of ice cream or water ice arranged in horizontal layers; the mixture is sliced across for serving; the name is also applied to a gelatin dish arranged in layers of different colors

nectarine   A variety of peach; it is smooth and looks like a cross between a peach and a plum

nesselrode   "Containing chestnuts"; Nesselrode pudding: a frozen dessert with a custard foundation to which chestnut puree, fruit, and cream have been added; it has been termed the most perfect of frozen puddings

Newburg   A form of creamed dish with egg yolks added; originally flavored with lime or sherry; most often applied to lobster but may describe other foods

parfait   "Perfect"; a mixture containing egg and syrup; may also refer to a layered dessert of fruit, syrup, whipped cream, and ice cream; frozen without stirring; may be molded but is more commonly served in parfait glasses

paté   A rich, well-seasoned blend of finely ground meat, poultry, or fish often baked in a crust

pawpaw   A green melonlike North American fruit

pectin   A substance found naturally in certain fruits, especially apples and currants; when boiled with sugar, it acts as a gelling agent

petit fours   Small fancy cakes

pilaf   A rice preparation in which the rice is first cooked briefly in fat and then braised in a seasoned liquid; fish, meat, poultry, or vegetables may be added to make a more substantial dish; another name for this preparation is pilau

pistachio   Nuts from a small tree of the cashew family, used in flavoring ice creams and other desserts

plank   A hardwood board designed for use in cooking and serving broiled meat or fish, thought to give the meat a superior flavor; planked steak is served on a board and is attractively garnished with a border of suitable vegetables or fruits

poach   Cooking in water or other liquid

praline   Usually a flat sugar candy flavored with nuts

quiche   A pie shell filled with an egg mixture and baked until puffy and brown; quiche Lorraine is a combination of eggs, bacon, cream, and Swiss cheese

ragout   A rich, highly seasoned, thickened stew frequently made of sweetbreads but more often with meat and vegetables

ravioli   A mixture of ground meat, cheese, or other foods cooked inside folded pieces of noodle paste and served with a variety of sauces

remoulade A highly seasoned dressing of egg yolks, vinegar, chopped pickles, olive oil, barley, and mustard

render To slowly heat pieces of solid fat to obtain liquid fat

rissole Usually a seasoned meat, fish, or vegetable mixture enclosed in pastry and then deep-fried or baked; sweet rissole may be filled with jam, fruit, and nuts; may also refer to foods cooked to a golden brown crispness

roux A cooked mixture of flour and butter; a common thickening agent in many sauces and gumbo

sauté Small amount of oil used to heat and brown foods

scallion Any onion that has not developed a bulb

shallot A form of onion with a stronger but mellower flavor than the common varieties

smorgasbord Swedish appetizers, including pickled fish, salads, cheeses, celery, pickles, and the like

soufflé A fluffy baked preparation of a flavored sauce or base into which is folded stiffly beaten egg whites; it is served hot either as an entree or as a dessert, depending on the ingredients

succotash A concoction of corn and lima beans; native to North America

sweetbreads The pancreatic glands of calf or lamb

terrine An earthenware dish in which meat, poultry, or fish patés are cooked

timbale A mixture of meat or vegetables cooked in a cup-shaped mold, or a paste crust fried in cup shapes and filled with any variety of meat or vegetable mixtures

tortilla Thin fried cornmeal pancake

truffle An underground fungus somewhat like a mushroom but very rare, used as a garnish for other foods or as a delicate seasoning in egg dishes, patés, and some sauces; truffles are either black or white and are available canned; also a chocolate confection

tutti frutti Referring to a mixture of "all fruits"

vinaigrette An oil and vinegar dressing with salt and pepper to which other seasonings and herbs are sometimes added; it is used as a salad dressing, as a marinade, or as sauce for vegetables, meat, and fish

Yorkshire pudding An English dish usually served with roast beef; this popover-like mixture may be baked with the meat or separately with some of the drippings from the roast

zest Outer rind of clean lemons, limes, oranges, grated to add flavor to a variety of foods, may also be purchased dry

zwieback A twice-baked bread that is usually sliced and toasted, now used largely in feeding small children

CHAPTER 21

DISTRIBUTION AND SERVICE

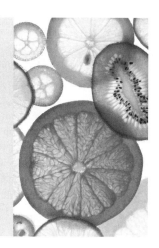

LEARNING OBJECTIVES

- Analyze various methods for assembly, distribution, and service of food to customers.
- Know the needs, wants, and perceptions of customers.
- Determine factors affecting distribution systems, equipment needs, and styles of service.
- Calculate tray delivery time and tray accuracy.
- Use a patient satisfaction form to determine how well the customer grades the service and food.
- Set up a *sensory assessment* for a test tray.
- Complete a plate-waste study for both patient and non-patient customers.

HOW MENU ITEMS are presented to customers has as much, or more, effect on the success of a health care foodservice operation as the menu itself. The department director may plan and the operation may produce menu items that customers want, but unless items are served in a manner they find satisfactory, customers will rate the operation as unacceptable.

Advances in technology have provided many options in patient, resident, and nonpatient meal service systems for health care facilities. Several factors affect the design of the system: the physical layout of the health care operation, customers' nutrition and social needs, the type of food production system used, the operation's standards (for food quality, quality monitoring systems, and *microbiological* controls, for example), the timing of meal service, skill levels of service personnel, and the cost of equipment. Most health care meal service systems include tray service to patients' rooms and cafeteria service for visitors, staff, and (in extended-care facilities)

ambulatory residents. Other services may be offered to meet customer needs.

Generally speaking, meal service systems are designed to satisfy three functions: assembly, delivery, and service. *Assembly* involves portioning and plating menu items for specific customers. The items are then delivered to the point of service. Service is the actual presentation of menu items to customers. Depending on the nature of the operation, the service function may be a simple process (such as providing over-the-counter service) or a complex activity (such as providing patient trays). Because most menu items are at peak quality immediately following food preparation, efficient meal service systems rely on the accessibility of appropriate personnel and suitable equipment. The various components of each meal service system should be considered apart from the production system components because many of the meal service systems can be combined with any or all of the alternative production systems, as illustrated in Table 21.1. Figure 21.2 shows carts that may be used to serve for both the cook-serve and cook-chill.

In this chapter, assembly, delivery, and service of meals to three customer groups—patients, residents in long-term care facilities, and nonpatients—are discussed. Certain advantages, and in some cases disadvantages, of specific delivery systems are pointed out. Major delivery systems covered in the chapter include centralized and decentralized tray service, cafeteria service, and table service. Service refinements and expansions such as over-the-counter, catering, vending, and off-site meal service operations are addressed with a view toward their revenue-generating potential.

CUSTOMERS

Distribution and service constitute the third functional subsystem. The distribution of the produced food to the customer depends on:

TABLE 21.1   Alternative Systems for Foodservice to Patients

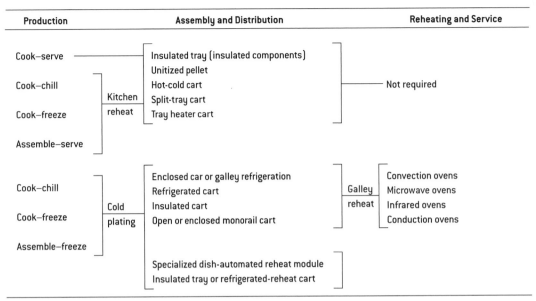

Production	Assembly and Distribution	Reheating and Service
Cook–serve Cook–chill — Kitchen reheat Cook–freeze Assemble–serve	Insulated tray (insulated components) Unitized pellet Hot-cold cart Split-tray cart Tray heater cart	Not required
Cook–chill — Cold plating Cook–freeze Assemble–freeze	Enclosed car or galley refrigeration Refrigerated cart Insulated cart Open or enclosed monorail cart	Galley reheat: Convection ovens Microwave ovens Infrared ovens Conduction ovens
	Specialized dish-automated reheat module Insulated tray or refrigerated-reheat cart	

Source: Adapted from Herz, 1977.

- The type of production system used
- The time and effort of meal assembly before service
- The distance between the production and service areas
- The amount of time between completion of production until service to the customer

Equally important is knowing who the customers are. A *customer* is someone who purchases the goods offered by foodservice, such as food, or receives services offered, such as nutrition counseling. Customers are classified as external customers and internal customers. *External customers* are the end users of the products made by an organization. In a health care system, external customers are the inpatients and outpatients and their families.

Internal customers are the individuals who provide direct service to the external customers; they belong to the organization that produces the service. Internal customers in health care are employees, suppliers, physicians, nurses, and other health care providers. Another type of customer, the captive cliental, is rare today because of our mobile society. *Captive clientele* are customers who must use a product or service because they have few to no other options. Customers, both internal and external, have other choices of where to purchase goods and services.

Health care facilities exist to provide services to their customers. As a result, the foodservice department, in concert with nursing and other interdisciplinary professionals, needs to ascertain:

- What is the best time to serve meals that will not interfere or delay other provided services?
- How many meals should be served: three, four, or five?
- What is the best type of service to offer the customers: tray, dining room, or buffet?
- What types of food should be served to meet the nutritional needs of the customers as well as religious, cultural, and other needs?
- Where will the meal be served?

- What department personnel will serve the meal? Nursing? Foodservice? Others?

Health care foodservice may be in competition with other retail and commercial operations that are vying for the same customers. Employees may eat in the facility cafeteria, at an outside foodservice operation such as a fast-food outlet, or may call out for services such as pizza. It is important for health care foodservice operations to maintain a certain percentage of participation. The participation rate refers to the proportion, usually a percentage, of a potential customer group that actually uses the facility's foodservice operations. The participation rate has a significant effect on the operation's revenue. Providing products and services that meet the needs of the customer also means that customers are loyal to the operation. When they enjoy the product and service, it means repeated patronage.

What are the needs of customers? What do customers need, want, or like? The answer varies but includes some of the following:

- *Cost of product.* The product must be priced to meet the financial capability of the largest majority of customers.
- *Preferences.* Preferences, as the word implies, are personal and they change with age, health, or financial status.
- *Choice, variety, and expectations.* Customers want a choice of food items made by a variety of food production methods as well as a variety of methods of service, such as buffets, self-service bars, and the like. Customers rate food against what they expect to purchase.
- *Medical conditions.* Customers' medical conditions can change their needs. Medical conditions may affect appetite, taste, and the enjoyment of the food. Special attention needs to be given to these customers.
- *Religious, cultural, and ethnic needs.* Other factors besides hunger play a role in customers' expectations and

perceptions of the foodservice. It becomes the foodservice director and the dietitian's job to provide food and service that may affect customers' religious, cultural, and ethnic needs. Foods that will meet these needs should be incorporated into the menu.

- *Lifestyle and personal values.* Personal values play a role in accepting food and service. Because of the hectic pace of today's lifestyles, many customers eat in their automobiles while traveling from one place to another. The "grab-and-go" lifestyle needs to be addressed. Personal values such as vegetarianism, which is not based in religious beliefs but may based on health reasons, moral beliefs, or other reasons, have increased with the baby-boom generation. These preferences need to be addressed.
- *Comfort foods.* Other preferences that may need to be addressed include the need for comfort foods to meet the emotional needs of customers, especially when they are stressed, afraid, or ill.
- *Language barriers.* Language barriers may present a problem if a customer does not understand the menu items, has a problem hearing or seeing or other illness, or does not read or speak the language.
- *Other changes.* Illness, medication, or age can cause changes in taste or food preferences.

It is difficult to meet all the needs and expectations of all customers. However, foodservice directors need to recognize that providing food and service that meets the needs, wants, and perceptions of customers and does not harm them is not only their job but should also be considered a privilege.

MEAL SERVICE SYSTEMS

As indicated earlier, most health care foodservice operations serve a variety of markets or customer groups. Typically, these are patients, residents, and nonpatients (staff, visitors, and guests). The wants and needs in terms of meal service characteristics differ for each of these markets. Therefore, the foodservice director must design a variety of approaches to meal service to meet the various demands of these three groups.

Patient Meal Service

Patients are the primary target market of health care foodservice operations. Because most patients are unable to dine in a central location and because they are located on different floors or in different buildings, the director must devise a meal service system that incorporates the three broad functions mentioned earlier. That is, they must devise a system that provides food to patients' rooms by means of assembly of individual trays, delivery of trays to patient locations, and service of trays to patients.

Tray Assembly

Two major systems are used to assemble patient trays. In one, *bulk food* is distributed to patient areas, where it is then plated (*decentral-*

ized assembly system). In the other, food is assembled at a central location that uses various delivery methods to transport it to individual patients (*centralized assembly system*).

Decentralized Assembly Systems In *decentralized assembly systems*, most of the food is prepared in the food production area. Bulk quantities are then conveyed in food trucks with heated and unheated compartments to serving galleys in the patient areas, where individual trays are then assembled. For example, breakfast items (coffee, toast, eggs, and special food items) are prepared in the serving galley, which may be equipped with a hot plate, a microwave or convection oven, a coffeemaker, a toaster, a cabinet for heating dishes, and a refrigerator. Trays, dishes, and service ware are returned to the galleys for cleaning and storage. Alternatively, the dishes and flatware can be washed in either an adjacent area or a central dishwashing room. In either case, they are returned to the serving galleys and stored there until the next meal. Decentralized assembly requires less space in the foodservice department but more in the patient areas. When compared with centralized systems (discussed below), this approach generally results in less time between assembly and the actual service of trays to patients but utilizes valuable patient floor space. This system has seen a reduction in the last few years due to the expense and duplication of efforts. In a small operation, about four employees are needed. They include the starter, who places tray, silver, condiments, napkin, menu, and cup and saucer and sends the tray down the conveyor to the hot food server (cook), who places both regular and modified foods on a plate, while the cold-food server adds all cold foods, including milk, tea, salads, and desserts, and a checker who checks the tray for accuracy, places dome covers on hot food, and places the completed tray on a cart. The tray line is about 15 feet long and closely resembles L-2 in Figure 21.1.

Centralized Assembly Systems *Centralized assembly systems* are used in most health care foodservice operations today because they permit better control of food quality, portion size, food temperature, and diet modifications. They also reduce overproduction and waste, require less equipment, and greatly diminish labor time. In a centralized assembly system, foods are plated and trays are made up in a central location in or near the main kitchen. Because centralized assembly requires more tray preparation time than is the case with decentralized assembly, the department director must give special attention to this function of the meal service system. Centralized assembly usually is accomplished by means of a tray line.

Tray lines are composed of several stations, each of which is supported by equipment and staffed by a foodservice employee. Figure 21.1 depicts a number of straight-line serving lines. For the smallest operation, four employees are assigned stations. In a large hospital, as many as 14 employees may be assigned to specific duties. Most tray lines require at least three types of equipment. Temperature maintenance equipment helps preserve the aesthetic and microbiological quality of menu items. Accessibility of trays, dishes, service ware, and a variety of condiments requires a variety of dispensing equipment. Finally, the trays are moved from one station to the next usually by means of a conveyor.

FIGURE 21.1 Typical Tray Makeup Lines

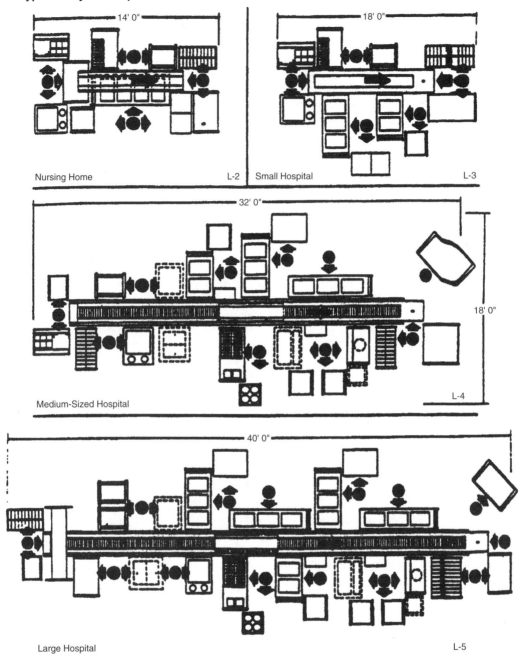

Nursing Home   L-2   Small Hospital   L-3

Medium-Sized Hospital   L-4

Large Hospital   L-5

Note. Plans show suggested work assignments (as described by various companies). The Level 1 (L-1) system is not shown because it does not involve a tray assembly system; that is, food is served from pots on the stove to plates and placed on carts to be delivered to patients (usually found in small facilities). Tray assembly systems are designed to meet the needs of the facility and the number of trays to be assembled and served. Hence, in a large hospital, a longer, more complicated tray assembly system is needed, as well as more personnel to assemble and serve. Scale: 3/16 inch = 1 foot.

Maximizing tray line efficiency is an important goal for operations that use centralized assembly systems, especially where management is challenged to do more with less, provide quality service, and a safe work environment. This system is called the *pod* and/or *work cell* system (see Figure 21.2). This system uses a small-size tray line assembly work cell using less space than a straight tray line. The system was developed by Toyota and has been successfully implemented in foodservice operations.

The work cell system allows the foodservice director to provide quality service to patients using fewer employees. Using the work cell system eliminates the traditional long straight tray line and replaces it with a flexible work cell design that can be configured into an array of work cell formats (Figure 21.2). The system is made up of mobile equipment that can be used and placed where needed for a continuous flow of work. Depending on the meal and the complexity of the menu a variety of equipment can be configured

FIGURE 21.2 B-Lean—Fully Configurable, Fully Mobile, Modular Meal Assembly System

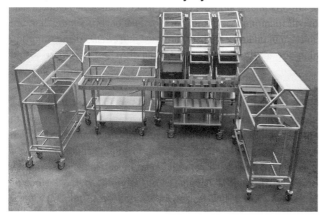

Source: Used with permission, Burlodge USA, 2011, www.burlodgeusa.com.

into a work cell. Using this system four to seven employees can prepare the same number of trays as 10 to 14 employees using a straight tray line system, The objective of this system is getting the right things to the right place, at the right time, in the right quantity to achieve perfect flow while minimizing waste and being flexible and able to change.

The system has seven principles:

1. Equipment must be flexible in order to be easily broken down and reconfigured.
2. Must be ergonomically correct and support safe work habits.
3. The flow of work must produce faster outcomes.
4. All equipment is constructed to support a system that can help reduce maintenance.
5. The equipment must allow restocking while the system is in use without interrupting service.
6. The cost must be reasonable and fit in existing or proposed space.
7. The equipment must be mobile, easily cleaned.

The latest centralized system is *room service*. Implementation of room service has improved patient satisfaction and in many cases reduced food and labor cost. The work cell or pod system works well with room service. Room service uses the following seven steps for service to the patient:

1. Patient orders meals, when *they* are ready, within the set hours of service (some health care facilities offer the service from 7 A.M. to 8 P.M.; others have 24-hour service—hours of operation vary). When admitted, a patient may be given a menu or there will be a preexisting menu in the patient's room for the patient to make selections. The menu may stay the same offering multiple choices of all items. The patient may order his or her service by telephone, computer, or in person from a foodservice patient associate. The nutritionist or dietitian checks the order to determine if the food ordered meets the medical nutrition therapy order.

2. If the system is a cook-chill rethermalization the food is retrieved from the food bank.
3. Using the work cell/pod system cold plating is completed.
4. Food is rethermalized using a compact oven.
5. When food is ready to serve, it is placed on a hot/cold cart.
6. Food is delivered to patient room.
7. The total time from order to delivery is 22 to 24 minutes.

Other systems for foodservice follow this route. 1. Same as above → 2. Order is called to the diet office which checks to determine if food ordered is allowed on patient's diet order → 3. Food order is sent to production staff who prepares the hot food, the foodservice room service personnel secures/prepares cold food. Secures trays, china, and so on → 4. Production sends hot food to assembly area and room service personnel adds hot food (using a heat retention system such as a wax pellet) and cold food to prepared tray → 5. Finished tray is placed on a room service transport cart and delivered to patient room. (A number of meals may be prepared at one time and delivered when all trays have been completed.) → 6. From order time until tray reaches patient may take as long as 45 minutes. The time depends on how much production—both hot and cold must be made at the last minute. Using sous vide individual portion packed foods helps to reduce the time. More information on sous vide may be found at *A Practical Guide to Sous Vide Cooking*, http://amath.colorado.edu/~baldwind/sous-vide.html.

Before implementing room service it is important that an objective evaluation is made of the department to determine the effect of room service on production—especially if there are numerous food outlets such as a cafeteria, self-operated vending, C-stores, other nonpatient off-site foodservice.

- Equipment needs—will existing work?
- Labor—will it reduce staff or add staff?
- Will food cost increase?
- Will there be a need to renovate the department?
- Will the increased cost improve patient satisfaction and meet the needs of the patient?
- Menus will need to be revised.
- Refrigerated and freezer space evaluated to determine if the existing space is available for an extended menu.
- Some management systems will need to be revised—job descriptions, salary scale, approval of unions, union changes, policies and procedures.
- Administration must approve the concept (see business plan, Chapter 3) and provide the funds needed for the change.
- Nursing and other health care providers must be involved to determine how meal service at all different hours will affect medications, tests, and other therapies.

Some health care facilities implement room service, using their existing staff, after they perform the necessary evaluation; others hire "room service consultants" to perform the evaluation, plan the menu, and implement the system. When consultants are used, the cost must be included in the total cost for the change.

There are varying reports of cost and satisfaction of room service. Most operators agreed and are pleased with switching to room service as the patient satisfaction results have increased, staff is motivated as more of the staff have an opportunity to see and talk face-to-face with patients. Another advantage is that food cost controls are easier to monitor and there is a reduction in the "peaks and valleys" of production and service.

Tray Line Requirements

Although the specific requirements of a tray line vary from operation to operation, several common questions should be considered:

- Is the spacing between menu and tray sufficient to allow tray line employees time to read the menu and place correct items on trays? (Room service and work cells can limit this.)
- Is the spacing between trays appropriate to achieve proper pacing of the work?
- Is there a smooth workflow at each station? (In the lean work cell/pod system the flow is much smoother.)
- Is the menu format consistent so that similar items are always located in the same place on every menu?
- Is the workload balanced between each station so that each employee contributes about the same effort on each tray? (This is vital when using a long straight-line system.)
- Is there a means of resupplying food and acquiring missing items (for example, a "floating" employee) so that the tray line is not delayed or stopped? (This system can eliminate some of these problems.)

Observation of each workstation will identify work methods that require improvement. To further enhance productivity of the tray line, the foodservice director can employ a variety of industrial engineering techniques, such as assembly line balancing. *Assembly line balancing* is a technique that reassigns tasks so that tray line work assignments are more evenly distributed in terms of time and work.

The following are the steps required in patient meal service in health care facilities:

- Patient or resident is admitted.
- Diet orders written by physician.
- Order relayed to food and nutrition service by nursing personnel.
- Menu provided to patient or resident (room service menu may be in room). If spoken menu is used nutrition hostess will visit patient/resident to discuss menu ordering; if selective menu food is selected a day in advance, menu may be place on patient meal tray, or passed out by the nutrition associate.
- Patient selects food using selective menu, spoken menu, or room service.
- Menus are "picked up," called in, or relayed by touchscreen computer to the foodservice central clerk's office.
- Dietary staff reviews request against written diet order, allergies, and patient or resident "write-ins."

- Food choices are tallied for hot and cold production (this would be true for all types of diet orders/menu selection system).
- Menu selections for each meal are filed in order of meal delivery to the patient unit; just before meal service, menus are adjusted for discharge, transfer, or new admission and approved for dietary changes. (This is not true for room service as room service can be at any time.)
- Menus are placed on tray at start station for assembly—if traditional tray line is used.
- Requested items are added by personnel at each station of the tray assembly system.
- Menu is checked against food on tray by manager.
- Trays are placed on delivery carts—room service uses a special room service cart and may hold up to 10 to 12 trays.
- Carts are delivered to patient's unit.
- Trays are served to patient or resident by foodservice staff, nursing staff, or others.
- After trays are served, additional patient requests are phoned in or sent electronically to main clerk's area for later distribution.
- Once the patient completes meal, tray is retrieved by foodservice personnel and sent to the dishwashing area.
- Dishes are washed, stacked, and heated for next meal.
- Meal carts are cleaned and stored.
- Garbage, trash removed; dishwashing area is cleaned and sanitized.

Tray Delivery

Because the point of decentralized tray assembly is in close proximity to the patient, trays are normally delivered by small carts, which are wheeled directly to patient rooms. Temperature maintenance does not pose a particular problem, but food items transported from the tray assembly area should be covered.

If centralized tray assembly is used, trays are transported to patient units for service, which depends on some means for serving food at the proper temperature through either temperature maintenance or rethermalization. The first five delivery systems shown in Table 21.1 are appropriate for use with any of the food production systems described in the previous chapter. The delivery systems are all designed to maintain the hot and cold temperatures of food cooked or reheated in the kitchen. Each delivery method has different characteristics that must be considered in relation to the physical layout and other features of the facility.

Insulated Tray The *insulated tray system* uses a lightweight thermal tray with individual molded compartments that hold both hot and cold foods. Specially designed china or disposable tableware is placed in the tray compartments, and the entire tray is covered with an insulated fitted cover. An insulated cup is used for beverages. No external heat or refrigeration sources are used in delivery or holding, so the foods must be at proper serving temperatures when plated. Food temperatures can be maintained up to 30 minutes by the insulating properties of the tray. Meal trays are delivered to the patient areas, either stacked or individually, on an open cart. No specialized carts are needed. It is somewhat difficult, however, to wash the trays and covers in most conveyor dishwashers, and special racks may be needed. Insulated tray systems can be purchased or leased.

Keep It Simple System   A temperature maintenance system that uses a dome that is constructed with a temperature reflecting materials to encapsulate the temperature generated from the food. The plate has been engineered with a temperature retaining technology to preserve food temperature. The system does not use a heated base or pellet. It is considered maintenance-free (www.randrfoodservice.Info).

Unitized Pellet   The *unitized pellet system* calls for the assembly of all hot items in a meal on a preheated plate. The preheated plate is placed on a preheated pellet base and covered with a preheated stainless steel or plastic lid that may also contain a metal or *wax-filled pellet* to retain heat and moisture. Cold items are placed on a tray simultaneously with the covered hot foods. The trays are delivered to the floor in an uninsulated cart. Insulated cold ware for beverages, cold salads, and cold desserts also may be used. Maximum holding time is about 45 minutes. Either china or disposable tableware can be used. Careful monitoring of pellet, plate, and lid temperatures is necessary.

Hot and Cold Cart   The *hot and cold carts system* uses a tray cart with electrically heated and refrigerated compartments to maintain proper food temperatures during transport. Standard trays are assembled with cold food plated and placed in the refrigerated compartment. Simultaneously, hot foods are plated and placed on a separate smaller tray and stored in the hot food compartment. Standard or disposable tableware is used. In another variation of this system, plated hot foods are placed in heated drawer compartments. Both versions require that the tray be reassembled at the point of service. Holding time before service can be longer because the temperatures are electronically controlled. These transport carts are heavy, but they can be motorized for use in large facilities or in facilities with ramps. Considerable cart storage space is required, and more labor time is needed for cleaning and maintaining the carts than in most other systems. Newer type carts are available that have been designed as multiportion point-of-service carts, for cook-service, cook-chill, and cook-freeze. Dual-oven carts that are heated by forced air convection allow simultaneous heating of foods with different densities and texture. (For more information see your equipment dealer.)

Split-Tray Cart   The *split-tray system* is similar to the hot-cold cart system, except that hot and cold items are loaded on opposite sections of the same tray. The trays are slotted to allow placement of one side of the tray in a heated compartment and the other side in a refrigerated compartment. Special carts are needed, as are electrical outlets for plugging them in on the patient unit. With this system, tray reassembly is unnecessary.

Tray Heater Cart   The *tray heater system cart* uses specially designed disposable tableware on which hot and cold foods are placed at serving temperatures. Trays with resistance heaters built in at the dinner plate and bowl locations keep hot foods hot. When the loaded trays are placed into the battery-powered cart, the resistance heaters are activated. The heating of individual food items is regulated by preset push-button controls. The tray heaters do not affect the temperatures of cold foods, but no refrigeration is provided in the cart. The heaters are automatically disconnected as each tray is removed from the cart. Hot beverages are delivered in insulated containers. The cart's batteries, which provide the electricity for heating and moving the cart, must be recharged between uses. This system is more complex than the others described and may require more maintenance. Because specialized disposable tableware is used, operating costs may be higher than for some of the other heat-maintenance systems.

Chill-Delivery and Food-Rethermalization Systems   The next four delivery systems listed in Table 21.1 are available for use with cook-and-chill, cook-and-freeze, or assembly-and-serve production systems in which foods are portioned cold and reheated in galleys in the patient areas. These delivery systems are designed to maximize food quality by reheating the food just before service, without extended hot-cold conditions required in the heat-maintenance systems. Labor time and costs may be reduced due to the system's greater scheduling flexibility in food portioning and tray assembly.

Foods held and delivered cold can be **rethermalized** (heated) by using a heat-support cart or insulated trays or components. The heat-support cart controls the amount of energy needed to rethermalize the food on the plate and in the bowl. However, foods must be plated in a specific way. The cart keeps the food hot until the tray is removed from the cart. Each cart has an insulated drawer for ice cream and other frozen products. However, the temperatures of other cold foods cannot be properly maintained. Insulated trays and tray components may be used for heating dinner plates. Mugs for hot and cold beverages also are available.

The features common to most of these systems include the transport of chilled or frozen foods on fully assembled trays to floor galleys. The types of carts used include enclosed nonrefrigerated, insulated, refrigerated, and carts on monorails. When nonrefrigerated carts are used, refrigeration is provided in the floor galley.

Several types of specialized equipment can be used for the rethermalization of foods: convection ovens, microwave ovens, tunnel microwaves, infrared ovens, and conduction ovens. Microwave ovens currently are the most commonly used rethermalization equipment. Service personnel must be trained in proper reheating procedures to attain the best food quality possible.

Several factors should be evaluated in selecting a tray delivery system:

- The system's ability to maintain the desired level of food quality
- The system's compatibility with the existing production system and facility layout
- The number of work hours and level of skill or training needed to operate the system
- The space requirements and mobility of system equipment
- The initial costs for equipment, maintenance, and leasing

- The costs associated with the purchase of specialized or disposable tableware
- The cost of renovating an existing facility to accommodate the system
- The flexibility of the system to accommodate a change in production system, number of meals served, or menu pattern
- The system's energy requirements

Seek assistance from a consultant in determining the best delivery system for the facility. There are numerous new systems on the market and many more are being proposed. Consultants can provide the facility's foodservice the latest trends. In many cases consultants can save the facility money.

Tray Service

Tray service for health care patient meal service is a joint responsibility between nursing and foodservice. Once the tray has been delivered to the patient unit it must be presented to the prescribed patient for whom it was assembled. For many years nursing department employees delivered the food trays directly to the patients' bedside. It was found that this approach resulted in delays in meal service, which had a negative effect on temperature and food quality. Today most foodservice department employees deliver food trays directly to the patient's bedside, resulting in a reduction of time between the delivery of the tray to the appropriate patient unit and presentation of tray to the patient. Regardless of which department delivers the tray the following needs to be accomplished: To provide continuous quality improvement, each department personnel will need training in customer service. Nursing will need to know the importance of delivering food at a safe temperature and foodservice personnel must realize that nursing may be in a crisis situation, involved in a clinical procedure they need to finish. It is important for each department to work together to ensure that the quality of the food is not deteriorating or that the temperature is not in the danger zone. The following points should enhance mealtime:

- Nursing staff needs to have the patient ready for the delivery of the tray by foodservice—this usually includes some form of hand washing, bed raising (if applicable), and the overbed table positioned over the bed or the patient in a comfortable sitting position in a chair.
- Foodservice staff (or nursing personnel) serving the trays need to verify that the name on the tray card is the same as the name of the patient. Due to the Health Insurance Portability and Accountability Act (Privacy Act), each facility must have a procedure in place to verify that the correct patient is receiving the correct meal (procedures, medicines).
- Nursing staff (or auxiliary personnel, such as trained volunteers or paid workers) will need to provide meal service assistance to patients who may need it. This may include opening packages, cutting food, and feeding.
- If the patient is having difficulties with the meal due to an inability to chew or has a complete dislike of the food being served and refuses to eat, another meal of equal nutrition must be offered.

- Foodservice personnel are well groomed without any perfume or aftershave or body odors.
- Personnel should distribute the trays promptly once they are received on the unit.
- If a patient has a question or request, refer to nursing staff or dietitian.

Regardless of the approach, there must be cooperation between nursing and foodservice departments to minimize delays and provide quality service.

Additional Tray Line Concerns

In a health care organization, challenges always occur in providing the patient meal service. The type of menu system, changes in diet orders, and lengths of stay all influence patients' satisfaction. The selective menu system can be a problem, especially for the written and spoken menu. Patients may be too sick to select, they cannot read the menu, they are unavailable to select because of being out of their room when menus are retrieved, they have been newly admitted and missed the advanced selection time, or their diet order has been changed. When any of the above happens, patients receive a meal tray that may not meet their expectations. When the likes, dislikes, and allergies of a patient are known, the clerk's office will complete a menu based on this information, which helps in patient satisfaction.

In hospitals, the average length of stay has steadily decreased from 7 days to 4.5 days or less. Some patients may be in longer or others for just a day. Some of the shorter-stay patients may not receive any meal service other than liquids, and others may not have the opportunity to select their food items because of reasons previously mentioned.

Patients can become confused when using a written selective menu because of the advanced selection required, which is usually for the next day. They select a meal in advance, and when the tray is received, patients are disappointed because they did not receive what they thought they had selected. This colors their perception of the operation because they think a mistake has been made. When using the written selective menu system, the clinical staff needs to communicate effectively to patients how the system works. When the spoken menu is used, this problem is reduced and room service further reduces the problem.

Patients may have been told that their diet order has been changed or that an ordered test will interfere with meal service. They may perceive that when they do not receive the food they selected that a mistake has taken place. Because of some last-minute changes, patients may receive a late tray. Late trays are usually served after all other patients' meal trays have been served.

Monitoring for Performance (Another Continuous Quality Improvement)

Accuracy, quality, and productivity for patients' meal service can be objectively measured. One method that is frequently used is trays per minute. *Trays per minute* is defined as how many trays are produced during each minute of a tray assembly process. The simple calculation would be as follows: the time the tray line started, the time the tray line ended, and the total number of trays assembled.

To calculate, determine the time in minutes and divide the number of trays by the total number of minutes. For example, the tray line starts at 11 A.M. and was finished at 12:30 P.M. This would be a total of 90 minutes, during which 400 trays were assembled. Trays per 90 minutes (400) are divided by 90, equaling 4.4 trays per minute. This figure can be used as a benchmark among peers. When this figure is higher than the peer group the foodservice director will need to investigate all steps of the operation to determine if/where changes need to be made.

Tray delivery time is another objective measure. *Tray delivery time*, or turnaround time for delivery, measures the time from the assembly of trays until the trays are received by the patients. For example, measure the time a preselected number of trays begin (add time to tray card) and complete the assembly (add time to tray card) and the time it takes to deliver the trays to the patients.

All times are recorded and added together for the total time. (Tray line started at 12:05, tray line ended at 12:20, and tray arrives at patient bedside at 12:32; from start to patient receives tray, 27 minutes). These data can be used to evaluate the system to determine if there is a problem—equipment or personnel—and to make appropriate changes.

The delivery of quality hot and cold food to the patient/resident is the goal and all procedures/methods need to be evaluated to meet this goal. Variables in turnaround time that must be considered are transportation delays, patients not ready for meal service, a patient's room changed, and emergencies that may be occurring on the patient unit. Measures should be made for a range of times. The longest period of time will need to be evaluated and possible changes made.

The accuracy of the tray is another objective measure. *Tray accuracy* is defined as how accurately the tray line employees followed the patient's selections in assembling the tray. The most effective method to use is to add several "dummy trays" to the total meal service. Once these trays reach their designated area, the manager compares the items on the tray with what had been selected. Calculate the error rate in the following way:

- Count the total number of selected items for each dummy tray; add all these numbers together: for example, 60 items for 6 trays.
- Count errors that were found: 4 missing items.
- Divide the number of errors (4) by the total number of items (60) = 0.07, or a 7 percent error rate.

To determine the accuracy rate, subtract the total number of errors from the total number of items served. This is the number of items accurately serviced: 60 − 4 = 56. Divide the number of items served correctly (56) by the total number of items (60), for an accuracy rate of 93 percent. This rate is important because it relates to patient satisfaction; the need for additional training; and a review of balancing the work on the tray line, especially if all errors occurred at the same station and the same employee. Routine monitoring is necessary to determine if the process needs to be changed and if more training is needed.

Special Patient Meal Services

In addition to providing basic meal service to patients, a facility may offer a number of optional patient services that can produce additional revenue. Examples include gourmet meal service, wine service, fruit baskets, or in-room foodservice for patients' family and guests. For each optional service offered, an efficient delivery method must be developed to ensure customer satisfaction.

Resident Meal Service

In response to the environmental changes described in Chapter 1, many hospitals have incorporated skilled-nursing units, long-term care facilities, or rehabilitation centers into their organizations. One such change relates to the social aspects of group dining areas, of particular importance for residents in such extended-care facilities. Also, proper implementation of the Omnibus Budget Reconciliation Act (OBRA) requires new, more flexible and appealing dining facilities. Therefore, the dining areas used by ambulatory persons in these facilities should be comfortable and attractive and provide enough space for wheelchairs and service personnel to move freely. Having one or several dining rooms may be desirable, depending on the needs and capabilities of residents. Several types of service can be used, each of which has advantages and limitations.

Cafeteria or Buffet Service

Cafeteria service is common in facilities whose residents are sufficiently ambulatory. Some assistance from food servers may be needed for persons who have difficulty carrying their filled trays to the table. With cafeteria service, attractive food displays, temperature control and portion control, are possible. Diners may make their own selections. In some instances a *buffet service* is available. A buffet service is a display of food that customers serve themselves with what they want to eat in the amount they think they can eat. Service ware is available for customers to serve themselves. The buffet bar, such as a salad bar, may be two-sided. Multi-units are usually used for hot food, sauces, and soup, or this may be one small unit. A separate area is set up for desserts and beverages, or in other instances the waitstaff will serve water and all beverages, including alcoholic ones if a liquor license has been granted. Buffets can be elegant with service ware, displays, and quality food that is well presented. There are two important rules governing buffet service: monitor the buffet area for cleanliness and safety (no food on the floor), and monitor each food bin for the appropriate amount of food.

Dining Room Service or Group Dining

Dining room service is where patients or residents and in some instances families go to the dining area for meals. In some facilities, the patients or residents may be served a prepared tray or they may order from a menu.

Table Service

The service provided by full-service restaurants, referred to as *table service*, may be appropriate for some types of health care foodservice operations. Table service, another option for dining room service, presents some difficulties when a selective menu is offered, but restaurant-style menus may be used. Because foods are portioned in the kitchen or service area, residents may not be able to modify their portion sizes or choose sauces, gravies, and condiments as easily as in a cafeteria. Unless portion sizes are carefully tailored to the residents' needs, plate waste may be higher than expected. In facilities where table service is customary, an occasional buffet, such as a Sunday brunch for residents and their families, makes a pleasant change in routine.

In some facilities that use a more formal method of service for patients, residents, and family members, waitstaff may be used to serve the meals. The waitstaff has been trained to provide a variety of services. This service can be expensive but can be used for special holidays.

The waitstaff should be trained in the four basic service styles: French, Russian, English, and American.

1. The *French* style of service is often used in exclusive and expensive restaurants. Portions of food that may be fully or partially cooked are brought to the dining room on serving platters and placed on a small heater called a *rechaud*, which is placed on a portable cart called a *gueridon*. The cart is wheeled to the table where the *chef de rang* completes the preparation. The chief waiter then serves the plates, which are carried by a *commis de rang*, who is an assistant waiter to each guest. This is the most expensive service because of the number of personnel involved and the leisurely pace of service. The service is gracious and individual.

2. The *Russian* style is the most popular, especially in better restaurants and hotel dining rooms. In this service, the food is completely prepared and portioned in the kitchen. The needed number of portions for the guests at a table are arranged on serving platters by a chef. The waitstaff brings the platters to the dining room with heated plates and places them on a tray stand near the guests' table. A heated plate is placed in front of each guest, and the waitstaff carries the platter of food to each guest and serves each a portion using a spoon and fork as tongs in the right hand and serving from the left side. The service is speedy. The disadvantage is that the last person served may receive a different-size portion from an unattractive serving platter. If all guests order a different entrée, many platters would be necessary.

3. The *English* and *American* styles of service are similar. In the English style, all food is prepared in the kitchen, but meat is carried into the dining room. The chef places portions of meat on plates and passes them to waitstaff to deliver to each guest. The service uses family-style dishes, and platters of food are passed among guests at the table.

4. The *American* style service is basically used in the United States and is the oldest. In this style of service, a maitre d' or headwaiter greets and seats the guests and gives them a menu for the meal. Waitstaff takes their orders, brings the food from the kitchen area, serves each guest from the left side, and may remove soiled dishes from tables. Employees who are known as bussers may set up tables, pour water, serve bread and butter, and remove soiled dishes from the dining room.

Family Style

Family-style service is rarely used in extended-care facilities and is not recommended for several reasons. Portion control is difficult: considerable handling of foods at the table increases microbiological hazards and the danger of burns or spills, and food waste can be significant. More tableware is needed because bulk serving bowls and platters are used, and the amount of dishwashing is increased. More labor is needed in the dining room to clear tables than with the other styles of dining room service.

Group dining in long-term care facilities provides a pleasant, home-like atmosphere and social interaction. Many facilities that provide group dining offer a beautifully appointed table using linens, fresh flowers, and seasonal decorations. Most of these dining rooms have no television or radio but do play music for dining. The service may be table service or buffet. Employees who work in this area are well trained and dedicated.

Regardless of the style of service used, some basic rules need to be followed:

- The *cover* or place setting is made up of linen, china, flatware, and glassware to be used by each person at the table. When a tablecloth is used, it should be smooth and should drop evenly on all sides.
- The table must be *balanced* (when possible, the same number of guests on each side of the table).
- The *centerpiece* should be in the middle of the table and low enough that diners may see other diners at the table; when candles are used, they should burn above or below eye level. Do not put candles on the table unless they are to be lit.
- Each *place setting* should be set at equal distances, allotting 24 to 36 inches of the table edge space for each guest.
- *Utensils* should be balanced (same place setting for all guests).
- Dinner plates and handles of flatware should be placed 1 inch from the edge of the table, and the dinner plate is placed directly in front of the guest.
- The waitstaff uses the *left hand* and serves the food from the left side of the guest.
- Beverages are served using the *right hand* from the *right side* of the guest.
- Dishes and beverage containers are removed from the *left*.

Napkins are normally placed so that the open corner is at the lower right. The lower edge of the napkin should be even with the end of the flatware and the rims of the plate. Although usually placed beside the fork at the left of the cover, napkins may be placed in the center (between knives and forks for family service). When napkins are monogrammed or embroidered, they should be folded to display the design.

Flatware should be placed in the order in which it is to be used from outside toward the plate. Place knives to the **right** of the plate with the cutting edge toward the plate. Place spoons to the right of the knife with bowls up. Place forks to the **left** of the plate with tines up. Place butter spreader on the bread-and-butter plate across the upper edge. A butter spreader is not necessary when a dinner knife is on the cover. Place the salad fork to the **left** of the dinner fork. A salad fork is necessary only when the salad is served as a separate course. Place the dessert fork to the right of the dinner plate if a salad fork is included.

Glassware should never be more than three glasses. Place the water glass at the top of the knife. Place the milk or ice beverage glass to the right and slightly in front of the water glass. Place a juice glass to the right and in front of the last glass. Use an underliner beneath an iced beverage glass or hot beverage to accommodate the spoon. For wine service, a variety of glasses may be used. Wine glasses are placed to the right of the water glass.

China or *dinnerware* varies depending on the style of service. For American style of service, place the dinner plate in the center of the cover; for family service, place stacked plates in front of the server. Place bread-and-butter plates to the left near the top of the fork. Place the salad plate slightly to the right of fork tip above the dinner plate; place to left if a bread-and-butter plate is not used. Place coffee or tea cups to the **right** of the knife with the cup handle forming a straight line parallel with the edge of the table. Do not put cups on the table if the beverage is to be served with dessert only.

Patient Meal Tray Service

Trays for persons confined to their rooms should be attractively arranged for convenience and eye appeal. For patients who must be fed, sufficient time should be allowed so that the person doing the feeding is not hurried. The staff members who feed patients should be familiar with menu items so that they can answer questions and encourage reluctant eaters to eat at least some of every food item. Persons with limited vision find that eating is more enjoyable when the foods they are eating or being fed are described to them. Regardless of the type of service system used, residents eagerly await meals, and it is especially important that they be served on time and at the appropriate temperature.

Nonpatient Meal Services

In most hospitals and in many extended-care facilities, the number of nonpatient customers (visitors, staff, and guests) exceeds the number of patients. Therefore, meal service for these customers becomes a significant part of foodservice. A variety of approaches to meal service may be necessary to meet the wants and needs of this consumer group.

Cafeteria Service

The cafeteria may be designed as a traditional straight-line system or a modified version of a free-flow system in which employees, staff, visitors, and guests serve some food items themselves. The number of menu choices, the physical layout of serving equipment, the serving speed, the number of lines, and the number of cashiers affect the rate of customer flow in the cafeteria. When a large number of diners are to be served in a limited period, special attention to line speed may necessitate setting up additional lines, offering fewer choices, and adding more cashiers. Business during slow periods, typically evenings, weekends, and holidays, may be increased with strategies such as offering special discount prices for senior citizens' meals.

Limiting the operating hours of the employee cafeteria has become necessary due to the downsizing of staff and the expense of operating for a smaller number of customers. However, some foodservice departments have seen the profit potential in cafeteria operations that provide varied menu choices for employees and visitors over an extended period. The cafeteria should offer high-quality, attractively merchandised items. Employees of both the foodservice department and the health care operation as a whole usually enjoy special theme days for cafeteria service.

How can the foodservice department respond appropriately to the trend toward more ambulatory and outpatient care? In reviewing cafeteria operations, it is appropriate to examine the particular dietary needs of these patients. Specifically, the cafeteria's accessibility to ambulatory patients, appropriateness of menu offerings, price range of foods, and hours of operation should be evaluated. If the cafeteria is viewed as a profit center as well as a service center, the needs of all persons using the health care facility, including nonpatients, can be met in a fiscally responsible manner.

Payment methods need to be designed for nonpatient meal service. Four methods are commonly used:

1. For à la carte service (basically cafeteria service), individually purchased items are *paid with cash*.
2. A *debit card* is where a customer pays in advance for a specified dollar value card, and each purchase is subtracted from the balance. Periodically a customer adds more funds to the account. This is an electronic payment for meals.
3. Colleges and universities usually use *meal plans*. The plan provides meal service that is paid in advance for a given number of meals.
4. *Payroll deduction* is when an employee uses his or her identification badge that contains an encoded number. The employee purchases a meal, swipes the card through a reader, and the dollar value is charged and recorded in a database. The amount of all the charges is deducted from the employee's net paycheck.

Over-the-Counter Service

Because of the speed of *over-the-counter-service*, this type of operation is popular with several of the customer groups served by health care foodservice operations. After placing their orders with service personnel, customers expect quick service. Therefore, careful menu planning is essential to meeting this demand, and only foods that can be prepared or consumed quickly should be offered. Offering special meals of the day at discounted prices also may speed service.

Once customers receive their orders, several dining options may be available. Most over-the-counter operations have on-site seating and disposable service ware for on-site dining or carryout service. Counters may be designed to offer take-out services for bakery items and special holiday foods. Other over-the-counter options may include delivery of orders to customers. *Kiosks* may be mobile carts, which can be wheeled to other high-customer-traffic areas such as lobbies or patios, also have proved successful. Kiosks may be located in fixed areas and offer a larger variety than a cart. Kiosks provide specialty services such as coffee, desserts, and other items. A kiosk may be used as a carving station or a beverage station for buffet service. *Convenience stores* combine the elements of a grocery store with convenience food, especially cold canned/bottled beverages, snacks, premade sandwiches, salads, and some breakfast items. The store may also include a deli, freezer case for ice cream and/or prepackaged meals, coffee service, and microwaves, as well as snacks. *Home-replacement meals* (HRM) are meals a customer can purchase and take home to eat. Home-replacement meals may include a full meal or specialty items such as baked goods. They may be purchased in the C-store, the cafeteria, or the main kitchen. *Food courts* are popular in large facilities and may be operated by the foodservice operation or a franchised company. They may offer such items as pizza, fast food, ice cream, bakery, and local favorite food such as barbeque or a local ethnic food. A food court is a cluster of quick-service outlets that allow customers to go to the service area they choose. A common dining area is provided for all food court customers. Because many of the customer groups served by the foodservice department rely on quick meal service, these types of operations are popular. *Boxed meals* and *snack shops* may be located in a kiosk where boxed meals may be sold or an order for a number of boxed meals for a meeting could be offered through catering. Snack shops may be available in an area where families gather. Box lunches or other fast/snack foods may be offered.

Display, Service, and Transport

Foods must be handled according to specific local, governmental, and surveying agencies' rules/standards/guidelines. The following procedures should be enforced for displaying, serving and transporting food:

- Potentially hazardous food (PHF) should be kept at internal temperature of 41°F (5°C) or lower or at 140°F (60°C) or higher during transportation, display, and service.
- Milk and milk products for drinking purposes should be provided to the customers in unopened commercially filled packages no larger than one pint in capacity, or should be drawn from a commercially filled container stored in a mechanically refrigerated bulk milk dispenser. If such a dispenser is unavailable and portions less than a half-pint are required for service, the milk products may be poured from a commercially filled container no larger than one-half gallon.
- Cream and half-and-half should be provided in individual service containers or protected pour-type pitchers, or they

should be drawn from refrigerated dispensers for such service.
- Condiments for self-service use can be served in individual packets, from dispensers, or from original containers. Seasonings and dressings for self-service use can be served in the same manner or from counters or salad bars that are protected from contamination.
- To avoid unnecessary manual contact with food, suitable dispensing utensils (for example spoons, ladles) should be used by employees or provided to consumers who serve themselves. Between use, dispensing utensils should be stored in the food or stored clean and dry, under running water, or in a running water dipper well.
- Food on display should be protected from contamination by being supplied in appropriate packaging; by being displayed on easily cleaned counters or serving lines; or being protected by salad bar protector devises, display cases, or other shielding devices. Enough hot-or-cold-holding equipment should be available to keep PHF at safe temperature levels.
- Self-service customers should not be allowed to serve themselves with soiled service ware or utensils previously used by the customer. Beverage cups and glasses may be refilled without contaminating bulk supplies when served by the waitstaff. (Check local/state standards.)
- Leftover food on a customer's plate should not be served again, although packaged food that is still sealed and in sound condition may be salvaged (e.g., individual packets of condiments).
- Ice for customers use should be dispensed only by employees who use scoops, tongs, or other ice-dispensing utensils or through automatic self-service ice-dispensing equipment. Between uses, utensils and receptacles must be cleaned and stored in a way that protects them from contamination.
- Reuse of soiled tableware by self-service customers returning to the service area for additional food is prohibited. Reusable mugs and beverage containers may be used. (Check local and state regulation. Always check the latest issue of the *Food Code*.)
- During transportation, including transport to other locations for service, food must be held under the conditions specified for hot and cold holding.

Something New

"Food truck food" comes from a drivable commercial kitchen that provides foodservice that is not "inside of a brick and mortar building." These food trucks are mobile kitchens that can be driven from spot to spot. The kitchen is fully furnished, usually measuring 16 feet in length of kitchen space and approximately 24 feet from bumper to bumper. Cost varies from $130,000 to $150,000, depending on the equipment. Fryers, ovens, grills, freezer, refrigerators, dry storage space, three-compartment sinks, under-the-counter ice bin, coffee service, air-conditioning, ventilation, fire suppressants,

hand-washing sinks, generators, and liquid propane tanks. As in all foodservice operations, the menu is key to what equipment will be included in the truck. All local codes for a foodservice operation must be followed, and when the truck is in motion all employees must be wearing seat belts. Watch for one of these food trucks coming to your neighborhood soon. These trucks can be parked outside of your facility as another method of feeding staff and visitors.

Catering Services

In today's competitive environment, more and more health care facilities are seeking ways to expand their service lines and generate additional revenue. Catering is one way to accomplish this goal. Catering may take place on or off the premises (as discussed in Chapter 3). The event may be as simple as a coffee and tea setup for a meeting or as elaborate as a reception or banquet.

Before a full-scale catering program can be implemented, its feasibility should be studied. A number of questions need to be answered and logistics planned:

- What type of catering will be done?
- What kinds of menus will be offered?
- Will table decorations be needed?
- Can the existing staff handle the added workload?
- Does current staff have the necessary skills?
- What will additional equipment, supplies, and labor cost?
- Does the facility have space for this additional activity?
- How will start-up costs be covered?
- How will costs of the program be calculated?
- Will the foodservice department receive the revenue generated from the program?
- Can the revenue generated significantly enhance existing programs?

The food production system generally can accommodate the demands of catering with minor adjustments in its preparation equipment in terms of both type and capacity or volume. With careful attention to the scheduling of food production employees, the effect on production labor requirements (for example, in regard to both regular work hours and overtime) can be minimized. The type of meal service specified for a particular catered event will most certainly vary. For customers with limited budgets, buffets can be suggested. For customers who desire more elegant meal service, full table service with waitstaff can be provided.

Although the activities described above vary from one catered event to another, proper food handling is always critical. To implement the guidelines discussed in Chapters 13 and 14 the operation must provide transportation and holding equipment to ensure that food remains healthful. A variety of such equipment is available on the market.

Aside from being an excellent means of service expansion, special-events catering helps promote the foodservice department and enhance the larger facility's image. However, this specialized service requires dedication, creativity, expertise, labor, special equipment and serving components, funds to purchase needed food and supplies, savvy marketing research and complete support from administration. Policies and procedures must be developed that relate to menus available, hours of service, cost (and tax if applicable), and who receives the leftover food. (Refer to Chapter 3 for catering details.)

Vending Operations

Vending operations are a popular alternative for meeting the needs of employees, guests, residents, and outpatients on a round-the-clock basis in many hospitals and long-term care facilities. Compared with cafeteria service, vending services are less labor-intensive and require little space for the typical bank of machines. Vending machines maintain chilled food items at more appropriate temperatures than when they are displayed for cafeteria service. Potential customers generally are familiar with the operation of a microwave oven, the primary method for heating cold or frozen food items purchased from vending machines. Wherever chilled or frozen foods are vended, microwave ovens usually are provided. Some machines use debit card systems that eliminate the use of coins and cash. A cash machine may be available for changing bills up to $5.

In planning a vending service, a number of options are available for how to control and operate this type of meal service. The foodservice director can contract with a vending company to provide selections ranging from snacks and hot and cold beverages to full-scale offerings of hot canned foods, preplated convenience foods, sandwiches, pastries, snacks, and frozen desserts. Vending space can be rented on a per-square-foot basis, for a set amount for each item sold, or as a percentage of gross sales. Another option could allow the foodservice operation to provide food for the machines and contract with the vending company to provide other items (such as candy and beverages). A number of foodservice departments establish their own self-operated services. This decision, however, should be based on careful analysis of all capital and operating costs, along with close scrutiny of forecasted revenues.

Regardless of who controls the vending operation, food quality, equipment operation and maintenance, and vending area sanitation, temperature control, safety of food, and out-of-date products are major concerns that mandate attentive planning. Several factors must be considered, such as electricity sources, ease of restocking (review the security measures covered in Chapter 14), environmental amenities (comfortable and aesthetically pleasing furnishings), and waste disposal. If sanitation of the vending area is not a term of a contractual agreement with an outside service, this responsibility must be assigned to an appropriate department, such as maintenance or housekeeping.

Off-Site Meal Service

In addition to providing meal service to patients, residents, and nonpatients, many health care foodservice operations provide services to market segments in their surrounding communities. For example, *off-site meal service* to child-care centers, to elder-care centers, and to congregate feeding sites (churches or community centers, for example) is not unusual. Meal service also may be provided to home-confined individuals who require special diets or who cannot prepare nutritious meals for themselves. Sometimes health care foodservice operations are perceived throughout the community as the organizations best able to meet this need. As with catering special events, responding to the needs of the community can have a positive effect on the operation's public image and that of the health care facility as a whole.

Off-site meal service is another route to service expansion. However, as is true of catering services, meal prices must be determined carefully to cover food, labor, and supply costs and yet remain affordable for the customers. In many communities, additional funding is available from federal, state, or local sources. Prices and the extent of service for government-supported programs are contracted in advance.

Other factors must be considered when studying the feasibility of or planning for the implementation of off-site meal service. Appropriate operational standards for each functional area, such as menu planning, production, and sanitation, must be maintained. Therefore, to provide high-quality service to off-site locations, it is necessary to develop policies and procedures specific to this type of service. Many of these will depend on whether the food is to be provided to the customer in bulk quantities or as individual meals.

Quantity Meals

If the operation's menus are carefully integrated, providing bulk food for other health care facilities in the group or for congregate groups, such as community centers, does not require the preparation of additional menu items, just larger quantities. Next, a means for maintaining food temperature during transport is needed for all systems unless immediate delivery can be ensured. Many operations use insulated carriers or carts. The assembly of meals and the loading of delivery vehicles must be carefully integrated into the department's total work schedule.

The potential problems of providing food in bulk include the failure to return service ware and the excessive expense of disposable bulk food containers. Cost of operating a vehicle, gas and maintenance of the vehicle must be considered **before** any off-site programs are considered. Portion control at service time is more difficult to achieve, and it may be more difficult to monitor special dietary needs among community center attendees.

Individual Meals Many communities attempt to provide direct home meal service to individuals who are unable to prepare their own meals. One meal per day, which provides one-half to two-thirds of the adult daily requirements five days a week, is the most common service provided. A cold meal for later consumption also may be delivered at the same time as the hot meal. Mostly, meals are pre-plated in the foodservice department on disposable insulated tableware.

Volunteers or other community agencies—in which case training for the volunteers is required—often provide transport and delivery of meals to clients' homes. They need to understand the policies of the meal service program, details about special diets, food-handling procedures, emergency procedures, and techniques for assessing a client's general physical and mental well-being at the time of meal delivery. Home-delivered meal programs not only provide nutritional benefits for recipients, but they also play an important role in providing social contact for isolated persons and in serving as a check on their well-being.

Another type of individual meal service implemented at some operations is the sale of frozen meals for both normal and modified diets. These meals were originally developed for customers with special nutritional needs, such as weight-control patients, the elderly, or patients recently discharged from a facility. Operations that stock the meals for sale have found that they also may appeal to consumers who typically buy microwavable meals. To provide this service efficiently, foodservice directors need to help design mechanisms for the sale of these products as part of the meal service system. For instance, sales to nonpatients may require a location in the building with easy access to in-and-out parking. Other issues related to the feasibility of such a venture include estimating consumer demand, determining operational costs and capital requirements, and selecting an appropriate pricing method for the products. These and other related factors should be thoroughly explored before the implementation of such a venture.

STANDARDS

Quality standards pertain to the evaluation of the quality of service and satisfaction of customers. Certain standards must be monitored and, as appropriate, changes made when the standards are not met.

Standards that should be monitored include the serving temperature of food to patients, the trays per minute, the serving time, the acceptable number of negative responses to surveys, and employee hygiene, as well as other measurable objective criteria. Standards for customer services must be communicated to employees. They will need the proper tools, equipment, and training to meet the standards.

Customer Satisfaction

Customer satisfaction is difficult to accurately measure due to a number of variables such as age, education, socioeconomic and cultural levels, food habits, food preferences, and degree of illness of customers. Customer satisfaction provides an excellent means of learning more about customers even with the initial problems. A *customer satisfaction survey* is a series of questions designed to secure feedback from customers on the food and service. These surveys may be informal or formal, oral or written. An informal survey may include meal rounds, talking to the interdisciplinary staff, talking to peers in similar types of facilities, and observing food servers. Most of the informal surveys involve an oral approach. A formal survey may include written comment cards given to customers at mealtime or sent through the mail, suggestion boxes, formal interviews with customers, or a committee to provide suggestions, feedback, and monitoring.

When a written survey is used, the written questions should be clear and use plain language (Exhibit 21.1). This type of survey may be difficult to administer because some customers find it inconvenient or may not be able to read or write well enough to answer questions. Customers who answer this type of survey usually have strong positive or negative feelings.

Please answer each of these questions to help us provide you with better service. If additional space is needed, please write on the back of this sheet. Thank you for taking the time to help us meet your needs.

1. What is your diet order?
   - Regular
   - Medically modified
   - Don't know
2. Which meal did you enjoy the most?
   - Breakfast
   - Lunch
   - Dinner
3. What menu service did you use?
   - Selective
   - Spoken
   - Room service
4. Did you receive the meal items you requested?
   - Always
   - Frequently
   - Seldom
5. Have your meals been served at about the same time every day?
   - Yes
   - No
6. Please rate the following:
   Knocked on door before entering
   - Always
   - Frequently
   - Seldom
   - Never
   Checked arm band for name or ask patient name
   - Always
   - Frequently
   - Seldom
   - Never

7. How do you feel about the following? Please comment below
   Quality of food
   - Excellent
   - Good Average
   - Below Average
   - Poor
   Hot foods hot
   - Excellent
   - Good Average
   - Below Average
   - Poor
   Cold foods cold
   - Excellent
   - Good Average
   - Below Average
   - Poor
   Appearance of tray
   - Excellent
   - Good Average
   - Below Average
   - Poor
   Variety of foods
   - Excellent
   - Good Average
   - Below Average
   - Poor
8. What was your favorite menu item?

9. Menu items meet your needs, perceptions?
   - Yes
   - No
10. Were the foodservice personnel
    - Friendly
    - Helpful
    - Willing to answer your questions
    - Well groomed
11. If you were the foodservice director what would you do to change or improve the foodservice operation?

Other comments or suggestions:

Thank you for your help.

Optional _____

Date _____

Source: Developed by Ruby P. Puckett©, Revised 2010©.

EXHIBIT 21.2 Sensory Assessment for Test Tray (Another Continuous Quality Improvement)

Directions: Circle any negative comments for example

Sense	Food Item	Food Item	Food Item	Food Item
Color: Are the colors true? Are the greens bright, whites white, reds bright, or yellows a true yellow? Are all colors natural?				
Taste: Sweet, salty, sour, bitter, combination?				
Texture: Crisp, moist, dry, smooth, mushy, grainy?				
Aroma: Pleasant, unpleasant?				
Appearance: Looks the way it should, or unnatural, unacceptable?				
Temperature: Hot-hot, cold-cold, lukewarm?				

Person Testing Tray _____   Date _____

Source: Developed by Ruby P. Puckett©.

EXHIBIT 21.3 Plate-Waste or Food-Return Record (Another Continuous Quality Improvement)

When trays are returned from patient and nonpatient areas, check the amount of food returned.

Menu for Day   Date: _____

Name of Employee: _____

	Food Items Returned	What Percentage (Approximately) of the Serving Remains?	Why? Check Room Number or Time of Day for Nonpatient, When Possible
Patient tray			
1.			
2.			
3.			
Nonpatient tray			
1.			
2.			
3.			

Source: Developed by Ruby P. Puckett©.

With the oral method, customers realize that the foodservice department is interested in what they have to say and may provide too much information or too little because of the desire to be polite or to not hurt anyone's feelings.

When customer satisfaction surveys are used, efforts should be made to effectively select a cross-section of customers from all ages, sexes, and groups. All customers may be selected or those who have used the dining service during a specific period.

When developing questions, do not word the question to elicit a particular response or lead customers to a desired answer. Use open-ended questions because they cannot be answered with a "yes" or "no." They allow customers to answer honestly and truthfully.

After all surveys have been completed, the results need to be calculated and evaluated and, where appropriate, changes in food, menu, or service implemented.

Other Methods

Test trays are an effective way to determine if standards are being met. A *test* or *dummy tray* is a tray assembled as part of the usual tray line process specifically for the purpose of determining if the established standards are met. Test trays need to be evaluated by the director, dietitians, cooks, and meal servers. Exhibit 21.2 shows some of the items on a test tray that could be assessed.

Plate-Waste Studies

Plate-waste studies involve the calculation of the food that is left on plates after customers have completed their meals. The amount of uneaten food is systematically calculated to determine the percentage of uneaten food for each menu item (Exhibit 21.3). Trays should be selected randomly for a given meal. If the percentage of uneaten food is more than 50 percent, a study should be done when this same item is served again. If the percentage remains high, the menu, recipe, or production process (or all three) needs to be reevaluated.

ENHANCING CUSTOMER SATISFACTION

Whichever meal service system and customer group is targeted, to be truly customer-oriented and to operate competitively and cost-effectively, the health care foodservice operation must develop a marketing plan (described in Chapter 3) that allows room for customer feedback. As mentioned earlier, distributing customer surveys or conducting focus group meetings on proposed and actual menu items, publishing menus in advance, making questionnaires available, and offering daily specials at reduced prices and with evaluation forms are proven incentives for eliciting satisfactory ratings.

Both the design of a service system and how it is marketed are critical to the success of the foodservice department and to the larger facility. Both activities define the means by which products and services are presented to customers and how future demand for services is affected. A number of strategies described in Chapters 3 and 4 can be implemented to enhance satisfaction and demand.

Department Review

The department needs a formal system to self-evaluate to ascertain whether standards are being met. Checklists that evaluate the opera-

tion standards with "yes" or "no" answers assist in the evaluations. A section for comments should also be included. Once the checklist is completed, the results need to be evaluated. Compare the most recent survey results with those of several previous surveys. Have some standards been scored differently for the past several surveys? Does there appear to be a trend? Can unacceptable results be corrected by a change in procedure? Is the same employee responsible for making the same mistakes? How did the failure to meet the standards occur? What steps need to be taken to prevent this from happening in the future? Was the employee trained to carry out the function? Did the employee know the standards? Was "faulty" or broken equipment the cause? The department review can be used for retraining and counseling. It can also be used to determine if the standards are realistic and achievable.

SUMMARY

Health care meal assembly, delivery, and service to patients, residents, and nonpatients present a discrete set of demands for foodservice directors who must design meal service systems. Room service, a centralized service, is being implemented in many health care facilities, which has improved patient satisfaction. The length of time required for a tray to reach a patient's room from its assembly point is one of the most important factors in determining the selection and quality of food to be served. A wide variety of tray delivery equipment helps maintain the quality of food during this process. Numerous factors (such as the physical layout of the health care facility, the timing of service, and the cost of equipment) must be considered when planning an on-site or off-site meal service system.

Meal service for residents of extended-care facilities is usually provided by cafeteria, table, or tray service in a setting that takes into account the residents' social needs and ability to participate in group dining. The variety among nonpatient customers in terms of service preferences and expectations necessitates a variety of approaches. These range from cafeteria service to catering services to vending operations.

Many health care foodservice operations provide off-site meal service to community organizations, which can expand the service line, improve the facility's public image, and generate revenue. Regardless of the targeted customer group, it is important to implement marketing principles and customer relations strategies to enhance customer satisfaction.

American table service style

Assembly line balancing

Buffet

Centralized tray assembly

Convenience store

Customer satisfaction questionnaire

Customers

Debit card

Decentralized assembly system

Delivery time

English table service style

Food

Food court

Food truck food

French table service style

Home-replacement meals

Insulated tray

Kiosks

Meal plan

Plate-waste studies

Pod system

Rethermalization system

Room service

Russian table service style

Sensory assessment

Split-tray cart

Surveys

Tray

Tray lines

Trays per minute

Unitized pellet

Vending

Wax-filled pellet

DISCUSSION QUESTIONS

1. What are some methods that foodservice directors and staff can use to meet the needs, wants, and perceptions of customers? Include a comparison of various systems discussed in the chapter.

2. What are the advantages of the decentralized assembly method to the centralized assembly method?

3. What are the advantages and disadvantages of the pod system in comparison to the traditional straight tray line?

4. How would you calculate trays per minute, tray delivery time, and tray accuracy?

5. How do you use a customer satisfaction form and interview patients?

6. Complete a plate study for the same day, same meal for patient- and nonpatient-returned food.

7. Develop a self-evaluation form to determine if standards are being met.

CHAPTER 22

FACILITY DESIGN, EQUIPMENT SELECTION, AND MAINTENANCE

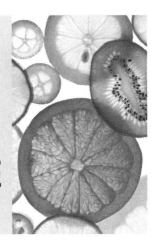

LEARNING OBJECTIVES

- Participate as a team member in a department renovation or new construction.
- Gather data on sustainability and "going green" and determine if this new environmental movement is cost-effective and will be of value to foodservice operations.
- Evaluate existing equipment needs and make recommendations for replacements.
- Develop a system for maintaining records on maintenance, repairs, and replacement of equipment.
- Follow the standards as described in the Americans with Disabilities Act in equipment selection.
- Write a specification for a large/major piece of equipment used in foodservice.
- Know the decibel and foot-candle of light regulations.

THE UNIQUE NATURE of individual health care organizations presents a challenge in planning and equipping a foodservice operation that is both functional and efficient in physical design. Several common problems plague some departments: wasted or underused space, inadequate or improper storage facilities, inflexible equipment arrangements, energy-wasting equipment, inappropriate equipment capacity or type, excessive cross-traffic, labor-intensive layout, and inadequate ventilation or lighting. The application of a systematic approach to facility planning and equipment selection can improve existing health care foodservice operations and guide the design of new ones.

This chapter explains some of the activities involved when health care foodservice directors are confronted with providing input on renovating current facilities or constructing new ones and

with helping select the right equipment to do their facilities' work. Depending on the mission, goals, and objectives involved, any number of activities go into the major task of project design. These include appointing a planning team to study project feasibility, gathering retrospective data, and writing a purchase contract.

How the roles of the foodservice director and the design consultant complement one another, how the team performs its initial research, and how layout plans for various departments and work areas are conceived are only some of the topics discussed. Others include how the planning team, of which the director is a member, arrives at a proposed layout for the operation's physical plant and facilities. The implications of the Americans with Disabilities Act on facility design also are discussed.

Guidelines are given for how to arrive at equipment specifications for purchase contracts. Guidelines also direct purchasers in buying items, from construction materials to security systems that ensure that the food preparation equipment received is of the quality ordered. Then an extensive list of food-processing equipment and devices is described. Some of these include ovens and ranges, refrigerators and freezers, compactors, mixers, dispensing equipment, and coffee makers. Maintenance of equipment is also discussed.

FACILITY PLANNING AND DESIGN

For this book an assumption was made that the money needed for the renovation or new construction and new equipment has been approved by the governing board and space allocation has been defined by engineering and the foodservice director. In some instances renovations and new construction are accomplished in the existing space, perhaps with some additional adjoining space. When a project is accomplished in this manner it is vital that policies, procedures, timetables, and above all communications of progress and changes are provided to all departments within the facility and to nonpatient members. This is a team effort and it takes planning, cooperation, and time to complete task and keep personnel motivates.

Planning and design of foodservice facilities is a complicated process because, generally speaking, no one individual has all the necessary data needed to produce an effective and efficient plan. Therefore, most organizations (whether renovating or constructing a new) form a facility-planning team to carry out this function. A *prospectus*, a written description of all aspects of the renovation or new construction under consideration should be developed to help other team members on the planning team understand the exact needs of the foodservice department. It should contain information that will help guide the proposed design and that will present a clear picture of the physical and operational aspects of the proposed new facility or renovation. The team should also develop a program evaluation and review technique (PERT) and Gantt charts for the project and meet routinely to discuss project status, changes in the plan, timelines for activities, and the like. The viewpoint of each team member should be carefully considered before making decisions regarding the project. Ample time should be allocated for team meetings and the overall planning process.

Composition of the Planning Team

The composition of the facility-planning team varies according to the scope of the project, availability of specialists, and expertise of the foodservice director. Depending on the individual organization and its resources, members of the team should include the foodservice director, an outside food facilities design consultant, an architect, a contractor or builder, a public health representative, facility engineer, an interior designer (for decor and furnishings), and a representative of administration and the finance or business department on an as-needed basis. The director's role and the consultant's role are summarized in the following subsections.

Foodservice Director

Foodservice directors are not expected to be experts in design and construction. Rather, their role is to represent the interests of the health care facility and foodservice operation by developing the operational standards to be supported by the project, providing critical information to other team members, contributing to planning decisions, and evaluating the plans that emerge for the foodservice operation.

For new construction or major renovations, decisions to be made and conveyed to other team members include identification of the foodservice operation's target markets, the volume requirements for each market, and the quality standards for food production and service. The director participates in the development of the overall concept, which specifies the type of production and meal service systems to be implemented. A critical function of the director is to evaluate proposed designs in terms of spatial allocation, layout of work areas and their relationship to one another, and the equipment proposed. The planning process is time-

consuming, but the director's careful study of each aspect of the operation is critical to successful project outcome.

Food Facilities Design Consultant

If the budget allows, the services of a food facilities design consultant should be considered for major changes in foodservice production or tray service, major renovations in the kitchen or cafeteria, or construction of a new foodservice department. The consultant's role varies depending on the director's own level of design expertise. Ideally, the design consultant should specialize in food facility design, construction, and foodservice equipment selection and be expected to make significant contributions during all phases of the project. Typical contributions to a construction or remodeling project include developing work-flow schemes, preparing drawings of equipment layouts, writing equipment specifications, and following up with the builder to ensure that all items on the punch list are resolved. A *punch list* is a detailed checklist that points out any defective, substitute, or inferior equipment so that corrections can be made before the opening or training date. The company or person installing the equipment should prepare the list, and each piece of equipment should be tested to ensure that it meets specifications and claims and that it has been installed correctly. The design consultant and foodservice director should review competitive equipment bids for accuracy, award-winning bid(s), and assure that the equipment specified is supplied in the final installation. The design consultant should have a thorough knowledge of current laws and regulations (such as the Americans with Disabilities Act) that may affect the project.

One expert quoted in the *FoodService Director* indicates that a food facilities design consultant should provide expertise, objectivity, creative solutions, and a return on investment. Despite these contributions, the foodservice director must become as knowledgeable as possible about these issues to fulfill his or her responsibility for the project, which may include being the project manager.

Planning Process

The planning team (Figure 22.1) should establish a systematic approach to the food facility planning process. The scope of the project is the first step in the planning process. The foodservice director and consultant define the type of facility, size, budget, and general ideas about the look of the area. At this point a decision must be made regarding:

- Safety of personnel during the construction/renovation
- Adherence to local, state, federal regulations related to construction
- Whether the department will "go green" (implementing practices that increase our sustainability and reduce the impact on the environment, and whether a Green Seal certification will be sought)
- The use of locally grown products
- Whether the facility will have a garden where some products are grown

FIGURE 22.1 Flow of Planning Process

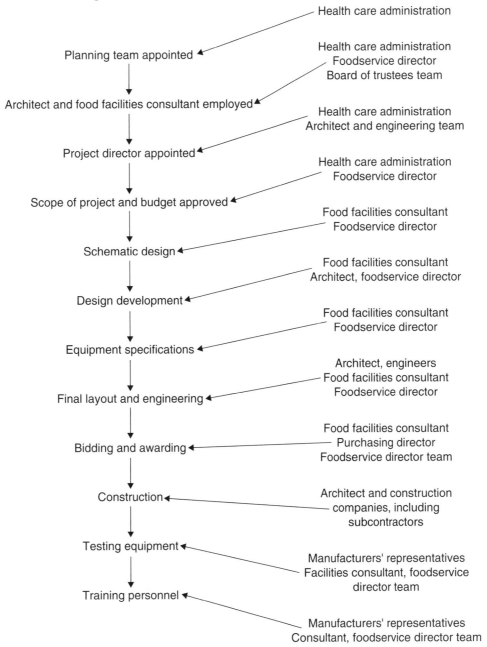

Source: Developed by Ruby P. Puckett©.

- Methods to reduce the chemical pollution that foodservice contributes to the environment
- Whether cooking oil will be used for fuel
- The use of disposables versus reusables
- Establishing a recycling program
- The tipping fees for landfill
- Energy, fuel, water cost
- Noise level and temperature control
- Storage—on-site, off-site
- The use of technology
- Products that will maintain/reduce the sanitation and cleanliness of the department

- The purchase of equipment that will reduce the use of water and electricity
- The team will need to give much thought and time to the four **Rs—Reduce, Reuse, Recycle,** and **Rethink**.

Other areas that need to be considered are:

- Purpose, space constraints, capital budget
- Menus, operational hours
- Number of customers to be served—patients, visitors, staff, and so on
- Whether the foodservice will be cook-from-scratch, heat-and-serve, or self-service

A major concern is how much technology will be used. Many improvements in technology, especially in equipment, have been made to reduce the need for human efforts, improve ergonomics practices, reduce energy consumption, and improve safety and sanitation of the entire area, equipment, and staff.

The amount of space required is directly related to the functions required of the department, such as the menu system, patient/nonpatient foodservice, hours of operation, and so forth. The amount of space needed varies with each organization. There must be enough space to meet the department objectives. As a rule of thumb, space needs will vary for a small operation serving 100 or more meals per day to approximately 600 to 800 square feet plus fixed space, compared to a large operation serving 1,500 to 5,000 meals per day to approximately 7,500 to 15,000 square feet plus fixed space. (This amount of space does not include a food mall, cafeteria, vending operation, patient feeding, doctors' dining, or classrooms. Again, there is **no set rule** for space needs as there are too many variables.)

Typically, the planning process is initiated by collecting background information from internal and external sources and analyzing operational factors for the specific operation. Then the work areas can be planned and the flow of work between areas considered. At this point, a scale drawing or layout of the operation should be developed and evaluated. The team also should provide input regarding general building features and materials, outside areas and safety of employees.

Collecting Background Information

Before a layout is designed, the team must gather background information about the proposed operation:

- Mission, vision, goals, values, and objectives of the health care operation and the foodservice department and the health care facility expectations from foodservice
- Long-range plans and philosophy of the parent organization
- Number of beds and spatial configuration of the health care operation
- Customer expectations
- Constraints on the budget and space allocation
- Number of daily meals served to patients and nonpatients, all in one building or will there be off-site facilities?
- Extent of services provided to nonpatients by the foodservice department
- Availability of labor and skill levels required and any limitations due to language or ability to read
- Safety and sanitation such as HACCP, *Food Code Standards,* TJC, OBRA, OSHA, and CMS that contain specific standards for temperature, humidity lighting, heat, ventilation, plumbing, air-conditioning, and much more
- Local and state building codes, especially as they apply to health care facilities
- Security as to the location of the loading dock, entrance, and exit doors for employees, need for cameras, questioning the security of food, supplies, and employees

The foodservice director and facility design consultant should work together as a team to provide information to the planning team. For example:

- The number of persons eating in the nonpatient area, the number of other food establishments within five miles of the facility, and the number of customers on regular and modified diets
- The cultural, ethnic, and socioeconomic makeup of staff and patients that will influence menu planning and service to the customers
- The concern of customers for fitness and wellness, healthy lifestyle, and the effects on the menu
- The need to conserve energy and water and other environmental considerations, whether the department will seek green approval, use local products, and implement the 4Rs (reduce, reuse, recycle, and rethink)
- The latest trend in equipment especially for ergonomic factors that will reduce fatigue help prevent injury
- The need for an efficient arrangement of equipment in the area to maintain or reduce the number of employees—pod system versus straight line, high-tech equipment, skills of employees
- The use of space for seating in nonpatient foodservice, offices, multipurpose areas, and classrooms
- The need for a safe environment for personnel, customers, food, and supplies
- Copies of all regulatory standards and local, state, and federal rules and regulations or laws
- Impressions by the foodservice director and members of the team after visiting other facilities, especially facilities where the consultant has previously completed a job
- Copies of equipment catalogs and advantages and disadvantages of the type of production and distribution system to be used

Such information is important because these factors affect the type of production and meal service systems to be used by the foodservice department. The optimum system should be compatible with the mission, goals, and objectives of the operation, with the final decision based on projected capital costs, operating costs, ease of administration, and subjective comparisons (such as the aesthetic characteristics of public dining areas).

In addition to internal background information, external sources of information also must be considered. Key among these are the local, state, and federal laws and regulations such as the Occupational Safety and Health Act and ergonomic needs that apply to facility design and equipment selection. The Americans with Disabilities Act, which guarantees civil rights protection for persons with disabilities, also must be considered.

When planning a renovation or new building project, the foodservice director should contact the human resources department and occupational therapy staff members who manages compliance with the Americans with Disabilities Act. These individuals can assist the planning team in determining appropriate accommodations for persons (both customers and employees) with disabilities.

In addition, the foodservice director and facility design consultant should have a working knowledge of this law so that its requirements can be incorporated into the facility plans.

In *Americans with Disabilities Act: Answers for Foodservice Operators*, the National Restaurant Association outlines the following steps necessary to accommodate persons with disabilities in eating establishments:

1. Understand the intent of the law.
2. Evaluate employment practices, customer service policies, and facilities to ensure that they are accessible and usable.
3. Implement changes primarily through employee training and removal of barriers.
4. Continue considering accessibility issues when planning renovation and new construction.

The book focuses on identifying barriers (with an easy-to-use checklist), removing common barriers and implementing low-cost solutions, and providing quality service to all customers. The appendixes detail Americans with Disabilities Act design requirements for restaurants, illustrate accessible design features, and provide references for technical assistance.

Analyzing Operational Factors

Other operational factors, past and future, also must be considered. The foodservice director can provide information about menu items and menu patterns, the department's production and meal service procedures, its purchasing policies and practices, systems that will be implemented, workload, and staff projections. The facilities designer will provide data on space availability, equipment requirements, cost estimates, and environmental impact.

Menu Information   Because the menu determines the equipment needed and the space required in the production area, further analysis should include the following information about each of the operation's menus:

- Menu pattern and number of selections within the pattern for each course or category of food served
- Complexity of menu items served
- Type, service, and number of modified-diet menu items served
- Type and number of meals prepared
- Use of convenience items versus on-site preparation
- Centralize or decentralize service, room service, sous vide and *cook-chill* or *freeze*

Types of Production and Meal Service   The type of production systems planned affects what equipment, space, and personnel are required in the central kitchen. (Food production systems—cook-and-serve, cook-and-chill, cook-and-freeze, and assembly-and-serve—were described in Chapter 21. The meal service systems described in this chapter also must be considered.) The planning process must weigh the following factors:

- Use of an ingredient room
- Total quantity of each menu item needed to yield the required number of portions
- Batch size preferred
- Amount of time required vis-à-vis the amount of time available for production
- Assembly, delivery, and service systems used

Certainly this list is not all-inclusive, and similar information must be gathered for other subsystems (such as receiving, storage, and ware washing) of the operation. An operational plan that states organizational constraints and projected needs can then be developed and used as a basis for designing functional work areas.

Purchasing Policies   The department's purchasing policies and practices determine the type of equipment and the amount of space needed for low-temperature and dry storage areas and production and meal service facilities. These considerations include:

- The market form in which food supplies are purchased (the amount of processing that has taken place before purchase, local, organic, or grown on-site)
- The state of food supplies at delivery time (canned, frozen, chilled, dehydrated, fresh, or freeze-dried)
- Frequency of delivery for all categories of food
- The volume purchased and the amount of inventory carryover from one purchase period to the next
- The department's issuing and inventory control procedures

Planning Work Areas

The location of each workspace and the amount of space allocated to the area within the department must be determined for each individual foodservice facility. The relationship of one work area to another is equally important. A good layout should provide a smooth, orderly flow of employees and materials through all parts of the operation in as straight, short, and direct a route as possible. Backtracking and cross-traffic increase labor time and decrease efficiency and productivity.

The same principle applies to the amount of space that should be allocated for each area. The trend has been to minimize the department's overall dimensions, particularly in the production area, but also in other areas because of the rising costs of new construction. This trend has been made possible in many institutions by changes in the types and forms of food purchased and the availability of slim-line, multiuse equipment, pod tray line, modular, and mobile equipment. The efficient movement of food, supplies, and people requires consideration of the essential tasks to be performed in each stage of production, assembly, delivery, and service; the number of employees involved; and the equipment required for the activities. In an existing facility, improvements in space often can be made by identifying points of congestion and rearranging equipment or tasks to alleviate them.

To ensure that the best arrangement of work areas has been planned, a chart that illustrates the flow of work can be developed (Figure 22.2). At this point, the actual amounts of space and

FIGURE 22.2 Flow of Work and Materials

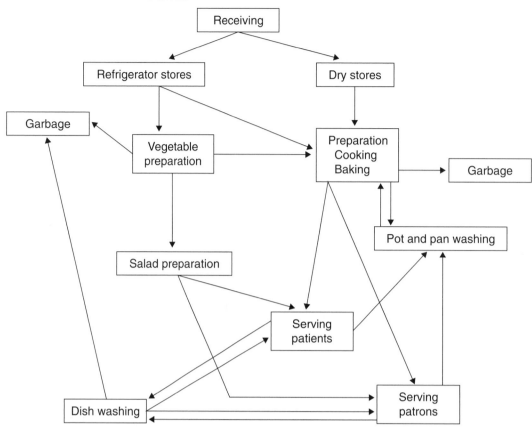

Note: Foods should flow from receiving to service in as short and as straight lines as possible; the design should keep food flowing in the same direction to avoid as little cross-contamination and handling as possible.

equipment are not needed. The chart is merely a diagram showing what happens when food and people travel from the receiving area to the point of service and cleanup area. Once the ideal, or at least the best possible, space relationship has been determined, a scale drawing can be made to show the approximate size of each work area and its location relative to other departments. The architect would perform this task in conjunction with the foodservice design consultant.

The next step in the planning process is to draw a schematic plan, based on all the important data gathered earlier, that shows work areas, traffic aisles, and the location of specific pieces of equipment. At this point, it is important for the foodservice director to evaluate the proposed layout. Charting the workflow for typical menu items on the scale diagram is an excellent way to assess the plan's feasibility. It is possible to pinpoint traffic problems that can result from misplaced or inadequate equipment, too little or too much space, and generally poor work-flow patterns. The foodservice director should suggest improvement before actual construction begins. Changes after construction has begun, or after it is finished, are costly and sometimes impossible to make. The foodservice director should also be aware of the department's basic requirements for location, building materials for interior surfaces, lighting, utilities, and ventilation.

Location The foodservice department should have ready access to receiving, storage, and dining areas and to elevators. The distance from the foodservice department to patient areas is a factor in determining the method of food delivery, but new technology in tray distribution systems has helped to reduce temperature control problems. An area located away from the primary traffic patterns of other departments is recommended.

Receiving The receiving area's location and space requirements depend on the health care operation's purchasing policies. For example, if a materials management department is responsible for procuring all goods used by the facility, a central receiving point should be provided for all deliveries. Because materials used in the foodservice department account for a large proportion of the total deliveries, a location close to foodservice is desirable.

In designing a new facility, the traffic flow that surrounds the facility, the space needed for parking delivery trucks, and building constraints should be taken into account. Some states require that foodservice receiving areas be separated from the central docking area. The receiving dock should be covered, if possible, to protect receiving clerks and supplies from inclement weather. The size of the receiving area depends on the delivery schedule, the volume of goods in each shipment, the time lapse between receipt and storage, and proper receiving equipment. For safety and security reasons, storerooms should be designed with walls that extend from floor to ceiling and with ceilings that cannot be entered from adjoining room(s). The ingredient room should be adjacent to the receiving and storage area. A rule of thumb is to not make an area too large as it may become a dumping ground for broken equipment and other debris.

Storage   Space for nonperishable foods and supplies may be shared with other departments in the institution, or the foodservice department may have its own storeroom. In either case, a location reasonably close to the kitchen and service areas reduces transportation time. Usually, a short-term dry storage area is provided near or within the kitchen or as part of an ingredient control center. The space needs of the system are based on procurement policies related to product volume, purchase frequency, inventory level, and delivery schedule.

General construction features to consider when evaluating current facilities or planning new ones include materials used for floors, walls, and ceilings; ventilation and temperature controls; lighting; and safety and security and the ingress and egress, preferably one door in and out.

To prevent contamination by rodents and insects, the floor, walls, and ceiling of dry storage areas should be smooth, moisture proof, and free from cracks. Light colors are preferable. Floors should be level with the surrounding areas to facilitate the use of mobile equipment in moving supplies. Floors should be made of nonslip, easily cleaned material.

Good ventilation is essential to retard the growth of bacteria and molds, to prevent mildew and rusting of metal containers, and to minimize the caking of ground or powdered foods. Ventilation and air circulation help maintain proper temperature and humidity. Temperatures should be kept between 50°F and 70°F (10°C and 21°C). Several methods can be used to accomplish this. The installation of doors with louvers at the floor level allows fresh air to enter the storeroom, and louvers at ceiling level enable warm air to escape. However, this simple system is not adequate in many warm-weather locations, and so mechanical means such as intake and exhaust fans or air-conditioning must be used (see Chapter 20).

Water heaters, compressors, motors, and other heat-producing equipment should not be located in the storeroom. All steam or hot water pipes should be insulated, and condensation from cold water pipes or cold walls must be controlled. One or more wall thermometers should be placed strategically in the storeroom and checked at regularly scheduled intervals to ensure compliance with state and local health codes. When humidity seems to be a problem, a recording hygrometer can be installed to determine its extent.

Adequate lighting is needed for good housekeeping and inventory control. A level of 15 foot-candles is recommended, with fixtures centered over each aisle for best light distribution. Windows should have frosted glass to protect food from direct sunlight.

A security sash, screen, or bar should be installed on windows in storerooms located at ground level. Other security measures include provisions for locking doors from the outside but allowing them to open from the inside without a key for safety purposes.

The storage area should include space for nonperishable food as well as refrigerator and freezer space for storing perishable goods. The dry storage space should be close to the receiving area as well as to the ingredient preparation and control area. Storage space needs are based on procurement policies related to product volume, purchase frequency, inventory level, and delivery schedule. A separate storage area should be provided for cleaning supplies, chemicals, paper goods, and other nonfood materials; space needs, equipment requirements, and sanitary construction features are just as important for these goods as for food supplies.

Space requirements for standard and low-temperature walk-in units vary considerably among foodservice operations. Specific needs depend on menu offerings, the amount of preparation done before purchase, and the volume of perishables and frozen foods purchased and delivered at specified times. Analysis of these factors and the usable space provided by stationary or mobile shelving can be used as a guide.

Standard and low-temperature, self-contained refrigerator units provide convenient storage at point of use. Where space is limited and in small facilities, self-contained units should be considered in place of walk-ins. Many options are available, so construction features, size, and where and how the unit will be used should be considered before the purchasing decision is made.

Food Production   The production area should be close to raw ingredient storage areas, the ingredient control area, and on a direct route to assembly and service areas. The size and shape of the area allocated to production influence equipment arrangement and work-flow patterns. The shortest possible route from one area to the next with a minimum of backtracking or cross-traffic is preferred. In large rectangular kitchens, work and materials can flow in parallel lines by using an island arrangement for cooking equipment. In square or small kitchens, a U-shape, L-shape, or E-shape arrangement for equipment may be more efficient.

A well-laid-out kitchen should focus on three areas for food production—hot food, cold food, and bakery. In smaller kitchens these three functions may be all together and either used for bakery and hot food with a separate space for cold food. In large kitchens the space is more defined and the equipment needed to operate the kitchen is grouped together according to function. Consideration needs to be given to the safety of the employees, their job satisfaction, and above all the efficiency of the operation.

Major cooking equipment such as ranges, ovens, braising pans, and fryers usually are grouped together. Steam-jacketed kettles and compartment steamers are placed close by for convenience. Compact central arrangements of such equipment facilitate construction of effective exhaust hoods over all cooking surfaces and steam equipment. The aisles between equipment should be wide enough to park carts, turn them around, and permit employees to use them without blocking traffic (hot production).

Space for vegetable and salad preparation, baking, and food preparation should be allocated within the main production area; when ingredient control rooms are used, a smaller space may be allocated for vegetable preparation. Dividing the open space into operational areas by equipment arrangement rather than by partitions is an effective way to create a sense of spaciousness, improve air circulation, simplify cleaning, permit more effective supervision, and allow greater flexibility for equipment additions and use of mobile equipment.

Space will also be needed for work surfaces such as metal cooks' tables and at least one metal table with a cutout with a sink that has both hot and cold water, and space to store utensils (ladles, knives, measuring/weighing equipment, and so forth). Space will be needed to store raw ingredients, drawers for smaller equipment, mitts, pot holders, rags, recipes, and computers and carts, in addition to space to place the finished product to be delivered to patient or nonpatient areas. Adequate aisle space is a must to carefully move/store carts and for personnel to carry out their tasks.

Meal Service The work space, equipment, and layout needed for the assembly of food for patients or residents requiring tray service all depend on the type of delivery and service systems selected (as detailed in Chapter 22). All assembly areas require careful planning to achieve maximum efficiency and to ensure delivery of high-quality meals at a reasonable cost to consumers. In a centralized service system, the assembly area should be close to production areas, storage areas, dishwashing facilities, and tray-cart storage areas. Easy access to food and materials and minimization of transportation time greatly improve quality and help control costs. Analysis of the basic functions to be performed and the equipment needed to simplify tasks helps determine space requirements. Factors to consider during the planning stage for patient meal service are:

- Number of patients or residents served at each meal, meal hours, foodservice or nursing serve the trays
- Menu composition (the number of food components offered and selected for normal and modified diets), room service versus traditional service
- Type of tray assembly, delivery, and service—straight or pod system
- Time limitations for tray assembly—trays per minute
- Amount and dimensions of the space available or planned for tray assembly and support equipment, such as storage of meal carts, lowerators, and other needed equipment

Some hospitals and most extended-care facilities provide dining space for ambulatory patients or residents either within the patient care area or near the central kitchen. Service arrangements and dining room furnishings are affected by the type of service (for example, table or cafeteria), the number of diners served at each meal, menu variety, the location of the dining room, health and mobility factors (for example, residents' disabilities), and the activities other than serving food that take place in the area.

Because of its potential for speedy service and food presentation possibilities, cafeteria service is the most popular way of serving employees, staff, visitors, and guests. Foodservice managers must bear in mind food quality as well as cost components related to service. Location of the service area, layout of the service line, equipment availability, and the employees' work methods affect consumer satisfaction as well as the efficiency and economy of the foodservice system.

Locating the cafeteria (preferably on the same floor as the main kitchen) close to the central kitchen reduces transportation time and can help control food quality. For the sake of preserving quality, batch cooking of vegetables and other foods that suffer from overcooking is recommended, but this technique is difficult if the service area is too far from the production center. Close access to dishwashing facilities is preferred.

Service lines can be of various sizes and configurations, depending on the number of people served, the service time allotted for each meal, menu complexity, and the dimensions of the available space. Conventional service lines may be straight or L-shape; variations in new and large facilities include circular, scatter, and open square designs (Figure 22.3). The flow of traffic is important in whatever configuration is chosen.

The length of the service counter depends on the size of the menu and the amount of food displayed. Adequate space should be provided for attractive display and preservation of food quality. Sneeze guards that meet local sanitation codes should protect all hot and cold sections.

Additional space is needed on or near the line for trays, tableware, napkins, beverage containers, and so forth. These materials should be located for easy accessibility by the customer but not where traffic flow will be interrupted or slowed. The same principle applies to the location of cash registers: A line can form easily when there are not enough cashiers; meanwhile, the customers' food gets cold.

Overall space requirements for the employees' dining area must be carefully analyzed to ensure efficient movement of customers and service workers. Today, foodservice directors prefer more self-service in the cafeteria because labor is saved and customers prefer it because they have more control over the amount and kinds of food they can choose. The space behind the line should be wide enough for transportation equipment and for efficient movement by employees. The customers' side also must be wide enough for bypassing others in the line, if this is allowed, and for easy access to the dining area. A periodic check of waiting times at various stations and customer counts per minute will indicate bottlenecks that can be eliminated by equipment rearrangement or menu changes.

Once customers have been served, adequate space in a pleasant, attractive dining room is needed. Because health care personnel usually have little time to relax at meal breaks, waiting and overcrowding are not conducive to good morale. The size of the dining area should depend on the number of people expected to be seated during a given time and the rate of turnover. Generally, a minimum of 10 to 14 square feet per person is recommended.

Ware Washing The cost of labor, equipment, and supplies required for sanitizing pots, pans, and service ware makes the ware-washing area one of the most important areas of the foodservice department. Centralized washing located close to the tray assembly area, cafeteria, dining room, and production areas eliminates duplication of equipment and personnel. The supervision and control of sanitation can also be more effective when all ware washing is performed in one location.

A location close to the main production and service areas is convenient. The dish room's layout should be planned to provide

FIGURE 22.3   Cafeteria Service Line Configurations

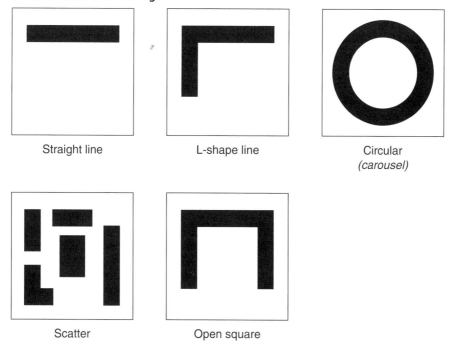

Straight line

L-shape line

Circular
(carousel)

Scatter

Open square

good workflow, minimize labor time, and ensure efficiency and safety. The arrangement of equipment can take any form: straight line, L-shape, oval, square, rectangular, or triangular. The shape depends on the equipment used, the space available, and the methods of soiled dish return and clean dish removal and storage. Before the type and arrangement of equipment are planned, the department's policies, practices, and needs should be analyzed. Factors influencing the space arrangements include:

- *Type of service:* Is it tray, cafeteria, table, or a combination of these? Each style requires different types and quantities of service ware.
- *Number of persons served:* Are there fluctuations from meal to meal and from day to day? Service demand will affect the type and amount of service ware used and the space requirements.
- *Type and number of menu items served:* Are there variations among the types of service at one meal and from meal to meal? The style and quantity of dishes, trays, and so forth affect the space needed. Storage space for carts and dollies also will vary with these requirements.
- *Length of meal service and time:* Is service ware used more than once during each meal, or is it stockpiled and washed later? Service-ware inventory, dishwasher capacity, and space requirements vary according to these practices.
- *Space consideration for parking patient delivery carts:* Delivery cart used for removing the soiled wares.

Adequate space is needed for scraping, sorting, and racking soiled dishes. Tables that are 2 to 2½ feet wide, the same height as the dishwasher (34 inches high is convenient) and long enough to hold the prewash and waste disposal unit, should be provided. Some

dish-room arrangements include slanted overhead shelves for holding glass and cup racks while they are being loaded. Convenient placement of these shelves can help to reduce employee fatigue, to utilize space efficiently, and to maintain a high degree of productivity.

Table space is needed for air-drying clean dishes held in racks, carts, and dollies. Table heights and widths should be the same as those mentioned in the preceding paragraph. Length varies according to the type of dishwasher used and the washing load. Flight-type machines require less table space because dishes are removed from the conveyor and placed in storage units almost immediately. Specialized equipment may be used, such as portable soak sinks, a glass washer, and a pulper-extractor waste disposer. All these require space and should be carefully planned for in the overall design.

Trends for Work Area Design   The trend to minimize the department's overall dimensions, particularly in the production area but also in other functional areas because of the rising cost of new construction, has been made possible in many operations by changes in the types and forms of food purchased and in the availability of slim-line, modular, and mobile equipment. Once the ideal, or at least the best possible, space relationship and arrangement have been determined, a scale drawing of the work area can be produced.

Planning the Flow of Work

After all data are collected, the next step is for the designer to begin to block out a layout (the arrangement of equipment on a floor plan, giving special attention to process and flow). The orderly flow of employees and materials, the workflow, deserves special consideration by the planning team. Therefore, the location of each work area in relation to other areas in the department must be determined to minimize backtracking and cross-traffic. The efficient movement of food, supplies, and people requires consideration of the essential tasks to be performed at each stage of production and meal service (assembly, delivery, and service), the number of employees involved, and the equipment required for the activities. To ensure that the best arrangement of work areas has been planned, a chart that illustrates the workflow can be developed (see Figure 22.2). At this point, the actual amounts of space and equipment are not needed. The chart is merely a diagram showing what happens when food and people travel from the receiving area to the point of service and cleanup area.

Developing the Layout

The next step in the planning process is to draw a schematic plan, based on all the data gathered earlier, that shows work areas, traffic aisles, and the location of specific pieces of equipment. The architect usually performs this task in conjunction with the food facilities design consultant and the foodservice director. A new concept called the *disposable prototypes* is being used by some fast-food chains but can be adapted to other types of foodservice operations. This approach is to build a "movie-set style" prototype in a space, such as a warehouse, where design, equipment placement, and decor can be seen and tested *before* investing in the actual building. This allows the foodservice director, management staff, and employees to evaluate the proposed layout, decor, and materials that can/will be used in the building. It also provides for "buy-in" from the total staff and can reduce resistance to change. Charting the workflow for typical menu items on the scale diagram is an excellent way to assess the plan's feasibility. A good layout should provide a smooth, orderly flow in as straight, short, and direct a route as possible. It is possible to pinpoint traffic problems that can result from misplaced or inadequate equipment, too little or too much space, and generally poor work-flow patterns. The foodservice director should evaluate the layout before plans are finalized and blueprints are drawn.

The drawing to scale for mechanical, electrical, switch control boxes, gas, plumbing, telephone outlets, heat, and ventilation will need to be completed before the final blueprint is completed. These plans are drawn to scale with locations of doors, windows, and aisles using the architectural symbols to denote location. To-scale templates are used for placing equipment. Each template is labeled with the name of the equipment and space requirements, noting the swing of the doors (to right or left) and any special installation needs. The architect may make these drawings or a computer program called a computer-assisted design (CAD) may graphically design them. A newer program entitled "Autodesk® Revit® Architecture Conceptual Design Modeling" is replacing CAD. Autodesk® Revit® is a software program that allows visualizing a form in the earliest stages, to help the designers to communicate ideas and evaluate these forms that yields an advantage in predicting and optimizing real world performance of the built projects. As you work with the architect you may want to ask about using this new system.

After the team has thoroughly checked the preliminary plans, the architect prepares a complete set of drawings that are called **blueprints**. Blueprints always contain:

- Name and address of the facility
- Name and address of the architect
- For some states, the approval of the state and local health department
- Scale used for the drawing (for example, ½ inch equals 1 foot)
- Date the plan was drawn
- Details of the construction
- Materials for inside and outside (stone, brick, concrete block, and so forth)
- Plumbing, heating, and ventilation
- Electrical wiring, connections, fixtures, fuse boxes, and the voltage needed for equipment, and so forth
- Side elevations, including doors to and including the direction in which the doors will open, window finishes, stairwells, and built-in or attached equipment
- Dimensions of rooms and their use (office, locker, and so forth)

The architect prepares written documents to accompany the blueprints that include the general conditions and scope of the work to be accomplished; schedules of when work is to be done; penalties for failure to meet deadlines; the responsible party for installation of equipment and inspection and how often inspections are to be done; specifications for all aspects of the work to be done; and other information, which may include the type of base construction, mix of cement, conduits, drains, vents, hardware, doors, and windows.

Before the actual work begins, contract documents must be presented for bids. Notices of bids are usually printed in the newspaper and mailed to contractors or builders who may have the skills, equipment, personnel, and finances to complete the job. These bids contain specific instructions concerning the time to return a bid, name and address of person to receive the bid, the opening date, and the location where the bids will be opened. Once the bids are awarded, a starting date for construction is set.

The foodservice facility consultant and the foodservice director prepare the specifications and bids for equipment, and the same procedure is followed as for the construction bid. This is frequently referred to as **request for proposal (RFP)**, which is a formal document stating the requirements for the purchase (see Chapter 19 purchasing bid openings). The RFP needs to include (1) whether the cost includes installation of equipment, (2) foodservice personnel training, (3) training for maintenance personnel, (4) manuals, (5) warranties, (6) discounts for all, and (7) whether the bid is for one or more pieces of equipment. It is suggested that if brand names are specified then equivalent bids not be accepted.

There may be instances where a *justification* or *cost-benefit analysis* will need to be made. A justification or cost-benefit analysis compares cost with benefits to determine value. For example, what will Equipment A provide that Equipment B is unable to do. Cost analysis must be an objective evaluation using the same criteria to evaluate similar pieces of equipment—Brand A dishwasher/Brand B dishwasher. The lowest price may not be the best buy.

Once the bids have been opened, a flow sheet will need to be completed with the supplier name; cost of items; instructions to follow, such as one or all; specified brand name as outlined in bid; additional cost for installation and training; evaluated an all bid and other data that the supplier has included to make an objective evaluation. It may be necessary to complete a cost-analysis. The bids/flow sheets will need to be evaluated by the foodservice director, consultant, and administrator for an objective decision in choosing the supplier. The foodservice director, working with the purchasing department, will issue purchase orders to the accepted suppliers. The consultant/foodservice director will meet with the construction team to establish a date when plumbers, electricians, and other personnel will be on site to coordinate installation and training. The foodservice director and engineering will schedule training on use and maintenance of equipment for engineering and foodservice personnel. Manuals will be provided to each department with telephone numbers or e-mail addresses for service. Warranties will be discussed and for some equipment a maintenance contract will be signed.

The contracts for construction and equipment may not always go to the lowest bidder. Other circumstances may determine the choice, such as the reputation of the contractor, ability to handle the specific job, the location of the company, "free on board" of equipment delivery, a training program offered by the equipment company, any discounts for early or complete payments, and so forth.

Budget

The design consultant should provide the foodservice director an approximate cost of all the needed equipment. This does not include plumbing, electrical, and mechanical work.

Specifying General Building Features and Materials

In addition to developing the layout, the planning team must make decisions related to general building features and types of materials to be used in construction. The foodservice director should be aware of the requirements for interior surfaces, lighting, utilities, and ventilation.

The floors and walls of the dish room should be constructed of materials that are easy to sanitize. The distance between the walls and stationary equipment must be wide enough to accommodate easy cleaning and movement of mobile equipment. The floor is particularly important because it can be a safety hazard when water or other debris is allowed to accumulate. Nonskid flooring or mats that comply with local sanitation and safety codes can help alleviate the problem. Adequate floor drains should be strategically placed.

Floors, Walls, and Ceilings Floors should be durable, easy to clean, nonslippery, nonabsorbent, and resilient. It is difficult to satisfy all these specifications with one material, and the use of the same material throughout all areas is not aesthetically pleasing. For example, a quarry tile floor in the dining area is not conducive to a

relaxing atmosphere even though it meets most of the criteria. A hard-surface floor meets the basic requirements, particularly for preparation areas. However, it has two main drawbacks: it may be slippery when wet, and because it lacks resiliency, it tends to increase employee fatigue levels. Quarry or ceramic tile is usually used in kitchens, and vinyl tile or carpeting is used in dining areas. The various types of floor coverings available on the market should be examined before final selections are made because materials are constantly being developed and improved. Newer materials are available that reduce microbiological buildup and are nonslip and resilient.

Regardless of the floor material chosen for the kitchen, adequate drains installed near steam equipment, food cutters, and warewashing facilities will help reduce safety hazards and make housekeeping tasks more efficient. All floors should be finished with a baseboard, flush with the wall, for ease in maintaining sanitation.

Walls should be hard, smooth, washable, and impervious to moisture. Glazed tile to the ceiling, or at least to a 5- or 8-foot height (with plaster and washable paint above), is preferred for kitchen and service areas. Pleasing color combinations enhance the area's appearance and can even increase employee morale. Pipes, radiators, and wiring conduits should be placed inside the walls. In the dining area, it may be desirable to have tile wainscoting on the walls and around columns, with corrosion-resistant metal corner guards.

Ceiling heights vary widely from 14 to 18 feet. Ceilings should be acoustically treated and lighter in color than the walls. Ceilings must resist deterioration from changes in temperature, steam, humidity, and cooking odors. They should also contain a fire retardant and be easily removed and washable.

When the daily noise exposure is composed of two or more periods of noise exposure at different levels, their combined effect should be considered, rather than the individual effect of each. Exposure to impulsive or impact noise should not exceed the 140-*decibel* peak pressure level. When employees are subjected to sound levels exceeding those in Table 22.1, administrative or engineering

TABLE 22.1 Permissible Noise Exposure

Duration per day, hours	Sound level, dBA[a] glow response
8	90
6	92
4	95
3	97
1.5	100
1	102
0.5	105
0.25 or less	110
	115

[a]dBA refers to decibels on the A scale of a standard sound-level meter at a slow response.

controls should be used. If such controls fail to reduce sound levels within the levels of Table 22.1, personal protective equipment should be provided and used to reduce sound levels within the levels as stated above.

Soundproofing should be considered carefully in planning construction and before selecting equipment. Kitchens and especially dishwashing rooms can be noisy, and excessive noise can result in fatigue and low productivity among employees. The Occupational Safety and Health Administration has set standards for permissible noise exposure. The use of acoustical materials in ceilings appreciably reduces the noise level. However, the selection of ceiling materials should be based on their ease of cleaning as well as their noise-reducing characteristics.

Lighting The proper amount and kind of lighting in all work areas are important for cleanliness, safety, and efficiency. Natural lighting should be used as much as possible. When energy conservation is the only lighting consideration given, fluorescent lights are used. Because the natural color of foods is enhanced when displayed under incandescent light, however, high-intensity incandescent lighting should be used in display and merchandising areas. Low-intensity incandescent lighting is used in dining areas for mood enhancement. A lighting expert should be consulted for special requirements. Table 22.2 lists lighting guidelines for foodservice areas.

Utilities and Ventilation In some areas, both natural gas and electricity are available and are used as the power sources for various pieces of equipment. The selection of gas as a heat source for cooking equipment should be coordinated with the health care operation's engineering department. Foodservice directors should be familiar with the power requirements of various pieces of equipment and evaluate the electrical plans to make sure that enough outlets are available and that they are appropriately located. In most operations, the form of energy most often used is electricity. Two voltage systems are used: 110 to 120 volts and 200 to 240 volts. Correct voltage must be available for the particular piece of equipment.

As stated elsewhere, equipment purchasing decisions should evaluate EPA-sponsored ENERGY STAR rated equipment. ENERGY STAR equipment identifies energy efficient equipment. There are many new-generation pieces of equipment that use technology and less energy, including combination microwave-light wave convection ovens, steam-powered griddles, and improved refrigeration that are presently being used in Europe and some of which are available in the U.S. market.

Proper heat, ventilation, plumbing, and air-conditioning systems are important for food-quality preservation, employee comfort, and building maintenance. The department director should work with the project engineer to identify areas of excessive heat and humidity to ensure that space is properly ventilated. Excessive moisture or heat can ruin walls and ceilings as well as employees' dispositions. Therefore, heat must be provided in the winter, and during the summer the air should be cooled and dehumidified to acceptable comfort levels. Plumbing must meet all health codes as well as local codes.

Ergonomic Considerations The need to reduce physical fatigue, variations in climate, and repetitive motion injuries need to be considered when selecting flooring; machines; small equipment; heights of equipment; any job that requires repetitive action, such as cashiering; travel distance; locker rooms; restrooms; and dining facilities. Employees need accessibility to products, supplies, and other frequently used items and clean, clear, and sufficient traffic areas. A new line of adjustable ergonomically friendly workstations have been designed to improve the workplace environment by being easily refigurable to proper task height for the individual worker. These tables can be adjusted for the height for the individual worker's comfort as well as raised for precision work or light- and heavy-duty work.

A new line of ergonomically designed kitchen tools is also available. These tools have been designed to match personal capabilities and should allow the worker to use good posture and avoid unnecessary motion or force. Many of the tools have pads on the handles for required grip, while handles on other tools are designed with ergonomic angles to keep hands in a more natural position.

Experts such as physical and occupational therapists can provide guidance.

General rules are as follows:

- Average height of worktable should be: for women, 37 to 39 inches; for men, 39 to 41 inches
- Light work, standing: 5-foot maximum reach
- Heavy work, best height is where wrist bends: about 36 inches standing and 28 inches sitting
- Personal protective equipment for wearing in freezers and walk-ins to protect against climatic changes
- Equipment that has been ergonomically designed for repetitive tasks

A minimum of 4 linear feet of workspace is recommended for each preparation employee, but 6 feet is preferable.

Safety, Sanitation, and Security All health codes, local and state rules, and regulations and laws must be met. Health regulations provide for temperature and humidity standards for dry storage,

TABLE 22.2 Effective Lighting Guidelines

Light Intensity, foot-candles	Activity
10–20	Walkways, halls, corridors
15–20	Dining area
15–35	Rough work
35–70	Food display
70–150	Reading computer printouts, measuring ingredients, inspecting, checking, record keeping

Note. Foot-candle, a unit for measuring illumination, is the amount of direct light thrown by a source of one candle on a square foot of surface, every part of which is 1 foot away from the source and facing directly toward the source.

lighting requirements, design, venting heat, ventilation and air-conditioning, toilets, restrooms, hand-washing sinks, and locker rooms. A representative from the health department should be part of the team, and the latest public health standards should be provided to the consultant, architect, foodservice director, and contractor.

At this point research needs to be made concerning the latest enhancements that have been made to equipment to inhibit the growth of various bacteria, mildew, and fungi. Some equipment companies have incorporated antibacterial materials into the construction of the equipment. The material is odorless, tasteless, and colorless and last for the life of the product; it cannot be washed off or removed.

Security for personnel and customers should be given a high priority. Doors in storerooms, walk-in refrigerators, and freezers should have a mechanism that allows someone to exit when the door is locked. Loading docks need to be secure; some doors should be designated as staff entrance doors and others as exits. Only authorized personnel should be allowed in the department. Department doors need to provide a protective barrier for employees.

Plumbing Water and waste management are discussed in Chapters 12 and 13. It is vital that a source of *potable water* be available for drinking, preparation, ware washing, hand washing, and sanitation. An approved source must be available.

Plumbing must furnish potable water to the facility and remove waste to a sewer or disposal plant. There are four major concerns that relate to plumbing and in most states these concerns are inspected by the local public health sanitarian:

1. *Cross connection:* Fixtures and equipment used in a foodservice department must not be cross-connected, which is a link between an outlet of drinking water system and unsafe water. This is a structural design issue and must be addressed during the project.
2. *Backflow:* When contaminated water flows into potable water.
3. *Backsiphonage:* Occurs after pressuring the water supply, water is siphoned back into the drinkable water supply.
4. *Air gap:* Helps prevent backflow. Air gap is an unobstructed air space between an outlet of potable water and the flood rim of a fixture or equipment.

EQUIPMENT SELECTION

Many kinds of equipment are discussed in this chapter to provide some basic information about the types of equipment and arrangements available that help achieve the standards necessary to provide high-quality and healthful food. Because equipment represents a large financial investment, it should be studied carefully before a purchase is made. Well-chosen equipment, used and maintained properly, provides many years of service.

Once the team has accepted the flow of product and people in the department and the budget has been approved, a detailed list is made of *needed new* equipment plus equipment on hand that is still usable. Multiuse of a piece of equipment and increasing productivity

are major concerns in equipment selection. After the list is completed, equipment specifications are developed for the exact pieces of equipment. Brand names may be used. The equipment selection process needs to be reviewed by the team.

Factors Affecting Equipment Selection

Because of the many variables associated with foodservice departments, the equipment buyer should fully understand the needs of the department and what equipment would best meet each of those needs. The amount and type of equipment needed depends on the operation's menu pattern, the facility's financial resources, its utility supply, equipment design and construction, and its safety and sanitation features and local codes. Other considerations include the saving of water and energy, the total life cycle of the equipment, maintenance, and sanitation features such as a coating on stainless steel that retards bacteria growth and ease of cleaning.

Menu Offerings

Because menu offerings influence the choice of equipment, one basic question that should be answered is why a specific piece is needed. If the equipment would save time and money and would improve quality and personnel performance, then further study to justify size, capacity, and space needs can proceed. Analysis of the items listed in the menu, the number of servings needed, the batch size followed, and the production time required provide the background information necessary for making decisions on equipment purchases. This is a vital consideration if room service is used and a pod system is used for tray assemble.

Cost

Another important aspect of the purchase decision is cost, and not just the initial cost. The costs involved with the installation, operation, maintenance, and repair of foodservice equipment also must be considered.

Utility Supply

Equipment requiring electricity or gas must be compatible with the facility's utility supply unless utilities are so outdated or inadequate that renovation is planned. For example, the facility's wiring and circuits must be able to supply the voltage required for operation of all electrical equipment. A piece of equipment designed for a 230-volt circuit will lose about 20 percent of its efficiency if connected to a 208-volt circuit. A motor designed for 208 volts may burn out at higher voltages. Consequently, the voltage (whether alternating or direct current) and phase (the source of alternating current in the circuit) available in the kitchen must be considered before equipment is ordered. Some equipment items require a single phase of alternating voltage, whereas others require three phases. That is, three separate sources of alternating current are arranged to handle larger power and heating loads. If gas equipment is preferred, an adequate gas supply must be available for peak operating periods, and convenient connections must be provided.

Design and Construction

The importance of design and construction to ensure proper performance without costly repairs cannot be overlooked. Equipment should be functional and durable as well as compatible with other equipment in the department/facility. Make sure equipment will fit into available space and can be moved through existing doors. The information supplied by manufacturers in catalogs, bulletins, brochures, and specification sheets should be studied carefully. Contact with other foodservice directors and equipment specialists is helpful. If standard stock items do not meet the facility's needs, custom-built equipment can be ordered, even though it is generally more expensive.

Safety and Sanitation Features

The safety and sanitation features of equipment are critical considerations in the selection process. All equipment should be constructed and installed in a manner that complies with the requirements of the Occupational Safety and Health Act of 1970 and other federal, state, and local regulations and codes. Several national not-for-profit organizations establish standards and controls to ensure the sanitation and safety of foodservice equipment and of the operating environment. Among them are the National Sanitation Foundation (NSF), the Underwriters' Laboratory, the American Gas Association, the National Board of Fire Underwriters, and the American Society of Mechanical Engineers. Choosing equipment bearing the seal of approval of any one or more of these organizations is recommended.

Saving Water and Energy

The newer foodservice equipment includes equipment designed for high efficiency and low water consumption. ENERGY STAR, a joint program of the U.S. Environment Protection Agency (EPA) and the U.S. Department of Energy currently certifies ware washers, refrigerators and freezers, ovens, ranges, holding cabinets, steamers, fryers, broiler, pasta cookers, griddles, and ice machines.

Selecting ENERGY STAR–rated equipment can optimize efficiency and save energy, up to 25 percent on some equipment and reduce the water consumptions as well as the cost. Rebates on energy-efficient equipment may be available from energy providers and the federal government.

Water-intensive equipment—combination oven-steamers, ware washers, and prespray nozzles contribute to the high use of and cost of water. Equipment needs to be evaluated for use of water specified as to what will reduce the amount of water and sewage bills.

Life Cycle of Equipment

All equipment is not always equal in cost, durability, and life. Durable, reliable, long-lasting pieces of equipment are worth the investment. To ensure the longevity of the equipment a preventative maintenance schedule must be followed to minimize the life-cycle cost resulting in greater efficiency of operation of the equipment.

Purchasing reliable equipment and properly maintaining it will result in preventing down time and save energy and money.

Keeping Equipment Clean

To increase the life cycle, reduce maintenance/service cost, and maintain efficiency of the equipment, the equipment must be kept clean. When developing specifications, ease of cleaning of equipment needs to be included. For example, specify the location of refrigeration coils and method for cleaning, the ability to unclog gas cook tops, the ease of removing racks from equipment, and so forth.

Equipment Specifications

Equipment is classified as small or capital. Capital equipment is defined as expensive, usually more than $500 with a long life. It is carried on the financial books and a percent of the cost of the equipment is **depreciated** (lessens the value) annually, until the life has reached zero years.

Once there is a determination of the need for the equipment, an investigation of the options of the equipment on the market is outlined. Compare brands to determine what is available and what might work best in the facility. Talk to other foodservice directors, visit other facilities. Talk to vendors. Check on discounts for multiple sales, a large scale, or for a government entity; check out equipment for size, energy use, read the vendor's spec sheet. Visit local vendors and trade shows to inspect the equipment. Check the warranty and if extended warranties are available, service contracts, and training for personnel.

Make a decision to purchase the equipment. Once the decision to purchase the needed equipment an advertisement is posted in newspapers, trade magazines, Internet and known suppliers stating that a *request for a proposal* (RFP) is being made for equipment for the newly renovated or new construction of the Foodservice xxx Hospital, located in City, USA. Bid materials may be picked up at the foodservice department or a request of a copy of the materials may be made in writing and sent to the company. The RFP states the requirements for purchase, with information about the type, size, capacity, and installation. All information must be very specific. This communication should be in writing to eliminate any possible misunderstanding of what should be delivered. Specifications can be brief or extended written documents, depending on the facility's procurement policies. The important point is that they be written simply and concisely, giving only those details that are necessary to ensure the delivery of the equipment desired.

Some procurement policies prohibit the use of trade names, a proscription usually specified in organizations that use a formal bid system. When this method is used, a great deal of care must be taken to ensure that the equipment ordered actually meets foodservice requirements. When brand names can be stated on the purchase order, the clause "or approved equal" may be included so that competitive bidding can be undertaken, other manufacturers with reputations for quality, dependability, and service should be listed. Another solution is to require that bidders submit complete, detailed specifications of what they propose to furnish and then compare these statements with the original specifications to be sure that they really are equal. The burden of proof should be placed on the seller. Too often, items are purchased on the basis of price alone. Equipment should be purchased primarily for its quality and performance. All equipment may be purchased from one supplier as long as all specifications are met.

Specifications should spell out whether equipment is delivered "free on board" to the dock or "free on board" from the factory and who will be responsible for moving equipment from the dock to the work site and for installing and testing the new equipment. Training personnel in the use and care of the equipment must be made a term of the written purchase contract. Follow up on the performance of each piece and appropriate utilization by foodservice employees is the responsibility of the foodservice director. A thorough understanding of what is stipulated in the warranty, particularly the warranty period, replacement of parts, and service included will save money in the future.

The next step is the opening of the bids and preparing a *justification* (Chapter 7) and *a cost analysis* to determine what benefits the preferred or more costly piece of equipment has over a less expensive one.

Using the cost-benefit analysis, knowledge from other users, and the total budget allocation, make a final decision on what to purchase. Cut a purchase order and alter the winning supplier of the result.

Receive the equipment, check to determine if what was specified was received, check for damage to product, and that all connection parts are with the equipment. Have the "contracted personnel" install the equipment with facility engineering present. Set up a time with the suppliers/manufactures, for training foodservice and maintenance personnel, on use, maintenance and cleaning of the equipment

Equipment for Receiving Area

The receiving area includes an outside area or a loading dock, preferably covered, and adjacent to space to check, examine, or count food that is being delivered. The floor of the dock should equal the height of a standard delivery truck bed: the height should be 8 feet. Accurate scales are needed for weighing all food purchased by weight, For most operations, platform scales with a maximum capacity of 250 pounds are adequate, however, for large operations and large orders an in-the-floor scale of 500 pounds capacity would be preferred, with a smaller platform scale for weighing smaller orders. A desk or table, clipboards, filing cabinets, bar code reader, and computers help increase productivity. In addition, closed-circuit television or a perimeter alarm system (or both) can be installed to increase security in the receiving area.

Heavy-duty two- and four-wheel hand trucks or semi-live skids are essential. (Semi-live skids are low platforms mounted on wheels on which materials can be loaded for handling or moving.) Skids are a good investment when large-quantity deliveries are received and storage space is available. Cases can be loaded on skids, wheeled to the storage area, and dropped in place, thus eliminating excessive handling.

Storage Equipment

The right equipment contributes to the maximum use of available space in storage areas. Equipment for dry, refrigerated, and low-temperature storage areas is summarized below. The storage area should be close to the receiving area. Dry storage area is space allocated to canned foods, staples, and groceries.

Dry Storage Equipment

Equipment for dry storage areas may include shelving, metal or plastic containers on wheels or dollies, and mobile platforms. Adjustable metal louvered or wire shelving is recommended to permit air circulation and to allow exact shelf spacing. For safety and convenience, the top shelf should be accessible without the use of a stool or stepladder. Local ordinances may specify at least 6 inches from the floor to the lowest shelf. At least a 2-inch space between the wall and shelf is needed for air circulation and cleaning access.

Shelving may be mobile or stationary. Selecting the right width and length of shelves is important. Widths range from 12 to 27 inches. If space allows, shelves can be placed back-to-back for easy access from both sides. Widths of 20 to 24 inches can easily accommodate two rows of No. 10 cans on a single shelf. The clearance between shelves should be at least 15 inches to allow the stacking of two No. 10 cans. The length of shelves can vary from 36 to 42 inches or more. Calculations of the dimensions of packaging for each item, the weight per unit, and inventory quantities should be used as a guide to determine the total number of linear feet of shelving needed.

Metal or plastic containers with tight-fitting covers are useful for storing broken lots of flour, cornmeal, other cereals and grains, and sugar. Food from packages that have been opened should be stored in food-grade containers with tight-fitting covers, with the contents clearly marked on the outside. When large amounts of dry food items are stored, mobile platforms and dollies are useful for moving and storing these goods until they are opened.

A separate storage area should be provided for cleaning supplies, chemicals, paper goods, and other nonfood materials. Space needs, equipment requirements, and sanitary construction features are just as important for these goods as for food supplies. For safety purposes, approved types of fire extinguishers should be located in or near all storage areas, and employees should be trained how to use them correctly.

Refrigerated and Low-Temperature Storage

Standard refrigeration, which operates between 32°F and 40°F (0°C and 4°C), and low-temperature units, with a temperature range of −10°F to 0°F (−24°C to 18°C), are needed. Standard refrigerated and low-temperature systems are available in walk-in and self-contained units. Refrigeration systems that can quickly chill, freeze, and thaw foods are needed when a cook-and-chill or cook-and-freeze production system is used. Selection should be based primarily on need, flexibility, and convenience.

Walk-In Coolers and Freezers Important features to consider when assessing coolers and freezers include the refrigeration system used, the construction materials and design, optional features, and the amount of usable space inside. In walk-ins, the condenser and motor usually are located in a remote area. They should be built to provide even temperature, balanced humidity, and good air circulation.

The floors, ceilings, walls, and doors of walk-in coolers and freezers should be constructed of durable, vapor-proof, and easily cleanable materials. The type and amount of insulation used on all these parts are important. Many cooler manufacturers use foamed-in-place or froth-type insulation, but the thickness may vary. Doors should be provided with an effective seal to prevent condensation and loss of energy. Hanging overlapping strips of clear, heavy vinyl inside door openings also reduces energy consumption by keeping cold air in when the door is opened. Locking hardware on the outside is needed for security. An inside safety release prevents entrapment when the door is locked from the outside.

Ideally, the floors of walk-in units should be level with adjacent flooring. However, models are available with built-in interior or exterior ramps. Nonskid strips on an incline are needed for added safety. Automatic audio and visual warning systems outside the unit or in a remote location will indicate significant temperature changes. Built-in thermometers on the outside of the unit should also be checked regularly.

Optional features on some walk-ins include reach-in doors and regular doors with view-through windows. If the walk-in is located in the production area, the reach-in feature could be convenient for in-process holding or obtaining frequently used ingredients. View-through windows should not frost or fog. Walk-in units constructed with modular panels assembled on the premises are recommended over permanently installed models because they allow for future relocation or expansion. The amount of food storage space needed in interior cubic feet can be calculated by dividing the total amount of food stored (in pounds) by 15 (the number of pounds that can be stored in a cubic foot of storage or total food stored). Approximately 1 cubic foot of refrigerated space could store 30 pounds of food. However, because of the amount of space needed for aisles between shelves in walk-in units, 15 pounds of food per cubic foot is the best rule of thumb.

The requirements for walk-in-freezers are similar to those for walk-in coolers, except that more insulation is needed. Freezer units installed with the door opening into a walk-in cooler eliminate storage space on one wall of the cooler, and access to the freezer can be inconvenient. All walk-in coolers and freezers should be equipped with recording temperature thermometers that can be easily read by foodservice personnel. Alarms should be installed in the engineering department that alert engineering staff to a problem.

Some facilities use blast chillers to control the growth of bacteria. Blast chillers may be a stand-alone piece of equipment that comes in a variety of sizes (some can fit undercounter) or a built-in chiller. Blast chillers should drop temperatures by 90°F in 90 minutes. In the stand-alone blast chiller, the blast chiller is automatic, and when the proper temperature has been reached, the single compressor runs to maintain the required temperature. As a safeguard the system indicates if the process of chilling has been interrupted by open doors or power failure. The self-diagnostic/warning also allows an automatic defrost mode with a manual override and remote hookup capability. Temperature probes are placed in the product, which is chilled to the preset temperature and held there. Chillers are available with printers, PC downloads, and mobile trolleys to work with a combi-oven.

Self-Contained Refrigerators and Freezers In self-contained units, the refrigeration system is mounted at the top or bottom. Bottom-mounted models reduce the amount of convenient space available. A compressor, condenser, and evaporator of the right size are needed for uniform temperature control regardless of the load. Foamed-in-place or froth-type urethane insulation of 2½ inches or more thickness is recommended for walls, ceilings, and doors. A one-piece, durable, seamless lining in the interior cabinet is needed to allow for easy cleaning. Exterior finishes vary among manufacturers; vinyl in a choice of colors, stainless steel, and other durable metals are used.

Refrigerators and storage freezers are designed as reach-in or pass-through and roll-in or roll-through units, which are convenient in areas between production and service. Solid or glass doors may be hinged on the right or left. One-piece molded door gaskets that provide a positive seal are recommended to conserve energy. Full- and half-door models with self-closing and safety-stop features are available. A system for locking all doors is needed for security. An exterior dial thermometer and audiovisual temperature alarm should be installed in all units. Adjustable legs facilitate leveling of reach-in and pass-through cabinets. Single units may be equipped with casters for mobility. Other design options include provisions for interchangeable interiors that accommodate adjustable rustproof wire shelving, tray or pan slides, rollout shelves and drawers, and flush-with-floor models for mobile carts and foodservice racks.

Quick-Chill and Freezing Systems Refrigeration systems capable of chilling precooked foods to 41°F (5°C) in less than four hours are available in one- or two-section roll-in units. Rapid chilling is accomplished by circulating fans installed within the cabinet. High-velocity air, forced horizontally over the surfaces of the food product, eliminates the formation of layers of warm air that can slow heat transfer.

Self-contained or remote quick-chill models can be purchased. Cabinet finishes, insulation materials and thickness, door gaskets, hinges, locks, and other features are similar to those found in conventional storage refrigerators. One model automatically reverts to a 38°F (3°C) storage refrigerator at the end of the quick-chilling process. Standard equipment includes a chill timer and several temperature probes. An external probe selector switch, temperature indicator, and audiovisual alarms should be requested.

Foods can be frozen by blast or cryogenic freezing systems. Self-contained roll-in models or large chambers with a conveyor belt are available. In blast freezing, the product's temperature is lowered to 0°F (−18°C) or lower by high-velocity circulating air and a mechanical refrigeration system. In cryogenic freezing, liquid nitrogen or carbon dioxide in a liquid or gaseous state and moving air quickly remove heat from the product. The design and construction features of the cabinet are similar to those of other refrigeration systems.

Comparisons of the capabilities of the mechanical parts used to lower temperatures and the time required in various models should be made before selecting a freezer.

Tempering Refrigerators Foodservice departments that use mostly frozen foods should consider specialized equipment for tempering (thawing) foods rapidly. Conventional refrigeration systems require a great deal of time for this process. Individual units are designed to thaw foods rapidly by using high-velocity airflow and a system of heating and refrigeration. Products are safe throughout the process because the cabinet air temperature never exceeds 45°F (7°C). When the tempering process is completed, the cabinet may be operated as a conventional refrigerator. Conventional refrigerator models also are available with accessories designed to convert them to tempering units by using special controls. This type may be more suited to foodservice departments that use a limited amount of prepared frozen foods.

Ice-Making Equipment

Ice can be made in blocks, cubes, crushed, or flaked form. Block machines produce more ice per day than do cube machines. Cubes last longer in drinks. Block ice cools drinks faster but melts faster. It is important to decide what kind of ice would best serve the operation. A different machine makes each type. Once the decision is made as to the type of ice to use, the next step is to calculate how much ice will be needed.

The production capacity depends on internal engineering but also on the temperature of the water coming into the machine and the ambient temperature around the machine. The major components of any icemaker are the compressor, condenser, evaporator, and water distribution system. A new special feature aided by technology includes sensors that detect potentially damaging changes in water and power supply, with the ability to trigger auto shutdown and restart, self-cleaning system for water lines; and microprocessors smart controls that require no seasonal adjustments. The machines also contain easy access air filters to protect condensers from grease, dust and dirt.

The location of the ice machine within the facility will affect its performance and efficiency. In some instances where sediment and scale buildup are a problem, the machine should be equipped with a water filter. Some models come with a self-cleaning system.

Food Production Equipment

In modern facilities, the food production center is designed to combine all preparation activities in the same area to save labor time, reduce space needs, and eliminate the potential for duplication of some equipment. Adequate space and equipment are needed for the production and holding of foods before assembly, delivery, and service.

Preparation Equipment

The types, styles, capacities, and construction features of various kinds of preparation equipment are chosen according to individual foodservice policies and standards. Other considerations include capability with existing equipment, ease of operation and of cleaning. The major pieces of preparation equipment commonly used in health care facilities are described in the rest of this section. Much of the production equipment is computerized and can be set for time and temperature for preparation. Some of the newer models contain a computer board with pictures and words that identify the product to be prepared. Setting the time and temperature using this identification system helps eliminate overcooking of products.

Oven cooking requires little attention from foodservice employees, can be energy efficient for large quantities of food, and is the only method efficient enough to achieve the quality desired for some products. New oven designs that incorporate microprocessor controls can be programmed for more carefully controlled cooking times. Some systems enable operators to vary the temperature in different parts of a single oven. More digital readouts indicating things such as elapsed cooking time, interior temperature push pads rather than dials or buttons, and instruction symbols allow for simpler operation.

Another oven is known as the *accelerated cooking oven*. This technology combines some of the best features of the convection oven, microwave oven, and the impingement (a conveyor type oven) oven to create some of the fastest quality food-producing units. This oven can cook a variety of products and cook faster than any other previously on the market. There are a number of combination of cooking types that can be specified. The ovens can be expensive. Check with your local equipment supplier.

The most common method of oven cooking is by radiation and convection. Microwave energy is used primarily for reheating individual portions of ready-prepared foods. Several types of ovens are available.

In small foodservice operations or those where space is limited, ovens may need to be located below the range top. If range ovens are used, doors should be counterbalanced and designed to support at least 200 pounds. Range sections can be joined together with other units in the food preparation work area.

A *convection oven* is versatile, efficient, compact, and has high-volume output. It has replaced traditional ovens in many foodservice departments. Because of rapidly moving air, it speeds cooking time by 30 percent and allows for a heavier load than conventional ovens. In addition, the convection oven can operate at about 50°F less power because the circulating heat is used more efficiently. Fuel use is lower than with other kinds of ovens for production of an equivalent volume of food.

In some convection ovens, two-speed fans can vary the rate of airflow or can be turned off to convert the oven to a conventional one. Others have a heat source control that regulates the rate at which air is reheated when the oven is partially or fully loaded. This feature affects the amount of fuel used. All of these ovens have thermostatic and timer controls.

Interior capacities are designed for volume production, with five or six shelves considered standard. Two convection ovens can be conveniently stacked to reduce space requirements. The door style can be selected to suit available space. Solid metal doors or doors with tempered glass to permit visual inspection of foods can be purchased.

Other criteria for selection include materials used for interior and exterior surfaces to facilitate cleaning; type and amount of insulation; ignition system for gas models; sturdiness of hinges and door handles; accessibility of components for inspection, adjustment, repair, and replacement; and temperature distribution throughout the oven cavity. Optional features of some large and compact models include provisions for roll-in mobile racks and baskets to minimize food handling.

Deck ovens require more space than other ovens but can be stacked in double or triple units. However, convenient and safe working heights should be maintained so that the top and bottom units are easily accessible without excessive reaching or stooping. Various oven widths and cavity heights are available to accommodate sheet pans, standard-size pans, and roasting pans. Individual thermostatic controls for each compartment are recommended. Heat balance within the oven is improved by having top and bottom heating units for each deck. Thermostats should be sensitive enough to provide quick recovery of the preset temperature. Interior and exterior finishes must be durable and easily cleaned. Gas ovens of all types should have ignition systems that eliminate the need for a constantly burning pilot light.

Rotary and reel ovens may be suited to facilities that produce large volumes of baked goods. Flat shelves are rotated horizontally in a rotary oven; in reel ovens, shelves rotate on a vertical axis. The conventional system of radiant heat transfer is used. Door openings are located at a convenient height for product removal. Various sizes and capacities are available to fit the needs of users. Careful analysis of energy requirements, space, projected use, and cost versus other types of ovens is necessary before this type of equipment is chosen.

High-volume foodservice operations may wish to consider ovens that accept one or more upright mobile racks of food products. These units combine the features of a convection oven with enhanced labor savings made possible by loading and unloading in rack-size batches. The basic versions accept one rack (2 by 2 feet, 5 feet high), which remains stationary in the oven cavity. Other units accept a full rack and slowly rotate it in the oven cavity so that the food bakes more evenly. Larger units are available that accept two racks or four racks.

Infrared and *microwave* ovens are considered radiation ovens, in which energy waves are transferred from the source to the food. Infrared ovens are used for broiling. High-density infrared ovens cook food rapidly. Infrared heating lamps are used to keep food hot once it has been prepared. Microwave ovens are rarely used for cooking foods but are frequently used to reheat foods in vending areas and in galleys in patient areas. Microwave ovens may also be used as a part of the thawing process; once food is thawed it needs to be cooked following the recipe.

Broilers use radiated heat energy to cook. Most broilers heat the product from above; others use the bottom of the unit.

Ranges Traditionally, designers of foodservice facilities planned the layout of the food preparation center to include several utility ranges. With the choices of cooking equipment available today, a limited number of surface cooking units are used in renovated and new facilities. However, if space is needed for the preparation of small batches of food for modified diets or ingredients used in some recipes, modular units, either gas or electric, should be considered. Modular ranges in 12- to 36-inch widths and mounted on casters can be placed side-by-side or used alone. In addition, they can be relocated easily. Most ranges are mounted on the floor, with cooking done in pots directly on the range top. Ranges should have removable drip pans for ease of cleaning. From one to four ranges may be needed, depending on the total number of meals served daily. *Hot-top ranges* require 20 to 30 percent more energy than open burners. Burners are limited to one pan; hot tops are more flexible. Cleaning methods must be considered in the choice.

Electric utility ranges are available in two styles: solid tops that are heated uniformly and tops that have round heating elements with individual controls. Combinations of solid tops or round units with griddles or broilers also are available. On a solid-top range, it should be possible to heat only a portion of the top at a time. High-speed heating capacity is important for all types of utility ranges. Heating elements, along with the drip pans underneath them, should be removable for cleaning. As mentioned in the previous section, units may have roasting ovens or pan storage beneath the cooking top. All units should be constructed of durable metals that can be cleaned easily.

The construction of *gas ranges* is similar to their electric counterparts: solid tops, open burners, and combinations of the two are available. The solid top should be capable of heating the entire surface uniformly, whereas the open burner directs the flame to the bottom of the cooking utensils. In selecting gas ranges, construction materials, ignition systems, thermostatic controls, safety features, and ease of cleaning should be evaluated.

Induction heating, widely used in Europe, is available for cooking surfaces. This system uses magnetic fields to heat the food in the pan without heating the pan or the air in it. According to operators, induction heating is faster and more even than traditional approaches. In addition, the surface of an induction heat range is flat and therefore easier to clean.

There are a number of different types of dry-heat cooking equipment besides ranges:

- Convection ovens
- Infrared ovens
- Mechanical and pizza ovens
- Microwave ovens
- Deck ovens
- Broilers
- Griddles

Combination Oven-Steamer A *combination oven steamer* puts steam energy and hot-air convection together. In the convection mode, the oven has a water-injection button, which is ideal for pastries, bread, and glazing. The steam mode perfectly steams fish, shellfish, rice, vegetables, and meats. In the combination mode the oven controls humidity in the cooking chamber to maintain a perfect atmosphere for meats, rethermalizing meals, and general cooking results. This type of oven provides all the settings necessary for several styles of cooking. An additional advantage is the savings due to the decreased shrinkage of product and reduction in labor. The combinations come in gas and electric models; a variety of sizes, cooking modes, and capabilities; touch-pad controls; digital timers; probes for temperature measurement; humidity control; and artificial intelligence, which measures food product temperatures at internal points and adjusts cooking processes automatically for optimum finish. They can be programmed for 99 menu items times nine cooking stages, with hazard analysis critical control point tracking options.

Tilting Braising Pans or Skillets The *tilting braising pan* one of the most versatile pieces of cooking equipment. Braising pans have replaced or reduced the need for ovens, range tops, grills, and other surface cooking equipment in many facilities because they are designed to grill, fry, sauté, stew, simmer, bake, boil, or just warm an endless variety of foods. The rectangular, shallow, flat-bottomed vessel, made of heavy-duty stainless steel with welded seam construction, may be heated by electricity or gas. Pans are designed with a contoured pouring lip, and most models have a self-locking tilt mechanism to facilitate removal of cooked products and cleaning. Units range in capacity from 10 to 40 gallons. Small units may be table mounted, whereas larger sizes can be wall-mounted or supported by tubular legs with or without casters. Braising pans are energy efficient, reducing cooking time by as much as 25 percent on many combination food items. Human energy also can be conserved because a significant volume of pot and pan washing is eliminated.

Steam Equipment Energy-conscious foodservice directors have found that steam equipment, properly used, results in significant fuel savings as compared with surface or oven cooking. Equipment operated by steam includes *low-pressure, high-pressure*, or *no-pressure (convection) compartment steamers*, and *steam-jacket steamers*. Any of the compartment steamers may be purchased as individual units, as combination units, or with steam-jacketed kettles. Each classification is discussed separately.

In most models, steam is injected into the compartment at 5 to 7 pounds of pressure per square inch (psi). This means that food is cooked at a temperature of 227°F to 230°F (108°C to 110°C). The models available offer many choices in size, capacity, and special features such as controls, shelving, and heat source. One-, two-, or three-compartment steamers are available as self-contained units or for connection to a remote steam source. Self-contained units generate their own steam through the use of a boiler powered by gas or electricity. Selection should be based on energy sources available in the operation. Self-contained units have the advantage of greater mobility if rearrangement of the layout becomes desirable. However, a self-generating unit should be limited to two compartments for ease of handling cooked products. The height of a three-compartment steamer makes it inconvenient and unsafe to use for most employees.

Steamers are equipped with either metal grate shelves or multipan supports to hold standard full-size, half-size, or smaller pans in each compartment. Manual or automatic timers for each compartment are needed. An automatic timer cuts off the steam supply at the end of the preset cooking period, and the steam and condensate are then exhausted. If a manual timer is selected, the bell or buzzer should be loud enough and sound long enough to be easily heard in a busy kitchen. Doors should be equipped with one-piece, easily replaceable gaskets. Self-engaging latches are needed for ease of opening and closing doors. Interiors should be of stainless steel and exterior finishes of baked enamel or other durable material for ease of sanitation.

High-pressure steamers are suitable for cooking small batches of fresh or frozen foods. Energy is conserved because cooking time is reduced by forcing steam directly into foods at a high velocity. High-pressure steamers operate at 15 psi and at a temperature of 250°F (121°C). Sizes and capacities range from compact countertop or freestanding single units to multiunit combinations of large, medium, and small compartments for large-volume operations. Like low-pressure steamers, they can be purchased as self-generating units or units that require a direct steam source. All models come equipped with automatic timers and shutoff valves and safety features that prevent personnel from opening the door before the interior pressure is reduced to zero. Other features to consider before purchasing a high-pressure steamer include doors that can be opened easily, replaceable gaskets, removable or easily cleaned pan holders, and finishes that are durable and easily sanitized.

A *convection steamer* forces unpressurized steam around the food, vents out, and then replaces it continuously with freshly heated steam. Because a layer of cold air is not allowed to form above the food product, rapid and uniform cooking takes place. The general design features are similar to those for compartment steamers. The steam supply may be generated in self-contained units by gas or electricity or come from a remote source. Single- or two-compartment units and countertop or freestanding models are available. Some are convertible to low-pressure cooking units. Overall dimensions, capacity, pan racks, slides, timers, and construction materials are other features to be considered before purchasing.

Steam-jacketed kettles are suitable for most foodservice operations because they can be used for browning, simmering, braising, and boiling—just about any type of cooking except frying and baking. Stainless-steel double walls through which the steam flows may extend to the full height (fully jacketed) or to a partial height (partially jacketed) of the kettle.

Steam-jacketed kettles are of two types: stationary kettles, from which food must be ladled or drawn off through a valve at the base of the kettle, and tilting kettles, from which food can be poured. Tilting or trunnion kettles can be manually operated, or they can have a power-tilting mechanism, which is especially useful for large-capacity models. Capacities range from 2½ to 120 gallons. The depths of the kettles also vary. In larger sizes, such as 40 and 60 gallons, broader, shallower depths may make the kettles easier to use and clean. The smaller sizes, up to 10 gallons, are convenient for use in vegetable- and bakery-preparation units and in small operations. In general, the capacity that best suits the batch sizes needed in the foodservice operation should be selected.

Manufacturers offer many optional features, such as removable or counterbalanced lids, automatic stirrers and mixers (20- to 80-gallon sizes), basket inserts for cooking several different products at the same time, and pan holders for ease of removing products for service. Steam-jacketed kettles may be purchased as self-contained or direct-connect steam models, individually or in combination with other steam equipment.

In some kettles, foods can be cooled after cooking. A cold-water line is connected to the kettle, and when the steam is turned off, water circulates in the jacket. Foodservice operations using a cook-and-chill system may want to consider making use of this feature to reduce microbiological hazards. A steam-jacketed kettle that has this feature along with a mixer can lower the product temperature from the cooking zone to a chilled state in one to two hours, thus shortening the product's exposure to temperatures at which rapid bacteriological growth occurs.

The newest steamers are connectionless steamers. These steamers require no hookup to a water line, which eliminates maintenance for lime buildup. These steamers are not high-volume steamers, but they work well in medium production use. The cost advantage includes no hookup to a water line and units use steam more efficiently and produce less of it than high-powered, plumbed models. There is no drain hookup. These steamers use 10 percent or less as much water as a conventional unit. Models may use three to six 2½-inch deep pans.

Griddles Griddles may be gas or electric, freestanding or countertop. The size depends on the use of the griddle. Manufacturers can help calculate the need. Burners are usually placed one per foot of griddle surface. Cast iron is the cheapest material used in griddles, but the weight makes them the least-used of all griddles. Aluminized steel is the most standard of the shelf griddles.

The newest griddle on the market is an infrared burner. Infrared offers energy advantages. The griddle plate is between ¼ and 1 inch thick. The thicker the plate, the more heat it retains, but the 1-inch-thick plate takes longer to heat up. Cold spots are a problem with some griddles. It is important that the griddle provides even heat.

Deep-Fat Fryers Properly prepared deep-fried foods provide menu variety and can increase volume in nonpatient cafeterias and snack bars. Several kinds of gas-fired or electric fryers are available with a wide range of capacities and features. Freestanding counter models or built-in single or multiple units are available. Capacities range from 15 pounds to 130 pounds. The type of fat—solid or liquid—that may be used varies in each.

Accurate thermostats and fast heat-recovery features are essential for product quality and the prevention of fat deterioration. Fryers should be made of nonporous materials. Some models provide a cool zone at the bottom of the kettle where crumbs and other sediment can collect, thus prolonging the life of the fat. An easily accessible drain for removing and filtering the fat and cleaning the fryer also is an important feature. Other features are automatic timers and basket lifts.

Specialty fryers, such as pressure fryers, are available for more rapid cooking of foods. Pressure fryers are equipped with tightly sealed lids. The moisture given off by the food or steam under pressure is retained during the cooking process to yield a tender yet crispy product in less time than in conventional fryers.

Mixers The time- and labor-saving attributes of mixers make them essential pieces of equipment for producing baked goods, desserts, and some entrées. Mixer sizes range from 5- to 20-quart bowls in bench models to 140-quart bowls in floor models. Capacity should be selected on the basis of volume needs, handling convenience, and product quality level. Bowls are raised or lowered by hand lifts on small-capacity mixers or by power lifts on larger ones. Timed mixing controls with automatic shutoffs are available. Some models have transmissions that allow speed changes while the mixer is in operation. Speed controls range from three to four or more changes in large models.

Standard equipment with most mixers includes one bowl (either heavily tinned or stainless steel), one flat beater, and one wire whip. Optional accessories include bowl adapters to accommodate smaller bowl sizes, splash covers, bowl extenders, bowl dollies, and mixer agitators such as dough hooks, pastry knives, and other specialty whips and beaters. To make this equipment even more versatile, mixers are constructed with a hub on the front of the machine. Attachments such as a slicer, dicer, grinder, chopper, strainer, and shredder can be purchased to increase productivity and reduce human labor. When purchasing more than one mixer or kitchen machine, the same hub size should be selected so that attachments are interchangeable.

Food Cutters Various types of specialized *dough cutters* and *choppers* can supplement mixer attachments or perform functions not otherwise possible. High-speed vertical cutter-mixers perform cutting, blending, whipping, mixing, and kneading functions. The capacities of these floor machines range from 25 quarts to 130 quarts. The unit can be mounted on locking casters or permanently installed. Various cutting and mixing blades are available. One model is equipped with an easily removable plastic bowl inserted into the outer metal bowl to facilitate removal of food; the metal bowl also tilts for easy emptying. Bowl covers can be made of solid metal or transparent plastic. Counterbalanced bowl covers interlock with the motor for safety. Because of the extremely high speed of the knife blades, large amounts of food can be prepared in seconds. Vertical cutter-mixers should be located near a hot and cold water supply and convenient floor drain for cleaning.

Several other types of food cutters are available to make production jobs more efficient. Careful study of the construction features and the functions that can be performed by each must be undertaken before a selection is made. Capacities vary considerably, so food-processing requirements must be analyzed carefully. Food cutters can be obtained in table or pedestal models. Attachments for grating, dicing, slicing, and shredding also are available for some brands. Good safety features are built into every reputable manufacturer's models. However, this does not eliminate the need for the continuous training and supervision of personnel.

Food Slicers *Food slicers* are machines designed to slice meats and other foods uniformly. Manual or automatic models come in various sizes, and models are available with gravity or pressure feeds. In gravity-feed machines, the food carriage is slanted, and the weight of the food pushes it against the blade. Most automatic machines have more than one carriage speed and can be operated manually. A dial for adjusting cut thickness is standard on slicers. Optional features include chutes for such foods as celery and carrots that are to be cut crosswise or fences for the carriage that allow placement of two or three rows of similar items for simultaneous slicing. Heavy-duty slicers should be driven by a ½-horsepower motor, and cutting blades should be 12- to 14-inch stainless steel. All machines should have a minimum and maximum slice thickness and be certified by the NSF.

The machine's safety features and ease of operating and cleaning should be checked before a slicer is purchased. Safety features should ensure maximum protection against contact with the knife when the slicer is in use and when the blade is being sharpened. Food slicers should be easy to disassemble for cleaning.

Toasters The preferred serving temperature and texture of toast is difficult to achieve in foodservice departments where the time lapse between preparation and service is considerable. If toast must be made in the production or central assembly area, a rotary toaster capable of producing large quantities in a short time is preferable. Gas and electric models are available for toasting both bread and buns. An automatic sensing and compensating device is helpful for maintaining desired color during consecutive cycles and voltage fluctuations. Employees must be made aware of preheating and production times to avoid serving cold, dry, or soggy toast.

Toast is better made at the point of service using a heavy-duty conventional toaster. Two-slice units, four-slice units, or a combination of these can provide more flexibility and certainly a better product with a little extra labor time. Models are available to accommodate bread and buns of varying thickness. All types of toasters should have good controls and be made of materials that are durable and easy to clean.

Baking Equipment A separate baking unit may not be necessary in small facilities or in large operations where most bread and pastry items are purchased ready to serve. However, if any baked goods are produced on site, some basic equipment is needed, including portable bins, scales, mixers, baker's table, pan storage, cooling racks, small steam-jacket kettle, dough divider, proofing cabinet, reel ovens, hand sink, preparation sink, and storage space for dry and refrigerated goods and other appropriate small equipment. In addition, cooling racks and equipment for storage of products are needed as well as space to store all the racks when not in use. Whether specialized bakery equipment is needed depends on the type and volume of goods produced. If a great deal of baking is done, the purchase of such labor-saving devices as a dough divider-rounder, electric dough rollers, and sheeters that can handle various types of dough should be considered. Proofing cabinets are available in various sizes. Units may be manually or automatically controlled to maintain proper temperature, humidity, and air movement around the dough.

Ventilation Equipment

A good ventilation system is essential for maintaining a clean, comfortable, and safe working environment. Any equipment that produces heat, odor, smoke, steam, or grease-laden vapor should be vented through an overhead hood with a blower (fan) to move air through exhaust ducts that lead to an area outside the foodservice facility. Fire protection equipment also is essential.

Hoods are made in canopy or back-shelf styles. Canopy hoods are either wall-mounted or hung from the ceiling over a battery of equipment. They extend only partway over the surface rather than over the entire piece. Careful design and placement of either type are important for convenience and safety as well as operating efficiency.

The size of a canopy hood is determined by the overall dimensions of the equipment to be covered and by local health and fire safety code requirements. A 6-inch overhang is adequate. A practical rule of thumb is 2 inches of overhang for each foot of hood clearance. The clearance between the surface of the equipment and the lower edge of the hood must be sufficient for employee safety and yet exhaust air effectively. A minimum of 6 feet 3 inches and a maximum of 7 feet are recommended for the distance between the floor and lower edge of the hood.

The *back-shelf hood* does not require an overhang. It extends the width of the equipment and is about 18 to 22 inches deep, as measured from the back of each piece. Clearance above the work surface varies according to the type of equipment needing ventilation, the hood design, and the exhaust air volume. Because this type of hood is smaller and closer to the cooking equipment, fire hazards may be reduced and maintenance made easier. Both styles of hood are built with a filtering or extracting system to prevent grease deposits and other suspended particles from accumulating and creating fire and health hazards (see Chapter 14).

The design and construction of exhaust fans and ducts are extremely important in energy conservation. To maintain a balanced ventilation system, proper air movement is necessary. A continuous supply of makeup air for comfort, cleanliness, and preservation of equipment must replace any that is expelled through the system. However, if makeup air is withdrawn too rapidly, drafts can occur, and energy usage increases. Filters should be cleaned at least once a week because clogged filters reduce airflow and the efficiency of the system.

Technological advances continue to be made in systems design for reducing energy consumption. The basic premise behind these energy savers is to reduce the amount of air drawn from the kitchen. Separate air-supply ducts and exhaust ducts are placed in the hood; untempered air flows down the ducts, draws off heat and fumes under the hood, and is expelled. Some air from the kitchen is used, but much less than by conventional methods. A design specialist should be consulted so that the most economical, efficient, and safe ventilating and heat recovery system can be selected for the operation.

Plumbing and Electricity

The foodservice director should work closely with the architects and engineers to plan for adequate floor drains in the kitchen, dish room, and steam equipment area; the location of sinks in the main area and in restrooms; and adequate drains to sewer lines for water disposal equipment. Potable drinking water fountains may be located in the main kitchen. (Check local codes.)

The amount of voltage needed for equipment should be supplied to the architects and engineers. All pipes and wiring going into the kitchen should be enclosed and out of sight. Fuse boxes should be conveniently located.

Worktables

The types and sizes of worktables needed in the food production center are based on the specific tasks to be performed, the number of employees using the space available, optional work heights, and the amount of storage needed for small equipment or food supplies. Well-planned and properly located tables can save time and reduce employee fatigue. A 12- to 14-gauge stainless-steel work surface is preferred because lighter weights are not as durable.

Tables equipped with locking heavy-duty casters provide greater flexibility for rearranging the work center and facilitate cleaning. In determining the length and width of tables needed, consider employees' normal reach and need for space in which to arrange supplies or pans. Tables 6 feet long or shorter are recommended if they are to be on wheels. Standard 30-inch widths accommodate most preparation tasks. Tables with straight 90-degree turned-down edges can be placed together without gaps that collect food particles and fit tightly into corners. For wall arrangements, tables are available with a 2-inch turn-up on the back. Adjustable feet, under-shelves, tray slides, roller-bearing drawers that self-close, sink bowls, and overhead shelves or pot racks can be selected as optional features. Under-shelves and drawers may be made of galvanized metal, painted or anodized metal, or stainless steel. Because of the high cost of specially designed tables, the many options available in standard models should be thoroughly investigated.

Portable stainless-steel or less-expensive but durable plastic or fiberglass bins are convenient for bulk storage in food production centers. Worktable designs should be planned so that bins can be rolled beneath work surfaces where needed. Also available are portable drawer units that offer convenient storage for small utensils and tools.

Sinks

The exact number of compartment and hand sinks needed in the foodservice department depends on the extent and complexity of the kitchen layout and local health code requirements. Several recommended construction features include:

- Stainless-steel (14-gauge) sinks with coved corners in each compartment and integral drain boards on each side
- Ten-inch splashboards over drain boards and sinks
- Hot and cold faucets for each compartment unless a swing faucet is provided
- Separate drain systems for each compartment, with an exterior activated-lever drain control and a recessed basket strainer for the drain
- Variable compartment size (but pot and pan sinks should be at least 11 to 14 inches deep and capable of accommodating 18-by-25-inch pans)
- Approximate sink height of 34 to 36 inches to the top of the rolled rim for convenience
- Rear or side overflows for each compartment

- Garbage disposal in one compartment or on adjacent drain board for sinks used in preparation or ware-washing area (the drain-board location is more desirable for pot-and-pan sinks to avoid loss of one compartment for waste disposal)
- Tubular legs with adjustable bullet feet
- Rack or under-shelf if space permits

The number and location of hand sinks depend on the size and shape of the kitchen and the number of employees. The sinks should be conveniently located near entrances to production and service areas and within work centers to help prevent employees from using sinks in the preparation and ware-washing areas for washing their hands. The sink size should be small enough to discourage use for cleaning small foodservice equipment. Foot- or knee-operated controls are recommended and may be required by local health codes. Hands-free electronic faucets use an electronic eye to enable employees to wash their hands without touching the faucet. No-touch soap dispensers and electronic paper dispensers are also available. Newer models that automatically dispense soap for hand washing and a system for drying are available. Newer standards from the Centers for Disease Control and Prevention and The Joint Commission should be considered when requesting hand-washing sinks.

Waste-Handling Equipment

All foodservice operations need an efficient method for disposing of waste materials for economic and sanitary purposes (see Chapter 12). The equipment available to simplify cleanup tasks includes *mechanical waste disposal, pulper extractors,* and *trash compactors.* The type or types selected depend on the volume of waste materials generated and local codes and ordinances. For example, mechanical waste disposers that grind and flush solid waste through drain lines into the sewage system are prohibited in some communities. The number of disposer units needed and their placement should be considered carefully before they are purchased. Operations that produce large quantities of food in an extensive amount of space may need disposers in several work areas such as preparation, salad, cooking, and ware washing. Small facilities can get by with one located in ware washing and another in some other production area.

Mechanical Disposers *Heavy-duty disposers* range in size from ½ to 5 horsepower or more; the size selected should be based on the intended use. A 1½- to 3-horsepower unit is recommended for the dishwashing center; smaller units may be acceptable in other areas where the load is smaller. However, horsepower is not the only factor to consider when purchasing a new unit. Because disposers can jam, one that has a reversible rotor turntable that can be operated by a manual switch is recommended to increase the life and efficiency of the grinding elements. Easy-access cutter blocks and replaceable cutter blocks also are desirable features.

Disposers can be table mounted with cones or installed in sinks or trough arrangements as in dishwashing areas. Sink installation is the least desirable option, particularly when sink space is at a minimum. Resilient mountings between the disposer and the cone are needed to prevent vibration and reduce noise. In all disposers, an adequate water supply is necessary to flush waste. Some models feature a dual-directional water inlet for this purpose. Accessory components that may be desirable include a silver-saver splash guard and an overhead prerinse spray.

Pulper Extractors   A pulper extractor is designed to reduce the volume of solid waste and trim handling costs if the volume of meals exceeds 1,500 per day. The cost varies: they can be expensive. A pulper can be freestanding or installed under the counter. Food scraps and disposable materials, excluding glass and metal, are pulped by rotating discs and shearing blades in a wet-processing unit. A mechanical steel screw that extracts the water picks up the pulp slurry. Waste material is forced into a discharge chute and dropped into waste containers. The water used to wash waste is recycled through the pulping unit. An automatic water-level control allows replacement of the small amount lost in the operation. The machine should be all stainless steel with a silverware saver. All stainless-steel panels need to be insulated to aid in reducing noise. This type of waste system may be used in combination with or instead of other disposers in situations in which sewage and refuse disposer systems are inadequate. Some models are freestanding, and others can be installed under counters. Capacities, in terms of pounds of waste handled per hour, vary by manufacturer and should be studied before a selection is made. Employees must be adequately trained in how to use the system. Support service should also be available because they require regular periodic maintenance (see Chapter 13).

Compactors   Another type of waste disposer used in some facilities is the compactor. Solid waste, including paper, glass, and metal containers, is reduced in size by crushing under pressure. Compression ratios vary from 4 to 1 to 20 to 1. The type and density of waste materials affect the actual amount of reduction. The volume of trash generated in a facility should be determined before capacity is selected because several sizes are available in either portable or stationary units. Whatever type of unit is used, trained employees who follow written instructions are the best insurance that the unit will be operated safely.

Meal Service Equipment

Meal service needs to be determined early in the planning of a new or renovated area. Chapter 20 provides full information on the various types of tray assembly systems. This chapter discusses the space and equipment needs for tray assembly.

Equipment should be provided for the service areas of the food-service operation to maintain the quality of the finished products. The type of equipment required to accomplish this goal depends on the type of production and service in place. In addition, the locations of the meal service areas and dining facilities should be considered when selecting meal service equipment.

To ensure that each tray is properly prepared, the components of a centralized assembly line should include a conveyor or tray makeup table; hot and cold food-serving carts or tables for temperature maintenance; and auxiliary equipment for holding and dispensing trays, dishes, utensils, covers, condiments, and so forth.

In some cases, preparation equipment for hot beverages and toast is needed. Individual equipment needs vary from one facility to another. Mobile units are recommended for easy rearrangement and cleaning.

Tray makeup lines may be long or short, in a pod design but ample space should be provided to accommodate peripheral equipment and service personnel. The key elements of the line are the conveyor (if one is used) and the peripheral equipment. Traditionally, straight-line conveyors have been used because they are economical to operate. When space is critical or the configuration of the available area is unusual, carousel conveyor systems or units with one or more turns can be purchased (see Chapter 21).

Conveyors   *Conveyors* are either powered or gravity operated. Small hospitals and extended-care facilities may find gravity-operated conveyors adequate. Powered conveyors have a continuous solid or slatted belt made of sturdy material that is resistant to animal fats, oils, and acids. An adjustable speed control and an automatic shutoff are used at the checker's end of the conveyor to prevent trays from piling up. Gravity conveyors are available with skate wheels or rollers in a variety of lengths. Conveyors must be easily cleanable. Heavy-duty, noncorroding, removable scrap pans make cleaning easier, and some conveyors are equipped with a built-in wash system.

Single- or double-stationary or movable overhead shelves can be added to some tray lines to reduce the floor space required for peripheral equipment. Side work shelves of various lengths also can be added. Individual tray carriers attached to a continuous-drive chain mechanism revolve around a rectangular table. The number of tray holders varies according to tray size and length of the assembly system. Flat or sloped shelves placed above the revolving trays hold the food to be assembled within easy reach of personnel and reduce the needed floor space.

Assembly Support Equipment   The assembly and serve system is the system most often used and is found in kitchens that are 20 to 30 years old. The type and arrangement of support equipment can make or break the operation, regardless of how sophisticated the belt line may be. The key position on the line is the *tray starter station*. Equipment for holding such items as trays, paper supplies, eating utensils, menus, and condiments should be within easy reach if a continuous supply of trays is to advance. Various starter units are made up of several component parts. Self-leveling tray dispensers and mobile carts or stand-type stations for holding flatware and condiments are helpful. The configuration of these stations can be adapted to a variety of requirements. These units should be the right height for visual control of the line.

Temperature maintenance equipment is required to maintain both the microbiological and aesthetic quality of the food served to patients, residents, and staff.

Serving tables or carts for hot food with heated pan wells, necessary for optimum performance, may be placed at right angles or parallel to the conveyor. Electrical outlets on the conveyor should be conveniently placed and wired to accept the voltage, cycle, and phase of the support equipment. Slim-line units that are easy to reach over are better for the parallel arrangement. All wells should be sized to hold standard 12-by-20-by-2-inch or deeper pans and should be designed to hold inserts for smaller pans needed for a variety of modified-diet foods. Mobile units with two, three, or more wells are available. Each well should have its own temperature control to keep each type of food at the proper serving temperature and to eliminate energy waste if all the units are not needed at each meal. Wells should be of the dry-heat type for better control. The size and number of units purchased should be based on menu requirements, such as the meal at which the greatest number of hot food items will be held, easy reach for placement of food by personnel, and balanced workload by servers.

Backup equipment for keeping hot foods is also needed in most facilities because batch cooking of all foods is not possible or practical. Steam-and-hold and cook-and-hold equipment cooks food at a lower temperature by creating a pressureless vacuum. Once the food reaches the desired setting it is automatically held. Cook-and-hold cooks food at a specified temperature for a set time to produce desired doneness of the product, once complete, the equipment switches to the holding mode that stops the cooking and holds the temperature above the danger zone.

Some units for holding are enclosed with heated compartments underneath. Steam-and-hold and cook-and-hold equipment, if space permits, *hot-holding cabinets* placed directly behind the service line are more convenient. All hot-holding equipment must be well insulated and have accurate temperature controls. The employees responsible for turning on the units should know the preheating time and follow good practices to reduce energy waste. Too often, hot-food wells are preheated far in advance and left uncovered, resulting in heat loss in the unit and higher temperatures in the kitchen.

Cold-keeping equipment is just as necessary as hot-holding equipment. In fact, cook-and-chill foodservice requires only cold-holding equipment to keep food microbiologically safe. Although the same principles of construction and arrangement previously mentioned apply to chill systems, the type and style may vary according to menu requirements. Some foodservice departments may use carts with refrigerated wells, chest coolers for beverages and frozen desserts, or portable cold tables for holding cold prepared salads and other foods placed on 18-by-26-inch trays. Reach-in or roll-in refrigerators located close to or adjacent to the serving line help keep cold foods cold and reduce labor.

Mobile Equipment

Equipment on wheels can increase kitchen efficiency, reduce labor costs, and lend flexibility to work-center arrangements. Manufacturers offer a wide variety of mobile equipment with general and specialized functions. The exact quantity, type, and size of the various pieces must be selected with the specific needs, layout, and budget of the operation in mind. The following is a partial list of the mobile equipment available:

- Bowl stands for hand-mixing bowls that come with or without a pan rack below
- Heavy-duty utility carts with two or three shelves (available in many sizes)

- Open or enclosed pan and tray racks with angled or channel supports for 12-by-20-inch or 18-by-26-inch pans
- Food-holding cabinets, insulated or uninsulated, with optional cooking-plate insert or heater-humidity unit
- Equipment stands with optional attachment storage below or on accessory poles or racks
- Pot-storage racks with slatted or solid metal shelves
- Tray and flatware carts, separate or in combination, with a varying number of openings for silverware cylinders, in stainless steel or stainless steel with vinyl laminates
- Dollies for dish racks, cup racks, garbage cans, mixer bowls, and case lots of food
- Dish carts, open or enclosed, unheated or heated, with or without self-leveling features
- Hand trucks or platform carts for moving heavy, bulky items to and from storage areas
- Tray carts for patients' meals
- Mobile steam tables

Construction features to be considered in selecting mobile equipment include durability of construction, load-carrying capacity, size relative to aisle width and space within the work centers, quality of wheels and casters, provision of bumpers, and ease of cleaning. Construction materials are either aluminum or stainless steel, depending on the type of mobile equipment needed.

Dispensing Equipment Other support equipment used in food assembly includes units for holding cups, saucers, glasses, dishes, and covers, if these are necessary for the delivery system. Open and enclosed carts or self-leveling enclosed dispensers are available in various sizes and capacities. Heated units are recommended for dinnerware used for hot foods; unheated carts are suitable for dish storage at room temperature. Heated units equipped with a separate thermostatic control for each section are energy efficient. When not all dishes in a unit are needed in a meal, they do not have to be heated. The control mechanism should be capable of warming dinnerware to a minimum of 165°F (74°C) or higher depending on the type of material used. Access to the thermostat and temperature controls should be convenient for regulating and repairing the equipment. The electrical supply cords on mobile dispensers should be retractable for safety. Polyurethane tires are best for equipment carrying heavy loads.

Self-leveling plate nits should be equipped with springs adjustable to the weight of the dinnerware. A manual control on top of the units makes adjustment easier, although some models are difficult to adjust. Strong guideposts at the top help prevent dish breakage when dispensers are moved.

Unheated open carts are practical and less expensive for dishes used in the salad and dessert portioning area. Single or double carts, with or without plastic-coated dividers, accommodate various sizes and shapes of tableware. If open carts are used, plastic covers should be provided to keep dishes sanitary when not in use. Cups and glasses can be stored on mobile carts or dollies that hold the racks in which they were washed. Self-leveling units are more convenient for employees, but they are also more expensive.

The principles for equipment selection and efficient use of space in a centralized tray assembly area also apply to a *decentralized system*. The type and capacity of equipment vary with the service system selected and the number of patients or residents served from a floor galley. Space for storage of food trucks, tray carts, dinnerware, trays, and the other equipment needed for limited preparation or service must be planned for efficient use of personnel and for quality assurance.

DINING AREAS

Dining areas in health care institutions should provide an attractive, relaxing atmosphere. The selection of colors for walls, window treatments, lighting, floors, tables, and chairs can set the tone for the dining area—bright and stimulating or subdued and relaxing. Extended-care facilities and rehabilitation centers usually have patient dining areas. The foodservice director should consult with the medical staff about the type of atmosphere best suited for the institution's patients. The designs for employees' dining rooms should also be discussed with other departments to determine the dining atmosphere most suitable for the institution. This discussion should include the use of live or artificial plants, artwork, music, and other factors that contribute to the atmosphere.

For Patients or Residents

Some hospitals and most extended-care facilities provide dining space for *ambulatory patients* or *residents* either within the patient care area or near the central kitchen. The service arrangements and the dining room furnishings are affected by the type of service—for example, table or cafeteria; the number of diners served at each meal; menu variety; the location of the dining room; health and mobility factors—for example, the disabilities of the residents; and the activities other than serving food that take place in the area.

A study published in the *Journal of Clinical Nutrition* found that a group of male Alzheimer's patients ate about 24 percent more food and drank 84 percent more liquids when served with bright red tableware than when served on white plates and cups and stainless steel silverware. The study suggests that vision problems may be a factor as color diminishes with age and people with Alzheimer's may have a hard time seeing contrast, which makes it difficult to distinguish food from a plate or cup.

Regardless of the type of service system used, mobile hot- and cold-holding carts or tables are more versatile and flexible than stationary equipment. Adequate space is needed for holding trays, dishes, utensils, and beverage containers. Having some on-site preparation equipment—toasters, beverage makers, egg cookers, and so forth—may be desirable for quality control. If cafeteria service is used, height and width of the counter and tray slides affect the convenience and safety of the diners. Residents who use wheelchairs will need a low tray slide if a self-service system is used.

Attractive, colorful furnishings help boost patients' and residents' morale. Tables suitable for seating two, four, or more persons are suggested. The space between the tables should allow easy movement of people and cleanup equipment. The height of the tables should be comfortable and yet suitable for wheelchairs. Chairs should be comfortable and sturdy but not too heavy for diners to move.

For Employees and Guests

Cafeteria service is the most economical way of serving a large number of people when personnel and time are limited. The speed of service and the presentation of high-quality food are two major concerns of consumers. Foodservice managers must share this concern as well as be aware of the costs related to service. The location of the service area, the layout of the service line, the equipment available, and the employees' work methods affect consumer satisfaction and the efficiency and economy of the foodservice system.

Locating the cafeteria close to the central kitchen reduces transportation time and can help control food quality. Batch cooking of vegetables and other foods that suffer from overcooking is recommended for quality reasons, but it is difficult if the service area is far from the production center. Close access to dishwashing facilities is also recommended.

Service lines can be of various sizes and configurations, depending on the number of people served, the service time allotted for each meal, the complexity of the menu, and the dimensions of the available space. Conventional service lines are straight or L-shape. Variations in new and large facilities include circular, scatter, and open-square designs. The flow of traffic is important in whatever configuration is chosen.

The length of the service counters depends on the size of the menu and the amount of food displayed. Adequate space should be provided for attractive display and preservation of food quality. Sneeze guards that meet local sanitation codes should protect all hot and cold sections. Mobile hot- and cold-food holding units lend themselves to rearrangement when greater efficiency and speed are needed.

Whether stationary or mobile, the hot-food holding section should contain an adequate number of wells to receive 12-by-20-inch pans to a depth of 6 inches. Dry-heat wells provide superior control. Individual, accurate temperature controls for each unit also help to conserve energy.

The cold-food section should provide appropriate storage bins or dispensers for salads, desserts, bread, butter, condiments, and beverages. Mechanical refrigeration may or may not be needed in this section. For example, if the facility is small and a small number of people are served in a short time, a service refrigerator nearby could provide adequate sanitary conditions for holding foods at the proper temperature up to a serving time.

Additional space is needed on or near the line for trays, tableware, napkins, beverage containers, and so forth. These materials should be located for easy accessibility by the customers but not where traffic flow will be interrupted or slowed. The same principle applies to the location of cash registers. A line can easily form when there are not enough cashiers. In the meantime, the customer's food gets cold.

Behind the service line, adequate space and equipment must be provided for dishes, food storage, and food setup. Mobile self-leveling dispenser units for dishes help reduce labor, handling, and breakage. Some should have the capability of being heated; others are merely dish storage units. Hot-food holding cabinets or drawers within easy reach of servers save time and help maintain the quality of foods held for short periods. Pass-through units from the kitchen are convenient. Likewise, pass-through, reach-in, or roll-in refrigerators are needed for cold foods.

In facilities serving fast-food items, grills and griddles are available for short-order cooking. Short-order cooking requires more labor, but the benefits are better food quality and customer satisfaction. If this type of service causes delays in the main service line, a separate station could be set up away from the general traffic flow, or fast-food production methods could be instituted.

The overall space requirements for the employees' dining area must be carefully analyzed to ensure the efficient movement of customers and service workers. Today, foodservice directors prefer more self-service within the cafeteria facility because labor is saved and customers have more control over the amount and kind of food they can choose. The space behind the line should be wide enough for transportation equipment and for efficient movement by employees. The customers' side must also be wide enough for bypassing others in the line, if this is allowed, and for easy access to the dining area. A periodic check of waiting times at various stations and customer counts per minute will indicate bottlenecks that can be eliminated by equipment rearrangement or menu changes. A decision must be made concerning the payment method to be used. Payroll deduction, debit cards, or cash may be used separately or in combination. Once this decision is made, the type and sophistication of cash register(s) must be decided.

Numerous types of registers are available. The foodservice director, the financial officer, and the information manager will need to determine which one meets the needs of the facility. Depending on the policies of the organization, it may be necessary to purchase a safe for the foodservice operation. The safe needs to be heavy duty and to store coins and paper money.

Once customers have been served, adequate space in a pleasant, attractive dining room is needed. Because health care personnel usually have little time to relax at meal breaks, waiting and overcrowding are not conducive to good morale. The size of the dining area should depend on the number of people expected to be seated during a given time and the rate of turnover. Generally a minimum of 10 to 14 square feet per person is recommended.

Also, the type of furnishing should be considered. Tables usually accommodate two, four, or more persons. Attractive booths similar to those used in commercial establishments can add to the decor and provide good space utilization. Instead of having one large room, the room can be divided by partitions, sliding or accordion doors, or large healthy plants or dwarf trees to create an atmosphere of seclusion and relaxation. Wall color and flooring materials are also important. Employees who use the facility can suggest suitable colors and materials. Professional decorators and foodservice employees are other good sources for decorating ideas.

Beverage Equipment

Beverage-making equipment for dispensing hot beverages, carbonated beverages, juice, and other noncarbonated drinks such as tea, along with ice makers, are important because these products are popular with customers and are among the highest profit generators on the menu. These machines may be located near the end of the assembly line or in the cafeteria, dining room, or floor galleys. For serving beverages, the main feature needed is temperature control. Therefore, beverages should be served last, in insulated servers or cups.

Coffeemakers are available in a wide variety of makes, models, and sizes. An important consideration in selecting a coffeemaker is the amount of coffee needed within a certain period. If all coffee is made in a central location, one or more urns with a capacity of several gallons may be needed. When a small quantity of fresh coffee is called for in continuous or intermittent service, half-gallon-batch brewers are ideal. Other key factors in balancing equipment and demand are the personnel available to make coffee, the physical dimensions of existing facilities, and the capital allocated for the initial investment.

Coffee urns come in three basic types: manual, semiautomatic, and fully automatic. The more sophisticated models help control quality by eliminating human error and reducing personnel time. However, trained personnel can produce good coffee with less expensive equipment. Precision controls that regulate brewing time and brewing and holding temperatures are important features.

In semiautomatic models, the water that is siphoned and sprayed over the coffee grounds and the replacement water for the urn jacket are controlled automatically. Timing of the brewing cycle and drawing off and repouring of a portion of the brewed coffee for proper blending must be done manually. Fully automatic urns control the entire process. Water spray, water refill, brew time, temperature, and agitation are accomplished through a simple push-button action.

Urn capacities range from 3 to 10 gallons in single or twin units with a hot-water faucet for making tea. Faucets may be placed on one side or both sides of urns or even on the ends to accommodate any serving arrangement. Urns can be permanently installed either above or below the counter, or mobile units may be selected. The source of heat can be gas, electricity, or steam, depending on the make and model of the urn.

Batch brewers are capable of making superb coffee in a short time through automatic controls that accurately measure both the time and the temperature of the brewing cycles. Some models require both water and electrical connections; others are the simple pour-over type that requires manual addition of water above the coffee grounds. These drip brewers are made in single units that hold a decanter on the base or have modular add-on warmer units beside, above, or as part of the base. Whatever type of coffeemaker is chosen, high-quality construction is necessary for ease of cleaning and maintenance.

Postmix carbonated beverage dispensers come in a wide variety of sizes and configurations. Common features include a storage vessel for flavored syrup, a source of chilled water, the carbonation element, and a dispensing head. Dispensers are available with different types of control units. The type appropriate for use on the cafeteria line is simply a mechanical lever that releases the flow of water and syrup when a cup is pressed against it. Control systems that activate the dispensing head at the touch of a button also are available.

For dispensing noncarbonated drinks, such as juice and iced tea, premix and postmix systems are available. Premix systems have the advantage of displaying the product in a clear tank but require more labor because the tank must be refilled frequently. Several postmix dispensing systems for noncarbonated beverages are available. In some machines, the concentrate must be placed in a tank. Other machines are designed to draw the concentrate directly from the container in which it is delivered. Some bag-in-box systems offer added convenience, reduce labor, and positively affect product quality.

Many of the beverages described earlier are served over ice. Ice makers should be selected on the basis of the purity of ice produced, sanitation features, insulation, volume of the storage bin, and capacity to produce ice. Capacities range from 40 to 4,000 pounds per day. Cube ice is the most appropriate format for beverages, but flake machines produce more ice per day. Ice dispensers in the service area should be located before the beverage-dispensing equipment.

Ware-Washing Equipment

The production and service of meals to customer groups of the typical health care foodservice operation requires a large number of utensils and silverware. After production and service is completed, these items must be washed and sanitized. A variety of equipment is available to make this process more efficient and effective. There is a continuous improvement in ware-washing equipment. Most of the improvements are the reduction of water and energy use. Before purchasing this expensive equipment work with consultants, manufacturers, and suppliers to determine which machines will best meet the needs and finances of the department. The following information is applicable, but many changes have been and continue to be made.

Equipment for Washing Cooking Utensils

Space should be provided for washing or at least scraping and presoaking pots, pans, and other preparation equipment, even though a dishwasher is used for the final wash and sanitizing cycle. A location close to the main production area is convenient. Basic equipment for washing cooking utensils includes a three-compartment sink with drain boards on each side, a waste disposer, an electric or mechanical pot scraper, and portable carts or racks to hold soiled and clean ware. Providing adequate space promotes good workflow.

The sink compartments must be large enough for washing, rinsing, and sanitizing utensils and equipment. However, some equipment is too large to fit into any sink. In this case, provisions should be made for cleaning through pressure-spray methods. All equipment washed manually must be allowed to air-dry. Stainless-steel wire racks with adjustable shelves are ideal for this use. Mobile racks and carts are recommended for transporting clean ware to the point of use when storage space is not available or when it is more convenient to store clean ware elsewhere.

Large facilities serving many meals a day may find that a mechanical unit capable of washing and sanitizing production

equipment is valuable. Such equipment is available in single-tank, stationary, moving-rack models. The necessity of purchasing such a machine should be carefully scrutinized because of the space it requires and the initial cost involved.

The use of mechanical conveyors saves time by transporting soiled dishes from dining areas to the dishwashing area. When mechanical conveyors are used, they need to be installed so as not to interfere with the normal service or cross-through work area.

The comfort and sanitation of employees are essential. Areas need to be well lighted, well ventilated, and acoustical materials used to help reduce the noise. Hand-washing facilities should be conveniently placed to prevent contamination of clean tableware and to safeguard employees' health. One of the most important considerations in planning this area is the ventilation system. Dishwashing is not the most pleasant job, but excessive heat and steam make it worse. Dishwashers with exhaust hoods attached at each end allow steam and hot air to be carried away from the dish room. An air-conditioning system should be included in plans for renovated and new facilities.

Dishwashing Machines

Many kinds and sizes of dishwashing machines are manufactured to meet the varying volume, labor, and space demands of foodservice departments. There are many new and innovate machines available to support saving the environment, such as recycling the final rinse water to wash dishes and to a machine that has a self-contained hood. Check with your supplier for additional information. Cleaning and sanitizing of utensils and equipment may be done mechanically by spray or immersion dishwashing machines. Institutional foodservice departments use spray machines. Some commercial operations use immersion machines. Most machines use hot water for sanitizing. Models designed to reduce energy consumption use chemical sanitizers. Spray dishwashers are classified as single-tank stationary rack, single-tank conveyor, and multitank conveyor units.

Single-Tank Stationary Rack Machines Single-tank stationary rack machines have revolving wash arms above and below the wash racks to distribute water thoroughly over, under, and around every dish. Separate rinse sprayers above and revolving rinse arms below are available in some models. Others that use the same nozzles for the wash and rinse cycles are known as single-temperature washers. Wash water and rinse water are dumped after each cycle. Chemical sanitizing machines are single-tank models that use approved chemicals in the rinse water rather than 180°F (82°C) hot water. Wash and rinse cycles for single-tank machines may be automatically or manually controlled. Standard equipment includes easily monitored dial thermometers for wash and rinse. Doors may be located on both sides for straight-through operation or on the front and one side for corner installations. Many other standard and optional features are available. Because of their limited capacity, single-tank models are suitable only for small operations.

Single-Tank Conveyor Machines Single-tank conveyor machines are similar to the stationary variety except that a drive mechanism carries the tray rack over the sprays and through the machine at a timed rate. Left-to-right or right-to-left operation can be specified, and an integral prewashing unit can be built in.

Multitank Conveyor Machines Multitank conveyor units have two or more tanks for prewash, wash, and rinse cycles. They can be built to receive dish racks, or a continuous conveyor with pegs or rods can be used to hold dishes upright as they travel through the machine. Racks may also be used for cups, bowls, and tableware to reduce labor time. Each tank increases the length of the unit. Flight-type dishwashers are the longest because of the space needed at the loading end of the machine for soiled dishes and at the drying end for the clean ones. Larger units also include a final rinse and a power rinse. Some models have drying mechanisms at the exit. As with single-tank machines, many additional features are included as standard or optional equipment. Most multitank conveyor dish machines are large enough to handle most cooking utensils and other equipment and thus can reduce labor costs and ensure sanitary conditions. Most dishwashing areas may include pulpers, compactors, and disposals (discussed earlier), tables for soiled and clean dishes, storage carts or lowerators, and carts to transport clean dishes to the proper area. The usual space allocated to dish tables is 60 percent for soiled dishes and 40 percent for clean. At least a 4-foot aisle is suggested on either side of the dishwasher.

For both single-tank and multitank machines, a booster heater is usually necessary to generate the required final rinse-water temperature. The energy supply may be gas, water, or steam. Placing the booster heater as close to the machine as possible and insulating water lines helps to eliminate line temperature loss. All machines have an attached data plate indicating the temperatures required for wash and rinse water and the water pressure to be maintained at the manifold of the final rinse. Frequent checks of temperature and pressure gauges are necessary to keep dishwashers in good operating condition. Minimum temperature requirements for clean wash water and pumped rinse water in spray machines are discussed in Chapter 13.

All dishwashing machines should carry the approval of the NSF. Once they are installed and in operation, preventive maintenance is necessary to continue to meet federal, state, and local codes and regulations.

A great deal more information than is presented here is needed before a decision on purchasing a dishwasher can be made. Equipment experts can help foodservice directors with the technical aspects and preferred features of dishwashing machines. However, directors must be fully familiar with the department's needs and space requirements to make the best selection.

Cart-Washing Equipment

The growing use of mobile equipment has created the need for space and cleaning devices to ensure compliance with the sanitation standards for this class of equipment. An area close to the dish room is usually convenient for washing carts. Space is needed for easy access to all sides of carts, food trucks, and other delivery equipment. Hot- and cold-water connections and a steam supply for sanitizing the equipment are needed. The area should be provided with adequate

drains and with walls and floors impervious to cleaning compounds and water. The employees assigned to this job require training and supervision to prevent damage to electrical equipment, to maintain a sanitary environment, and especially, to ensure safety in the handling of chemicals.

Can Washing

A space needs to be included for can washing. The enclosed room will need hot and cold water, floor drains, can washing machine, sanitizer and air-drying equipment. The floor will need to be able to withstand lots of water and sanitizer.

Equipment Advances with the Use of Technology

The National Association of Equipment Managers has developed an online kitchen protocol that will radically change kitchen management. This protocol represents an "industry-standardized electronic language" and, when combined with sensors and electronics in practically all kinds of kitchen equipment, it will allow that equipment to communicate in nearly real time with a hub in the form of the manager's computer. This new protocol will provide monitoring and recording of temperatures, energy consumption, maintenance history, and equipment performance or mechanical conditions of the equipment. Using these data, the manager can track preventive maintenance, labor schedules, and the like.

Technology has been used to develop a new combination convection-microwave oven that has become the number one oven of its type in the European market and is now available in the United States. It is used for batch cooking but is also large enough to hold two half-size sheet pans and small enough to fit on a countertop. Many of these ovens do not require vent hoods. Some of the units can store as many as 100 programs to cook different menu selections, have 10 power levels, and are easily cleaned. Another oven that is available is a convection microwave that cooks up to five times faster than other ovens. The convection heating and recirculation of hot air within the oven cavity thaws and cooks items in just a few minutes. The oven contains an advanced computerized program panel with at least 10 programs.

Technology is being introduced and used in blast chillers that provide self-diagnosis and warning for defrost, open doors, power failure, a defrost-mode with automatic manual override, and remote alarm hookup capability. The chillers are available with printers, a personal-computer download, and a mobile-rack trolley to work with a combination oven.

Ice makers are adding special features aided by technology to include sensors that detect potentially damaging changes in water and power supply, with the ability to trigger automatic shutdown and restart, a self-cleaning system for water lines, and microprocessor "smart" controls that require no seasonal adjustment. The machines also contain easily accessible air filters to protect condensers from grease, dust, and dirt. There are other changes such as cold tabletops or pans that will maintain a temperature of 41°F, as recommended in the Food and Drug Administration's *Food Code* and the NSF, who has a rule stating it will make no requirements contrary to the *Food Code*.

Low-temperature dishwashing machines are also making a comeback because of the ability of foodservice departments to lease these machines through their chemical company. An additional savings is the cost of energy and water and the reduced need for the use of vents and hoods because some municipalities do not require them for low-temperature dish machines. The need for air-conditioning can be lowered because of the reduction in steam that is produced by a traditional machine. The chemical company maintains a supply of parts that can be readily and easily replaced by the company on a short notice. Preventive maintenance is done on a regular basis, and the machine can be preset to use the minimum required water and chemicals.

Much of this technology is used to reduce dependence on human effort. Many culinary delights may be prepared by the push of a button, eliminating the dependence on skilled personnel. Labor costs and the availability of personnel have been responsible for operators and manufacturers rethinking how best to provide quality food with fewer personnel and using less energy.

Hood systems are now available that can monitor cooking equipment and increase exhaust-fan speed as needed. A new system is also available that uses ultraviolet light to clean hoods and ducts.

Many new-generation pieces of equipment use technology and less energy, including combination microwave-light wave-convection ovens, steam-powered griddles, improved refrigeration, and many new and improved pieces of equipment available in Europe that will soon be available in this country.

Robotics is being tested for fast-food outlets. A one-armed robot that "reportedly" can operate four griddles, four fryers, and a steamer at the same time is being tested. The robot can cook 500 hamburgers and 300 orders of fries with a failure rate of one mistake every 10,000 orders.

To kept informed on "what's new" attend local dietetic and restaurant shows as well as state and national meetings. Read trade magazines and talk to peers and suppliers for all of the latest trends.

Housekeeping Equipment

The need for sanitation is never fully met. Trash collection and removal, floor sweeping, mopping, waxing, sealing, and numerous other tasks must be carried out continuously to keep the foodservice department environment in perfect condition. Adequate space for cleaning supplies and equipment, close to or within the immediate kitchen vicinity, makes the job easier. A janitor's sink for washing mops and a separate one for air-drying mops should be provided. The same area can be used for cleaning trash containers. A separate room may be better when cans are used to collect garbage.

Equipment Selection and Purchasing

Many kinds of equipment are discussed in this chapter to provide some basic information about the types of equipment and arrangements available that help achieve the standards necessary to provide high-quality food. Because equipment represents a large financial investment, it should be studied carefully before a purchase is made. Well-chosen equipment, used and maintained properly, provides many years of service. Manufacturers are constantly upgrading equipment. The information on the needs addressed is general. Before selecting and purchasing equipment it is imperative that the manager and buyer has completed a thorough analysis of the available equipment on the market.

Because of the many variables associated with foodservice departments, the person responsible for planning and selecting equipment should fully understand the needs of the department and what equipment would best meet those needs. Selecting too much equipment or the wrong kind of equipment is a poor management practice that contributes to unnecessary and excessive costs. The amount and type of equipment needed depend on several factors, including the type and size of the facility, the menu pattern, the style of service, the facility's financial resources, and its plans for future expansion.

The menu influences the choice of the equipment in numerous ways. One of the basic questions that should be answered is why a specific piece is needed. If the equipment would save time and money and would improve quality and personnel performance, then further study to justify size, capacity, and space needs can proceed. Analysis of the items listed in the menu, the number of servings needed, the batch size followed, and the production time required provide the background information necessary for making decisions on equipment purchases.

Another important aspect of the purchase decision is cost, and not just the initial cost. The costs involved with the installation, operation, maintenance, and repair of foodservice equipment must also be considered

Other Information

It is not always feasible to construct a new facility, completely renovate the existing area or purchase new capital equipment. When new equipment is needed a cost analysis report will need to be developed. A *cost analysis* is a written report that compares the cost of replacing the item to the cost of repairing. When making the comparison include:

- Frequency of equipment breakdown
- Total cost for labor plus parts
- Depreciation value
- Disruption of service (such as increased costs for supplies such as disposals)

If the cost of repairing is equal to or greater than the cost of a replacement, then it would be wise to replace it. If costs have occurred over a period of time and the equipment has reached the life (depreciation) of the item it would also be wise to replace.

When purchasing new equipment the director should be aware of the nationally recognized organizations that review, approve and certify foodservice equipment. They are:

- National Sanitation Foundation (NSF): an NSF seal is placed on equipment that they approve
- Underwriters Laboratories (UL): a UL seal is placed on equipment that they approve
- American Gas Association

Other considerations include:

- A method to store electrical cords, especially mobile electrical equipment
- Safety issues, such as blade guards on slicers and other high-power cutters and mixers
- Automatic shutoff for electrical equipment
- Protective coverings for machines that are computerized
- Exhaust hoods that cover all production equipment—water, chemicals, or a newer method
- Handles on equipment are always cool to the touch

Training Employees on Safety and Sanitation

Employee training is essential to maintain a safe work place and protection for employees. In-services may need to be held department-wide or for specific areas such as production. In-services need to be planned and conducted that would include at least the following:

- Use of personal protective equipment (Chapter 15)
- Safety tips and features (Chapter 15)
- Electrical operations of equipment—shutoff, operating methods
- Cleaning of equipment (Chapter 13)
- Cross-contamination (Chapter 13)
- Other safety issues—employee injury, maintenance, and so on

EQUIPMENT MAINTENANCE AND RECORD KEEPING

Each piece of major equipment needs preventive maintenance from the time it arrives. It is the responsibility of the manufacturer, foodservice director, and engineering to keep equipment operating at top efficiency. When new equipment is purchased, the manufacturer must provide an operator's manual. The information contained in this manual should include the principles of operation; instructions for cleaning and maintenance; long-term preventive maintenance procedures and schedules; descriptions of problems that may occur, with suggestions for solving them; and a parts list with the location of service centers where replacements can be obtained. A second responsibility of the manufacturer is to see that a qualified representative explains and demonstrates the proper operation and care to the manager, maintenance personnel, and employees when the equipment is installed. The buyer should specify these obligations in the purchase contract.

The responsibilities of foodservice directors are more extensive. They include keeping equipment records, establishing preventive maintenance procedures and schedules, assigning and training employees to perform activities according to directions, and supervising inspection and follow-up procedures. Setting up a preventive maintenance program includes the following steps:

- Pertinent information related to the equipment purchased is recorded on a permanent record card or sheet, as shown in Exhibit 22.1, or on a computer flow sheet. When this record is complete, accurate, and up-to-date, it will prove invaluable in ordering new parts, having repairs made, checking warranties, making the decision to replace the equipment, and performing equipment inventories.
- The instruction manual on the operation and care of the equipment is studied thoroughly.
- Written operating instructions are developed for the employees who will be using the equipment. The instructions should be simple and easy to understand. Instructions for cleaning the equipment and the supplies to be used should also be included. After employees are trained, these instructions should be posted near the equipment for easy reference (Exhibit 22.2).

EXHIBIT 22.1 Equipment Record Card

Name of equipment: _____

Name, address, and telephone number of manufacturer: _____

_____

Date of purchase: _____

Price: _____

Model No.: _____

Serial No.: _____

Warranty (what parts): _____

Length of time of free service: _____

Preventive maintenance necessary to keep equipment in good running order: _____

Repairs: _____   Repairs: _____

Date: _____   Date: _____

Cost: _____   Cost: _____

Keep an extra copy of the operator's manual and parts list number on file.

Source: Developed by Ruby P. Puckett©.

EXHIBIT 22.2 Equipment Cleaning Record

XYZ Hospital

Name of equipment: _____

Location in department: _____

Who is authorized to use: _____

_____

Operating instructions:

Safety precautions:

Cleaning Procedure

Daily _____

Weekly _____

(Include after each use)

Source: Developed by Ruby P. Puckett©.

- A maintenance and inspection schedule is developed. Instructions should be explicit and complete and should include diagrams that indicate the location of key points or parts. The schedule should also indicate what, when, and how activities are to be performed.
- The employees responsible for performing maintenance tasks are trained. It is important that the employees understand the instructions and time schedules.
- A follow-up method of inspection is developed. A master check-off sheet that lists the equipment, the activities to be performed, and the employees responsible is useful. However, other types of systems also work well. The key is to devise a system that works best for the institution (Exhibit 22.3).
- Review records periodically and take action before a malfunction occurs. If service is required too frequently for any piece of equipment, the records should be checked. Repair costs may far exceed replacement costs in the long run. Accurate records provide management with data that can be presented to administrators in requesting new equipment.
- File manuals and other information received from the manufacturer in a location convenient to the foodservice director and engineering department personnel. Such materials should be part of the permanent equipment file for the life of the equipment. If the engineering department is in charge of routine inspection and care, an up-to-date file may also be located in that department. Files should be reviewed periodically and outdated materials discarded.

Preventive maintenance circumvents the effects of equipment breakdowns, and employees trained properly in the operation and care of equipment can be a valuable asset to management in this respect. The malfunctioning of equipment not only can damage product quality, it also is frustrating and possibly unsafe for employees. After training, many employees can practice preventive maintenance on the equipment they use (Exhibit 22.4). All employees should learn to report suspected malfunctions, unusual noises, and any other problems with equipment to the foodservice director.

In many health care institutions, maintenance department personnel are trained in routine inspection, care, and minor repairs. Large institutions may have a staff member who is specially trained to perform these duties. Enhanced diagnostics permit operators to more easily locate the source of equipment problems and begin repairs.

Having skilled personnel within the organization helps equipment repair times. However, additional salaries are involved, and money and storage space may be tied up in an inventory of spare parts. Alternative methods for equipment maintenance and repair are contract service agreements with the equipment manufacturer or vendor or informal agreements with a local repair service. Whatever the arrangement, it is important that factory-trained repair people and spare parts be available within a reasonable distance of the foodservice operation to eliminate lengthy delays in equipment repair. The cost, convenience, and delay time for each service should be evaluated before a maintenance decision is made.

EXHIBIT 22.3 Equipment Management Inventory

| Equipment Name | Acquisition Date | Identification Number | Location | Classification | | | Safety | Frequency of Repairs | |
				E	S	G		By Whom	Cost

Note: E indicates electrical; S, steam; and G, gas.
Source: Developed by Ruby P. Puckett©.

EXHIBIT 22.4 Preventive Maintenance Schedule

| Preventive Maintenance Schedule | Date of Work Order | Repairs | Responsible for Maintenance | | Education of Personnel | |
			Facility Engineering	Outside Contract	Orientation	Follow-Up*

*Has this piece of equipment caused any problems? _____

*What was the resolution? _____

*Was it equipment failure? _____

*Was it user error? _____

*If it was user error, was additional in-service training given to employee? _____

Source: Used by permission of R. P. Puckett©.

SUMMARY

Well-planned and efficiently designed receiving, storage, food production, meal service, and ware-washing areas for the foodservice department are essential for ensuring a smooth workflow and controlling labor costs. The planning stage requires a great deal of time and investigation of the many options in systems and equipment to make the best decision for the institution. When faced with the task of renovating or planning for a new facility, the foodservice director should consider using a food facilities design consultant. Professional design consultants are familiar with the various foodservice systems and equipment, workflow, and design of work units as well as space requirements. In addition, they can help the foodservice director develop basic objectives and cost estimates.

Accelerated cooking oven
Back-shelf hood
Combination oven-steamer
Convection oven
Decibels
Induction heating
Infrared cooking

Prospectus
Pulp extractor
Punch list
Request for proposal (RFP)
Rotary and reel ovens
Tilting braising pan

DISCUSSION QUESTIONS

1. Explain the role of the foodservice director in the facility design and equipment selection.
2. What are some of the newest trends in equipment?
3. What safety and security measures must be included in the planning?
4. Why is the planning process important?

5. Briefly explain RFP, the bidding process, and the reason for these steps in the planning process.
6. What methods are used to ensure that the flow, equipment selection, and concerns for patient foodservice meets all applicable codes and standards?

REFERENCES

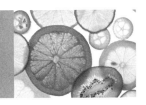

10 Must-Try Exotic Fruits. Accessed 8/02/2010. http://blog.hotelclub.com/10-more-must-try-exotic-fruits/

12 Dangerous Food Additives: The Dirty Dozen; Food Additives You Really Need to Know. Accessed 2/02/2010. www.sixwise.com/newsletter/06/04/05/12-dangerous-food-additives-the-dirty-dozen

20 Questions on Genetically Modified Foods. World Health Organization (WHO). Accessed 8/02/2010. www.who.int/foodsafety/publications/biotec/20questions/en/

A Matter of Record. Food Safety 1(4):8–11, 2001.

Able Dairies Product Specification—Dairy. Accessed 8/02/2010. www.abledairies.com/index.php?mid=2696

Albrecht, K., and R. Zemke. *Service America*. Homewood, IL: Dow Jones-Irwin, 1985.

Alexander, J. Selecting and Acquiring a Computer System for the Food and Nutrition Services Department. In F. A. Kaud (Ed.), *Effective Computer Management in Food and Nutrition Services*. Rockville, MD: Aspen, 1989.

Allen, S. D. Professional Practice Standards: Calculating Food Cost and Estimating Staffing Needs. *Dietary Manager* 10(6):11–15, 2001.

Allison, M., and J. Kaye. *Strategic Planning for Nonprofit Organizations: A Practical Guide and Workbook* (2nd ed.). Hoboken, NJ: John Wiley & Sons, 2005.

Almanac of the Canning, Freezing, Preserving Industry (99th ed.). Westminster, MD: Judge & Son, 2001.

The Almanac of Canning, Freezing, Preserving Industries, 2008/2009. Two-volume set. Can be ordered at www.foodinstitute.com/almanac.cfm

American Bar Association. Commission on Domestic Violence. Retrieved 6/06/2010. http://new.abanet.org/domesticviolence/Pages/Statistics.aspx

American Dietetic Association. *House of Delegates Task Force for Emergency Preparedness*. www.eatrighr.org/cpc/rde/xchg/ada/hs.xsl/nutritiob_17403_ENU-HTML.htm

American Dietetic Association. *House of Delegates Sustainable Food Systems Report*, August 2006.

American Dietetic Association. *2002 Dietetic Compensation and Benefit Survey*. Chicago: American Dietetic Association, 2003.

American Dietetic Association. *Job Descriptions: Models for Dietetic Profession*. Chicago: American Dietetic Association, 2003.

American Dietetic Association. Position Statement: Food and Water Safety. *Journal of the American Dietetic Association* 109(8):1449–1460, August 2009.

American Dietetic Association. Position Statement: Biotechnology and the Future of Food. *Journal of the American Dietetic Association* 93(2):189–192, 1995.

American Dietetic Association. Position Statement: Food and Water Safety. *Journal of the American Dietetic Association* 109(9):1203–1218, 2009 (content advisor).

American Dietetic Association. Position Statement: Food Irradiation. *Journal of the American Dietetic Association* 100:246–253, 2000.

American Dietetic Association. *Standards of Professional Responsibility*. Chicago: American Dietetic Association, 1985.

American Egg Board. *A Scientist Speaks about Egg Products*. Park Ridge, IL: American Egg Board, 1981, reviewed 2010.

American Heart Association. *Critical Pathways*. Accessed 3/05/2010. http://circ.ahajournals.org/cgi/content/full/101/4/461

American Nurses Association. *Nursing World: Workplace Violence*. Accessed 4/29/2010. http://nursingworld.org/workplace violence

American Red Cross. *Taking Hold of Stress: A Fact Sheet*. Gainesville, FL: American Red Cross, 1996.

American Red Cross Urges Caution During Heat Wave: The Elderly and the Very Young Are the Most Susceptible to Heat Illness. Accessed 6/24/2009. http://arcgbw,wordpress.com/2009/06/24american-red-cross-urges-caution-during-heat-wave

Americans with Disabilities Act of 1990. *Selected Regulations*. Chicago: Commerce Clearing House, 1991.

Americans with Disabilities Act of 1990. *EEOC Technical Assistance Manual*. Chicago: Commerce Clearing House, 1992.

Are Women Paid Less Than Men for the Same Work? *Straight Dope*, August 23, 2002. Accessed 2/29/04. www.straightdope.com/columns/0220823.html

Autodesk® Revit®. *Architectural Conceptual Design*—A White Paper 2010. Accessed 11/20/10. www.autodesk.com/revitarchitecture

Babines, M. Revitalizing Your Information System. *Dietary Manager* 17(10), November–December 2008, 12–15.

Bad Bug Book: Foodborne Pathogenic Microorganisms and Natural Toxin Handbook. Bacillus cereus and other *Baccillus* spp. U. S. Food and Drug Administration, U.S. Department of Health & Human Services, Washington, DC.

Potatoes in Foil Can Be Deadly. Accessed 11/02/2010. www.encognitive.com/node/4373

Barron, F. H. *Food Safety Inspections: Basic Compliance Checklist for GMPs, GAPs, SSOPs, and HACCP*. Clemson University, Department of Food Science and Human Nutrition, College of Agriculture, Forestry & Life Sciences. Publication EC 708, April 2002.

Beasley, M. No Magic Bullets for Patients' Satisfaction. *Innovator*, Summer 2000.

BEEF. Accessed 4/27/2010. http://en.wikipedia.org/wiki/Beef

Bendall, D. Exhaust Hoods and Fire Protection Equipment. *Food Management* 34(2):57, 1999.

Bendall, D. High Speed Cooking. *Food Management* 45(7):46, 48, July 2010.

Bennett, L., and L. Slavin. *Continous Quality Improvement: What Every Health Care Manager Needs to Know.* Accessed 6/18/2010. www.cwru.edu/med/epidbio/mphp439/CQI.htm

Berman, K., and J. Knight, with J. Case. *Financial Intelligence. A Manager's Guide to Knowing What the Numbers Really Mean.* Boston: Harvard Business School Press, 2006.

Black, J. S., and L. W. Porter. *Management Meeting New Challenges.* Upper Saddle River, NJ: Prentice Hall, 2000.

Blackburn H. Olestra. *New England Journal of Medicine* 334:984–986, 1996.

Blake, R. R., and J. S. Mouton. *The New Management Grid.* Houston: Gulf, 1978.

Blanchard, K., Carew, D., and E. Parisi-Carew. *The One Minute Manager Builds High Performing Teams.* New York: Morrow, 1990.

Blanchard, K. *Leadership at a Higher Level.* Upper Saddle River, NJ: Pearson/Prentice Hall, 2007.

Blue Goose Buying Guide for Fresh Fruit, Vegetables, Herbs and Nuts (9th ed.). Fullerton, CA: Castle and Cook, 1990.

Blue Goose Purchasing Guide to Fresh Fruits and Vegetables. Fullerton, CA: Blue Goose, 2000.

Boss, D. Disposable Prototypes. *FCSI-The Americas Quarterly* 1(1):36–38, 40, 42, February, 2010.

Boss, D. Waste Oil Wonder. *FCSI-The Americas Quarterly* 1(2):45–46, 48, February 2010.

Brown, K. R. Safety & Health Consultant, College of Public Health, University of South Florida. OSHA Consultant. Materials provided on latest OSHA materials.

Brown, L. P. *Don't Be Afraid of Computers: How to Use Them.* (Class). Gainesville, FL: Santa Fe College, 2000.

Brown, L. P., and R. P. Puckett. Ways Foodservice Operations Can Impact the Environment. *Market-Link* 26(3), Summer 2007, 4–6.

Brown, R. B., and D. Harvey. *Human Resource Management: An Experimental Approach.* Upper Saddle River, NJ: Prentice Hall, 2001.

Brunner, B. *The Wage Gap: A History of Pay Inequity and Equal Pay Act.* Accessed 6/26/2010. www.infoplease.com/spot/equitypayact1.hmtl

Buchanon, P. W. *Quantity Food Preparation: Standardizing Recipes and Control Ingredients.* Chicago: American Dietetic Association, 1993.

Buckingham, M., and C. Coffman. *First Break All the Rules.* New York: Simon & Schuster, 1999.

Bureau of Labor Standards. *Causes of Accidents.* Washington, DC: Bureau of Labor Standards, U.S. Department of Labor, 2001.

Bureau of Labor Statistics. *Fatal Cases Added on the Revised 2005 File.* Washington, D.C. Bureau of Labor Standards, U.S. Department of Labor, 2007.

Bureau of Labor Statistics: Economic News Release: Employment Situation Summary. Accessed 6/07/2010. www.bls.gov/newa.release/empsit.nr0.htm

Calibrate Electric for Better Controls. Tel-Tru Manufacturing advertising materials more information. Accessed 1/20/2010. www.teltru.com

Carosell, M. *Leadership Skills for Managers.* New York: McGraw-Hill, 2000.

Catalog of Food Specifications: A Technical Assistance Manual. Vol. 1. (5th ed.). Dunnellon, FL: Food Industry Service Group in cooperation with the U.S. Department of Agriculture, Food and Nutrition Service, 1992.

Causey, W. B. *An Executive's Pocket Guide to QI/TQM Terminology.* Atlanta: American Health Consultants, 1992.

Causey, W. B. Business Coalitions Pushing Deming-Style "Bonding" with Hospitals. *Quality Improvement Through Total Quality Management* 2(9):129–131, 1992.

Causey, W. B. Clinical Guideline Movement Merging with Supporting TQM. *Quality Improvement Through Total Quality Management* 2(12):179–180, 1992.

Causey, W. B. Converting Patients to Customers a Hard Struggle in Health Care. *Quality Improvement Through Total Quality Management* 3(1):8–10, 1993.

Causey, W. B. You Can't Separate Administrative, Clinical Systems, TQM Experts Say. *Quality Improvement Through Total Quality Management* 3(1):1–8, 1993.

CBORD Group. *Information Packet on CBORD Computer Information Systems for the Administration of Institutional Foodservice.* Ithaca, NY: CBORD, 2010.

CDC Commentary Series Healthcare Needs of the Older Adult: Profile of the Older Adult. Accessed 2/28/2010. www.medscape.com/viewarticle/408415

CDC Guidelines for Disinfection and Sterilization in Healthcare Facilities, 2008. Accessed 7/20/2010. www.cdc.gov/hicpac/Disinfection_Sterlization/3_3inactivBioAgents.html

CDC-Food Irradiation. Accessed 8/02/1–010. www.cdc.gov/ncidod/dbmd/diseaseinfo/foofirradiation.htm

Centers for Disease Control and Prevention, National Center for Infectious Diseases. *Questions and Answers Regarding Bovine Spongiform Encephalopathy (BSE) and Creutzfeldt-Jakob Disease (CJD).* Accessed 12/31/2003. www.cdc.gov/ncidod/diseases/cjd/bse_cjd_eqa.htm

Centers for Disease Control and Prevention. *Frequently Asked Questions about Food Irradiation.* Accessed March 2003. www.cdc.gov/neidod/dbmd/diseaseinfo/foodirradiation.htm

Certo, S. C. *Modern Management* (8th ed.). Upper Saddle River, NJ: Prentice Hall, 2000.

Certo, S. C., and S. T. Certo. *Modern Management: Concepts and Skills* (11th ed.). Upper Saddle River, NJ: Prentice Hall, 2009.

Cha, J. Keep on truckin'. *FCSI-The Americas Quarterly* 1(4):46–48, 50, 52, 54, 4Q 2010.

Charney, C. *The Instant Manager* (Rev. ed.). New York: AMACOM American Management Association, 2004.

Chen, J. Future of Phones. *Readers Digest*, May 2010, 95.

Chilton, J. Making HACCP a Reality. *Dietary Manager* 10(2):10–13, 2001.

Clean Air Act (United States). Accessed 4/27/2010. http://en.wikipedia.org/wiki/Clean_Air_Act

Clemson Cooperative Extension: Foodservice Operations Inspections. Accessed 4/08/2010. www.clemson.edu/extension/hgic/food/food_safety/other/hgic3862.html

Closed Shop. Accessed 5/09/2010. http://legal-dictionaty.thefreedictionary.com/Closed+shops

Clostridium Difficile—C. diff. Mayo Clinic Staff. Accessed 11/2/2010. www.mayoclinic.com/health/c-difficile/DS00736/DSECTIONS=causes

Code Green: Reconciling Green Cleaning with the Food Code. Accessed 7/20/2010. www.foodservicewarehouse.com/education/going-green/code-green.aspx

Cohen, A. R., Fink, S. L., Gadon, H., Willits, R. D., and N. Josefowitz. *Effective Behavior in Organizations* (4th ed.). Homewood, IL: Irwin, 1988.

Cohen, D. S., with foreword by J. P. Kotter. *The Heart of Change: Field Guide.* Boston: Harvard Business School-Deloite Development LLC, 2005.

Cohen, M. W. Arguments for and against MBO. *Hospital and Health Service Administration,* special issue, January 1980.

Coltman, M. M. *Cost Control for the Hospitality Industry* (2nd ed.). New York: Van Nostrand Reinhold, 1989.

Coltman, M. M. *Hospitality Management Accounting* (5th ed.). New York: Van Nostrand Reinhold, 1993.

Commercial Fishing-Fish Farms, PCB, Environmental Damage & Healthy, Safe Alternative. Accessed 8/05/2010. www.dulabab.com/food-medicine/commerical-fishing/

Common Questions on Food Safety. Accessed 4/09/2010. www.fsis.usda.gov/help/FAQs-Food_Safety/index.asp

Cooking Tips and Guide: Classification of Poultry. Accessed 6/10/2010. www.allcookingtips.com/2008/01/19/poultry-classification/

The Cook's Thesaurus Edible Flowers. Accessed 8/09/2010. www.foodsubs.com/Flowers.html

Cool Running with Ice Makers. *Foodservice Equipment Report* 7(3):42–46, 2003.

Cooper Instrument Corporation. *Professional Foodservice Quality Assurance Foods.* Middlefield, CT: Coopet Instruments. (Brochures available for various types and uses of thermometers.)

The Cost of Foodborne Illness. Accessed 4/09/2010. www.fightbac.org/content/view13/19

The Cost of Medicare/Medicaid Have Outpaced Health Cost by 1/3 Since 1970. Accessed 6/07/2010. www.weeklystandards.com/weblogs/TWSFP/2009/07/costs_of_medicaremedicaid_ha

Costa, A. D. Diversity Training as an Investment. *Consultant* 36(1):89–91, 2003.

Costello, T. The Work in Teamwork: Observations and Perspectives. *Consultant* 36(1):71–72, 75, 77, 79, 2003.

Covey, S. *7 Habits of Highly Effective People.* New York: Simon & Schuster, 1989.

Coyle, D. Blogging and Social Networking Aren't Just for Tweens. *NAFEM in Print* 8(2):12–15, Summer 2009.

Cross, E. W. Implementing the Americans with Disabilities Act. *Journal of the American Dietetic Association* 93(3):273–275, 1993.

Culinary Institute of America. *The Professional Chef* (7th ed.). New York: Wiley, 2002.

Culture Shock: The Language of Food Safety Must Speak to Many Cultures in Today's Foodservice Kitchens. *Food Safety Illustrated* 3(3):8–10, 12, 2003.

Cummings, L. E., and W. T. Cummings. Foodservice and Solid Waste Policies: A View in Three Dimensions. *Hospitality Research Journal* 14(2):163–171, 1991.

Cummings, L. Foodservice Solid Waste Wars: The Solid Waste Audit. *Consultant* 24(4):37–38, 1991.

Dalton, L. What's that Stuff? Food Preservatives. *Science & Technology*: 80945 (November 11, 2002).

Define "Cleaning" and "Sanitizing" and the Difference Between the Two Procedures. Accessed 7/20/2010. www.foodsafetysite.com/educators/competencies/foodservice/cleaning/cas1.html

Deming, W. E. Improvement of Quality and Productivity through Actions by Management. *National Productivity Review* 2(1):12–22, 1982.

Design Packaging and Merchandising. Accessed 3/08/2020. http://samsales.com.au/design-packaginf-merchandising.html

Dessler, G. *Human Resource Management* (8th ed.). Upper Saddle River, NJ: Prentice Hall, 2000.

Dessler, G. *Leading People and Organizations in the 21st Century.* Upper Saddle River, NJ: Prentice Hall, 2000.

Dessler, G. *Management Leading People and Organizations in the 21st Century.* Upper Saddle River, NJ: Prentice Hall, 2001.

Diagnosis (MSD). *Merck.* Accessed 5/19/2010. www.merck.com/mmhe/sec05/ch059/ch059c.html

Difference Between Advertising and Promotion. Accessed 6/14/2010. www.differancebetween.net/busines/difference-between-adertisin-promotion/

Dimitri, C., and C. Greene. *Recent Growth Patterns in the U.S. Organic Foods Market.* Publication AIB-777. Washington, DC: Economic Research Service, U.S. Department of Agriculture, 2002. Accessed December 2003. www.ers.usda.gov/publications/aib777/aib777c.pdf

Dlugacz, Y. D., and A. Greenwood. *The Quality Handbook for Health Care Organizations: A Managers' Guide to Tools and Programs.* San Francisco: Jossey-Bass, 2004.

DMA website www.DMAonline.org or the office of Pam Himrod RD, MS, Director of Education, 406 Surrey Woods Drive, St. Charles, IL 60174.

Donhauser, K., and M. Braunbach. Smart Purchasing Practices for Foodservice Supplies. *Dietary Manager* 18(10): November–December, 2009, 28–29.

Drucker, P. *The Practice of Management.* New York: Harper & Row, 1954.

Eccles T. *Succeeding with Change.* New York: McGraw-Hill, 1996.

Edible Flowers—How to Choose Edible Flowers. Accessed 8/09/2010. http://whatscookingamerica.net/EdibleFlowera/EdileFlowersMain.htm

Educational Foundation of the National Restaurant Association. *Serv-Safe.* Chicago, 2010.

Employer: Job Applicant and Interview FAQS. Accessed 6/26/2010. http://labor-employment-law.lawyers.com/human-resources-law?Employer-Job-Application

Ethics. Accessed 3/05/2010. Josephsoninstitute.org/michael/index.html

Evaluation of the Joint Commission Emergency Management Standards. www.nvha.net/bio/posting.jcstandards.pdf

Exotic Vegetables. Accessed 8/02/2010. http://foodlorist.blogpot.com/2007/06/exotic vegetables.html

The Extent of Foodborne Illness in America. Accessed 4/09/2010. www.fightbac.org/content/view/12/20

The Facts about Food Irradiation. Accessed 8/02/2010. http://uw-food-irradiation.engr.wisc.edu/Facts.html

Fact Sheet: *Use a Food Thermometer: Why Use a Thermometer.* Accessed 7/09/2010. www.fsis.usda.gov/factsheet/Use-a-foodthermometer/index,asp

Fannin, W. R. Making MBO Work: Matching Management Style to MBO Program. *Supervisory Management* 26:20–27, 1981.

Fat Content of Fish (Selected varieties). Accessed 8/05/2010. www.weightlossforall.com/fat-content-fish.htm

FDA Regulations for Bottled Water (Use FDA website and add bottled water.)

FDA U.S. Food and Drug Administration, U.S. Department of Health & Human Service. *Hazard Analysis and Critical Control Point Principles and Application Guidelines.* Accessed 4/05/2010. www.fda.gov/Food/FoodSafety/HazrdAnalysisCriticalControlPointsHACCP/HACC

Federal Emergency Management Agency Library. *Emergency Food and Water Supplies.* FEMA 215, 1992. Updated February 12, 2003. Accessed 3/20/2003. www.fema.gov/library/emfdwtr.shtm

FEMA. *Terrorism*. Retrieved 5/26/2009. www.fema.gov/hazard/terrorism/index.shrm

Ferraro, R. The Step by Step Series: How to Hire Good People. *Trade Talk*, March 2001, 3–36.

Fight Back: About Foodborne Illness—Booklet. Accessed 04/09/2010. www.fightbac.org/content/view/12/20

Fire Emergency Initial Response and Evacuation. Virginia Beach, VA: Costal Training Technologies Corporation, 2007.

FireProTec—Your Authority for Fire Codes. Code Updates. Accessed December 2003. www.fireprotec.com_updates.html

Fish. Accessed 8/05/2010. www.answers.com/topic/fish-food

Fitzpatrick, T. Composting Solutions: From Garbage to Black Gold. *Food Management* 45(6):34, 36, 38, 40, 42, June 2010.

Florida Agricultural Experimental Station, Office of Dean of Research. *New Plants for Florida*. Gainesville: Institute of Food and Agricultural Sciences, University of Florida, 2003.

Florida Department of Business and Professional Regulations. *Guide to Hazard Analysis and Critical Control Point*. Accessed 4/08/2010. www.MyFlorida.com/dbpr

Floyd, J. M. Biometrics—The Future Competitive Edge. *Foodservice Equipment and Supplies* 56(1), 2003.

Food Additives. Accessed 2/02/2010. www.foodadditivesworld.com/preservatives.html

Food Additives—Are they Safe? *Food safety, Preparation and Storage Tips*. Cooperative Extension, College of Agriculture & Life Sciences, University of Arizona.

Food and Drug Administration, U.S. Public Health Service. Food Code 2009. Washington, DC: U.S. Department of Health and Human Services, 2001.

Food Code 2009, Department of Health and Human Services, FDA Food and Drug Administration. Accessed 7/10/2010. www.fda.gov/Food/FoodSafety/RetailFoodProtection/FoodCode/FoodCode2009/uc

Food Purchasing. Green Seal™ Guide for Restaurants and Foodservices. Based on GS-46.

Food Safety Glossary. Accessed 4/09/2010. www.fightbac.org/content/view12/22

Food Safety Illustrated 3(3):8–10, 12, 2003.

Food Safety: Food Storage, Preparation & Handling. Accessed 8/22/2010. www.fsis.usda.gov/help/faqs_hotline_preparation/index.asp

Foodservice Inspections—Public Health. Accessed 6/06/2010. http://phdmc.controlpanel2.donet.com/index.php?/programs/protection/foodserviceinspectio

Food Storage Guidelines for Consumers. Virginia Cooperative Extension. Accessed 8/22/2010. www.pubs.ext.vt.edu/348/348–960/348–960.html

Foodborne Illness: Its Origin and How to Avoid It. Accessed 4/08/2010. www.eufic.org/article/en/page/RARCHIVE/expid/review-foodborne-illness

Foodborne Pathogenic Microorganisms and National Toxins Hand Book. May secure from the web at www.cfsan.fda.gov/~mow/intro-html

Food-Borne *Staphyloccus aureu*. Division of Environmental Health, Florida Department of Health. 2010 pamphlet.

Foodservice and Packaging Institute. *Foodservice Disposables: Should I Feel Guilty?* Washington, DC: Foodservice and Packaging Institute, 1991.

For Your Next Renovation: How to Take Charge. *FoodService Director* 5(8):152, 1992.

Frequently Asked Questions—Foodborne Illness. Centers for Disease Control and Prevention. Accessed 4/08/2010. www.cdc.gov/ncidod/dbm/diseaseinfo/foodborneinfections_g.htm

Fresh Produce Marketing Association. *Produce 101*. Newark, DE: Bill Communication, and Fresh Produce Marketing Association, 2010.

Gaines, R. Buy Fresh, Buy Local. *Dietary Manager* 14(8): 2005.

Gardner, J. Legal Matters—How to Hire Without Getting Sued. *Outfront*, Fall 2000.

Garvin, D. A. *Managing Quality: The Strategic and Competitive Edge*. New York: Free Press, 1988.

Gatley, R. F. Why Training Fails. *Consultant*, third quarter, 2000.

Geile, R. Latest Trends in Commercial Foodservice Equipment. *MarketLink* 28(1):5, Winter 2009.

Gsworth, M. D., Shanklin, C. W., Gench, B., and M. Hinson. Composition of Waste Generated in Six Selected School Foodservice Operations. *School Foodservice Research Review* 16(2):125–130, 1992.

Gibbs, N. A. Special Report on Women. *Time* 174(16):24–33, 2009.

Gibbs, N. What Women Want Now: A *Time* Special Report. *Time* 174(16):5, 24–35, 2009.

Gilbert, N. Bioterrorism: Better Safe than Sorry. *Provider* 26(6), 2002.

Giuliani, R. W. *Leadership*. New York: Miramax Books, 2005.

Gómez-Mejía, L. R., Balkin, D. B., and R. L. Candy. *Managing Human Resources* (3rd ed.). Upper Saddle River, NJ: Prentice Hall, 2001.

Greathouse, K. R., and M. B. Gregoire. Variables Related to Selection of Conventional, Cook–Chill, and Cook–Freeze Systems. *Journal of the American Dietetic Association* 88:476–478, 1988.

Greathouse, K. R., Gregoire, M. B., Spears, M. C., Richards, V., and R. F. Nassar. Comparison of Conventional, Cook–Chill, and Cook–Freeze Foodservice Systems. *Journal of the American Dietetic Association* 89:1606–1611, 1989.

Green and Bearing It. *Food Management* 46(3):30–32, 36–38, 40, March 2010.

Green Seal. *Energy Conservation*. 2-page handout, 2010,

Green Seal. *Waste Management*. 2-page handout. Relates to Green Seal™ Guide for Restaurants and Foodservice Standards GS-46. The entire GS-46 is at http://greenseal.org/certification/standards/gs46_restaurantsfoodservice.cfm

Green, D. L. Going Backwards: Bush Expected to Weaken Portions of Clean Air Act: Issue Revisited Amid High Approval Rating. Common Dreams News Center NOW. *Baltimore Sun*, December 23, 2001. Accessed 12/23/2003. www.commondreams.org/headlines01/1223–01.htm

The Greenwash Brigade: Define "Sustainability" Please. Accessed 7/02/2010. www.publicradio.org/colums/sustainability/greenwash/2008/01/define_sustainability

Greer, I. W. *Glossary of Weather and Climate Related Oceanic and Hydrologic Terms*. Boston: American Meteorological Society, 2000.

Grossbauer, S. Learn about Your Customers through Satisfaction Survey. *Dietary Manager* 11(9):11–15, 2002.

Gryna, F. M. *Quality Circles: A Team Approach to Problem Solving*. New York: AMACOM, 1981.

HACCP for the Foodservice Worker. Accessed 6/06/2010. www.aces.edu/pub/docs/H/HE-0726

HACCP. Accessed 4/15/2010. www.cabicompendium.org/ahpc/Library/HTML/Production/fsdq_haccp.htm

Haggerty, D. *Getting It Done: Communicate Better*. Milwaukee, WI: Credit Union Management, 2002.

Haimann, T., Scott, W. G., and P. E. Connor. *Management* (4th ed.). Boston: Houghton Mifflin, 1982.

Hand, B. *All about Artificial Sweeteners*. Accessed /29/2010. www.sparkpeople.com/resource/nitrition_articles.asp?id=289

Harvard Business School. *Managing Projects Large and Small*. Boston: Harvard Business School Press, 2004.

Hazard Communications 1910.*1200 OSHA Safety and Health OSHA Standards-29CFR.HC*. Accessed 4/15/2010. (Information from OSHA consultant, Keith Brown.)

The Health Care Affordability Act H.861. Committee of Conference—May 5, 2006. Accessed 3/05/2010. www.leg.state.vt.us/healthcare/H861_Two_Pager.htm

Health Care Financing Administration. Survey, Certification and Enforcement. *Long Term Care Survey Regulations, Forms, Procedures, Interpretive Guidelines SOM: 274*. Effective July 1995. Washington, DC: Health Care Financing Administration, 1995.

Healthcare Bill to Cause U.S. Hyperinflation by 2015. Accessed 4/29/2010. www.prnewswire.com/news-releases/healthcare-bill-to-cause-us-hyperinflation-by-2

Heib, F. Colored Dishware May Increase Residents Intake. *Dietary Manager* 15(1):30, January 2006.

Heimen, A. M. *What Is BHA and BHT?* Accessed 2/02/2010. http://chemistry.about.com/od/foodcookingchemistry/abba-bht-presevatives.hmt

Hellmich, N. Z-Trim Is the New Fat Substitute. *Gainesville (Fla.) Sun*, Section D, 1, November 6, 2003.

Henkel, J. Sugar Substitutes: Americans Opt for Sweetness and Lite. *FDA Consumer*, November–December 1999.

Hennenman, A. Nuts for Nutrition. *Food Reflections Newsletter*, University of Nebraska Cooperative Extension in Lancaster County (Free monthly e-mail newsletter available lancaster.unl.edu/food/foodtalk.htm)

Hernandez, J. Supplier Relationship Are Key to Safe Food Receiving. *Food Management*, 2nd Quarter 2009, 57–62.

Hersey P., and K. H. Blanchard. *Management and Organization Behavior*. Englewood Cliffs, NJ: Prentice Hall, 1988.

Hersey, P., and K. H. Blanchard. *Management of Organizational Behavior: Utilizing Human Resources* (4th ed.). Englewood Cliffs, NJ: Prentice Hall, 1982.

Herz, M. L. *Analysis of Alternative Patient Tray Delivery Concepts*. Natick, MA: U.S. Army Natick Research and Development Command, 1977.

Herzberg, F. One More Time: How Do You Motivate Employees? *Harvard Business Review*, January–February, 1968, 54–63.

Herzberg, F. *The Managerial Choice: To Be Effective or to Be Human* (new ed.). Salt Lake City: Olympus, 1982.

Herzberg, F. *Work and the Nature of Man*. Cleveland: World, 1966.

Holaday, S. Green House–front and back. *The Consultant*, 2nd Quarter 2009, 57–62.

Hollinworth, N. D., Shanklin, C. W., and E. W. Cross. Waste Stream Analyses in Seven Selected School Foodservice Operations. *The Consultant* 19: 81–87, 1995.

Holpp, L. Making Choices: Self-Directed Teams or Total Quality Management? *Training* 29(5):69–76, 1992.

Hopkins, R. Defend the earth, start in the kitchen . . . then feed it! *The Consultant*, 2nd Quarter 2009, 63, 65.

Hospital Emergency Management: Meeting the Joint Commission's New Environmental Management Standards. Accessed 1/30/2010. www.ecri.org/Conferences/Pages/Hospital_Emergency_Management.aspx

Howard, R. J. Bioterrorism and Our Food: What Are the Dangers? What Can We Do? *Dietary Manager* 10(19):24–25, 2001. Accessed 4/27/2010. www.1.eere.energy.gov/femp/newsevents/fempfocus_article.cfm/news-id=8306

Hudson, N. R. *Management Practice in Dietetics*. Belmont, CA: Wadsworth, 2000.

Hysen, P., and J. Harrison. Facilities Design. In J. C. Rose (Ed.), *Handbook for Health Care Foodservice Management*. Rockville, MD: Aspen, 1984.

Ingle, S., and N. Ingle. *Quality Circles in Service Industries*. Englewood Cliffs, NJ: Prentice Hall, 1983.

Inman-Felton, A., and M. S. Rops. *Ensuring Staff Competence: A Guide for Meeting JCAHO Competence Standards in All Settings*. Chicago: American Dietetic Association, 1998.

Introduction to Clean Water Act. Accessed 4/27/2010. www.epa.gov/watertrain/cwa/leftindex.htm

Irradiation in Action. *Food Safety Education* 7(3):8, 2002.

Is an Avocado a Fruit or a Vegetable? Accessed 8/09/2010. http://wiki.answers.com/Q/Is_an_avocado_a_fruit_or_a_vegetable

ISO 22000 2005. *Plain English Introduction*. Accessed 4/15/2010. www.praxiom.com/iso-22000-intro.htm/

Iverson, K. M. *Managing Human Resources in the Hospitality Industry: An Experimental Approach*. Upper Saddle River, NJ: Prentice Hall, 2001.

Jackson, R. Information Technology: High-Tech Solutions Improve Care, Reduce Costs. *Health Care Food and Nutrition Focus* 20(11): 1–8, 2003.

Jeary, T., with K. Dower and A. Fishman. *Life Is a Series of Presentations*. New York: Simon & Schuster, 2004.

Joint Commission. *Accreditation Manual*. Oak Brook Terrace, IL: Joint Commission, 2009.

Joint Commission on Accreditation of Healthcare Organizations. *Accreditation Manual for Hospitals*. Vol. I: Standards (178–188). Oak Brook Terrace, IL: Joint Commission on Accreditation of Healthcare Organizations, 2010.

Joint Commission Resources. *Assessing Hospital Staff Competence*. Chicago: Joint Commission on Accreditation of Healthcare Organizations, 2002.

Jones, J. M., and K. Elam. Sugar and Health: Is There an Issue? *Journal of the American Dietetic Association* 103(8):1058–1060, 2003.

Jones, K. H., and J. Adler. Time to Reopen the Clean Air Act: Clearing Away the Regulatory Smog. *Cato Policy Analysis* No. 233. July 11, 1995. www.cato.org/pubs/pas/pa-233.html

Juran, J. M. *Quality Control Handbook*. New York: McGraw-Hill, 1951.

K & A First Aid: Training and Safety Compliance. Monthly Safety Updates: February 2002. *Fire Extinguisher Use*. Accessed December 2003. www.kafirstaid.com/febo2.htm

Kahan, B., and M. Goodstadt. *Continuous Quality Improvement and Health Promotion: Can CQI Lead to Better Outcomes?* Oxford, UK: Health Promotions International, Oxford University Press, 1999.

Kaiser, J., and F. J. DeMicco, with R. N. Grimes. *Contemporary Management Theory Controlling and Analyzing Costs in Foodservice Operations*. Upper Saddle River, NJ: Prentice Hall, 2000.

Kanungo, R. New Deli Metallo-Beta-Lactamase1: Is There a Need to Worry? *Indian Journal of Medical Microbiology* 28(4): 275–276, 2010. Accessed 11/03/2010. www.ijmm.org/article.asp?issn=0255–0857;year=2010;volume =28;issue=4;spages=2

Karash, J. A. MRSA: Hospitals Step Up Fight. Will It Be Enough? *H&HN; Hospitals l& Health Network* (July 2010), 50, 52, 54.

Kasavana, M. L. *Computer Systems for Foodservice Operations*. New York: Van Nostrand Reinhold, 1984.

Kasavana, M. L., and J. J. Cahill. *Managing Computers in the Hospitality Industry* (2nd ed.). East Lansing, MI: Educational Institute of the American Hotel & Motel Association, 1992.

Katcher, B. L., with A. Snyder. *30 Reasons Employees Hate their Managers: What People May Be Thinking and What You Can Do About It.* New York: AMACOM American Management, 2007.

Katzenbach, J. R., and D. K. Smith. *The Wisdom of Teams.* New York: Harper Business, 1994.

Kaufer, S., and J. W. Mattman. *Workplace Violence: An Employer's Guide.* Accessed 5/19/2009. www.workviolence.com/articles/employees_guide.htm

Kearney, V. Sanitary Conditions F371 and Beyond. *Dietary Manager* 18(3): March 2009, 25–27.

Keiser, J., and F. J. DeMicco, with R. N. Grimes. *Contemporary Management Theory: Controlling and Analyzing Costs in Foodservice Operations* (4th ed.). Upper Saddle River, NJ: Prentice Hall, 2000.

Kistner, W. C. *Obra'89 Brings Few Changes to Individual Tax Bills-Omnibus Budget Reconciliation Act-Column.* Accessed 6/07/2010. http://findarticles.com/p/aeticles/mi_m3257/is_n2_v44/ai_8346861/

Kitchen Companion: Your Safe Food Handbook. *USDA, Food Safety and Inspection Service.* U.S. Government Printing Office, Washington, D.C., 2008.

Know Your Seafood. Florida Foodservice. Gainesville, Florida. www.ffsinc.com/OFE/KnowYourSeafood.pdf

Koontz, H., O'Donnell, C., and H. Weihrich. *Management* (7th ed.). New York: McGraw-Hill, 1980.

Kosher Shopping. Accessed 1/15/2004. www.erewhonmarket.com/shopguid/kosher.html

Kotler, P., and G. Armstrong. *Principles of Marketing* (9th ed.). Upper Saddle River, NJ: Prentice Hall, 2001.

Kotler, P., and R. N. Clark. *Marketing for Health Care Organizations.* Englewood Cliffs, NJ: Prentice Hall, 1987.

Kotschevar, L. H. *Standards, Principles, and Techniques in Quantity Food Production* (4th ed.). New York: Van Nostrand Reinhold, 2000.

Koury, J. Green Tips. *The Consultant,* 2nd Quarter 2009, 68.

Krzyzewski, H. M., with D. T. Phillips. *Leading with a Heart: Coach K's Successful Strategies for Basketball, Business and Life.* New York: Warner Business Books, 2000.

Kuppersmith, N. C., and S. F. Wheeler. Communication between Family Physicians and Registered Dietitians in Outpatient Setting. *Journal of the American Dietetic Association* 102(12):1756–1763, 2002.

Lambert, H. R. Partnerships Needed to Create Customer Value. *Institutional Distribution* 28(1):16, 1992.

Langley, R. *Gender Wage Gap Widening, Census Data Shows* (2004). Accessed 6/26/2010. http://usgivinfo.about.com/od/censusand statistics/a/paygap.grows.htm

Laube, J. How to Select and Retain Good Employees. *Consultant,* Summer 1997, 43–46.

Lawn, J. Seven Mistakes Purchasing Managers Make. *Food Management* 38(3):8, 2003.

Lean Path Food Waste Flyer. *Latest Trend: Proving ROI from Waste Reduction Investment* Vol. 4, September 2009.

Lean Path Food Waste Flyer. *The Latest Trend: the Growing Importance of Food Waste Audits* Vol. 3, June 2009.

Lean Path Food Waste Flyer. *The Power of Prevention* Vol. 8, June 2010. Best address for all *LeanPath Food Waste* newsletter is LeanPath_Food_Waste_Newletter@mail.vresp.com

Lean Path Food Waste Flyer. *Zero Food Waste: Is It Possible* Vol. 7, March, 2010.

Lennox, B. Bacteria, the environmental warrior. *The Consultant,* 2nd Quarter 2009, 67.

Levitt, M. O. *Report to Congress Improving the Medicare Quality Improvement Organization Program.* Response to the Institute of Medicine study. Accessed 6/12/2010. www.medpac.gov/publication/congressialreport/June2006-ch07.pdf

Linn, A. *At Long Last, Food Labeling Law Set to Take Effect.* Accessed 6/07/2010. www.msnbc.msn.com/id/26890660/

List of Common Bacteria and Guardia Found in Creeks and Streams. Accessed 4/09/2010. www.livestrong.com/article/27152-list-common-bacteria-guardia-found/

Lombardi, D. M. *Handbook for the New Health Care Manager* (2nd ed.). San Francisco: Jossey-Bass, 2001.

Lombardi, D. M., and J. R. Schermerhorn Jr. *Health Care Management.* Hoboken, NJ: Wiley, 2007.

Lottis, H. Building or Remodeling a Facility? Three Words of Advice: Plan, Plan, Plan. *Dietary Manager* 7(6), 1998.

Louria, D. B. Food Irradiation: Unresolved Issues. *Clinical Infectious Disease* 33:378–380, 2001.

Lumay, J. L. *Lead, Follow, or Get Out of the Way—Leadership's Strategies for the Thoroughly Modern Manager.* San Diego: Advant Books, 1986

Marketing and Advertising Tips from businessballs. Accessed 6/14/2010. www.businessballs.com/market.htm

Marvin, B. Why Do Workers Leave? *Outfront,* Fall 2000, 8–14.

Maslow, A. H. *Motivation and Personality.* New York: Harper & Row, 1954.

Maxwell, J. C. *The 21 Indispensable Qualities of a Leader.* Nashville: Nelson, 1999.

Maxwell, J. C. *The 360° Leader.* Nashville: Thomas Nelson, 2005.

McClelland, D. C., and D. H. Burnham. Power Is the Great Motivator. *Harvard Business Review* February and June, 1995, 126–136.

McConnell, C. R. *The Effective Health Care Supervisor.* Rockville, MD: Aspen, 1998.

McCormick. *Spices for Health.* Packet. May also be secured from www.spicesforhealth.com

McCoy, J. T. *The Management of Time.* Englewood Cliffs, NJ: Prentice Hall, 1982.

McSwane, D., F., Rue, N., and R. Linton. *Essentials of Food Safety and Sanitation* (4th ed.). Upper Saddle River, NJ: Prentice Hall, 2008.

McSwane, D., Rue, N., and R. Linton. *Essentials of Food Safety and Sanitation* (3rd ed., rev.). Upper Saddle River, NJ: Prentice Hall, 2003.

McWilliams, M. *Food Fundamentals* (9th ed.). Upper Saddle River, NJ: Pearson/Prentice Hall, 2009.

Mead, P. S., Slutsker, L., Dietz, V., McCaig, L. F., Bresee, J. S., Shapiro, C., Griffin, P. M., and R. V. Tauxe. Food-Related Illness and Death in the United States: A Synopses. *Emerging Inspection Diseases* 5(5), September–October, 1999.

Megginson, L., Mosley, D., and P. Pietri Jr. *Management: Concepts and Applications.* New York: Harper & Row, 1986.

Melissa Kaplan's Vegetables and Fruits (Last update December 18, 2009). Accessed 8/09/2010. www.anapsid.org/resources/vegetablenames.html

Meno, K. Joint Commission Survey Readiness for 2009. *Today's Dietitian* 11(5):48–55, 2009). Accessed 3/05/10. www.todaysdietitian.com/newaechives/050409p48.shtml

Mentor: Expanding The World of Quality Mentoring—What Is Mentoring? Accessed 06/18/2010. www.mentoring.org/mentors/about_mentring/

Merritt, R. J. Dietary Compensation for Fat Reduction and Fat Substitutes. *Nutrition and the MD* 19(3):1–3, 1993.

Messersmith, A., and J. L. Miller. *Forecasting in Foodservice.* New York: Wiley, 1992.

Mill, R. C. *Restaurant Management: Customers, Operations and Employees.* Upper Saddle River, NJ: Prentice Hall, 1998.

Miller, K. C. *A Profile of Energy Use in Restaurants (Tampa Bay Area). Report to the Florida Energy Office, Energy Extension Services. IFAS.* Gainesville: University of Florida, 1992.

Mills, L. E. What's Cooking? Culinary Terms Defined. *Dietary Manager.* 16(9):22, October 2007.

Molt, M. *Food for Fifty.* Englewood Cliffs, NJ: Prentice Hall, 2000.

Mondy, R. W., Noe, R. M., and S. R. Premeaux. *Human Resource Management* (8th ed.). Upper Saddle River, NJ: Prentice Hall, 2002.

Montgomery, K. S. Soy Protein. *Journal of Parental Education* 12(3):42–46, Summer 2003.

Muller, F., and H. Schildkraut. Designed for food safety. *Food Safety Illustrated* 3(1):8–12, 2001.

Musculoskeletal Disorders. Accessed 5/19/2010. www.hse.gov.uk/msd/index.htm

Myers, L. B. *Introduction to Type: A Description of the Theory and Applications of the Myers-Briggs Type Indicator* (12th ed.). Palo Alto, CA: Consulting Psychologists Press, 1990.

Nagel, A. *Cultural Diversity in the Workplace: How a Diverse Workforce Can Contribute to the Bottom Line.* Business to Business. Accessed 3/05/2010. www.btobmagazine.com/Articles/2009/February?Cultural_Diversity_in_the_Workplace

National Association of Equipment Managers, Special Report by Data Protocol Steering Committee. Future kitchen. *Foodservice Equipment Report* 5(5):32–34, 35, 38, 2001.

National Association of Meat Purveyors. *Meat Buyer's Guide to Portion Control Meat Cuts.* McLean, VA: National Association of Meat Purveyors, 1997.

National Association of Meat Purveyors. *Meat Buyer's Guide to Standardized Meat Cuts.* McLean, VA: National Association of Meat Purveyors, 1997.

National Association of Meat Purveyors. *Meat Buyer's Guide.* McLean, VA: National Association of Meat Purveyors, 2010.

National Association of Purchasing Management. *Principles and Standards of Purchasing Practices.* Tempe, AZ: National Association of Purchasing Management, 1991.

National Center for Non Profit Boards. *Kit: 20 Ideas for Jumpstarting Your Board Meeting.* Washington, DC: National Center for Non Profit Boards, 2001.

National Fire Protection Association. Standards for Portable Fire Extinguishers. *NFPA Publication* 10, stock no. 1012. Deerfield, MA: Dray, 1990.

National Organic Standards. *Dietetics in Practice* 2(3):2, 2002.

National Restaurant Association Educational Foundation, *Food Production: Competency Guide.* Upper Saddle River, NJ: Pearson Prentice Hall, 2006.

National Restaurant Association. *Americans with Disabilities Act: Answers for Foodservice Operators.* Chicago: National Restaurant Association, 1992.

Nedland D., and R. Teixeria. *New Progressive America: The Millennial Generation.* Accessed 2/25/2010. www.americaprogress.org/issues/2009/05/millennial_generation.html

North America Meat Processors Association (NAMP) has a 2010 edition of NAMP Meat Buyer's Guide™. May be ordered through NAMP website: www.namp.com. Approximate cost $70.

Norton, L. C. Bioterrorism in Healthcare Foodservice. *ASHFA Trends* 8(1):6–7, 13–14, 2006.

Nursing Home Regulations: 483.75 (m) Disaster and Emergency Preparedness; F518 training/written plan, 483.75 (m) What to Do in Case of a Fire.

Occupational Safety and Health Administration, U.S. Department of Labor. *OSHA Inspection. OSHA 2098.* Washington, DC: U.S. Department of Labor, Occupational Safety and Health Administration, 2009.

Occupational Safety and Health Administration, U.S. Department of Labor. *Occupational Exposure to Bloodborne Pathogens: Precautions for Emergency Responders. OSHA 3130.* Washington, DC: Occupational Safety and Health Administration, U.S. Department of Labor, 1992.

Occupational Safety and Health Administration, U.S. Department of Labor. *All About OSHA. OSHA 2056.* Washington, DC: Occupational Safety and Health Administration, U.S. Department of Labor, 1994 [rev.].

Occupational Safety and Health Administration, U.S. Department of Labor. *Subpart W: 1910.900 Ergonomics Program Standards. 29CFR 1910 OSHA Code of Federal Regulations* (2nd ed.). Davenport, IA: American Safety Training, 2001, 381–390. www.oshacfr.com

Occupational Safety and Health Standards for General Industry (29 CRF Part 1910). Chicago: Commerce Clearing House, 1993.

Odiorne, G. S. *The Practice of Management by Objectives in the Eighties.* Westerfield, MA: MBO, 1981.

Olive Oil. Accessed 8/08/2010. http://en.wikipedia/wiki/Olive_oil

Olive Oil-Extra Virgin Olive Oil-Virgin Olive Olive-Cooking with Olive Oil-Buying and Storing Olive Oil-Olive Oil Tasting. Accessed 8/08/2010. http://whatscookingamerica.net/OliveOil.htm

Oncken, W. Jr., and D. L. Wass. Management Time: Who's Got the Monkey? *Harvard Business Review*, November–December 1974, 75–80.

Opus Environmental Introduces Innovative Food Waste Elimination Equipment to U.S. Market May 07, 2009. Accessed 4/8/2010. www.foodservicecentral.com/article.mvc/Opus-Environmental-Introduces_Innovative

OSHA Fact Sheet. What Is Workplace Violence? (May be secured by calling 202–693–1888.)

OSHA Proposal Cuts Workers' Right to Know about Chemical Risk (last update March 23, 2010). Accessed 7/26/2010. www.ombwatch.org/node/10858

OSHA Worker Rights under the OSHA Act of 1970 (current 3/30/2004). Accessed 7/26/2010. www.osha.gov/as/opa/worker/rights.html

OSHA-Occupational Health and Safety Administration (entry last updated May 06, 2010) Accessed 7/26/1010. www.ilpi.com/msds/ref/osha.html

Pacific Gas and Electric Company.® 10 Ways to Save Natural Gas 12949 Alcosta Blvd., Suite 101; San Ramon, CA. Accessed 4/27/2010. www.fishnick.com

Payne-Palacio, J., and M. Theis. *West and Wood's Introduction to Foodservice* (9th ed.). Upper Saddle River, NJ: Prentice Hall, 2001.

Pest Control. *Food Safety Monitor* 2(3):8–10, 2002.

Peters, T. *Essentials of Leadership—Inspire, Liberate, Achieve.* New York: Tom Peters, Doring-Kindersley, 2005.

Pew Research. Accessed 03/05/2010. www.pewinternet.org/

Polzini, B. Quality: If It's Going to Be, It's Up to Me. *Dietary Managers* 10(3):10–14, 2001.

Prickett, F., and V. White. *The Auburn Cookbook: The Alabama Cooperative Extension Services.* Auburn, AL: Auburn University, in cooperation with U.S. Department of Agriculture, 1987.

Pritchett, P., and R. Pound. *The Employee Handbook for Organizational Change.* Dallas: Pritchett, 1990.

Produce Marketing Association. *Produce 101.* Newark, DE: Produce Marketing Association, Foodservice Division, 1999.

Puckett, R. P. American Dietetic Association Standards of Professional Performance for Registered Dietitians (Generalist and Advanced) in

Management of Food and Nutrition Systems. *JADA* 109(3), March 2009, 540–543, e13.

Puckett, R. P. A Brief Overview of Productivity. *Market-Link* 20(4):2, 9, 2001.

Puckett, R. P. A Glimpse into the Future. *Healthcare Food and Nutrition Focus* 20(2): 1, 3–8. 2003.

Puckett, R. P. A Realistic Approach to Time Management. *Dietary Manager* 6(5):18–20, 22, 1997.

Puckett, R. P. Another Way to Look at Productivity. *Market-Link* 21(2):3–4, 2002.

Puckett, R. P. Are Meetings Necessary? *Contemporary Administrator* 6(6):18–20, 1983.

Puckett, R. P. Are We Managers or Leaders? *Market-Link* 28(2): 10–11, November 2009.

Puckett, R. P. Are You Ready for 2004? *Health Care Food and Nutrition Focus* 21(1):1, 3–7, 2004.

Puckett, R. P. Be Prepared for Possible Biological and Chemical Bioterrorism. *Healthcare Foodservice Trends* 4(3):14–16, 2002.

Puckett, R. P. Be Prepared: Disaster Planning. In J. C. Rose (Ed.), *Handbook for Health Care Foodservice Management*. Rockville, MD: Aspen, 1984.

Puckett, R. P. Continuous Quality Improvement: Where Are We Going in Health Care? *Topics in Clinical Nutrition* 7(4):60–68, 1992.

Puckett, R. P. Developing an Effective System for Inventory & Control. *Dietary Manager* 16(06), June 2007, 25–18.

Puckett, R. P. *Dietary Manager Training Guide*. Gainesville, FL: Division of Continuing Education, 2010. Lesson 5, pp. 143–157.

Puckett, R. P. *Dietary Manager Training*. Gainesville: University of Florida, Department of Correspondence Study, 2009.

Puckett, R. P. *Dietary Manager's Independent Study Course*. Gainesville: Department of Independent Study by Correspondence, University of Florida, 2009.

Puckett, R. P. *Dietary Manager's Independent Study Course*. Gainesville: University of Florida Department of Independent Study by Correspondence, 2010. Lessons 12–13, pp. 585–687.

Puckett, R. P. *Dietary Manager's Training Guide*. Gainesville, FL: Division of Continuing Education, 2010. Lesson 16, pp. 741–758, and Lesson 2, pp. 61–63.

Puckett, R. P. *Dietary Managers Training*. Chap. 15. Gainesville, FL: Division of Continuing Education, University of Florida, 2009.

Puckett, R. P. *Dietary Managers Training*. Gainesville: Division of Continuing Education, University of Florida, 2009.

Puckett, R. P. Disaster Planning: Addressing New Threats. *Dietary Manager* 10(10):18–20, 22–23, 2001.

Puckett. R. P. Educating Foodservice Employees on Disaster Preparedness. *Market-Link* 12(1), Winter, 2006, 1–3.

Puckett, R. P. Effective Foodservice Receiving and Storage Practices. *Dietary Manager* 16(2): February 2007, 12, 14–16.

Puckett, R. P. Estimating Productivity Levels. *Market Link* 21(3):3–4, 2002.

Puckett, R. P. et al. Topics in Practice: A Systems Approach to Measuring Productivity in Foodservice Operations. *Journal of the American Dietetic Association* 1(105):122–130, January 2005.

Puckett, R. P. Fine Dining at the University of Florida. *Market-Link* 26(3), Summer 2007, 3, 9.

Puckett, R. P. Future trends in menu planning. *Dietary Manager* 12(9):11–13, 2003.

Puckett, R. P. Healthcare Facilities Foodservice. Chap. 12. In L. Wolper (Ed.), *Healthcare Administration: Principles, Practice, Structure and Delivery* (2nd ed.). Gaithersburg, MD: Aspen, 1995.

Puckett, R. P. Healthcare Foodservice. *Topics in Clinical Nutrition* 17(3):10–22, 2002.

Puckett, R. P. Institutional Foodservice Operations. Chap. 27. In R. Schmidt (Ed.), *Food Safety Handbook*. Hoboken, NJ: John Wiley & Sons, 2003.

Puckett, R. P. Is Your Fish Diet Killing You? *Market-Link* 2003.

Puckett, R. P. JCAHO's Agenda for Change. *Journal of the American Dietetic Association* 91:1225–1226, 1991.

Puckett, R. P. Management Briefs: Benchmarking. *Market-Link* 2005.

Puckett, R. P. *Management by Objectives*. Presented at the American Dietetic Association–Health, Education, and Welfare Workshop 12, 1980. (Unpublished work for master's degree)

Puckett, R. P. Management Words and Their Meanings. *Market-Link* 28(2) 4, 10. November 2009.

Puckett, R. P. Optimizing Employee Productivity through Motivation. *Journal of Foodservice Systems* 1(3):205–220, 1981.

Puckett, R. P. Organic and Sustainable Foods. *Market-Link* 2008.

Puckett, R. P. Performance Outcome Descriptions

Puckett, R. P. Personal and Organizational Preparedness: The Key to Surviving a Disaster. *Hospital Care Food and Nutrition Focus* 22(1), January 2006, 1, 3–7.

Puckett, R. P. Pre-Work Shop at ADA Food, Nutrition Conference and Expo (FNCE). *Productivity in Foodservice Operations*. San Antonia, TX, October 25, 2003.

Puckett, R. P. Product Selection and Specifications *Dietary Manager*, February 2005.

Puckett, R. P. Productivity Measures for Foodservice—A Practice Paper. *Journal American Dietetic Association (JADA)* 105(1), January, 2005, 122–130 (Up for review/revision 2011).

Puckett, R. P. Recruiting and Retaining Employees. *Market-Link*, Summer 2000, 6–7.

Puckett, R. P. *Safe Handling of Food, HACCP, OSHA and Other Safety Precautions in Foodservice Departments*. Correspondence course. Gainesville: Division of Continuing Education, University of Florida, 2001.

Puckett, R. P. *Safe Handling of Food, HACCP, OSHA and Other Safety Precautions in Foodservice Department*. Correspondence course. Gainesville, FL: Division of Continuing Education, 2002.

Puckett, R. P. Surveys, Surveys, Surveys, What Is New? *Healthcare Foodservice TRENDS* 1(11).

Puckett, R. P. Sustainability in Foodservice Operations. *TRENDS* 11(3), Fall 2008.

Puckett, R. P. Tips for Improving Product Selection and Specifications. *Dietary Manager* 14(2): February 2005, 25–27.

Puckett, R. P. The 4 R's of Sustainability. *FCSI-The Americas Quarterly* 1(3) August, 2010, 8.

Puckett, R. P. Training: A How to Do It. In J. C. Rose (Ed.), *Handbook for Health Care Foodservice Management*. Rockville, MD: Aspen, 1984.

Puckett, R. P. What's New in Equipment. *Dietary Manager* 11(2):13–15, 2002.

Puckett, R. P. Yesterday, Today and Tomorrow: What Can We Expect Next in Healthcare? *Dietary Manager* 2(9):13–16, February 2010.

Puckett, R. P., and K. Drummond. How to Measure and Improve Patient Satisfaction with Foodservice. *Healthcare Foodservice Trends*, Spring 2000, 17–21.

Puckett, R. P., and R. Jackson. A System Approach to Productivity. Chap. 13. In R. Jackson (Ed.), *Nutrition and Foodservice for Integrated Health Care: A Handbook for Leaders*. Gaithersburg, MD: Aspen, 1997, 441–474.

Puckett, R. P., and R. A. Lucas. *Food, Nutrition and Medical Nutrition Therapy through the Life Cycle*. Dubuque, IA: Kendall/Hunt, 2009. 111 and Module 6, 406–422.

Puckett, R. P., and B. Miller. *Foodservice Manual for Health Care Institutions*. Chicago: American Hospital Association, 1988.

Puckett, R. P., and L. C. Norton. *Disaster and Emergency Preparedness in Foodservice Operations*. Chicago: American Dietetic Association, 2004. (Still available, being revised; available in 2011)

Puckett, R. P., and L. C. Norton. *HACCP: The Future Challenge: Practical Application for the Foodservice Administrator* (4th ed.). Gainesville: Division of Continuing Education, University of Florida, 2001. (Out of print)

Recommended Symbols (Kosher). Accessed 1/15/2004. www.kosherquest.org/html/Reliable_KosherSymbols.htm

Reed, L. *SPECS: The Comprehensive Foodservice Purchasing and Specification Manual* (2nd ed.). New York: Van Nostrand Reinhold, 2010.

Report from the House of Delegates of the American Dietetic Association, Task Force on Sustainability. *Definition of Sustainability*.

The Rising Cost of Medicare and Medicaid in the Years Preceding. Accessed 6/07/2010. www.examiner.com/x-11321-Newark-Independent-Examiner~y2009m6d13-The-risin

Rmgenberg, C. Breathing cleaner air. *Solid and Hazardous Waste News* 9: 3, 2003.

Robbins, S. P., and M. Coulter. *Management* (10th ed.). Upper Saddle River, NJ: Prentice Hall, 2009.

Robbins, S. P. *Fundamentals of Management* (3rd ed.). Upper Saddle River, NJ: Prentice Hall, 2001.

Robbins, S. P. *Managing Today!* (2nd ed.). Upper Saddle River, NJ: Prentice Hall, 2000.

Robbins, S. P. *Managing Today* (2.0 Edition). Upper Saddle River, NJ: Prentice Hall, 2002.

Robbins, S. P., and D. A. DeCenzo. *Fundamentals of Management* (3rd ed.). Upper Saddle River, NJ: Prentice Hall, 2001.

Rock, J. B., and E. Jacks. *Get Your People to Work Like They Mean It*. New York: McGraw-Hill, 2007.

Roloff, S. Equipment Trends: Helping Facilities with Safety Regulations. *Dietary Manager* 15(7):14–17, July–August, 2006.

Rosen, L. Criminal Records, Employment Application. Accessed 6/26/2010. www.esrcheck.com/article/crime_and employment_application.php

Runion, M., and J. Brittain. *How to Say It, Performance Reviews*. New York: Prentice Hall, 2006.

Rupp's Insurance & Risk Management Survey. *Resource Conservation and Recovery Act (RCRA)*. Accessed 12/23/2003. Nils, 2002. http://insurance.cch.com/rupps/resource-conservation-and-recovery_act.htm

Safe Food Handling. www.fsis.usda.gov/factsheeets/Basic_for_Handling_Food_Safety/index.asp

Safety: Workplace Safety and Employee Safety. Accessed 5/19/2010. http://humanresources.about.com/od/safetyworkplacesafety/Safety_Workplace_Safety_and_Employee_Safety.htm

Salkin, S. Why GPOs Are Booming. *Food Service Director* 59(3):60, 1992.

Sanders, B. C. Genetically Modified Foods. *Consultant* 33(3), 121, 123, 2000.

Satawa, L. *Women in Leadership: Do Gender Issues Still Play a Role? Maybe . . . But Maybe Not*. Accessed 6/14/2010. www.allbusiness.com/human-resources/employee-development-leadership/446884–1

Save Check FreLoc Temperature System. Accessed 1/20/2010. www.greenedgesystem.com

Scalise, G. (researcher). Tool for patient satisfaction. *Hospital & Health Network* 78(3), March 2004 [4-page suppl.].

Schermehorn, J. R. *Exploring Management* (2nd ed.). Hoboken, NJ: John Wiley & Sons, 2010.

Schmidgall, R. S., and W. P. Andrew. *Financial Management in the Hospitality Industry*. East Lansing, MI: Educational Institute of the American Hotel & Motel Association, 1993.

Schmidt, R. H. *Basic Elements of a Sanitation Program for Food processing and Food Handling*. University of Florida IFAS Extension. Accessed 4/09/2010. http://edis.ifas.ufl.edu/fs076

Schneider, K. R. and R. G. Schnider. *What Are Genetically Modified Foods?* University of Florida, Institute of Food and Agricultural Sciences (IFAS) Extension. (Document FSHN 02–2), 2009.

Schweitzer, D. Foodservice Kitchen Safety, A Model for Reducing Injuries. *Dietary Manager* 19(6), 20–24.

Scientific Cleaning Procedures and Sanitation for the Foodservice Industry. St. Paul, MN: Economic Laboratories (n.d.).

Seafood Selector Recommendations: TUNA. Accessed 8/05/2010. www.edf.org/page.cfm?tagID=16314&s_src=ggad&s_subscr=tuna&gclid=CJDzi7y7

Seelye, H. N., and A. James-Sellye. *Culture Clash*. Chicago: NTC Business Books, 1995.

Seunghee, W. Shanklin, C. W., and K-E Lee. A Decision Tree for Selecting the Most Cost-Effective Waste Disposal Strategy in Foodservice Operations. *Journal of the American Dietetic Association* 103(4), 475–482, 2003.

Shakman, A. Food Waste Tracking: What You Need to Know. *FCSI the Americas Quarterly* 1(1):31–34, 2010.

Shell Oil Company. *Meeting the Energy Challenge* (6-page brochure) 2009. More information available at www.shell.us/energytalk

Shigellosis. Accessed 7/09/2010. www.co.monroe.mi.us/government/departments_office/public_health/shigellosis.html

Short, L., and D. H. Kaye. NASA Ames Research Center Health Unit. *Quality Assurance in Occupational Health Setting* June 29, 2005. Accessed 6/15/2010. Slide presentation available at ohp.nasa.gov/conference_ info/conf_gen.../2005/...wed_np-short.pdf

Shortell, S. M., and W. A. Peck. Enhancing the Potential of QI Organizations to Improve Quality of Care. Accessed 6/19/2010. www.annals.org/content/145/5/388.full

Slips and Falls. Accessed 4/27/2010. www.fpcmat.com/Dirty%20Facts2.html

Smith, F. B. *RE: Comments Relating to Codex Committee on Food Labeling: Proposals for Section 5 of the Proposed Draft Recommendations for the Labeling of Foods Obtained Through Biotechnology*. Accessed 1/15/2004. www.consumeralert.org/issues/trade/fdacodex.html

Sneed, J., and K. H. Kresse. *Understanding Foodservice Financial Management*. Rockville, MD: Aspen, 1989.

Snyder, J. W. The US Food and Water Supply: A Target for Committing an Act of Bioterrorism. Presented at the Food and Nutrition Conference and Exhibition, American Dietetic Association, October 21, 2002, Philadelphia.

Snyder, P. O. HACCP in the Retail Industry. *Dairy Food Environmental Sanitation* 11(2):73–81, 1991.

Solomon, M. R., and E. W. Stuart. *The Brave New World of E-Commerce: For Marketing: Real People, Real Choices*. Upper Saddle River, NJ: Prentice Hall, 2001.

Solomon, M. R., and E. W. Stuart. *Marketing Real People and Real Choices* (2nd ed.). Upper Saddle River, NJ: Prentice Hall, 2000.

Spears, M. C. *Foodservice Procurement: Purchasing for Profit*. Upper Saddle River, NJ: Prentice Hall, 1999.

Spears, M. C. *Foodservice Organizations: A Managerial and Systems Approach* (4th ed.). Upper Saddle River, NJ: Prentice Hall, 2000.

Sprayberry N. K. *Update on Food & Nutrition Standards for the Joint Commission.* MedAssets Healthcare Business Summit 2010. Accessed 6/12/2010. www.medassets.com/HBS-2010/…Food-Nutrition-Joint-commission.pdf

Stair, R. M. *Principles of Information Systems: A Managerial Approach.* Boston: Boyd & Fraser, 1992.

Standards for Professional Performance for Entry Level Management Registered Dietitians. *Journal of the American Dietetic Association* 3:e1, 1–13, 540–543, March 2009. Dietary Manager Association of Food and Nutrition Association Professional Standards. http:dmaonline.ggnet.net/marketplace.dma/

Standards for RDs. Check ADA website www.eatright.org for Professional Performance for RDs in Management of Food and Nutrition Systems. *JADA* 10, 9(3):540–543; 543.e1– 543.e13, March 2009.

Steiner, G. A. *A Step-by-Step Guide to Strategic Planning: What Every Manager **Must** Know.* New York: Simon & Schuster, 1979.

Stier, R. F. The Dirty Dozen: Ways to Reduce the 12 Biggest Foreign Matter Problems. *Food Safety* 9(2):44, 46, 48–50, 2003.

Strutz, B. Getting a Handle on Food Waste. *Consultant* 35(4):111–115, 2002.

Studies Available on Cleaning and Maintenance of Dish Machines: How to Set Up a Pot-Washing Operation. White Plains, NY: Economics Laboratories, 2000.

Supplement to the 2009 Food Code. www.fda.gov/Food/FoodSafety/RetailFoodProtection?FoofCode?FoodCode2009/uc

Sustainable Foodservice: Disposable Foodservice Products. Accessed 4/9/2010. www.sustainablefoodservice.com/cat/disposable.htm

Thermistor. *Kitchen Companion, Your Safe Food Handbook.* USDA, Food Safety and Inspection Service. U.S. Printing Office, Washington, DC. (2008), 18.

Thermy™ Food Safety Education: Types of Thermometers. Accessed 7/09/2010. www.fsis.usda.gov/food_safety_education/types_of_food_thermometers/index.asp

Thomas J. Lipton Company. *Tea Time: A Guide from Lipton to the Resources of Tea.* Englewood Cliffs, NJ: Lipton, 1991.

Toczek, W. The Fruit Basket Approach to Evaluating Benchmarking. *Dietary Manager* 2(19), February 2010, 17–20.

Townsend, J. *Recycling in Hotels and Motels.* Gainesville: Energy Extension Service, University of Florida, 1993.

Trace, T. L., Lynch, J. F., Fischer, J. W., and R. C. Hummrich. Ethics and vendor relationships. In S. J. Hall (Ed.), *Ethics in Hospitality Management: A Book of Readings.* East Lansing, MI: Educational Institute, 1992.

Tucker, J. *Gender and Work Differences between Men and Women.* Accessed 6/14/2010. http://businessmanagement.suite101.com/article.cfm/gender_and_work

Tucks, R. S. Better to Engage a Professional Kitchen Planner. *Consultant* 35(3):103, 105, 107, 2002.

The Types of Coffee Beans and Their Difference. Accessed 8/08/2010. www.coffee-makers-et-cetera.com/types-of-coffee-beans.html

Types of Fruits. Accessed 8/08/2010. www.botancial-online.com/frutoscarnosangles.htm

U.S. Census Bureau News Census Bureau Estimates the Number of Adults, Older People and School-Age Children in States. Accessed 2/23/2010. www.census.gov/Press-Release/www/release/archives/population/001703.html

U.S. Census Bureau Population Profile of the United States. *Older Adults in 2005.* Accessed 2/23/2010. www.census.gov

U.S. Department of Agriculture, Agricultural Marketing Service. How to Buy Poultry. *Home and Garden Bulletin* No. 157. Washington, DC: U.S. Department of Agriculture, 1945.

U.S. Department of Agriculture, Agricultural Marketing Service. How to Buy Eggs. *Home and Garden Bulletin* No. 144. Washington, DC: U.S. Department of Agriculture, 1995.

U.S. Department of Agriculture, Food Safety and Inspection Service. *The Food Safety Educator* Vol. 7(2). Washington, DC: Food Safety and Inspection Service, U.S. Department of Agriculture, 2002. Accessed January 2003. www.fsis.usda.gov/oa/educator/educator.htm

U.S. Department of Agriculture. Food Safety and Inspection Service. *How to Use a Meat Thermometer and Take the Guess Work Out of Cooking.* Washington, DC: Food Safety Inspection Service Washington, USDA, 2000.

U.S. Department of Commerce, National Technical Information Services (5285 Port Royal Road, Springville, VA 22161) Report 2002100189. www.cfsan.fda.gov/~dms/fc01-int.html

U.S. Department of Energy: Energy Efficient and Renewable Energy: Federal Management Program: FEMP FOCUS-Fall 2004. *Clean Up with Water Savings.*

U.S. Department of Health and Human Services. *HCFC State Operational Manual.* Washington, DC: U.S. Government Printing Office, July 1999.

U.S. Department of Health and Human Services. *HHS to Require Food Labels to Include Trans Fat Contents: Improved Labels Will Help Consumers Choose Heart-Healthy Foods.* Accessed January 16, 2004. www.gov/news/press/2003pres/20030709.html

U.S. Department of Labor, Employment Standards Administration, Wage and Hour Division. Handy Reference Guide to Fair Labor Standards Act. Publication WH-1282, revised. Washington, DC: Employment Standards Administration, U.S. Department of Labor, 1998.

U.S. Department of Labor, Occupational Safety and Health Administration. Hazardous communication. Federal Register 48(228):53280–53348, 1983.

U.S. Department of Labor. *How to Prepare for Workplace Emergencies and Evacuations.* OSHA 3088, revised 2001. Washington, DC: U.S. Government Printing Office, 2001.

U.S. Environmental Protection Agency, Office of Solid Waste. *The Solid Waste Dilemma: An Agenda for Action.* Final Report of the Municipal Solid Waste Task Force. Publication EPA/530/SW-89–019. Washington, DC: Government Printing Office, 1989.

U.S. Environmental Protection Agency, Reduce, Reuse, Recycle. Accessed 4/27/2010. www.epa/epaoswer/non-hw/muncpl/reduce.htm

U.S. Food and Drug (FDA). *What Do You Know about Mercury in Fish and Shellfish?* Accessed 8/05/2010. www.fda.gov/food/foodsafety/product-specificinformation/seafood/foodborneppathoge

U.S. Food and Drug Administration, Center for Food Safety and Applied Nutrition. *Food Code 2009.* Springville, VA: U.S. Food and Drug Administration, Center for Food Safety and Applied Nutrition. *The "Bad Bug Book": Foodborne Pathogenic Microorganisms and Natural Toxins Handbook.* Revised 2008. www.cfsan.fda.gov/~mow/intro.html

U.S. Food and Drug Administration, Center for Food Safety and Applied Nutrition. *Guidance for Industry: Food Producers, Processors, Transporters, and Retailers: Food Security Preventive Measures Guidance.* January 2002. www.cfsan.fda.gov/~dms/secguid.html

U.S. Food and Drug Administration. *Revealing Trans Fats.* Accessed 1/16/ 2004. www.fda.gov/fdac/features/2003/503_fats.html

U.S. Health Care Cost, *Background Brief*. Retrieved 6/07/2010. www.kaiseredu.org/topics_im.asp?imID=1parentID=61&id=358

U.S. Public Health Service, Food and Drug Administration. *FDA 2010/Food Code*. Washington, DC: U.S. Department of Health and Human Services, U.S. Food and Drug Administration. Updated March 28, 2002. http://cfsan.fda.gov/ndms/fe01.html

Understanding and Helping with Personal Problems: Employee Assistance Program. www.dm.usda.gov/pdsd/Security%20DGuide/Eap/Intro.htm

Understanding Generational Differences in Today's Diverse Workforce. Accessed 2/28/2010. http://network.dversityjobs.com/profiles/blogs/understaning-generational

Underwriters Laboratories, Inc. Code Authority. *"K" Classification Fights Restaurant Fires*. Accessed December 1993. www.ul.com/auth/tca/v7n2/classk.html

United Fresh Fruit and Vegetable Association. *Fruits and Vegetables: Facts and Pointers*. Washington, DC: United Fresh Fruit and Vegetable Association, 1999.

United Nations Environment Programme. *More Action Needed to Guarantee Recovery of Ozone Layer: New Substances May Damage Earth's Protective Shield*. Environment for Development Press Release, September 2001. Accessed 12/23/2003. www.unep.org/Documents/?DocumentID=214&ArticleID=2933

United States Department of Agriculture, Agricultural Marketing Service, Grading, Certification and Verification. Institutional Meat Purchase Specification, Washington, DC, 2010.

United States Department of Agriculture, Marketing and Regulatory Programs, Agricultural Marketing Service, Livestock and Seed Program. Institutional Meat Purchase Specification (various meats). Washington, DC, 1996.

University of Florida, Environmental Engineering. *Conserve Florida Water*. One-page information sheet. 2008. More information at info@conservefloridawater.org

USDA. *Get the Facts: New Food Allergen Labeling Laws*. Accessed 6/07/2010. www.cfsan.fda.gov/~dms/wh-alrgy.html

Van Pelt-Higgins, K. Space Planning for a Comfortable and Efficient Kitchen. *Dietary Manager* 2(4):8–9, 11, 1993.

Vasilion, L. E. Food Purchasing—Not Just a Trip to the Market. *Dietary Manager* 10(7):13, 2001.

Vasilion, L. E. Ten Articles published in *Dietary Manager* 2006 and 2008 on various fruits and vegetables: (2006) Kiwi, apples, bananas, cranberries, (2008) Oranges, eggplant, strawberries, soy, cantaloupe, blueberries, zucchini, winter squash, and pecans.

Vibro vulnificus. Fact Sheet for Healthcare Providers. Interstate Shellfish Sanitation Conference (more information on web at www.issc.org).

Vickery, K., and J. Smokler. Hanging on in Tough Times: Providers Struggle to Hold Their Ground. *Provider* 29(1):23, 25, 26, 28, 31, 32, 35–36, 38, 2003.

Volsky, I. *Defining Affordability in Health Care Reform* (2009). Accessed 3/05/2010. http://wonkroom.thinkprogress.org/2009/06/18/health-reform-affordable/

Vroom, V. H., and A. G. Jago. *The New Leadership: Managing Participation in Organizations*. Upper Saddle River, NJ: Prentice Hall, 1988.

Vroom, V. H., and P. W. Yetton. *Leadership and Decision Making*. Pittsburgh: University of Pittsburgh Press, 1973.

Walton, M. *The Deming Management Method*. New York: Dodd, Mead, 1986.

Weese. HACCP for Foodservice Workers. Alabama Cooperative Extension. *ACES Publication*. Pub.ID HE 0726.

Weisberg, K., and B. Lorenzini. Going Green. *FCSI The Americas Quarterly* 1(1):26–28, 1Q 201020–2224.

Weston, N. *What Is Z Trim?* Accessed 4/29/2010. www.slashfood.com/2007/01/24/what-is-z-trim/

What Is a Mentor? Accessed 5/16/2010. www.wisegeek.com/what-is-a-mentor.htm

What Is Autism? Accessed 4/29/2010. www.autism-pdd.net?what-is-autism.html

What Is Mentoring? Accessed 6/04/2010. www.asha.org/students/gatheringplace/mentoring.htm

What Is Mentoring? Accessed 5/16/2010. www.mentoring.org/mentors/about_mentoring/

What Is Merchandising? Accessed 3/08/2010. wiki.answers.com/Q/What-is-merchandising

What Is Sustainability? Accessed 7/7/2010. www.epa.gov/sustainability/basicinfo.htm

Whitman, D. Genetically Modified Foods: Harmful or Helpful? *Digest*, Spring 2001, 1, 3–5.

Wildlife Management Institute, *Outdoors News Bulletin*. Recommendations on Lead in Game Meat. Accessed 8/02/2010. www.wildlifemanagementinstitute.org/index.php?option=com_content&view=article

Williger, D. The Different Types of Coffee from All over the World. Ezine @ articles. Accessed 8/08/2010. http://ezinearticles.com/?The-Differeny-Types-of-Coffee-From-All-Over-The-World&id=72

Witt, D. B. Foodservice Equipment Purchasing. *Dietary Manager* 16(07):16–18, July–August 2007.

Wixson, J. A. Recipe for Successful Kitchen Planning. *Trade Talk* March 2003, 29–31.

Workplace Injury Causes and Cost: Liberty Mutual Releases Study on Top 10 Workplace Injuries. Accessed 7/23/2010. www.wwdmag.com/workplace-injury-causes-and-costs (2002 data).

Zamora, A. *Hygiene Viruses, Bacteria, and Parasites—How to Prevent Infections*. Accessed 07/09/2010. www.scientificpsychic.com/health/hygiene.html

Zenk, C. It's Not Easy Being Green: Growing Trends for Sustainability. *Dietary Manager* 17(6):12–16, June 2008.

INDEX

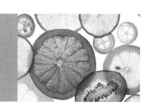

Association of Healthcare Food Service, 107

Association of Nutrition and Foodservice Professionals (ANFP), 107, 299; code of ethics, 14; education conventions, 16

At-risk groups, food-borne illness, 261–262

Atkinson, J., 32–33

Attendance, at team meetings, 135

Attentiveness, in communication, 140

Attitude objectives, 162

Audience, presentations, relating to, 136

Authority: as depicted on organizational chart, 102; distributing, 109–110; line and staff responsibilities, 110; of managers, 26

Authority decision, Vroom-Yetton-Jago model of, 22

Autism, 1

Autodesk® Revit® Architecture Conceptual Design Modeling, 516

Availability and cost, and revision of menus, 349

Avoidance, 33; and conflict resolution, 142

Awkward positions, in ergonomics, 340

B

Baby boomers, and the workforce, 7

Bacillus cereus illnesses, 272–273, 275

Back-shelf hood, 527

Backflow, 519

Background checks, 156–157

Backsiphonage, 519

Backup of data, 204

Bacon: and inhibitors, 266; and molds, 268; as processed meat, 376; recommended storage temperatures/times, 435; smoke point, 438; wrapping, 438

Bacteria: acidity/alkalinity, 266; aerobic, 267; facultative, 267; in food, 266; growth and reproduction, 263; inhibitors, 266; mobility, 263; moisture, 265–266; multiplication of, over time, 267; spores, 268; temperature, 263–265

Baked eggs, 474

Baked fish, 378

Baked potatoes, 269, 390, 476

Baking equipment, 527

Balance on hand, 441

Balance sheet, 233

Bananas, 391, 393

Bandages, 302

Bar-code reader, 204, 408, 431, 440, 521

Barriers: to communication, 128, 129–131; to diversity, 170

Base pricing method, 362

Basil, 484

Bay leaves, 484

Béchamel sauce, 480

Bedside charting, 11

Bedside menus, 358

Beef: canner grade, 373; choice grade, 373; cutter grade, 373; primal cuts of, 374; quality grades, 372; as ready-to-serve meat, 375; recommended storage temperatures/times, 435; roasts, 374; select grade, 373; standard grade, 373; utility grade, 373; yield grade, 372–373

Behavior, communication barriers due to, 129–130

Behavioral interviewing, 155, 157–158

Behavioral objectives, 162

Behavioral segmentation, 40

Belgium carrots, 389

Bell peppers, 390

Benchmarking, 24, 53; and clinical quality assessment, 60; defined, 68; delivery of care, 3, 65; external, 68; and monitoring for performance, 497; and quality programs, 61

Benefits administration, 186

Benefits programs, 31

Benzoates, 275

Bereavement time, 150, 176

Berries, 391

Best practice, 68

Beverage service ware, 402

Beverages, 353; alcoholic, 44, 333, 346; bottled water used in, 259; carbonated, 333; cocoa, 400; coffee, 399, 482; refilling cups/glasses of, 500; serving from dispensers, 242; specifications, 400; tea, 399–400, 482–483

BHA, 275

BHT, 275

Bias, as barrier to diversity, 170

Bid packet, 417

Bid request (form), 423

Bids, obtaining, 416

Bimetal probe/dial-instant read thermometers, 280–281

Binding arbitration, 187

Biodiesel fuel, 242, 258

Biohazard symbol, 325

Biological threats, 338–339

Biotechnology, 11–12, 370; defined, 11

Bioterrorism, 338

Bird droppings, 308

Biscuit method, for mixing quick breads, 480

Biscuits, 480

Bisques, 480

Black/African American population, 7

Blind receiving, 432–433

Blistering agents, 338

Blood agents, 338

Blue 1/Blue 2/Red 3/Yellow 6, 275

Blue cheese, 386

Blueberries, 393

Bluefin tuna, 379

Blueprints, 516

Board of commissioners, 73

Board of directors, 73

Board of trustees, 73

Body hair, covering by clothing, 301

Body language: of learners, 161; as nonverbal communication, 127, 130–131, 136, 139, 161

Body odors, 496

Bologna: and molds, 268; as processed meat, 376

Bona fide occupational qualifications (BFOQ), 147–148

Bonded employees, and cash, 216

Bottled water, 259

Botulism (*C. botulinum*), 339; and canned goods, 271

Bovine spongiform encephalopathy (mad cow disease), 339

Boxed meals, 500

Bracelets, 278, 326

Brainstorming: defined, 30; team, 62, 81; and team decision making, 91

Bran, 395–398

Branding, 9

Bratwurst, as processed meat, 376

Braunschweiger, as processed meat, 376

Breach of contract, and dismissal for cause, 182

Bread-and-butter plates, placement of, 499

Breads: delivery/storage, 420; fermentation/rising, 480; flour, 396; gluten, 396, 479–480; quick, 480; specifications, 398; unbaked dough, refrigerating, 480; yeast, 479–480

Breakeven point, 217

Breakfast cereals, 398

Breakfast menus, 353

Brick cheese, 386

Brie, 268, 386

Brisk cut of beef, 374

Broccoli, 362, 388, 389, 393, 419, 476, 478

Brochures, 43

Broiled fish, 469

Broilers, 524

Brown rice, 397–398, 477

Brown sauce, 480

Brown stock, 480

Brussels sprouts, 475, 476

BTUs (British thermal unit), 252

Bubble diagram, 106

Budget preparation, setting a timetable for, 213

Budgetary control, 221–225

Budgeted balance sheet, 211

Budgets, 118, *See also* Financial management; capital, 80, 211, 221; cash, 80, 211; department, 80; expense, 211; financial, 211; fixed, 214; food cost, 218; labor, 217–218; marketing plan, 48; master, 211; materials, 218; nonmonetary, 211; operating, 211–214; operating, food service department, 153; overhead, 218; project-based budgeting, 214; revenue, 211, 214–216; static, 214; traditional, 214; variable, 214; zero-based budgeting (ZBB), 214

Bulb thermometers, 280–283, 438

Bulk food, distribution of, 491

Bundling, 42

Bureau of Labor Statistics (BLS), 7

Bush, G.H.W., 4

Business etiquette, 142

Convenience system, 451
Convention oven, 523
Converted rice, 397
Cook-and-chill system, 450–451
Cook-and-freeze system, 450–451; procedures, 287
Cook-and-serve system, 448–450; with extended holding, 450; with limited holding, 450
Cooked breakfast cereals, 398
Cooked salami, as processed meat, 376
Cooking utensils, basic equipment for washing, 533
Cooperative vending, 9
Cooperatives, 420–421
Coordination, 26–27
Core values, 71
Coriander, 484
Corn, 390, 393
Corn/cornmeal, 397; recommended storage temperatures/times, 435
Corn oil, 395
Cornbread, 480
Corporate marketing, 47
Corrective action, taking, 210–211
Cost center, 214
Cost-of-living adjustment (COLA), 186, 218
Cottage cheese, 385–387
Counter wiping cloths, 305
Country-of-origin labeling, 369
Coupons, 41–43, 408, 425
Cover, 498
CQI, See Continuous quality improvement (CQI)
Cream, 384–385, 474–475, 500
Cream cheese, 386
Cream of tartar: and color changes in vegetables, 476; and scrambled eggs, 474
Cream soups, 480
Cream substitutes, 385
Credibility, in communication, 139
Credit memo, 430, 432
Credit records, and background check, 157
Criminal record, and background check, 157
Crisis management, 276–277
Critical incidents, 172
Critical limits, 294
Critical paths, 67, 97
Critical plan method, 84
Crosby, P., 52
Cross connection, 519
Cross-contamination, 262–263; preventing, 303
Cross-functional teams, 98
Cross-functional training, 2, 3, 30
Cross training, and process decentralization, 98
Cryptosporidiosis, 267
Cryptosporidum parvum, 339
Cucumbers, 390
Culinary glossary, 486–488
Cull grade lamb, 373
Cultural differences, 130; and participative management, 35

Cultural diversity, 9–10, 169–170; barriers to, 170; and menu planning, 345; in menus, 10; policies/procedures, 170; of workforce, 7–8
Cultural factors, in communication, 130
Cultural identity group, as barrier to diversity, 170
Culture audit, 29
Culture, communication barriers due to, 130
Culture inventory, 29
Cultured buttermilk, 383
Cultured nondairy sour cream, 385
Curdling of milk, 474
"Current good manufacturing practices" (CGMP) regulations, and bottled water, 259
Current marketing situation, marketing plan, 48
Customer awards, 186
Customer departmentalization, 97
Customer-focused service strategy, 60
Customer needs, identifying/leading, 9
Customer-oriented focus: aging population, 9–10; cultural diversity in menus, 10; demographic changes, 9–10; nutrition awareness, 9; quality-cost equation, value in, 9; women as primary decision-makers, 9–10
Customer satisfaction: and CQI, 54–55; enhancement of, 505; survey, 502
Customer service: moving from customer orientation to customer satisfaction, 60; moving from service plan to, 60; and satisfaction, 59–60
Customer survey results, and revision of menus, 349
Customers, 489–491; choice/variety/ expectations, 490; comfort foods, 491; cost of product, 490; defined, 490; language barriers, 491; lifestyle/personal values, 491; medical conditions of, 490; needs of, 490–491; preferences of, 490; religious/cultural/ethnic needs, 490–491; satisfaction, enhancing, 505
Cutter grade beef, 373
Cutting boards, 401
Cybernetic control systems, 209
Cycle menus, 352, 358
Cyclicity, 49
Cyclospora cayetanensis, 268

D
Daily coaching, 30
Daily production: schedule, 453; sheet, 456
Daily receiving record, 432–433
Daily schedule, 120
Dairy products, See Milk/dairy products
Data collection: decision making, 89; market research, 46–47; and organizational planning, 72
Data, defined, 189–190
Database, defined, 190
Database review, 204; and computers in foodservice operations, 204
Deadlines, 121
Debit card, defined, 499

Decaffeinated coffee, 399
Decaffeinated tea, 400
Decentralization, 109
Decentralized assembly systems, 491; equipment selection/storage space, 531
Decibels, 517
Decision making, See also Team decision making: action plan, activating to implement best choice, 90; alternative solutions/ outcomes, identifying, 89–90; alternatives, evaluating relative values of, 90; and availability of crucial resources, 89; and conflict resolution, 88; data collection, 89; defined, 88; elements essential to, 88; evaluating the decision, 90; follow-up, 90; and individual bias, 89; influences on, 89; and lack of clear objectives, 89; and lack of knowledge/ ability, 89; in menu planning, 352; obstacles to, 88–89; in planning process, 88; process, 89; team, 90–91; team meetings, 135
Decisional role, of leaders, 25
Deck ovens, 524
Deep-fat frying, 526; of fish, 471; oils/ shortening for, 395
Defensiveness, as communication interference, 128
Degermed cornmeal, recommended storage temperatures/times, 435
Delegation, 109–110, 125
Deliveries, 430
Delivery of care, 37; changes in, 2–3
Delivery slips, 431
Deming, W. E., 51–52
Demographic changes, to customer-oriented focus, 9–10
Demographical segmentation, 39
Demonstrations, and training, 163
Department: budget, 80; business plan, 80; objectives, examining, 213; policies and procedures manual, 76; review, of meal service system, 505; structure, factors influencing, 107; survey, 55
Departmental activity reports, 137
Departmentalization: customer, 97; as depicted on organizational chart, 102; functional, 96–97; geographic, 97; process, 97–98; product, 97; time, 98
Depreciation, 217
Dessert fork, placement of, 499
Desserts, 353, 480–482; cakes, 481; fruit, 482; gelatins, 482; pastries, 482; pies, 482
Detergents/soaps, 303–306; alkaline, 304; automatic dispensers for, 306; ordering, 250; reducing the cost of, 258; sanitizer, 305
Development, 160
Diabetes mellitus, 1, 129, 262, 346; and food-borne illness, 270; and listeriosis, 272; and nutrition dietitians, 108; and patient menus, 359; and V. vulnificus infection, 273
Diagnostics, and technology, 11
Dial-instant read thermometers, 280–281

Diet Coke®, 12

Diet spreadsheet, 353

Dietary manager (DM), 104, 107

Dietary Reference Intake (DRI), 347

Dietetic technician registered (DTR), 107

Dietitian Week, 186

Digital computerized thermometers, 431

Dill, 484

Dining areas: can washing, 534; cart-washing machines, 534; checking, 45; employee training in safety/sanitation, 536; for employees/guests, 531–533; equipment, 531–536; equipment selection and purchasing, 535–536; housekeeping equipment, 535; for patients/residents, 531; technology and equipment advances, 534–535; ware-washing equipment, 533–534

Dinnerware, 499; plates, placement of, 498

Direct issuing, 439

Direct labor costs, 218

Dirty food handler, 308

Disability: under the Americans with Disabilities Act, 147; under the Americans with Disabilities Act of 1990 (Title I), 147–148

Disasters, See also Foodservice department disaster plan: Disaster Assessment Checklist, 335; disaster committee, 334–336; disaster plan, design of, 334–335; disaster training programs, 336; drills, 336; external, 334; F Tags, 334; foodservice department disaster plan, 336–340; internal, 334; notification system, 336; signed memorandum of understanding (MOU), 336

Discipline: compared to coaching, 174; progressive, 182

Discounts, 41–42, 242, 359, 408, 417, 419, 420

Discretionary benefits, 150

Dish machines, 305–306

Dishwashing machines, 533–534

Dismissal, 182

Disorganization, and communication, 131

Dispensing utensils, 500

Disposable gloves, 302, 306

Disposable prototypes, 516

Disposables, reducing quantity of, 242

Dissatisfaction stage, group development, 100

Distracters: to communication, 129; keeping to a minimum, 140

Distributors' sales representatives (DSRs), 409

Diversity, 169–170; barriers to, 170; policies/procedures, 170

Divided loyalty, of contract company employees, 14

Divisional structure, as depicted on organizational chart, 102

Documentation, team meetings, 135

Double-hand-wash method, 301

Dough cutters and choppers, 526

Downer cow, 275

Downtime, foodservice operation computers, 204

Downward communication, 141

Dragon fruit, 393

Drained weight, 419

Dress code, 45

Dried beef, as processed meat, 376

Dried fruit, 393

Dried legumes, USDA grades for, 394

Driving record, and background check, 157

Drucker, P., 88

Drug abuse, 1

Drug screening, 152

Dry cereal, 398

Dry storage: facilities, 434; maintenance, 434–437

Dry storage equipment, 521

Du jour menus, 351

Dummy tray, 505

Durum wheat, 477

E

E-mail, 138–139; answering, 125; etiquette, 139

Earrings, 278, 326

Economic downturn, 2

Economical order quantity, 444

Economy of scale, of contract foodservice management, 14

Edam, 386

Edible flowers, 398–399

Edible portion (EP), 419

Edible price (EP price), 419

Edible yield factor (EYF), 419

Ednet, 299

Education coordinators, 160

Education record, and background check, 157

Effective Behavior in Organizations (Cohen/Fink/Gadon/Willits/Josefowitz), 22

Effective leadership, 25; behavior theories of, 21–22

Effluent, use of term, 258

Egg/egg products: baking, 474; chilled egg products, 472; cooking methods, 473–474; dehydrated egg products, 472; dried egg solids, 472; egg substitutes, 472–473; frozen egg products, 472; frying, 473; hard cooking, 473; medium cooking, 473; omelets, 474; poaching, 473; processed egg products, 472–473; scrambling, 473–474; soufflés, 474

Egg noodles, 397

Egg Products Inspection Act (1970; 1972), 380, 381

Eggnog, 383

Eggs/egg products, 380–381; delivery/storage, 420; egg products, defined, 381; Egg Products Inspection Act (1970), 381; price consideration in purchasing eggs, 381; recommended storage temperatures/times, 435; shell egg grades, 380; shell egg USDA size categories, 381; shell egg weight/size, 380–381; specifications, 381

Eggs, grade stamps/inspection marks, 372

Elderly population, 5; and food-borne illness, 270; and V. vulnificus infection, 273

Electrical fire, 330

Electricity, and food preparation/work areas, 527–528

Electronic data interchange (EDI), 408

Electronic receiving tools, 431

Emergency Medical Treatment and Labor Act, 5

Emergency preparedness planning, 334–340

Emergency room (ER), 1–2

Emerging pathogens, 272–276

Emotional behavior, 129–130

Emotional stress of daily living/working, 1

Emotions, as communication interference, 128

Employee as customer, 8–9

Employee assistance programs (EAPs), 175

Employee-centered behavior, 22

Employee chemical information request form, 320

Employee empowerment, 34

Employee grievances, 180

Employee hazard communication program, prospectus, written description of, 320

Employee involvement, 31

Employee morale, 153

Employee orientation program, 152

Employee relations department, See Human resource department

Employee restriction, 300–302

Employee Retirement Income Security Act (ERISA) (1974), 149

Employee skepticism, and participative management, 35

Employee stock option, 150

Employee training, See Training

Employee turnover, reducing, 182–183

Employees' level of development, and participative management, 35

Employer-employee relationship, 145–151

Employment at will, and dismissal for cause, 182

Employment process, 152–153

Empowerment, 26; of employees, 34; and foodservice, 34–35; high involvement, 34; job involvement, 34; levels of, 34; of personnel, 3; and positive reinforcement, 57; suggestion involvement, 34

Enclosed carts, 530

Endosperm, 396

Energy conservation, 252–258; fuel costs, saving on, 258; practices, 257

ENERGY STAR rated equipment, 518, 520

Energy utilization: energy management program, 252–253; measurement/rates, 252

Environmental intelligence, 46

Environmental issues, and sustainability, 237–249

Environmental Protection Agency (EPA), 258, 299, 520; drinking water standards, 258

Environmental sanitation, 302–307; cleaning compounds, 303–304; cleaning equipment, 305; cross-contamination, preventing, 303; equipment/utensils, storing, 307; germicides/sanitizers, 305; grease-extracting equipment, use of, 303; grills/griddles/deep-fat cooking equipment, 303; hand-washing facilities, 303; lighting, 303; maintaining high standards of, 302; manual ware washing, 306–307; mechanical ware washing, 305; overhead pipes, removing/covering with a false ceiling, 302; plumbing, 303; potable water, 303; rodent/pest/insect control, 303; toilets, 303; of utensils/service ware, 305–307; ventilation hoods, 303

Environmental trends, 6

Environments, communication barriers due to, 129

Equal Employment Opportunity Commission (EEOC), 115, 146; definition of harassment, 146–147

Equal employment opportunity legislation, 146–148

Equal Pay Act (1963), 148

Equal™, 12

Equipment: business meetings, 133; cleaning, 302, 305; departmentalization, 97–98; energy-efficient, rebates on, 520; food equipment/utensils, 300; grease-extracting, 303; and overhead budget, 218; personal protective, 326; portioning, 401; and procurement process, 413; recycling of, 242; refrigeration, 258, 438; repair, 211, 314, 519, 530, 535, 538; repair costs vs. replacement costs, 538; schedule for cleaning of, 304; small, 400–401; stationary, cleaning, 305

Equipment maintenance/recordkeeping, 536–539; equipment cleaning record (form), 537; equipment management inventory (form), 539; equipment record card (form), 537; preventive maintenance schedule (form), 539; preventive maintenance program, setting up, 536–538

Equipment maintenance, 536–539

Equipment management inventory (form), 539

Equipment on wheels, *See* Mobile equipment

Equipment record card (form), 537

Equipment selection, 519–531, *See also* Dining area equipment; cleaning of equipment, 520; and cost, 519; cost-benefit analysis, preparing, 521; design/construction, 520; food production equipment, 521–529; ice-making equipment, 523; justification, preparing, 521; life cycle, 520; and menu offerings, 519; receiving area equipment, 521; safety/sanitation features, 520; specifications, 520–521; storage equipment, 521–523; utility supply, 519; water/energy savings, 520

Equipment specification guidelines, 507

Equivalent meals, calculating, 117

Ergonomically friendly workstations, 518

Ergonomics: awkward positions in, 340; customization of work area for computer/cash register users, 341; force factors in, 340; repetitions, 340

Escherichia coli (E. coli), 271–272, 275, 279, 339; enterohemorrhagic, 274–275

Estimated Average Requirements (EAR), 347

Ethical violations, and dismissal for cause, 182

Ethics, 5–6; codes of, 14–15; defined, 14; in food purchasing, 426–427; and foodservice operation computers, 204

Ethnic slurs, 147

Ethnicity, 7

Ethnocentrism, 130

Evaluation phase, marketing management cycle, 49

Evaporated milk, 383–384, 474–475

Exchange cart process, 440

Executive Order 11246, 147

Executive Order 11375, 147

Executive search firms, 154

Executive summary: business plan, 82; marketing plan, 48

Executive's Pocket Guide to QI/TQM Terminology, An (Causey), 52, 54

Exemplary individual contributions, and high-performance teams, 99

Exempt employees, 148

Exit interviews, conducting, 182

Exotic fruits, 393

Expectancy theory, 33

Expense budget, 211

Expense journals, 234

Expense, of contract foodservice management, 14

Experience/experience stage, in supplier selection, 424–425

Expert power, 28

Expertise, of contract foodservice management, 14

Extended-care facilities, 4–5; length of stay, 5; observing image in, 45

External benchmarking, 68

External customers, 490

External recruitment process, 153

External security, 333–334

External stress, and staff, 15–16

Extinction, 33

Extrinsic motivation, 32

F

Facebook, 189

Facility planning/design, 507–519, *See also* Work area planning; background information, collection of, 510–511; food facilities design consultant, 508; foodservice director/manager, 508; meal service, 511; menu information, 511; operational factors, analyzing, 511; planning process, 508–510; planning process flow, 509; planning team composition, 508; production, types of, 511;

prospectus, 508; punch list, 508; purchasing policies, 511; space required, 510; technology, 510; work areas, planning, 511–515

Factor system (markup system), 359

Facultative bacteria, 267

Fair Credit Reporting Act, 157

Fair Labor Standards Act (FLSA) (1938), 148

Fair Packaging and Labeling Act, 369, 387, 407

Family and medical leave, 150

Family and Medical Leave Act (1993), 3, 149

Family physicians, lack of, 3

Farina, 398

Farm Security and Rural Investment Act (2002), 369

Fat substitutes, 12

Fats/oils: butter, 394; deep-fat frying, oils/shortening for, 395; margarine, 395; specifications, 395; trans fat/hydrogenated shortening, 394–395; vegetable oils, 395

Favoritism, avoiding, 140

Fear, as resistance to change, 91

Fear of failure/job insecurity, and participative management, 35

Federal Employee Polygraph Act (1988), 158

Federal labeling requirements, 369

Federal regulatory agencies, and food safety, 299

Feedback, 45, 46, 128–129, 140; in communication, 140; techniques, 49

Feedback phase, marketing management cycle, 49

Feedback tools, quality-control program, 58

Feigenbaum, A., 52

Fennel, 484

Feta, 386

Fiber-added milk, 383

Fight BAC™, 461

Fill, standards of, 369

Filled Cheese Act (1896), 387

Fillets, 378

Financial analysis methods, 49

Financial budget, 211

Financial control: defined, 209; model for health care foodservice operations, 208–211; types of, 208–209

Financial control and management, 211–233; allocated cost budget, 218; budgetary control, 221–225; budgets, 211–212; financial records and reports, 225–233; food cost budget, 218; journalizing, 234; labor cost budget, 217–218; materials budget, 218; operating budget, 211, 212–213; overhead budget, 218; processing activities, 234; processing components, 234; processing element of the foodservice operation, 233–234; productivity indicators, calculating, 219–221; profit-and-loss statement, 216–217; statistical indicators, determining, 219

Financial information, 207

Financial management, defined, 207–208

Financial strategy, 80–81

Financial woes, 2

Foodservice department: decentralization, 97; functional departmentalization, 96–97; functional organization of, 96; image, 35; inventory systems, 11; nutrition analysis, 11; operating budget, 153; operation of, 152, 237–238; organizing, 102–109; orientation to, 159; and process decentralization, 97–98; role of, 14; scheduling work in, 118–125; staffing, 110–118; waste removal, 249

Foodservice department disaster plan: biological threats, 338–339; bioterrorism, 338; blistering agents, 338; blood agents, 338; chemical agents, 338; choking agents, 338; cleanup, 337; communications, 337; coordination, 337; floods, 337–338; heat exhaustion, 338; hurricanes, 337–338; menus, 336–337; methods of alert of impending dangers, 336; nerve agents, 338; nuclear agents, 338; participation, 337; planning for disasters, 337–340; power failures, 337; sanitation, 337; security, 337; service priorities, 337; signed memorandum of understanding (MOU), 336; supplies, 337; volunteers/employees from outside of the department, 337; water procedures, 336; winter storms, 338

Foodservice director, 3, 8, *See also* Team decision making

FoodService Director, 508

Foodservice director: accidents/injuries, 312–313; allergens, knowledge of, 276; applicant interviews, 155–156; benefits administration, 186; budgets, 212–214, 221–223; business meetings, 132–134; buyer qualifications, 412–413; capital budget request, 221; chemical hazards, 278; committees, service on, 99; compensation administration, 185–186; composting, 242–243; continuing education, 16; control process, 207, 209; data collection, 46–47; department business plan, 80; department policies and procedures manual, 76; departmental plans, 26; dining areas, 531–536; disaster and emergency preparedness planning, 334–340; downward communication, 141; educational background, 107; and employee behavior/ motivation, 33; employee compensation/ benefits, 32; employment process, 152–158; energy management program, 252; environmental issues, 237; environmental waste, 241; equipment maintenance/record keeping, 536–539; equipment selection, 519–531; ergonomics, 340–341; ethics, 426–427; evaluation of formal meetings, 134; facility maintenance/waste hauler, 250; facility planning/design, 507–519; feedback to, 45; fire safety and prevention, 326–331; food-borne illnesses, 261–263, 269; food quality standards, 447–451; functional-hierarchical structure, 104; goals/objectives, 87; HACCP process, implementation of,

285–286; hazardous chemicals, 250; horizontal communication, 141; and human resource specialists, 151; and human resources department, 115, 145, 151; in-service training programs, 161–163; infection control, 250; inventory control procedures, 439–444; locally grown organic foods, purchase of, 370; make or buy decision, 410–411; management responsibilities of, 19; managerial ethics/ social responsibility, 14–15; meal count, 223; meal service systems, 491–502; menu evaluation, 362–364; menu planning, 352–359; menu specifications, 349–352; MIS system for analyses, development of, 189; monthly performance report/control reports, 231–233; networking, 16, 24; operating procedures/standards/expenses, review of, 225; operations data, evaluation of, 223–224; orientation, 159; performance evaluations, 170, 223, 225; performance measurement, 210; personal and professional development, 16; personal code of ethics, 15; persuasive communication skills, 137; and pest infestations, 309; plate waste and sales volume studies, 349; and power requirements of equipment, 518; pricing strategies, 359–362; procurement process, 411–417; product evaluation, 417–420; production forecasting, 452–453; production schedules, 453; production strategy, 80; productivity measurements, identifying/establishing, 118; professional organizations, membership in, 107; profit-and-loss statement, 216; purchasing methods, 420–424; and quality, 58; quality control, 58, 210; reduce/reuse, 241–242; refrigeration/refrigerants, 258; responsibilities of, 88, 107, 109, 262, 447; revenue, 216; as role model/mentor, 16; safety training, 326; sanitary food service, provision of, 300–303; scheduling, 118–125; security, 332–334, 434; service supplies, 402; standards, 67; statistical indicators, determination of, 219; storage procedures, 434–439; strategic planning, 27, 75; stress, 15–16; and stress, 15–16; supplier selection/ relations, 424–425; sustainability, 237–249; training, role in, 160; transporting, 409; units of service, estimating, 214; variance analysis, 223, 225; waste management, rethinking, 242–249

Foodservice Energy Management Survey, 254–257

Foodservice equipment, 12–13

Foodservice industry: background of, 13; classifications, 13–14; managerial ethics/social responsibility, 14–15

Foodservice manager, *See* Foodservice director

Foodservice operations: foodservice director's responsibilities, 262; and Obama health care plan, 1

Foodservice opportunities, 6

Foodservice organizations, systems approach to, 101–102

Foodservice staff, and food tray service, 496

Foodservice workers, availability/skills of, 347

Foot-candle, 518

Force factors, in ergonomics, 340

Forcing, and conflict resolution, 142

Forecasting, 414, 452–453; and computers in foodservice operations, 203

Forecasting in Foodservice (Messersmith/Miller), 453

Forecasting methods, monitoring, 242

Foreign language menus, 358

Foreshank cut of beef, 374

Forks, placement of, 499

Formal/informal surveys, and CQI, 55–56

Formal leaders, 25

Formal rewards, 30

Format: business plan, 82; menus, 359

4Rs (reduce, reuse, recycle, rethink), 241–242

401(k) plan, 150

Fowl, 379

Free-on-board (FOB), 417

Freezers, 519

French-fried potatoes, 390, 477

Freshwater fish, 375

Fried eggs, 473

Fringe benefits, 150

Frozen foods: delivery, 420; storage, 420, 437–439

Frozen meals, sale of, 502

Frozen vegetables, 389, 476

Fruit cocktail, 393

Fruit desserts, 482

Fruits: apples, 391; bananas, 391; berries, 390, 391; botanical types of, 390–391; canned, net weights of, 388; cherries, 392; citrus, 391; container size, 389; dehydrated, 393–394; delivery/storage, 419; dragon, 393; dried, 393; dupes, 390; exotic, 393; grades, 393; grades of, 387–388; guava, 393; intended use, 388; jackfruit, 393; kiwi, 392; kumquat, 393; mangoes, 392; melons, 391–392; oranges/ citrus, 392; passion, 393; peaches, 392; pears, 392; pineapples, 392; plums, 392; preparing/ serving, 479; rambutan, 393; recommended storage temperatures/times, 435; rose apple, 393; specifications, 393; tropical, 391; types of, 391; watermelons, 392

Full-function wholesalers, 410

Full-slip, use of term, 390

Full-time employee (FTE), 153

Full-time equivalency needs, calculating, 117–118

Functional departmentalization, 96–97

Functional organization, of the foodservice department, 96

Fungi: molds, 268–269; yeast, 268

Fuse boxes, 528

G

Game meat, 375

Gantt chart, 82–84, 85, 508

Garbage and refuse disposal, and health inspection, 300

Garlic, 484

Garnish, 353

Gelatins, 482

General ledger, 234

General-line wholesalers, 410

Generation X and Generation Z, and the workforce, 7

Genetic engineering, 11–12

Genetically engineered (GE) organism, defined, 369

Genetically enhanced ingredients, in food, 6

Genetically modified foods: cloned food, 370; health concerns, 369–370

Genoa salami, as processed meat, 376

Geographical location, and supply/price of foods in marketplace, 348

Geographical segmentation, 39

Geriatric medicine, 1

Germ, 396

Germicides, 305

Giardiasis, 267–268

Ginger, 484

Glass, as packaging waste, 240

Glass ceiling, 147

Glassware, 499

Global Harmonization Standards (GHS), 316

Gloves, use of, 302, 306

Gluten, 396, 479–480

Goals and objectives, marketing plan, 48

Goals, well-written, characteristics of, 85–87

Goat's milk, 383–384

Good Agricultural Practices (GAP), 370

Good grade veal, 373

Good Manufacturing Practice (GMP), 370

Goods, 38

Gorgonzola, 268, 386

Gouda, 386

Gourmet meal programs, 354–356

Gourmet meal service, for family members, 43

Governing board, 73

Grades, meat/meat products, 371–372

Grains/cereals, 477, See also Flour; barley, 396; breakfast cereals, 398; buckwheat, 396; cooking methods, 477; couscous, 396; flour, types of, 396; graham, 396; oats, 397; pasta, 395–396; rice, 396; wheat, 396; wheat germ, 396

Grapevine communications, 141–142

Graphic rating scale, 171

Graphology, 158

Grease-extracting equipment, use of, 303

Grease fire, 330

Green Seal™ Environmental Standards for Restaurants and Foodservices (GS-46), 409

Green tea, 399

Greenhouse gas (GHG) emission, 409

Greens, 390

Griddles, 526

Grievance, defined, 180

Grievance procedures, 180–181; record of employee counseling (form), 181

Gross profit method, 362

Group decision, Vroom-Yetton-Jago model of, 22

Group development stages, 100

Group performance, rewarding, 30

Group purchasing organizations (GPOs), 420–421

Gruyere, 386

Guava, 393

Gueridon, 498

Guest relations, 59–60

Gumbos, 480

H

HACCP, See Hazard Analysis Critical Control Point (HACCP)

Half-and-half, 500

Half-slip, use of term, 390

Halo effect, 171

Ham: and inhibitors, 266; and molds, 268; as processed meat, 376; recommended storage temperatures/times, 435; wrapping, 438

Hand antiseptic, 301

Hand trucks, 521

Hand-washing: facilities, 300, 303; habits, 301; procedures, 280

Harassment, EEOC definition of, 146–147

Hard drive, foodservice operation computers, 204

Hardware and telecommunications review, 204

Hazard Analysis Critical Control Point (HACCP): action plan for implementation, 298; CCP monitoring system, establishing, 294–295; control measures, 286–287; cook-and-chill procedures, 293; cook-and-freeze procedures, 287; cooling plan documentation, 298; corrective action, establishing, 295–296; critical control points, determining, 287; critical control points, flowchart for, 295; critical limits for each CCP, 287–294; decision tree for critical control points, 292; defined, 286, 298; documentation/record keeping establishing, 296–297; food hazard analysis, components of, 291; foodservice operation hazardous practices, 290; and foodservice systems, 287–294; implementing, 285–286; inspections, 299; and ISO 22000, 286; potential hazards, 286–287; principles of, 286–299; purpose of, 287; ready prepared foods, 287; recipe flowchart, 288–289; records to maintain, 297; verification procedures, establishing, 296

Hazard analysis critical control point programs, 419

Hazard Communication standards (OSHA), 316, 320

Hazard training programs, OSHA, 319

Hazardous communication standards, 250

Hazardous waste management: material safety data sheets (MSDSs), 250–251; Medical Waste Track Act, 249; "Standards for the Tracking and Management of Medical Waste," 249

HazCom Standards, Occupational Safety and Health Administration (OSHA), 316

Health and safety legislation, 150

Health care: affordability, 4; ambulatory care, 5; case management, 5; changes in, 2–6; extended-care facilities, 4–5; future of, 1; internal operations of organizations, 1–2; lack of access to, 1; patient-focused (patient-centered) care, 5

Health care foodservice operations, competition with other retail/commercial operations, 490

Health-care management levels, 26

Health care meal service systems, 489, 491–505; nonpatient meal service, 499–502; patient meal service, 491–497; resident meal service, 497–500; standards, 502–505

Health-care providers: factors faced by, 2; interdisciplinary, 3

Health inspections, 299–300

Health insurance, 150; lack of, 1

Health Insurance Portability and Accountability Act (HIPAA), 64, 496

Hearing, listening vs., 140

Heart disease/ heart disease patients, 1, 5, 10; potable water for patients, 258; and soy protein, 387

Heat-and-serve processed meat, 375

Hemochromatois, and V. vulnificus infection, 273

Hemorrhagic fever, 339

Hepatitis A, 274, 279

Herbal tea, 400

Herbs/spices, 399, 468, 469, 476; cooking with, 483–484

Herzberg, F., 32

Hierarchy of needs, 31–32

High involvement, 34

High-performance teams: building, 3; characteristics of, 99–100

High-pressure steamers, 525

High-ratio method, of mixing, 481

Hispanic/Latino population, 7

Historical data, reviewing, 214

HIV, 8

HIV/AIDS: and listeriosis, 272; and V. vulnificus infection, 273

Home care: and health care quality, 52; hospital-own services, 1, 5; transition to, 62

Home-replacement meal (HRMs), 500

Hominy, 397

Honey, 400

Horizontal communication, 141

Horizontal integration, 409

Hospital-owned home care services, 1

Hospitality industry, segments of, 13

Hospitalized children, menu planning for, 353–355

Hot and cold carts system, 495

Hot and cold holding conditions, 500

Hot stove rule, 178

Hot water temperatures, for cleaning/sanitizing dishes and utensils, 306

Hourly employees, 153

Housekeeping products, 278

Human resource control, 208–209

Human resource department, *See also* Personnel; Personnel policies and procedures; Recruitment; Training: applicant interviews, 152; compensation and benefits administration, 185–187; contract employees, 153; drug screening, 152; employee orientation program, 152; employer-employee relationship, 145–151; and fair treatment of all employees, 151; full-time employee (FTE), 153; functions of, 151; health care, areas of responsibility, 151; hourly employees, 153; job sharing/job splitting, 153; nonprofessional employees, 152; orientation to the organization, 159; part-time employee (PTE), 153; personnel requisition, 152–153; professional employees, 152–153; recruitment, 152; references, checking, 152; resolution of employee issues/problems, 151; role of, 151–159; salaried employees, 153; skilled workers, 153; structure of, 145; temporary employees, 153; training, 160–167; turnover rate, 153; unskilled workers, 153

Human resource management, 19–20, 145–168; absenteeism, reducing, 184–185; Age Discrimination in Employment Act (1967), 146; Civil Rights Act (Title VII) (1964), 146; compensation and benefits administration, 185–187; cultural diversity, 169–170; discrimination, interpretive guidelines on, 146–147; dismissal, 182; employee assistance programs (EAPs), 175; employee turnover, reducing, 182–183; equal employment opportunity legislation, 146–148; ethnic slurs, 147; exit interviews, conducting, 182; labor relations, 186–187; laws affecting, 145–146; personnel policies and procedures, 176; personnel records, 175–176; Pregnancy Discrimination Act (1978), 146; racial jokes, 147; resignation form, 184; sexual discrimination, 146–147; sexual harassment, 146–147; Vietnam Era Veterans Readjustment Assistance Act (1974), 146; Vocational Rehabilitation Act (1973), 146

Human resources management: Americans with Disabilities Act of 1990 (Title I), 147–148; benefits administration, 186; bona fide occupational qualifications (BFOQ), 147–148; Civil Rights Act (1991), 147; compensation and benefits legislation, 148–150; Executive Order 11375, 147; glass ceiling, 147; health and safety legislation, 150; immigration reform legislation, 150–151; performance evaluation systems, 170–175; Privacy Act (1974), 147; recognition and awards programs, 186

Humidity, and food quality, 438–439

Hydrochlorofluorocarbons (HCFCs), 253, 257–258

Hydrogenated vegetable oil, 275; smoke point, 465

Hydrogenation, 394–395

Hygiene, 300–301

Hygiene factors, 32

I

Ice, 259; dispensing, 500

Ice beverage glass, placement of, 499

Ice-making equipment, 523

Iced tea, 400

Identity, standards of, 369

Ignorance, and conflict resolution, 142

Illegal Immigration Reform and Immigrant Responsibility Act (1996), 150–151

Image: enhancement of, 41; foodservice department, 35

Imitation milk, 385

Immersion dishwashers, 306

Immigration Reform and Control Act (1986), 150–151

Impingement, 524

Implementation phase, marketing management cycle, 49

Improved skills, 186

In-service training, 30; group, 161–162; maintaining records of individuals/group training programs, 165–167; sessions, evaluating, 163; topics/resources, identifying, 163–164

Incentives, 8

Incident reports, and training, 163

Indirect labor costs, 218

Individual bias, as barrier to diversity, 170

Individual meal service, 502

Individual motivation, and high-performance teams, 99

Induction heating, 462

Industrial engineers, and standards, 210

Influencing function, 27

Informal buying, 423–424

Informal leaders, 25

Informal rewards, 30

Informal surveys, and CQI, 55–56

Information: defined, 190; measuring the value of, 190

Information control, 209

Information overload, and communication, 131

Information phase, marketing management cycle, 46

Information systems, 11

Informational role, of leaders, 25

Infrared ovens, 524

Ingredient control, 460–461; production system based on, 461

Ingredient file, 191

Ingredient room layout, 460

Ingredient substitution, in standardized recipes, 460–461

Injuries, defined, 312

Innovation, and CQI, 57

Input, 102

Inquiry/inquiry stage, in supplier selection, 424–425

Insect control, 303; and health inspection, 300

Insecticides, using around food, 309

Inspection, meat/meat products, 371

Instant coffee, 399

Institutional foodservice, 13; self-operated, 13–14

Institutional foodservice jobs, demand for, 7

Insulated tray system, 494–495

Intangible standards, 210

Integrated system, EPA definition of, 241

Integration of health care organizations, 2

Interactive computer training, 162–163

Interdepartmental teams, 56

Interdisciplinary health-care providers, 3

Interest, lack of, and communication, 130

Interest tests, 158

Interferences, 128

Intergraded pest management (IMP), 309

Intermediate-range planning, 73

Internal benchmarking, 68

Internal customers, 490

Internal records, 46

Internal recruitment, 153

Internal security, 332–333

International Classification of Diseases (ICD-9), 299

Internet, 125; education-based courses, 163; promotion using, 43; and recruitment, 154

Interpersonal power, 28

Interpersonal relationships, and high-performance teams, 99

Interpersonal role, of leaders, 25

Interpersonal skills, of leaders, 24–25

Interstate Certified Shellfish Shippers List, 273

Interviewing applicants, 155–156; behavioral interviewing, 157–158; effective sessions, 156; post-interview steps, 156

Intradepartmental teams, 56

Intrinsic motivation, 32

Inventory control: computerized inventory management system, 444–445; first-in, first-out (FIFO) method, 443; inventory turnover, 443; issuing process, 439–440; last-in, first-out (LIFO) method, 443; procedures, 439–444; record keeping, 440–442; shrinkage, 443; stores requisition, 439; weighted averages, 443

customer preferences, 363; customer survey form for a new menu item, 364; cycle, 352, 358; day-to-day distribution, 363; defined, 343; Dietary Reference Intake (DRI), 350; du jour, 351; facilities/equipment, 363; flavor combinations, 362; food shapes/sizes, 363; food temperatures, 363; foreign language, 358; form/presentation, 363; format, 359; nonpatient, 358–359; nonselective, 351; patient, 352–353, 359; patient menus, 352–353; pattern, 362; personnel/time, 363; planning factors, 344; popularity of foods, 363; preparation methods, 363; preselected, 357; as primary control of foodservice system, 343; printed, 351; revision of, 349; selective, 351, 359; single-use, 352; specifications, 343; spoken, 357; static, 351, 352; surveys, 363–365; table d'hote, 351; texture/consistency, 362; truth in, 349; types of, 351–352

Merchandising, 43

Mercury contamination, 379

Mergers, 2

Merit increases, 185–186

Method, of objectives, 87

Mettwurst, as processed meat, 376

Microbial hazards, contamination by, 262–269

Microbiological controls, 489

Microorganisms, defined, 263

Microwave ovens, 524

Middle-level management, 26

Military reserve, 150

Milk/dairy products, 381–385; acidophilus-cultured milk, 383; cooking methods, 474–475; cream, 384; cultured buttermilk, 383; delivery/storage, 420; dry buttermilk, 384; eggnog, 383; evaporated milk, 384; fiber-added milk, 383; flavored milk, 383; forms of, 383–384; goat's milk, 383–384; grades of milk, 383; ice cream, 384; ice milk/sherbet, 384; lactose-free milk, 383; nonfat dry milk, 384; 1% low-fat milk, 383; organic milk, 383; skin/nonfat milk, 383; sour cream/sour half-and-half, 384; specifications, 384–385; sweetened condensed milk, 384; 2% low-fat milk, 383; whole milk, 383; yogurt, 384

Milk glass, placement of, 499

Millennials, and the workforce, 7

Mineral water, 259

Mini-max system, of inventory control, 444

Minimum wage, 148

Minnesota Department of Natural Resources (MN DNR), 375

Minority workers, 7

Mint, 484

Mirroring, 140

Mistrust, as barrier to diversity, 170

Mixed message, 131

Mixers, 526

Mobile equipment, 530–531; dispensing equipment, 530–531; self-leveling plate units, 530; unheated open carts, 530

Moist-heat methods of cooking poultry, 469

Molded gelatin salads, 479

Molds, 268–269

Molluscan shellfish, and Vibrio infections, 273

Monterey Jack, 386

Monthly performance report, 231–233; example of, 232–233

Monthly supply costs, 230–231

Montreal Protocol, 257

Morbidity, and length of stay, 67

Mosquitoes, 308

Motivation: application of theories, 33–34; content theories of, 31–32; defined, 31; extrinsic, 32; intrinsic, 32; maintenance motivation theory, 32; process theories of, 32–33; reinforcement theory of, 33

Motivation factors, 32

Motivational theories, application of, 33–34

Mozzarella cheese, 386, 387

MRSA, 280

Muenster cheese, 386

Muffin method, for mixing quick breads, 480

Muffins, 480

Multidepartment management, 109

Multifacilities, 109

Multiple-sponsor service, 108–109

Multitank conveyor machines, 534

Municipal solid waste, 240

Musculoskeletal disorders (MSDs), 340

Mushrooms, toxic, 269

Mutual accountability, and high-performance teams, 99

My Plate, 346–347, 350

Mycolaxin, 278

Mycotoxins, 268

Myers-Briggs Type Indicator, 158

Mystery shoppers, 46

N

Napkins, 498

Natick Research Laboratories (U.S. Army), and the HACCP process, 285

National Association of Purchasing Management, Principles and Standards of Purchasing Practices, 427

National Electrical codes, 314

National Environmental Health Association (NEHA), 299

National Environmental Protection Agency (NEPA), 237

National Fire Protection Association (NFPA), 331

National Food Processors Association (NFPA), 11–12

National Guard service, 150

National Labor Relations Act (Wagner Act) (1935), 149–150

National Labor Relations Board (NLRB), 149

National Marine Fisheries Service (NMFS), 299

National Nutrition Month, 41

National Patient Safety Goals (NPSGs), 64, 66

National Restaurant Association: Americans with Disabilities Act: Answers for Foodservice Operators, 510–511; Education Foundation, 299

National Sanitation Foundation, codes, 314

National Science Foundation International (NSF), 299

National Shellfish Sanitation Program Guide for Control of Mulluscan Shellfish, 273

National Social Security Act, 64

Native Hawaiian/Pacific Islander population, 7

Naturally occurring chemical hazards, 278–280; chemicals, 278; housekeeping products, 278; new concerns, 279–280; pesticides, 278; physical hazards, 278–279; toxic metals, 278

Need, and planning time frames, 73

Need for achievement, 32–33

Need for affiliation, 33

Need for power, 33

Needs assessment: procurement process, 413; training, 161–162

Negotiation and selection stage, in supplier selection, 424–425

Nerve agents, 338

Net weight, 419

Networking, 16

Neutral compounds, 304

New Delhi Metallo-beta-lactamase-1 (NMD-1), 279

New employee training, See Training

New Silent/Generation Z, and the workforce, 7

Newsletters, 42, 186

Niche market, 40

Nits, 308

Noise exposure, and soundproofing, 517–518

Non-cybernetic control systems, 209

Non-unionized healthcare facility, 180

Noncommercial foodservice: defined, 13; in-house management of, 13–14

Noncontract purchasing, 423–424

Nondairy substitutes for milk and cream, 385

Nonexempt employees, 148

Nonfat dry milk, 384, 474

Nonmonetary budgets, 211

Nonpatient meal service, 499–502; boxed meals, 500; cafeteria service, 499; catering services, 501; convenience stores, 500; display/service/transport, 500; food courts, 500; food truck food, 500–501; home-replacement meal (HRMs), 500; kiosks, 500; off-site meal service, 501–502; over-the-counter service, 499–500; payment methods, 499; quantity meals, 502; snack shops, 500; vending operations, 501

Nonpatient menus: community residents, 358–359; employees/staff/visitors, 358; format, 359

Pancakes, 480

Panfrying fish, 469

Pans, 328, 337, 400–401; pan size yield, 462; panfrying fish, 469; sauce-, 401; sheet, 401; storage of, 307; washing/cleaning/sanitizing, 302, 305

Paperwork, reducing, 125, 140

Par stock system, of inventory control, 444

Parasites, 267–269; *anisakiasis*, 267–268; *cryptosporidiosis*, 267, 268; *cyclospora cayetanensis*, 268; food-borne illnesses caused by, 267; fungi, 268–269; *giardia lambia*, 268; *giardiasis*, 267–268; invasive, 267; noninvasive, 267; and pork, 267–268; *toxoplasma gonndii*, 268; transmission of, 267; *trichinella spiralis*, 267; trichinosis, 267

Parmesan cheese, 386

Parsley, 484

Part-time employee (PTE), 153

Participation, team meetings, 135

Participative culture: apprenticeship, 29; brainstorming, 30; communication, 31; compensation/rewards, 30; creating, 29; employee involvement, 31; job rotation, 29; management responsibilities in, 29–30; motivation, 31; obstacle removal, 31; on-the-job training (OJC), 29; shared decision making, 30; team building, 30; training and development, 30

Participative management, 29–35; and cultural differences, 35; and employee skepticism, 35; employee skepticism, 35; employees' level of development, 35; fear of failure/job insecurity, 35; positive effects of, 29; roadblocks to, 35–36

Passion fruit, 393

Passwords, foodservice operation computers, 204

Pasta, 353, 395–396, 477; durum wheat, 477; specifications, 397; types of, 397

Pasteurization, 263

Pastrami, as processed meat, 376

Pastries, 482

Pastry and cake flours, 396

Pathogens: defined, 263; emerging, 272–276; known to cause disease/death, 275

Patient care unit, 97

Patient-focused care, 5; units, 97

Patient meal service, 491–497; monitoring for performance, 496–497; special services, 497; tray accuracy, 497; tray assembly, 491–494; tray delivery, 494–496; tray delivery time, 497; tray line concerns, 496; tray line requirements, 494; tray service, 496; trays per minute, 496–497; written selective menu, patient confusion about, 496

Patient meal tray service, 499

Patient menus, 352–353; format, 359

Patient Protection and Affordable Care Act, 4

Patient Satisfaction Questionnaire, 503

Pay for performance, 186

Payroll deduction, defined, 499

Payroll stuffers, 43

Peaches, 392

Pears, 392

Pediatric patients, menu planning for, 353–355

Peer review, 172

Perception, as communication interference, 128

Performance coaching, 173

Performance evaluation, 185; 360° review/feedback, 172; appraisal performance, 172; coaching, 173; competence, 172–173; critical incidents, 172; defined, 170; graphic rating scale, 171; halo effect, 171; objective-based performance review, 172; ongoing review, 171; peer review, 172; performance appraisal form, 170–171; performance standards, 171; preparing for appraisal sessions, 171; recency error, 171; self-evaluations, 172; subordinate review, 172; systems, 170–175; verbal performance reviews, conducting, 171–172; verbal review, 170; written evaluation, 170

Performance planning, 27

Perfume, 301, 496

Periodic operational planning, 76–77; department budget, 80; department business plan, 80

Periodic plans, 72

Perishable resources, 38

Perpetual inventory, 441

Perquisite programs (PRPs), 286

Personal and professional development, 16

Personal appearance, presentations, 136

Personal appraisals, 170–171, *See also* Performance evaluation

Personal ethics, defined, 14

Personal perception, communication barriers due to, 129

Personal power, 28

Personal protective equipment, 326

Personality conflict, and communication, 130

Personality tests, 158

Personnel: empowering, 3; and health inspection, 300; policies and procedures, 176, 178–180; records, 20, 175–176; requisition, 152–153; review, and computers in foodservice operations, 204

Personnel department, *See* Human resource department

Personnel policies and procedures, 176; corrective action record (form), 179; grievance procedures, following, 180; hot stove rule, 178

Persuasion, 131

Pest control, 303, 307–309; checking for infestations, 309; intergraded pest management (IMP), 309; kitchen pests, 308; pest control employee/operator, hiring, 309

Pesticides, 278

Petty cash, 216

Phenotype group, as barrier to diversity, 170

Phenylketouria (PKU), 275

Physical environment, business meetings, 133

Physical inventory, 441–442; record, 442

Pick-up service, 43

Pickles, 400

Pies, 482

Pilferage of food/supplies, 332, 333, 440, 441, 446

Pineapples, 392

Pink (humpback) salmon, 379

Place, as element of the marketing mix, 40–41

Place settings, 498

Placement offices, 154

Plan-do-check-act (PDCA) cycle, 51–52

Planning, 19, 71–88, 207; business planning phases, 81–82; core values, 71; defined, 71; intermediate-range, 73; long-range, 73; as management function, 26–27; objectives, 71; operational, 72; and organizational agendas, 71–72; periodic plans, 72; purpose of, 71; short-range, 73; single-use plans, 72; standing operational, 75–78; standing plans, 72; strategic, 72; strategies, 71; types of, 72

Planning function, 27

Planning grid, 84–85

Planning phase, marketing management cycle, 47–48

Planning process, 47–48, 72–73; decision making in, 88; and time, 73

Planning team composition, 508

Plant food toxins, 269

Plastic, as packaging waste, 240

Plate waste and sales volumes studies, and revision of menus, 349

Plate waste, observing, 363

Plate-Waste or Food-Return Record, 504

Plate-waste studies, 505

Play and Make step, 339

Plumbing, 303, 518; and food preparation/work areas, 527–528; and health inspection, 300; work area, 519

Plums, 392

Poached eggs, 473

Poaching fish, 472

Pod system, 492

Point-of-sale items, 43

Point-of-sales (POS) cash register system, 215

Policies, 75–76

Political issues, 3–6; accountability/ethics, 5–6; health-care affordability, 4–5; regulation/legislation, 3–4

Politically correct terms, use of, 130

Pollock, 378–379

Polygraph test, 158

Pop-up timers, 283

Popovers, 480

Pork, 373; primal cuts of, 374; as ready-to-serve meat, 375; recommended storage temperatures/times, 435

Pork sausage, as processed meat, 376

Portion control, 455

Portioning equipment, 401

Positive reinforcement, 33; and empowerment, 57

Posting transactions, 234

Potable water, 303, 519; need for, 258–259

Potassium bromate, 275

Potatoes, 353, 390, 476–477; baked, 476; dehydrated, 394; French-fried, 477; mashed, 390, 476

Potentially hazardous foods (PHFs), 269, 462, 500

Pots, 401; storage of, 307; washing/cleaning/sanitizing, 302, 305

Poultry, 379–380; broiling, 468–469; class, 380; cooking methods, 467–469; deep-fat frying, 468; delivery/storage, 419; delivery unit, 380; dry-heat methods of cooking, 468–469; grade stamps/inspection marks, 372; grades, 379–380, 380; grilling, 468–469; handling of, during preparation, 467–468; inspection, 380; kind, 379; market forms of, 379; moist-heat methods of cooking, 469; oven frying, 468; recommended storage temperatures/times, 435; roasting, 468; and Salmonella bacteria, 468; specifications, 379–380; storage of, 468; style, 380; thawing, 468; weight/size, 380

Poultry Products Inspection Act, 407

Power, need for, 33

Power-purchasing strategies, 405

Practical Guide to Sous Vide Cooking, A, 493

Prebiotics, 12

Preceding year's budget, 214

Precooked rice, 397

Pregnancy, and food-borne illness, 270

Pregnancy Discrimination Act (1978), 146

Prejudice, as barrier to diversity, 170

Preliminary control, 209

Preselected menus, 357

Presentations, 135–136; adding variety to, 135; anxiety, using to advantage, 136; audience, relating to, 136; conquering your fears, 135; handouts/visual aids, 135; organizing information for, 135; personal appearance, 136; planning, 135

Pressure fryers, 526

Pretending to listen, 140

Preventive maintenance schedule (form), 539

Preventive maintenance program, setting up, 536–538

Price consideration, in purchasing eggs, 381

Price, promotions, 45

Price quotes, 416, 417

Pricing: base pricing method, 362; considerations, 359; gross profit method, 362; methods, 359–362; odd-cents, 362; by the ounce, 362; overhead-contribution system, 362; strategies, 359–362; "what the traffic will bear" method, 362

Pride in Foodservice Week, 41, 186

Prime grade veal, 373

Prime vendor agreements, 421

Principles of Information Systems: A Managerial Approach (Stair), 190

Printed menus, 351

Prions, 274–275

Prioritization, 123–125

Privacy Act (1974), 147, 157

Private employment agencies, 153

Proactive managers, 29

Probiotics, 12

Problem-solving teams, 98–99

Procedures, 75–76

Process control charts, 62–65

Process decentralization, 97–98

Process reengineering, 67–68

Process theories of motivation, 32–33

Processed meat, 375–376

Processing: activities of, 234; characteristics of, 233–234; essential components of, 234; journalizing, 234

Procter & Gamble, 12

Procurement, defined, 411

Procurement process, 411–417; approved vendor/distributor list, 413; availability of food items, 413; bid and price quotes, 414; bids, obtaining, 416; buyer's qualifications, 412–413; buyer's responsibilities, 411–412; closed bidding, 415; contract bidding, 415; equipment/space, 413; food budget, 413; inventory system, 413–414; labor budget, 413; needs assessment, 413; order placement, 414; order quantity, 414; price quotes, 416; purchase order, 415–416; purchase requisition, 414–415; purchasing method, selection of, 413; record keeping, 414, 417; steps in, 413–417

Product, as element of the marketing mix, 40

Product evaluation, 417–420

Product-line management, 26

Product receipt, 432–433

Product selection, 367–403; beverages, 399–400; defined, 367; edible flowers, 398–399; eggs/egg products, 380–381; grains/cereals, 395–398; herbs/spices, 399, 468, 469, 476, 483–484; meat/meat products, 370–375; milk/dairy products, 381–385; nuts, 398; poultry, 379–380; procurement subsystem flowchart system, 368; procurement system flowchart, 368; product standards, 369–370; seafood, 375–380; service supplies, 402; small equipment/utensils, 400–401

Product standards: food irradiation, 369; genetically engineered (modified) foods, 369–370; labeling, 370; legislation, 369–370; organic standards, 370

Product yield, 419

Production: forecast, evaluating accuracy of, 242; meetings, 453; methods, 242; monitoring, 453–454; production-related forms, 191–202; stage, group development, 100; strategy, 80

Production system, *See* Food production system

Productivity, 210; defined, 230, 233; levels of, estimating, 116–117; standards, 210; statistics, 230; and turnover rate, 153

Productivity form (sample), 119

Productivity indicators: calculating, 219–221; labor hours data, 219; volume-of-service data, 219–221

Professional associations, 154

Professional employees, 152–153

Professional organizations, participation in, 16

Profit-and-loss statement, 216–217

Profit, defined, 217

Profitability analysis, 45; and foodservice catering, 45

Profitability ratios, 234

Program evaluation and review evaluation (PERT), 84, 508

Progress reports, on objectives, 88

Progressive discipline, and dismissal for cause, 182

Project-based budgeting, 214

Project teams, 98

Promotion: catering, 44–45; defined, 41; as element of the marketing mix, 41; enhancement of, 41; feedback, 45; price, 45; public image, 45

Proofing cabinets, 527

Prospectus, 508

Provolone, 386

Prunes, 392

Psychographical segmentation, 39–40

Psychomotor skills, 162

Public employment agencies, 153

Public health, 2

Public Health Service, 273; Food Code, and fish inspections, 377; and product standards, 369

Public image, 45

Pulper extractors, 529

Punch list, 508

Punishment, 33

Punitive damages, 147

Punitive power, 28

Purchase: order, 415–416; quantity, 444; register, 234; requisition, 414–415

Purchased service, 108

Purchasing, 405–428, *See also* Procurement process; Supplier selection and relations; basic guidelines, 425–426; centralized, 422; common mistakes, 419; computer-assisted procurement, 426; continuous quality improvement (CQI), 408; contract, 422–423; distributors' changing product line, 408–409; distributors' sales representatives (DSRs), 409; ethics, 426–427; food marketing/wholesaling, 409; food supply buyer guide, 406; full-function wholesalers, 410; general-line wholesalers, 410; goal of, 406; group purchasing organizations (GPOs), 420–421; issuance of items, 419–420; just-in-time (JIT), 421–422; limited-function wholesalers, 410;

477; precooked, 397; recommended storage temperatures/times, 435; types of, 397; white, 397–398; wild, 398

Ricotta cheese, 386

Right to know, 250

Right-to-Work law, 150

Rings, 278

Risk taking, 99; and CQI, 57

Roaches, 308

Roadblocks to participative management, 35–36

Robotics, and foodservice equipment, 12–13

Robusta coffee, 399

Rodent control, 303, 308; and health inspection, 300

Role model, serving as, 16

Romano cheese, 386

Room service, 493–494; program/menu, 356–357

Roquefort cheese, 386

Rose apple, 393

Rosemary, 484

Rotanz business plan format, 82

Rotary and reel ovens, 524

Rotating master schedules, 120

Rotating shifts, 120

Rotaviruses, 274

Roth plan, 150

Round cuts of beef, 374

Roux, 480

Rules of courtesy, business meetings, 133–134

Rutabagas, 476

Rye flour, 396

S

Saccharin, 12

Safe clothing and shoes, 326

Safe lifting procedure, 326–327

Safety, 311–331; accidents, 312–313; basic safety tips for the kitchen, 313; defined, 311–312; foodservice safety checklist, 312; and health inspection, 300; injuries, 312–313; procedures, training employees in, 314; risk management, 314; working conditions, 314

Safflower oil, 395

Sage archetype, 484

Salad fork, placement of, 499

Salad plate, placement of, 499

Salads, 353; assembly of ingredients, 479; base, 478; body, 478; combination, 478; dressing, 478; garnish, 478; main-dish, 478; molded gelatin, 479; preparation of ingredients, 479; relishes, 478–479; salad bars, 479; underliners, 478

Salami: and molds, 268; as processed meat, 376

Salaried employees, 153

Salary/wages, See also Compensation: annual bonus, 186; cash awards, 186; cost-of-living adjustment (COLA), 186; improved skills, 186; increases in, 170; merit increases, 185–186; pay for performance, 186

Sales analyses, 49

Salmon, 378–379

Salmonella/salmonellosis, 270–272, 275, 279; and poultry, 468; symptoms of, 270

Saltwater fish, 375

Sandwiches: assembly, 477–478; ingredients, 477

Sanitation, 243; codes, 242; cost of disposing of food waste, 249; and energy conservation, 257; environmental, 302–307; and food-borne illness, 274; and health inspection, 518–519; implementing a program of, 262; in-service training, 16; inspections, 210, 237, 299–300; and parasites, 268; as part of CQI program, 261; and quality control, 58; scheduling, 120; self-evaluation of conditions/practices, 307; of surfaces coming in contact with food, 241; violations, 211; ware washing, 305–307; and waste storage, 243

Sanitizers, 305

Sanitizing, defined, 303

Saucepans, 401

Sauces, 480

Sausage (Thüringen style), as processed meat, 376

Savory, 484

Scales, 401, 430, 431; receiving area, 521

Scheduling, 118–125; cleaning of equipment, 304; computerized, 121–123; daily schedule, 120; defined, 118; flexible schedules, 120; job sharing/job splitting, 120; limits, setting, 125; log of daily activities, 123; master schedules, 120; prioritization, 123–125; shift schedule, 120–121; software, 121–123; techniques, 82–83; telecommuting, 120; workweek, 118

School, observing image in, 45

Scombroid poisoning, 269

Scombroid toxin, 269

Scoops: approximate yield from, 455; and standardized recipes, 460

Scope of service, 26

Scrambled eggs, 473–474

Screening and control, 209

Screening applicants, 154

Seafood, See also Fish/shellfish cooking methods: aquaculture, 377; butterfly fillet, 378; canned fish, 379; Chinook (king) salmon, 379; chum (keta) salmon, 379; cod, 378; Coho salmon, 378–379; cooking methods for fish and shellfish, 469–472; crab, 378; defined, 375–376; delivery/storage, 419; drawn, 378; dressed, 378; fillets, 378; fish farms, 377; fish names, 377; fresh fish, 377; freshwater fish, 375; frozen fish, 378; grade stamps/inspection marks, 372; inspection for sanitary conditions and wholesomeness, 377; mackerel, 377; market forms of fish/shellfish, 378; mercury contamination, 379; oily fish, 377; packed under federal inspection, 377; pink (humpback) salmon, 379; pollock, 378; portions/sticks, 378; product grading, 377; recommended storage temperatures/times, 435; salmon, 378–379; saltwater fish, 375;

shellfish, 378; shrimp, 378; Sockeye salmon, 379; specification, 378; steaks, 378; trout, 377; tuna, 379; use of term, 375–376; whole/dressed, 378; whole/round, 378

Seasonal change, and revision of menus, 349

Secret ballot election, 150

Security, 332–334; employee theft, causes of, 332; and employment process, 332; external, 333–334; food theft, 333; internal, 332–333; pilferage, 332–333; problems in receiving, storage, inventory control, 333; receiving, 434; in service areas, 333

Select grade beef, 373

Selective communication, 130

Selective menus, 351, 359

Self-branding, 42

Self-contained refrigerators/freezers, 522

Self-discipline, in listening, 140

Self-evaluations, 172

Self-leveling plate units, 530

Self-managed teams, 99

Self-managed work teams, 99

Self-operated institutional foodservice, 13–14

Self-rising flour, 396

Self-service customers, 500

Semantics, as communication interference, 128

Semi-live skids, 521

Semolina, 397

Semolina flour, 396

Senders, 128, 140

Sensory Assessment for Test Tray (form), 504

Separation, and departmentalization, 96

Service America (Albrecht/Zemke), 60

Service area, 39

Service, of contract foodservice management, 14

Service sector, 38

Service strategy, 60

Service supplies, 402

Service ware: cleaning/sanitizing, 305–306; environmental sanitation of, 305–307

Services: characteristics of, 38; defined, 38; inventories, absence of, 38, 49; simultaneous production and consumption, 38; uniform and standardized services, 38

Serving tables, 529–530

7 Habits of Highly Effective People (Covey), 124–125

Sexual discrimination, 146–147

Sexual harassment, 146–147

Shared decision making, 30

Shared food-production systems, 109

Shared food-purchasing systems, 109

Shared professional and managerial expertise, 109

Shared service systems, 108–109

Sheet pans, 401

Shelf-life milk, 384

Shellfish, toxins, 269

Shelving, 521

Shewhart, W. A., 51–52

Shift schedule, 120–121

Shigella spp., 261, 275, 279, 339

Shigellosis, 273

Shipjack tuna, 379

Shochet, defined, 371

Shoes, 136, 302, 326

Short plate cut of beef, 374

Short-range planning, 73

Shortening, smoke point, 438

Shrimp, 378

Shrinkage, 443, 463–464

Sick employees, 279–280

Sick leave, 150

Signed memorandum of understanding (MOU), 336

Simmering fish, 472

Simple service function, 489

Simplesse®, 12

SINE mnemonic, 424

Single-service disposable dinnerware, 402

Single sourcing, 421

Single-tank conveyor machines, 533–534

Single-tank stationary rack machines, 533

Single-use menus, 352

Single-use plans, 72

Sinigrin, 476

Sinks, 528

Situational diagnosis, 81–82

Situational leadership, 22–23

Situational leadership theory, 23

Skids, 521

Skill enhancement programs, 30

Skilled workers, 153

Skills objectives, 162

Skin/nonfat milk, 383

Small equipment/utensils, 400–401; cutting boards, 401; knives, 401; measuring devices, 400; pans, 400–401; portioning equipment, 401; scales, 401; thermometers, 401

Smallpox, 339

Smoky links, as processed meat, 376

Snack shops, 500; for nonpatient meal service, 500

Soaps, *See* Detergents/soaps

Social litigation, 2

Social responsibility, 15

Social Security, 150; Social Security Act (1935), 148

Socioeconomic changes, 2

Sockeye salmon, 379

Sodium nitrite/nitrate, 275

Software review, 204

Soiled tableware, reuse of, prohibition against, 500

Solid waste management, 240–241

Solvency ratios, 234

Solvent cleaners/degreasers, 304

Soufflés, 474

Soups, 480

Sour cream/sour half-and-half, 384

Source, considering, in communication, 140

Source of message, and communication, 130

Source reduction, 241–242

Sous vide cooking, 493

Sous vide process, 11

Soy flour, 396

Soy protein concreate, 387

Soy protein isolate, 387

Soybeans, 387

Spaghetti, 397, 477

Span of control, as depicted on organizational chart, 103

Special events, catering, 501

Special holiday takeouts, 43

Special reporting, computers in foodservice operations, 203–204

Special services, menu planning for, 354–356

Specialty fryers, 526

Specifications, defined, 374; meat/meat products, 374–375

Specificity, of objectives, 87

Spices, *See* Herbs/spices

Splenda™, 12

Split-tray cart system, 495

Spoken menu, 357

Spoons, 500; placement of, 499; two-spoon method, 302

Spores, 265, 268; mold, 268–269

Spray dishwashers, 306

Sprays, using around food, 309

Spring ware, 259

Staff employees, 110

Staffing: competencies, 113; defined, 116; foodservice department, 110–118; full-time equivalency needs, calculating, 117–118; job analysis, 111; job description, 113–115; job enlargement, 116; job enrichment, 116; job specification, 113–115; meal equivalent factor (MEF), estimating, 116–117; needs, determining, 110–111, 117; outside consultants, 118; overtime needs, 118; productivity levels, estimating, 116–117; work division, 115–116

Stakeholders, 14

Standard grade beef, 373

Standard grade veal, 373

"Standard of identity" regulations, and bottled water, 259

Standardized recipes, 455–460; batch size adjustment, 457; defined, 455; form of ingredients, 456; ingredient amounts, 458; ingredient substitution, 460–461; number of portions, 458; order of ingredients, 456; portion of ingredients, 456; portion size adjustment, 457–458; preparation procedures, 457; quantity of ingredients, 456; recipe evaluation sheet, 460; recipe files, 456; recipe format, 457; recipe standardization elements, 456–460; size of portions, 458; specific size portions, 458; use of, 455

Standards: defined, 209; implementing, 3; intangible, 210; setting, 209–210; tangible, 210

"Standards of quality" regulations, and bottled water, 259

Standing committees, 98

Standing operational planning, 75–78; department policies and procedures manual, 76; policies and procedures, 75–76; rules, 76

Standing order purchasing, 423

Standing plans, 72

Staphylococcal infection, 271

Staphylococcus aureus (MRSA), 270–272, 275, 280

Staples, delivery/storage, 419

Star K, and kosher/kashrut standards, 371

Starches, 476–477

Static budgets, 214

Static menus, 351, 352

Stationary equipment, cleaning, 305

Statistical data, 233

Statistical indicators, determining, 219

Status report, 49

Steam equipment, 525–526

Steam-jacketed kettles, 525

Steamers, 525

Steaming fish, 472

Stereotyping, 130; as barrier to diversity, 170

Sterilization, 263

Steroid use, and listeriosis, 272

Stews, fish, 472

Stilton, 268, 386

Stock, 480

Stockpots, 401

Storage, 435; dry storage facilities, 434; dry storage maintenance, 434–437; low-temperature storage facilities, 434; low-temperature storage maintenance, 437–439; procedures, 434–439; recommended temperatures/times, 435; refrigerated, 434–435

Storage equipment, 521–523; dry storage, 521; ice-making equipment, 523; refrigerated and low-temperature storage, 521–523

Storage space: for germicides and sanitizers, 305; and menu planning, 348

Storage tags, 431–432

Stores requisition: defined, 439; form, 440

Strategic control points, 210

Strategic planning, 27, 72, 73–75; data gathering/analysis, 73–74; goals/objectives/strategies/plans, establishing, 74–75; implementation/evaluating/modifying goals and action plans, 75; middle manager's role in, 75

Strategies, 71

Stress, 15–16

Structural behavior, 22

Styrofoam, as packaging waste, 240

Submissive resolution, 142

Subordinate review, 172

Subsidy, 217

Substitutes: cheese, 387; cream, 385; fats, 12

Subsystems, 101–102

Waste-handling equipment: compactors, 529; mechanical disposers, 528–529; pulper extractors, 529

Waste management, 6, 240

Waste materials storage containers (worksheet), 246–248

Waste removal, 249

Waste-stream analysis, 243–249; factors influencing success, 249; waste removal, 249

Waste stream, defined, 243

Wastewater, use of term, 258

Water: contamination, 339–340; and health inspection, 300

Water conservation, 258–259; bottled water, 259; Clean Water Act, 258; Safe Drinking Water Act, 258

Water conservation programs, goal of, 258

Water-flow alarms, 331

Water glass, placement of, 499

Water line-mounted indicating thermometers, 306

Watermelons, 392

Weather conditions, and supply/price of fresh produce, 348

Weighted averages, 443

Weights and measures conversion chart, 462

Well water, 259

Wheat germ, 396

Whipping cream, 475

Whistleblowing, and dismissal for cause, 182

White population, 7

White rice, 397–398

White sauce, 480

White stock, 480

Whole message, listening to, 140

Whole milk, 383

Whole wheat flour, 396

Wholesaling, 410

Wholesome Poultry Products Act, 407

Wild rice, 398

Wine glasses, placement of, 499

Winter savory leaves, 484

Winter storms, 338

Wiping cloths, 305

Women: and leadership, 23; as primary decision-makers, 9–10

Word interpretation, 130

Work area planning, *See also* Equipment selection: blueprints, 516; budget, 517; ceilings, 517–518; design trends, 515; equipment selection, 519–531; ergonomic considerations, 518; floors, 517–518; flow of work and materials (chart), 511–512; food production area, 513–514; general construction features, 513, 517–519; heat-producing equipment, 513; justification or cost-benefit analysis, 516–517; layout, 512; layout development, 516–517; lighting, 513, 518; location, 512; meal service, 513–514; plumbing, 519; receiving, 512–513; request for proposal (RFP), 516; safety/sanitation/security, 518–519; schematic plan, 512; scraping/sorting/racking soiled dishes/space for, 515; security, 513; soundproofing, 517–518; storage, 513; utilities, 518; ventilation, 513, 518; walk-in unit space requirements, 513; walls, 517–518; ware washing, 514–515; work flow, 515–516

Work cell system, 492

Work division, 115–116

Work process focus, 57

Work simplification, 110

Work status, verbal/written reports on, 210

Worker motivation, 31

Worker's compensation, 149–150; insurance, 149; laws, 2

Workforce: age of, 8; cultural diversity of, 7–8; infectious disease in, 8; issues, 6–8; and literacy, 8

Working conditions, fundamental requirements, 314

Working teenagers, 8

Workplace spirituality, 107

Workplace violence, 331; and dismissal for cause, 182

Workstations, ergonomically friendly, 518

Workweek, 118

World Commission on Environment and Development, on sustainability, 237

Written communication, 131, 136–139; business letter, 137; computer programs for, 136–137; departmental activity reports, 137; departmental policy and procedures manuals, 138; disadvantage of, 136; e-mail, 138–139; employee handbooks, 137–138; financial reports, 137; internal memorandum, 137; justification in, 137; to patients, 138; persuasion in, 137; proposals, 137; reports, 137–138; tone of, 136; types of, 137–139

Written evaluation, 170

Written hazard communication programs, 319–320

Written questionnaires, to discharged patients, 55–56

Y

Yams, 390

Yeast breads, 479–480

Yeast, budding, 268

Yellowfin tuna, 379

Yersinia enterocolitica, 275

Yersinia pestis, 339

Yield grades, 372–373; meat/meat products, 371–373

Yields, 419

Yo-yo dieters, 345

Yogurt, 384–385

Z

Z-Trim™, 12

Zero-based budgeting (ZBB), 214

Zero defects, 52

Zero waste, 241